Stereoscopic Anatomical Atlas of Ear Surgery

Pu Dai • Vincent C Cousins
Yue-shuai Song • Xue Gao
Editors

Stereoscopic Anatomical Atlas of Ear Surgery

PMPH PEOPLE'S MEDICAL PUBLISHING HOUSE

Springer

Editors
Pu Dai
College of Otolaryngology Head and Neck Surgery
Chinese PLA General Hospital
Beijing
China

Yue-shuai Song
Department of Otolaryngology Head and Neck Surgery
Beijing Friendship Hospital, Capital Medical University
Beijing
China

Vincent C Cousins
Department of Ear Nose and Throat Surgery
Alfred Hospital
Melbourne
Australia

Department of Surgery
Monash University
Melbourne
Australia

Xue Gao
Department of Otolaryngology Head and Neck Surgery
PLA Rocket Force Characteristic Medical Center
Beijing
China

ISBN 978-981-16-0929-9 ISBN 978-981-16-0927-5 (eBook)
https://doi.org/10.1007/978-981-16-0927-5

Jointly published with People's Medical Publishing House, PR of China

This Springer imprint is published by the registered company Springer Nature Singapore Pte Ltd.
The registered company address is: 152 Beach Road, #21-01/04 Gateway East, Singapore 189721, Singapore

Preface

Anatomy is the basis of medical discourse (Hippocrates, De locis in homine 2). Ear surgeons would be no more than armchair strategists if they lacked anatomical knowledge and practical experience. Even audiological physicians would find it difficult to understand the etiology and pathogenesis of audiological disease if they lacked anatomical knowledge. Commencing in the 1960s, otomicrosurgery, otoneurosurgery, and lateral skull base surgery have developed rapidly, greatly aided not only by research into the pathogenic mechanisms of ear diseases but also by detailed studies on temporal bone and skull base anatomy. Today, practitioners must absorb a great deal of information and keep up with the newest development in this field.

Otolaryngologists and scholars around the world have published many, exquisitely clear, ear surgery monographs over the past few decades. These publications support both younger ear surgeons and other ENT professionals. However, ear anatomy is so exquisite and complex that traditional two-dimensional (2D) media can only reveal basic morphological characteristics and spatial relationships partly; stereoscopic micrographs yield a true stereoscopic effect by perceiving depth, which are definitely better. In the 1990s, guided by Academician Si-chang Jiang, the College of Otolaryngology Head and Neck Surgery of the Chinese PLA General Hospital commenced research on 3D visual technology, initially presented in the book entitled *Stereoscopic Anatomical Atlas of Ear Surgery (You-jun Yu, Pu Dai, etc., People's Military Medical Press, Beijing, 2006).* We later published the first microsurgical stereoscopic atlas in China, entitled *Stereoscopic Surgical Atlas of Otomicrosurgery (Dong-yi Han and Pu Dai, People's Medical Publishing House, Beijing, 2009).* This was well reviewed at home, being one of the top 100 original books honored by the Chinese General Administration of Press and Publications in 2011. Springer purchased the copyright and published an English version in 2017.

For this book, we prepared sophisticated surgical and photographic devices including *Zeiss* OPMI *Pentero* and *NC4* microscopes, a double light path photography system with *Canon EOS 5D* cameras, a *Medtronic* dynamic system, *SPIGGLE & THEIS* microscopic surgical instruments. In addition, we collected models of a cochlear probe electrode, vibrational sound bridge, and artificial auditory prostheses (*MED-EL*, *Cochlear*, *AB*, *SPIGGLE & THEIS*, *Kurz*, *Medtronic*). Professor Pu Dai performed all dissections illustrated in the book; 262 stereoscopic images were carefully selected. We collaborated with Professor Hao-bing Wang (Eaton-Peabody Laboratory, Massachusetts Eye & Ear Infirmary), and published, with thanks, 31 stereoscopic 3D reconstruction images using her 3D model. Thus, the book features 293 stereoscopic images showing the internal and external structures of the temporal bone.

Assisted by readers' feedback of our earlier *Stereoscopic Surgical Atlas of Otomicrosurgery*, we carefully explain each image in the new book and we approach ear anatomy in a logical manner. The images are taken from better camera angles presented in a logical sequence and seek to be as informative as possible. However, some errors are inevitable; we again welcome your valuable feedback and advice. Thank you.

Beijing, China

Pu Dai

Acknowledgement

This work was supported by National Natural Science Foundation of China (61827805).

Contents

List of Contributors

Qing-ling Bi Department of Otolaryngology Head and Neck Surgery, China-Japan Friendship Hospital, Beijing, China

Chao-chan Cai College of Otolaryngology Head and Neck Surgery, Chinese PLA General Hospital, Beijing, China

Vincent C Cousins Department of Ear Nose and Throat Surgery, Alfred Hospital, Melbourne, Australia

Department of Surgery, Monash University, Melbourne, Australia

Pu Dai College of Otolaryngology Head and Neck Surgery, Chinese PLA General Hospital, Beijing, China

Ying Fu Department of Otorhinolaryngology, Qilu Hospital (Qingdao), Cheeloo College of Medicine, Shandong University, Qingdao, China

Bo Gao College of Otolaryngology Head and Neck Surgery, Chinese PLA General Hospital, Beijing, China

Song Gao Department of Otolaryngology Head and Neck Surgery, The 909th Hospital of PLA, South-East Hospital Affiliated to Xiamen University, Zhangzhou, China

Xue Gao Department of Otolaryngology Head and Neck Surgery, PLA Rocket Force Characteristic Medical Center, Beijing, China

Ping Gu Department of Otolaryngology Head and Neck Surgery, Shenzhen Children's Hospital, Shenzhen, China

Chang Guo College of Otolaryngology Head and Neck Surgery, Chinese PLA General Hospital, Beijing, China

Bing Han College of Otolaryngology Head and Neck Surgery, Chinese PLA General Hospital, Beijing, China

Ming-yu Han College of Otolaryngology Head and Neck Surgery, Chinese PLA General Hospital, Beijing, China

Sha-sha Huang College of Otolaryngology Head and Neck Surgery, Chinese PLA General Hospital, Beijing, China

Yu-bin Ji Department of Otolaryngology Head and Neck Surgery, Beijing Tsinghua Changgung Hospital, Beijing, China

Yi Jiang Department of Otolaryngology Head and Neck Surgery, Shanghai Ninth People's Hospital, Shanghai Jiao Tong University School of Medicine, Shanghai, China

Zhan-guo Jin Department of Otolaryngology Head and Neck Surgery, Air Force Medical Center, Beijing, China

Su Jeong Lee Department of Otolaryngology Head and Neck Surgery, Peking University International Hospital, Beijing, China

Jia-nan Li College of Otolaryngology Head and Neck Surgery, Chinese PLA General Hospital, Beijing, China

Jian-hui Li College of Otolaryngology Head and Neck Surgery, Chinese PLA General Hospital, Beijing, China

Qi Li Department of Otolaryngology Head and Neck Surgery, Children's Hospital of Nanjing Medical University, Nanjing, China

Xiao-hong Li Department of Otolaryngology Head and Neck Surgery, Beijing Children's Hospital, Capital Medical University, Beijing, China

Yun-juan Lin Department of Otolaryngology Head and Neck Surgery, Peking University International Hospital, Beijing, China

Jun Liu College of Otolaryngology Head and Neck Surgery, Chinese PLA General Hospital, Beijing, China

Ya-qing Liu Department of Otolaryngology Head and Neck Surgery, Children's Hospital of Nanjing Medical University, Nanjing, China

Kun Ma Department of Otolaryngology Head and Neck Surgery, Peking University International Hospital, Beijing, China

Li-li Ren College of Otolaryngology Head and Neck Surgery, Chinese PLA General Hospital, Beijing, China

Sen-yao Shao Department of Otolaryngology Head and Neck Surgery, Peking University International Hospital, Beijing, China

Yue-shuai Song Department of Otolaryngology Head and Neck Surgery, Beijing Friendship Hospital, Capital Medical University, Beijing, China

Yu Su Department of Otolaryngology Head and Neck Surgery, Chinese PLA General Hospital Affiliated Hainan Hospital, Sanya, China

Bao-chun Sun Department of Otolaryngology Head and Neck Surgery, The Fourth Medical Center of PLA General Hospital, Beijing, China

Yi Sun Department of Otolaryngology Head and Neck Surgery, General Hospital of Central Theater Command, Wuhan, China

Yi-chen Wan Department of Otolaryngology Head and Neck Surgery, Peking University International Hospital, Beijing, China

Guo-jian Wang College of Otolaryngology Head and Neck Surgery, Chinese PLA General Hospital, Beijing, China

Hui-bing Wang Department of Otolaryngology Head and Neck Surgery, The Third Medical Center of PLA General Hospital, Beijing, China

Meng-hang Wang Department of Otolaryngology Head and Neck Surgery, Peking University International Hospital, Beijing, China

Wei-qian Wang Department of Otolaryngology Head and Neck Surgery, PLA Rocket Force Characteristic Medical Center, Beijing, China

Feng Xin Department of Otolaryngology Head and Neck Surgery, Second Hospital of Shanxi Medical University, Taiyuan, China

Jun-fang Xue Department of Otolaryngology Head and Neck Surgery, Peking University International Hospital, Beijing, China

Xu-kun Yan Department of Otolaryngology Head and Neck Surgery, Beijing Tiantan Hospital, Capital Medical University, Beijing, China

Fei Yu College of Otolaryngology Head and Neck Surgery, Chinese PLA General Hospital, Beijing, China

Yong-yi Yuan College of Otolaryngology Head and Neck Surgery, Chinese PLA General Hospital, Beijing, China

De-jun Zhang Department of Otolaryngology Head and Neck Surgery, The Second Hospital of Jilin University, Changchun, China

Hong-lei Zhang Department of Otolaryngology Head and Neck Surgery, Air Force Medical Center, PLA, Beijing, China

Jian-dong Zhao College of Otolaryngology Head and Neck Surgery, Chinese PLA General Hospital, Beijing, China

Yu-hua Zhu College of Otolaryngology Head and Neck Surgery, Chinese PLA General Hospital, Beijing, China

About the Editors

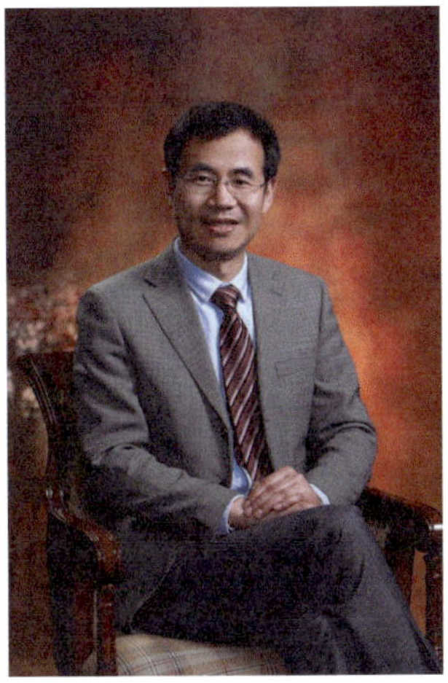

Pu Dai is a surgeon-scientist, full professor, and the Chair of the Scientific Committee, College of Otolaryngology Head and Neck Surgery, Chinese PLA General Hospital, Chinese PLA Medical School. Professor Dai specializes in otology, skull base surgery, and cochlear implantation surgery. His research has focused on minimal access and difficult cochlear implantation surgery, hearing preservation, and the genetics of hearing loss. Professor Dai initiated his pioneering three-dimensional (3D) morphological research on the temporal bone in 1990, and he authored the first *Stereo Anatomical and Surgical Atlas of the Temporal Bone* in China (2006) and a 3D atlas of micro ear surgery in the world (2017). Professor Dai has published more than 70 peer-reviewed journal articles worldwide and 160 journal articles in Chinese. He is the chief editor of four books in the field of otological surgery, anatomy, and inherited hearing loss. He is also the Principal Investigator for more than 10 grants, including those sponsored by the National Key Research and Development Project of China and the National Natural Science Foundation of China. His honors include two Second Grade Prizes in the National Science and Technology Progress Awards (for controlling birth defects causing severe-to-profound hearing impairment), one Seeking Truth Award, and a nomination as a National Distinguished Young and Middle-aged Specialist. He was the Chair of the Organizing Committee and the Conference Secretary for the Asia-Pacific Symposium on Cochlear Implantation and Related Science (APSCI) (2015) and is an APSCI board member.

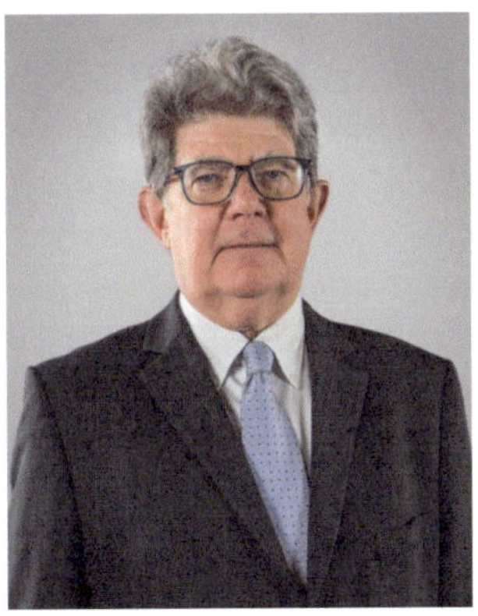

Vincent C Cousins graduated in Medicine from Monash University, Melbourne, Australia, in 1974. He completed his advanced surgical training in Otolaryngology Head & Neck Surgery in Melbourne (FRACS) in 1984. He then undertook a Head and Neck and Skull Base fellowship with Professor Donald Harrison in London, England, in 1984/1985, and an Otology fellowship with Professor Dietrich Plester in Tübingen, Germany, in 1986. He has practiced in Melbourne in otology and neurotology since then. He is currently Principal Specialist and Head of the ENT-Otoneurology Unit at the Alfred Hospital, Melbourne, and Adjunct Clinical Associate Professor in Surgery at Monash University. He is Past President of the Australian Society of Otolaryngology Head & Neck

Surgery. He has served the Royal Australasian College of Surgeons as Councilor, Chief Examiner (OHNS), and Board Chair of the Academy of Surgical Educators. He has been awarded Distinguished Service Awards from both of these organizations. He is a Past President and Life Member of the Neurotology Society of Australia. He was Visiting Professor in the Department of Otolaryngology, Sun Yat Sen University, Guangzhou, China, from 2003 to 2009. He was the Wong Hua Yuen Distinguished Scholar, Hong Kong University, in 2004. He was appointed as the JLO Visiting Professor of the Royal Society of Medicine Otology Section, London, UK, in 2007. He is a member of the Executive Board and Regional Secretary of the International Federation of Otolaryngological Societies (IFOS) for South East Asia, Western Pacific, and Oceania. His research interests include the management of acoustic neuroma, paragangliomas of the head and neck, facial paralysis, and temporal bone trauma as well as outcome measures and quality of life in otology and lateral skull base surgery. He has published more than 50 peer-reviewed journal articles and book chapters and is a member of Editorial Board or Peer Review Panel of multiple international surgical journals. He has a particular interest in surgical education and skills training in otology and lateral skull base surgery and has directed and instructed on temporal bone dissection and skull base surgery courses in Australia, Africa, and China over the last 30 years. He has been part of the Organizing and Scientific Committees and/or Invited Faculty member of more than 100 international Congresses or Courses on Otology and Skull Base Surgery.

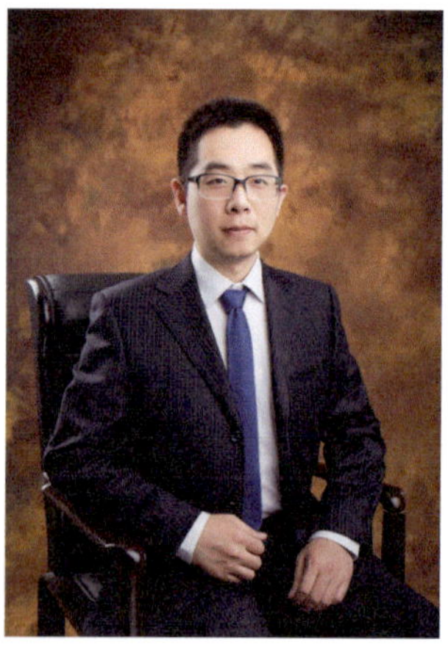

Yue-shuai Song is an associate chief physician of otolaryngology head-neck surgeon working in Beijing Friendship Hospital. He graduated from the Nankai University Medical School, in Tianjin, China, in 2009 and later completed his otolaryngology training and was awarded a doctoral degree from the Nankai University Medical School in 2012. He undertook a further 3 years of postdoctoral training at the Chinese PLA General Hospital from 2012 to 2015. He has practiced as an otolaryngology head-neck surgeon in Beijing Friendship Hospital since 2015. He has a great deal of experience in the anatomy of the temporal bone and skull base and has focused his research on cochlear implantation and the three-dimensional (3D) morphology of the temporal bone. He participated in the publication of the first 3D atlas of micro ear surgery and anatomy as vice and chief editor in 2009 and 2016, respectively. Yue-shuai Song has published 8 articles in SCI journals and 18 articles in Chinese journals. He holds seven national patents. He is in charge of the anatomy training program in ear surgery at Beijing Friendship Hospital.

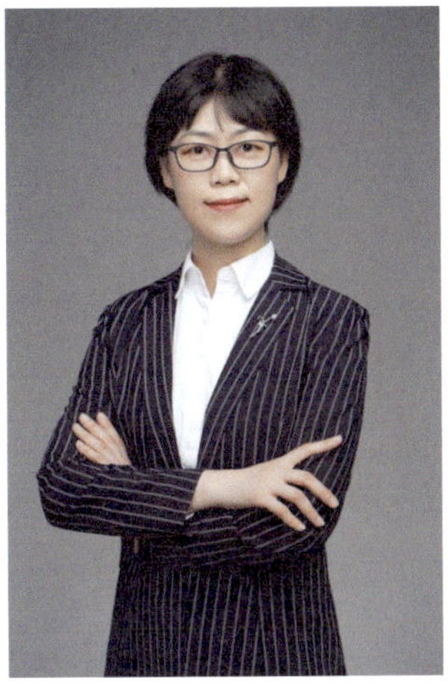

Xue Gao is an associate chief physician and Vice Chair of otolaryngology of Chinese PLA Rocket Force Characteristic Medical Center, with special interest in middle ear and cochlear implantation surgery. She graduated from the Fourth Military Medical University, in Xi'an, China, in 2002 and later completed her otolaryngology training and was awarded a doctoral degree from the Fourth Military Medical University in 2008. She undertook a further 5 years of postdoctoral training with Professor Pu Dai at the Chinese PLA General Hospital from 2011 to 2016. She specialized in otology, anatomy of the temporal bone, and the genetics of hearing loss and published 22 articles in international peer-reviewed journals. She is currently secretary of CSAH (Chinese Society of Artificial Hearing).

Overview

1

Yue-shuai Song, Song Gao, Pu Dai, Xue Gao, and Vincent C Cousins

Temporal Bone Dissection Instruments and Laboratory

Yue-shuai Song

Instruments

Temporal bone dissection covers the external, middle, and inner ear, and may extend to the occipital bone, parotid gland and cranial cavity. Therefore, a well-equipped laboratory and a broad range of dissecting instruments are strongly recommended.

Y.-s. Song (✉)
Department of Otolaryngology Head and Neck Surgery, Beijing Friendship Hospital, Capital Medical University, Beijing, China

S. Gao
Department of Otolaryngology Head and Neck Surgery, The 909th Hospital of PLA, South-East Hospital Affiliated to Xiamen University, Zhangzhou, China

P. Dai
College of Otolaryngology Head and Neck Surgery, Chinese PLA General Hospital, Beijing, China

X. Gao
Department of Otolaryngology Head and Neck Surgery, PLA Rocket Force Characteristic Medical Center, Beijing, China

V. C. Cousins
Department of Ear Nose and Throat Surgery, Alfred Hospital, Melbourne, Australia

Department of Surgery, Monash University, Melbourne, Australia

P. Dai et al. (eds.), *Stereoscopic Anatomical Atlas of Ear Surgery*, https://doi.org/10.1007/978-981-16-0927-5_1

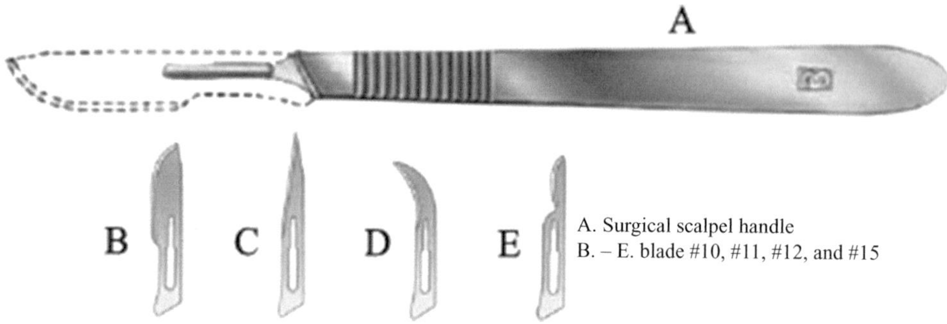

Fig. 1.1 Scalpels

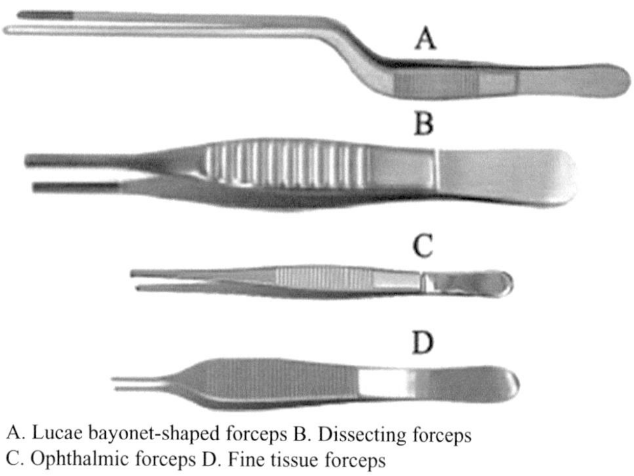

Fig. 1.2 Forceps

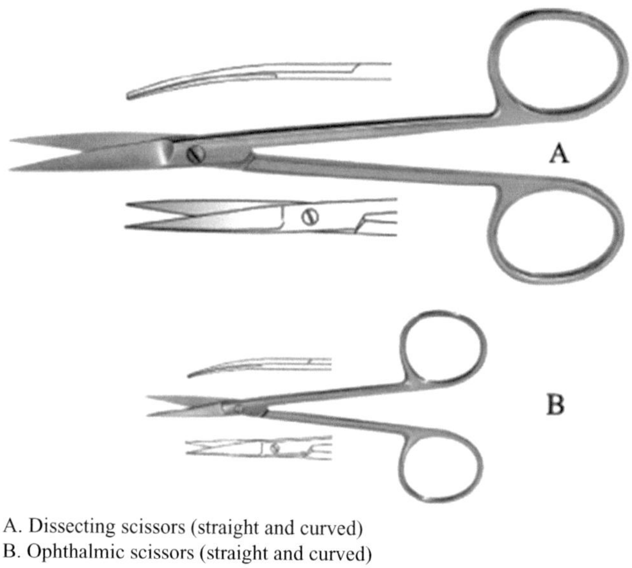

Fig. 1.3 Scissors

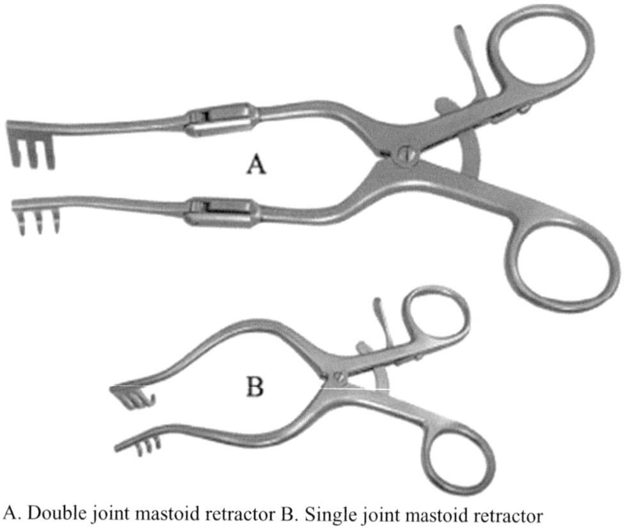

Fig. 1.4 Retractors

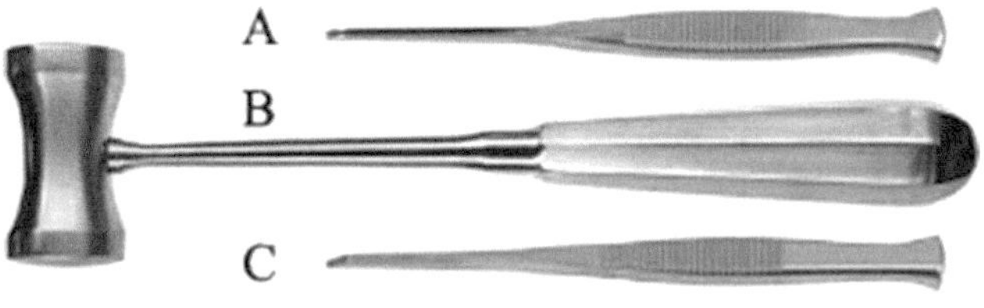

A. Round chisel B. Hammer C. Flat chisel

Fig. 1.5 Hammer and chisels

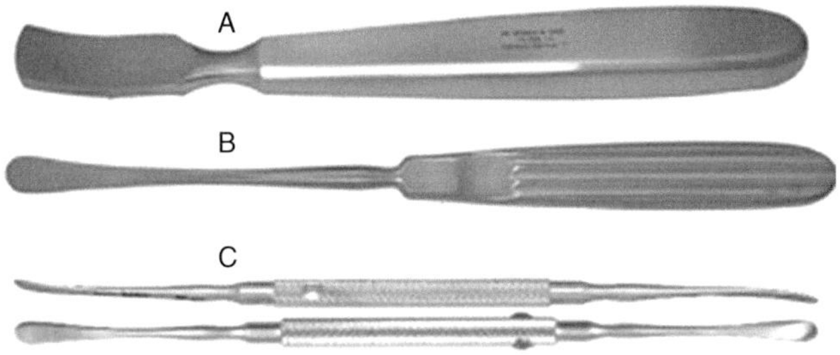

A. Faraboeuf periosteal elevator B. Cottle periosteal elevator
C. Freer elevator

Fig. 1.6 Elevators

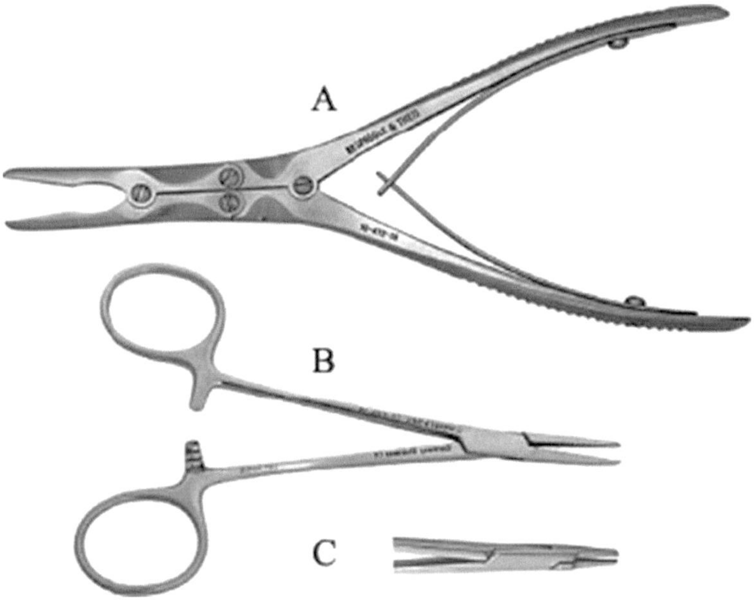

A. Beyer bone nibbler B. Vascular forceps C. Needle holder

Fig. 1.7 Forceps and needle holder

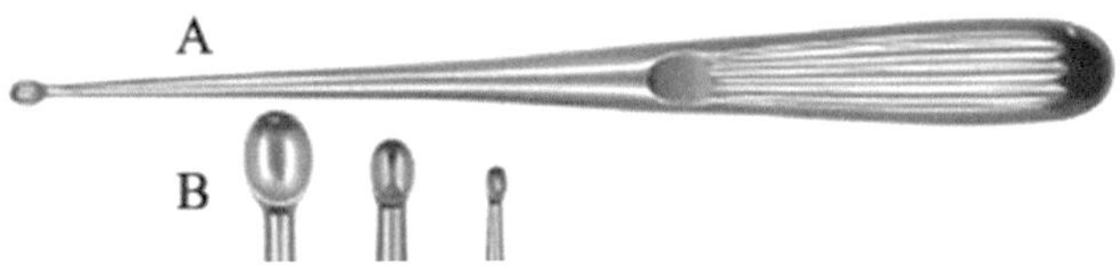

A. Handle
B. Heads of different sizes

Fig. 1.8 Curette

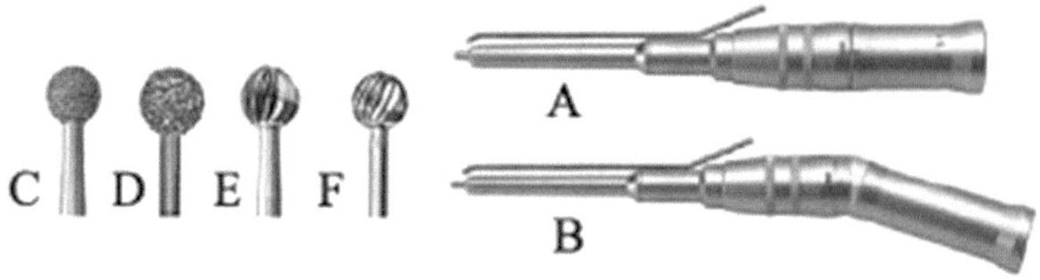

A. Straight handle
B. Angled handle
C. Fine diamond burr
D. Rough diamond burr
E. Cutting burr with large grooves
F. Cutting burr with fine grooves

Fig. 1.9 Drill handles and burrs (ϕ: 0.6–7.0 mm)

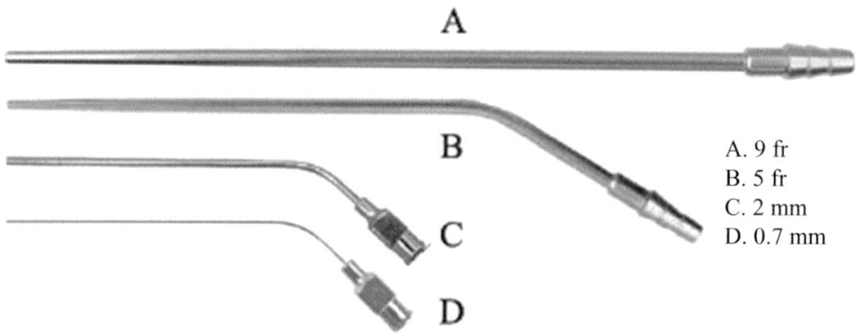

A. 9 fr
B. 5 fr
C. 2 mm
D. 0.7 mm

Fig. 1.10 Suction cannulas

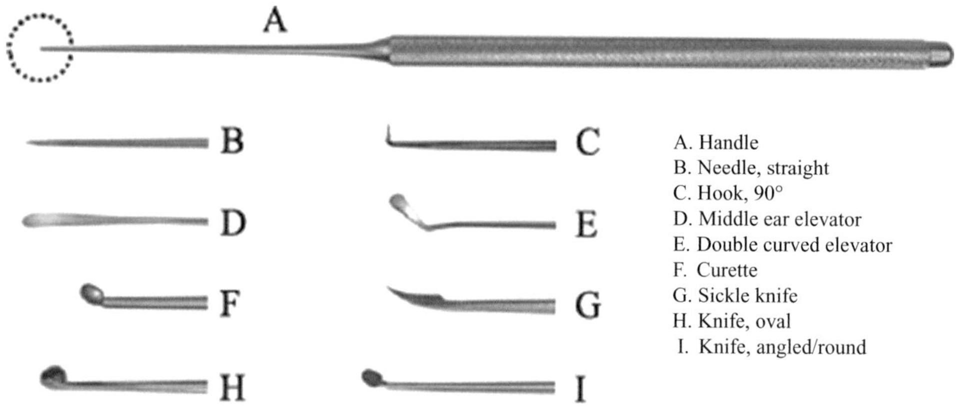

A. Handle
B. Needle, straight
C. Hook, 90°
D. Middle ear elevator
E. Double curved elevator
F. Curette
G. Sickle knife
H. Knife, oval
I. Knife, angled/round

Fig. 1.11 Microsurgical instruments (straight handle)

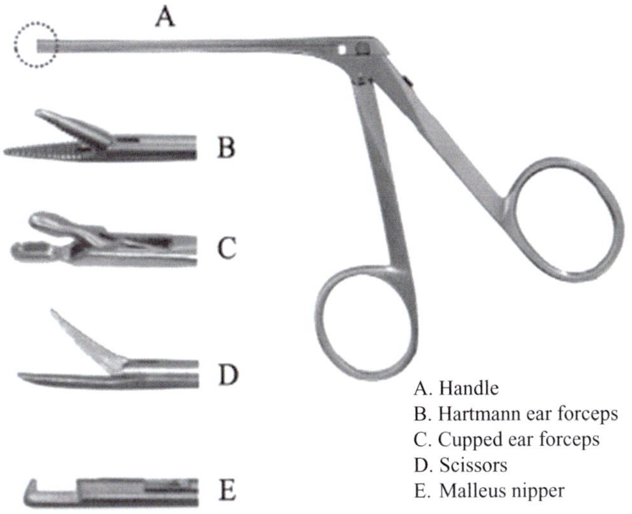

Fig. 1.12 Microsurgical instruments (forceps handle)

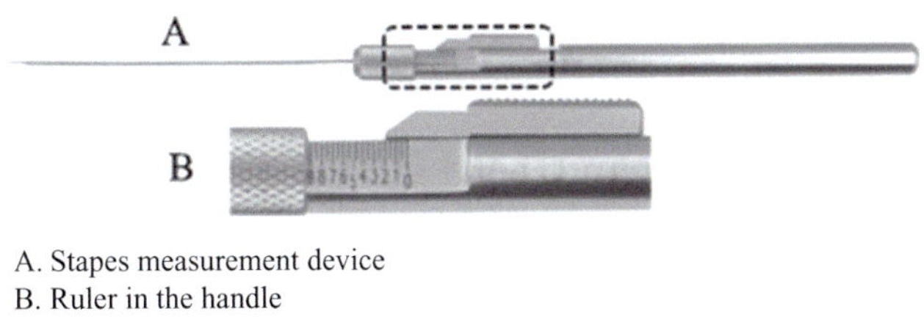

Fig. 1.13 Stapes measurement device

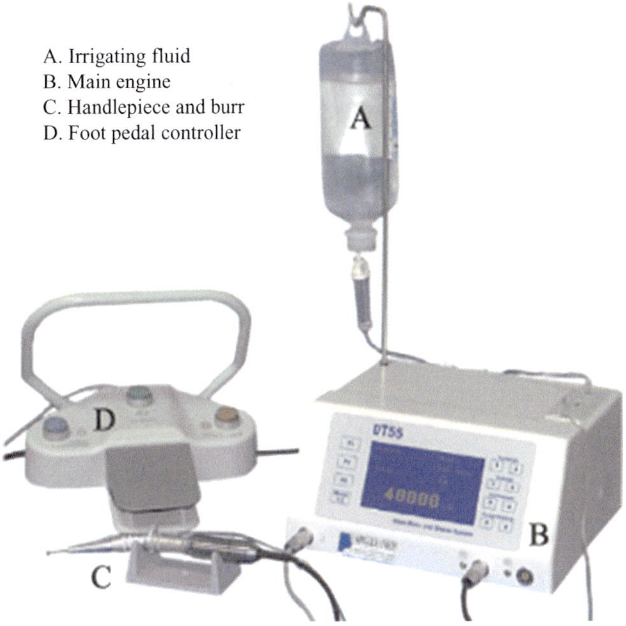

Fig. 1.14 Drill control system

Dissection Laboratory

The precise arrangements vary according to the available space. The items that should be taken into consideration are: (1) scale of the room; (2) number of dissection tables; (3) frequency of the anatomy program; (4) storage and management of specimens; (5) availability of equipment maintenance; (6) service staff; and (7) water, electricity, and cleaning systems.

Our laboratory has an area of about 100 m^2 and is equipped with water, electricity, and a cleaning system. There are 15 tables, each of which has a microscope (Carl Zeiss OPMI Pico or Kingtic YSX104) and a drill (Bien Air or XISHAN DK-ENT). There is a demonstration system, including a Carl Zeiss OPMI Universal S3 microscope and attached TV system. We have carried out temporal bone dissection courses in July and December every year since 1997.

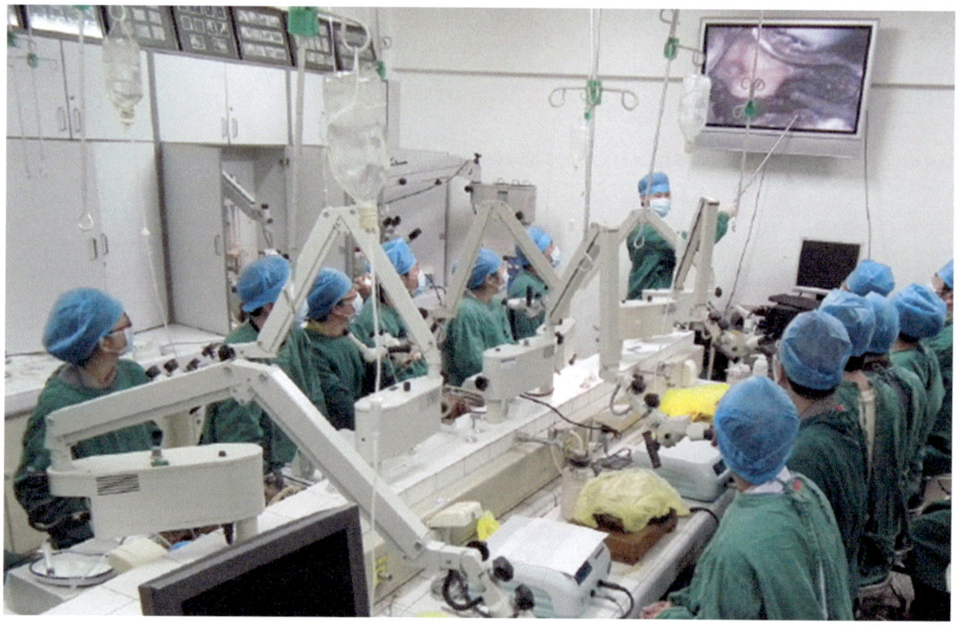

Fig. 1.15 Temporal bone dissection course, Chinese PLA General Hospital

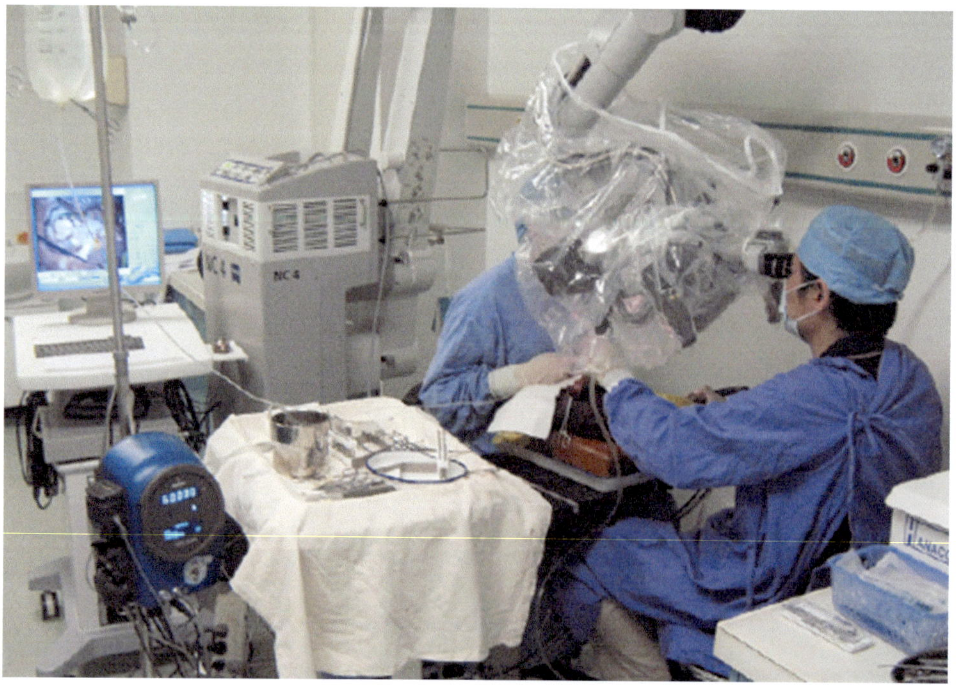

Fig. 1.16 Professor Pu Dai capturing three-dimensional pictures during temporal bone dissection for this book

Stereoscopic Anatomy of the Temporal Bone

Song Gao

Stereopsis and Stereo Images

The average adult inter-pupillary distance is 65 mm. The images on each retina are not exactly the same when we observe objects with both eyes at the same time, which is known as binocular vision. The perception of depth is created in the brain by the integration of the two different views, providing a stereoscopic vision of the objects being observed.

Stereo images mimic human binocular vision. A pair of photographs are taken from the left and right sides of an object at the same time and provide a stereo image when viewed through a stereoscope that preserves and reproduces the stereoscopic information.

Stereo images of microscopic ear and temporal bone surgery truly reproduce the surgical or anatomical field and provide more spatial information than two-dimensional (2-D) representations; such images help the observer or student better understand the spatial relationships between anatomical structures.

Brief History of the Development of Stereo Anatomy of the Temporal Bone

There is a temporal bone on each side of the skull, and each constitutes the floor of the ipsilateral middle cranial fossa and anterior wall of the posterior cranial fossa. Characterized by its small volume, irregular shape, subtle structure, and close proximity to a group of important structures, the temporal bone is the most complicated bony structure in the body. Its anatomy is the basis of otology.

A number of anatomical structures in the temporal bone are so small that they can hardly be observed with the naked human eye. Traditional anatomical images of the temporal bone are 2-D images, and it is difficult for beginners to gain an appreciation of the spatial arrangement of these anatomical structures in the temporal bone. The effective display of this 3-D spatial information is a challenge in the learning and studying of ear microsurgery. In the 1970s and 1980s, temporal bone tissue sections were used to develop three-dimensional (3-D) reconstructions. In China, Pu Dai took the first steps to depict the anatomy of the ear in three dimensions based on serial sections of celloidin-embedded temporal bones.

Pu Dai and colleagues published their *Stereo Anatomical and Surgical Atlas of Temporal Bone* utilizing a camera and stereo-photography. They achieved realistic stereovision when viewing the images through a stereoscope. At that time, the state of stereo photography technology was rudimentary and simulated binocular images by taking a pair of photos of the same anatomical areas from the left and right sides. Pu Dai later developed a stereo imaging system using an operating microscope (Patent No. *ZL200820078610.3*). The microscope has two image-collecting channels with two digital cameras mounted to record separate images during surgery. A pair of images are then viewed together using a stereoscope to provide a stereo image. This system provides real stereo vision of the surgical field. The *Stereo Operative Atlas of Micro Ear Surgery* published in 2009 by Dong-Yi Han and Pu Dai is the result of this research.

How to Achieve Stereo Vision Based for Use with the 3-D Atlas

Pu Dai, Yue-shuai Song, and Xue Gao

The most significant feature of this book is that all 293 anatomic and reconstruction images in the atlas contain 3-D elements. Readers can achieve stereo vision unaided or with the assistance of some simple tools. Here we introduce some methods to achieve the 3-D vision when viewing the images.

1. *Using presbyopia spectacles as an alternative stereoscope*

A set of +6.00D to +7.00D presbyopia spectacles (non-prescription reading glasses) can be used as a stereoscope. About 90% of readers can achieve 3-D vision with this system.

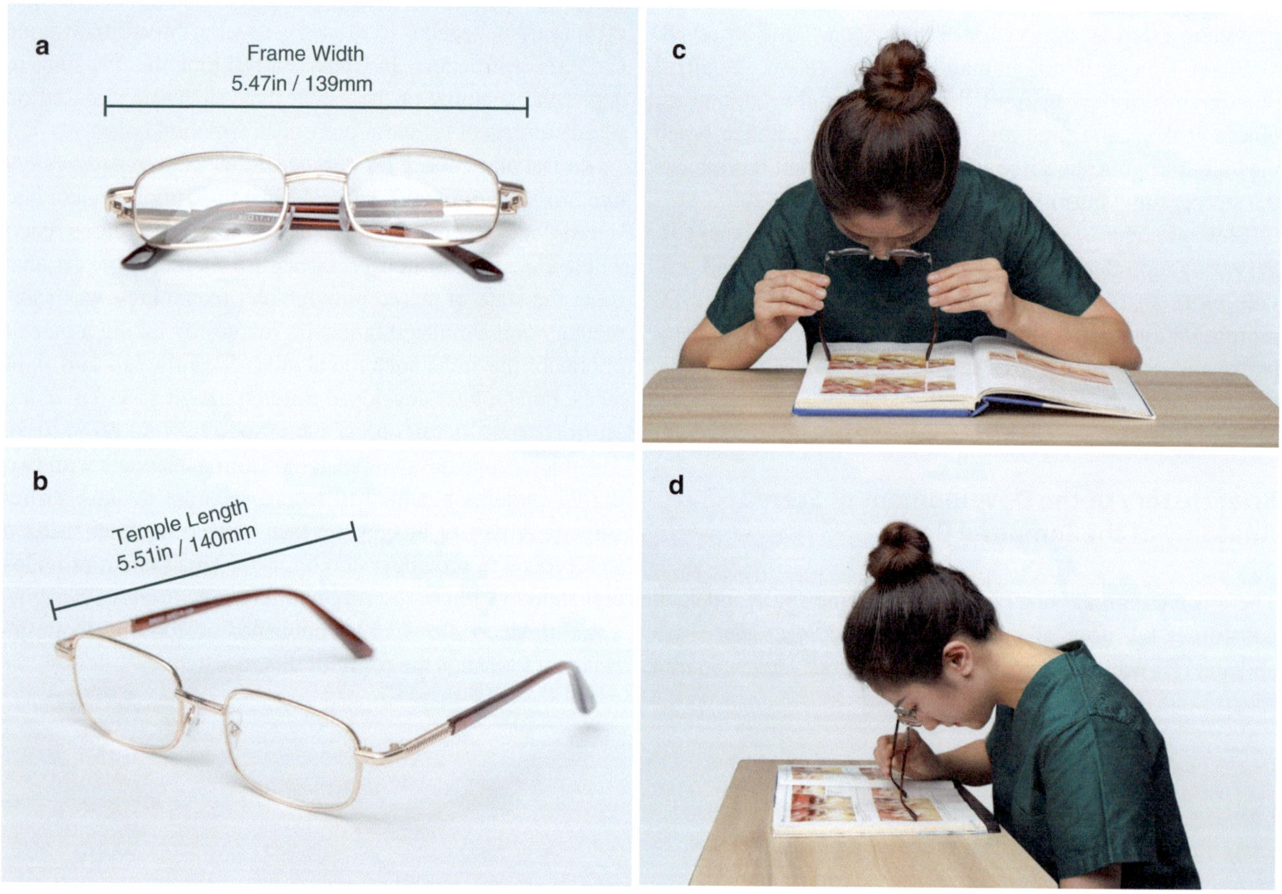

a. folded flat, b. unfolded for use, c. front view, d. side view

Fig. 1.17 Presbyopia spectacles and Viewing 3-D images of this book by presbyopia spectacles

Reverse the presbyopia spectacles so the lenses are close to the observer with the arms facing away, Place the frame over the images with the arms sitting on the outer edges of the images. Ensure each lens is centered over the corresponding image at a distance of approximately 15 cm. Some minor adjustments in positioning may be required to appreciate the 3-D view.

2. *Using a Loreo Lite 3-D viewer*

This is a simple folded card viewer with good quality lenses for viewing 3-D prints. These are made by Loreo Asia Ltd and generally easily obtained via the internet (http://www.loreo.com/pages/shop/loreo_products_online.html, amazon.com or other) and come with instructions: (1) This viewer may be used with or without eyeglasses. If you are severely long or short sighted, it is recommended that you keep your prescription glasses on. (2) The viewing panel still bulges a little in brand new viewers but settles in well after being erected and used. (3) Please note that this is not a "back-lit" viewer and works best when the 3-D prints are well lit but indirect light without reflection.

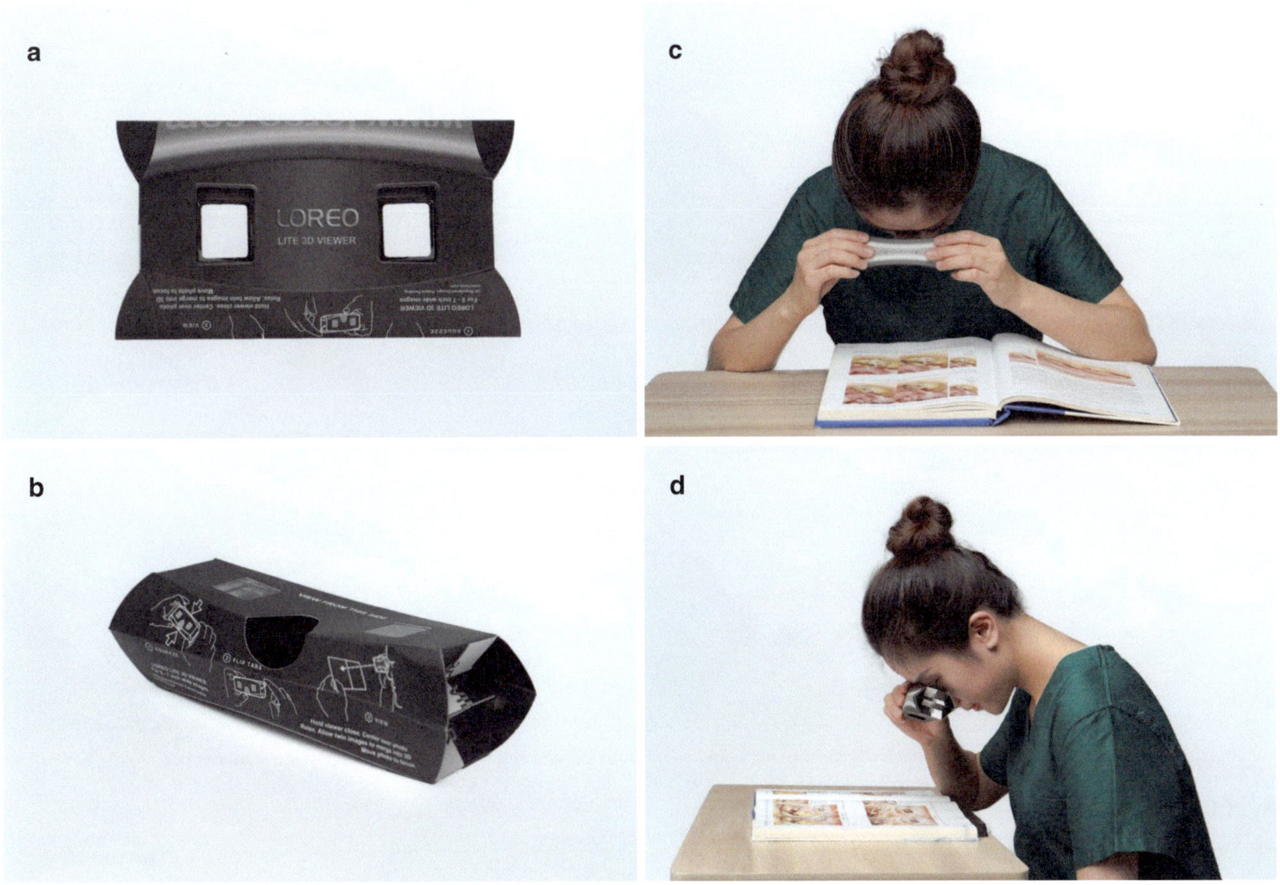

a. folded flat, b. unfolded for use, c. front view, d. side view

Fig. 1.18 Loreo Lite 3D viewer and viewing 3-D images of this book by Loreo Lite 3D viewer

3. *Using a foldable stereoscope*

The majority of readers can easily use the foldable stereoscope to yield the 3-D vision of anatomical scenes and reconstructed images of the temporal bone. In the Chinese version of this book, the foldable stereoscope is provided inside the back cover, see the below figures.

Inquiries about sourcing this viewer can be directed to mixueer0110@126.com.

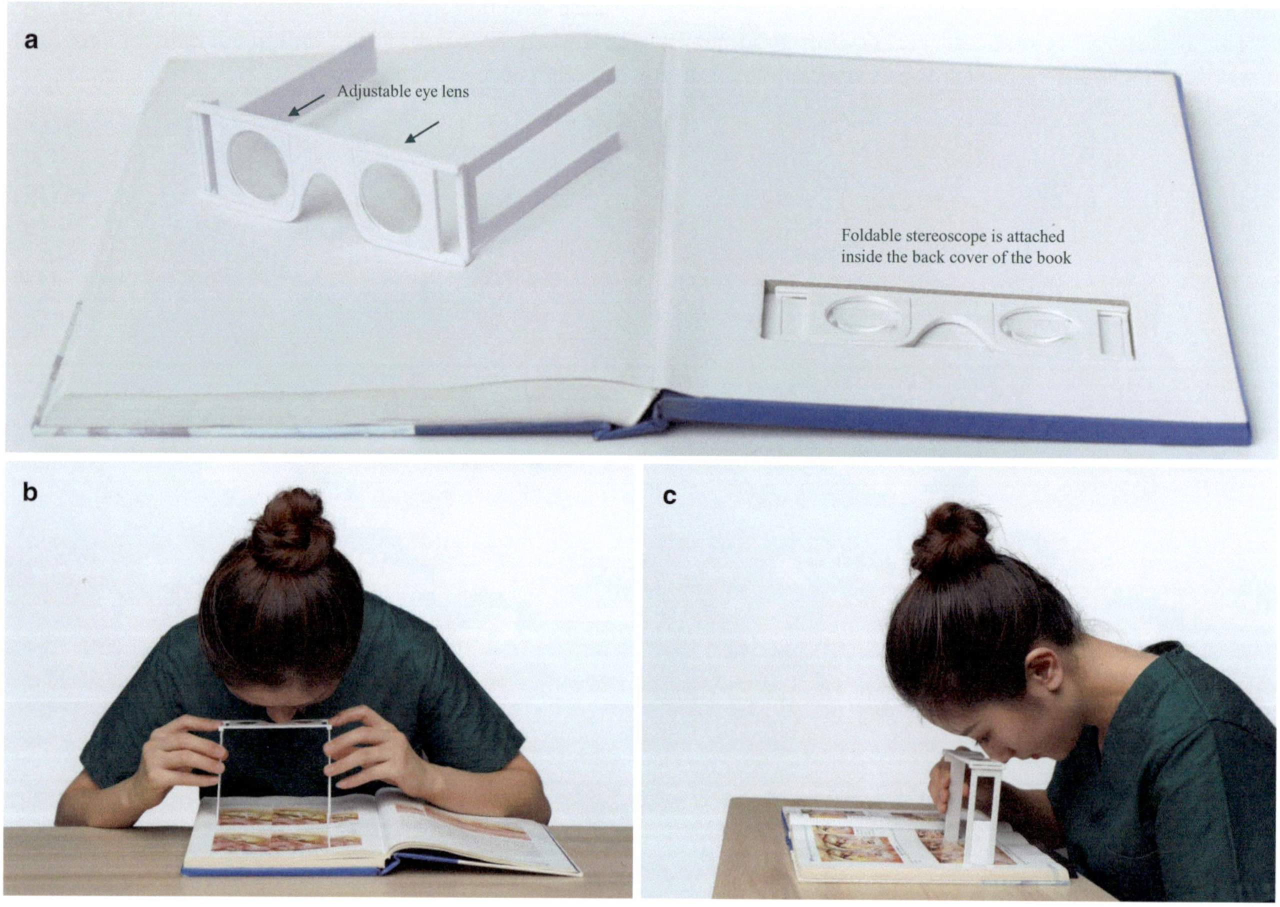

a. Foldable stereoscope is attached inside the back cover of the book. b, c. front view and side view of positioning of the stereoscope.

Fig. 1.19 Foldable stereoscope

Position the stereoscope with the lenses near the observer and the arms sitting in the middle of each side of the image pairs, the eye lenses are adjustable to accommodate interpupillary distance.

4. *Free-viewing with the naked eyes*

If none of the stereoscope systems above are available, you can try your naked eyes to achieve 3-D vision. This may be challenging but is an interesting way to appreciate the 3-D anatomic images unaided. Position your eyes equidistant from the center of the two images and defocus or attempt to focus beyond the images. Moving your head slightly toward or away from the image will often help the images to fuse and give you the intended 3-D view.

With practice, about 50% of subjects can succeed with this technique.

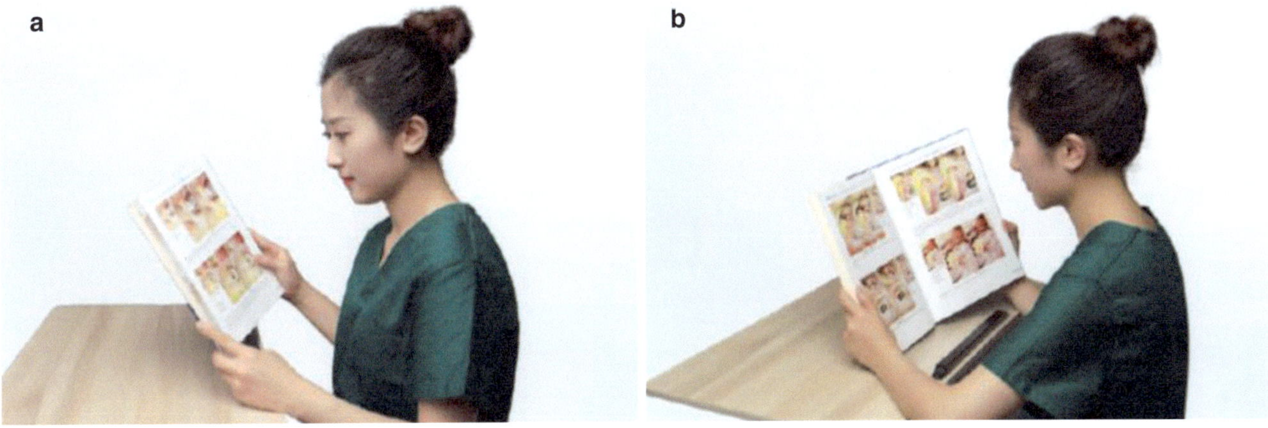

a. front-side view, b, back-side view

Fig. 1.20 Free-viewing the stereoscope image

View the stereoscopic image with naked eyes in a bright environment. The two important parameters are the distance from your eyes to the image (30~40 cm) and the diopter of your naked eyes; both can be varied. The eyes should be defocused and looking straight ahead. The fused image, or the central one if three are perceived, will appear in 3-D.

Note: Above four methods could also be applicable to our first 3-D atlas *Stereo Operative Atlas of Micro Ear Surgery* published in 2016 also by Springer.

Suggested Reading

Dai P, Han D-y, Cousins VC, et al. Stereo operative atlas of micro ear surgery. Singapore: Springer; 2017.

Dai P, Jiang S-c, Gu R. Computer assisted three-dimensional (3D) reconstruction and Mechanical model Establishment of Ossicular chain. Chin J Otorhinolaryngol. 1991;26(5):272–4.

Dai P, Shi L-y, Liu Y. The study and application of the three-dimensional anatomical atlas of temporal bone. Med J Chin People's Liberation Army. 2004;29(5):392–5.

Yu Y-j, Dai P, Liu Z. Stereo anatomical and surgical atlas of Temporal bone. Beijing: People's Military Medical Press; 2006.

2 Bony Landmarks of Temporal Bone

Ming-yu Han, Meng-hang Wang, Xue Gao, and Pu Dai

The temporal bone is composed of a squamous portion, a mastoid portion, a tympanic portion, a petrous portion, and a styloid process. The bony landmarks of these parts are described in detail as follows.

Squamous Portion

The squamous portion, also known as the temporal squama, is in the anterosuperior part of the temporal bone and has internal and external sides. It extends anteriorly to the greater wing of the sphenoid bone and posteriorly to the mastoid, abuts the upper parietal bone, and connects internally with the petrous bone.

1. The temporal line, also called the supramastoid crest, forms a continuous ridge from the superior border of the zygomatic arch anteriorly to the mastoid cortex posteriorly, which is the inferior limit of the temporalis muscle insertion. The temporal line provides an external landmark for the floor of the middle cranial fossa (tegmen of the temporal bone) which is the upper limit of a mastoid resection and the lower limit of the skull fenestration for a transcranial middle fossa approach.
2. The zygomatic process extends forward from the anterior portion of the squamous temporal bone to join the temporal process of zygomatic bone to form the zygomatic arch. There is a deep oval fossa, also called the mandibular fossa, located in the inferior surface of the front and middle of the zygomatic root. The zygomatic root and temporomandibular joint are important landmarks in middle ear and mastoid surgery and maybe the only ones discernable in some patients with congenital external auditory canal (EAC) atresia.
3. The sulcus for the middle temporal artery runs longitudinally backward from the outside of the squamous portion of the temporal bone.
4. The sulcus for the middle meningeal artery runs from the foramen spinosum and ascends along the inside of the squamous portion, and forms a deep indentation in the calvarium. The middle meningeal artery divides into anterior and posterior branches above the middle of the zygomatic arch.
5. Impressions of the cerebral gyri of the temporal lobe of the brain are seen on the inner surface of the squamous portion.

M.-y. Han (✉) · P. Dai
College of Otolaryngology Head and Neck Surgery, Chinese PLA General Hospital, Beijing, China

M.-h. Wang
Department of Otolaryngology Head and Neck Surgery, Peking University International Hospital, Beijing, China

X. Gao
Department of Otolaryngology Head and Neck Surgery, PLA Rocket Force Characteristic Medical Center, Beijing, China

P. Dai et al. (eds.), *Stereoscopic Anatomical Atlas of Ear Surgery*, https://doi.org/10.1007/978-981-16-0927-5_2

Mastoid Portion

The mastoid portion has a pyramidal shape with its base positioned posteriorly and inferiorly behind the squamous portion. The superior border of the mastoid portion is bounded by the temporal line with the squamous portion above and connected with the mastoid angle of the parietal bone in the parietal notch. The posterior border articulates with the occipital bone. Antero-inferiorly it is fused with the tympanic portion by the tympanomastoid suture. The most medial part of the mastoid portion forms the petrous pyramid. The mastoid portion has internal and external surfaces. The mastoid bone is filled with multiple sinuses called mastoid air cells. It may have one of four different forms depending on the degree of pneumatization: pneumatic, diploeic, sclerotic, or mixed.

1. The suprameatal spine, also called the Spine of Henle, is a small bony spur located under the temporal line and at the upper and posterior part of the orifice of the EAC. It is the major landmark for locating the cribriform area and the position of the tympanic antrum.
2. The suprameatal triangle, or Macewen's triangle, is the area between the posterior wall of the EAC, the suprameatal spine, and the posterior root of the zygomatic process of the temporal bone. The location of the triangle is constant. There are multiple small blood vessels passing through the bone surface forming the cribriform area.
3. The parietal notch is the angle formed posteriorly between the squamous and petrous parts of the temporal bone.
4. The mastoid foramen is positioned at the posterior edge of the temporal bone which allows passage of the mastoid emissary vein draining to the sigmoid sinus and the posterior meningeal branch of the occipital artery which supplies the dura.
5. The mastoid notch is a groove on the medial surface of the mastoid process of the temporal bone from which the posterior belly of the digastric muscle originates. It is also called the digastric fossa. The inside of the mastoid notch contains the occipital artery groove and at its anterior end is the stylomastoid foramen.
6. The digastric ridge is the curved bony eminence inside the mastoid bone where the digastric muscle attaches. It corresponds to the mastoid notch. It is the reliable marker for the facial nerve as its anterior limit abuts the vertical (mastoid) segment of the facial nerve passing inferiorly to the stylomastoid foramen.
7. The stylomastoid foramen sits between the mastoid and styloid processes of the temporal bone. It marks the lower end of the bony facial canal and is the point where the facial nerve and stylomastoid artery pass to and from the neck respectively.
8. The sulcus of the sigmoid sinus is an S-shape groove containing the sinus and is located medially to the mastoid and anteroinferiorly to the posterior cranial fossa. It is a long arching eminence when seen from a surgical mastoid cavity forming part of the posterior wall of the cavity.

Tympanic Portion

The tympanic portion is a U-shape curved plate of bone lying below the squamous part of the temporal bone, in front of the mastoid process. It surrounds the external part of the ear canal forming the anterior, inferior, and part of the posterior walls of the canal. The anteroinferior quadrate part of the bony plate constitutes the posterior wall of the mandibular fossa.

1. The tympanic sulcus is a groove on the tympanic ring where the tympanic membrane is attached.
2. The tympanic notch (Notch of Rivinus) is a deficiency in the posterior edge of the bony annular tympanic ring, approximately 5 mm in diameter. It is located just superiorly to the tympanomastoid suture line in the posterior EAC.
3. There is a fissure between the tympanic portion and the squamous portion of the temporal bone in which there is a thin piece of the tegmen tympani dividing it into two parts. The anterior part is the petrosquamous fissure and the posterior part is petrotympanic fissure which transmits the chorda tympani nerve, the tympanic artery and vein.
4. The tympanomastoid suture is the slit between the posterior tympanic portion and mastoid portion, which is closed in the adult, leaving a faint shallow groove.

Petrous Portion

The petrous portion of the temporal bone is pyramid-shaped and is wedged in the base of the skull between the sphenoid and occipital bones. Its base is positioned laterally. The apex is directed medially, forward, and slightly upward.

The pyramid has three surfaces, and three edges where the surfaces join (also called angles). It contains the whole inner ear. The petrous portion forms part of the skull base and is part of the endocranium.

Anterior Surface of the Petrous Portion

It forms the floor of the posterior part of the middle fossa. Laterally it is connected to the inner part of the squamous portion. From medial to lateral the important landmarks are as follows: foramen lacerum, trigeminal impression, groove for greater superficial petrosal nerve (GSPN), groove for lesser superficial petrosal nerve (LSPN), arcuate eminence, and tegmen tympani.

1. The foramen lacerum is a triangular hole in the base of the skull located between the sphenoid, the apex of the petrous temporal, and the basilar part of the occipital bone where the carotid artery transverses.
2. The trigeminal impression is a bony depression near the petrous apex, which accommodates the trigeminal ganglion.
3. Lateral to the trigeminal impression are two shallow trenches running parallel to the long axis of the petrous portion. The more medial is the groove for GSPN and the lateral is for the LSPN. The outer ends of the two grooves are the hiatus of the facial nerve canal and the superior aperture of the tympanic canaliculus respectively.
4. The arcuate eminence is an arch-like elevation seen on the anterior surface of the petrous part of the temporal bone in the middle cranial fossa. It has traditionally been regarded as a protrusion caused by the superior semicircular canal present in the petrous bone. This landmark is not always obvious.
5. The tegmen tympani is formed by a thin plate of bone lateral to the arcuate eminence as the roof of the tympanic cavity separating it from the cranial cavity. When performing a decompression of the facial nerve via a middle cranial fossa approach, the tegmen tympani can be drilled away to expose the malleus, incus, and cochleariform process to locate and track the facial nerve especially if the anatomical landmarks are unclear from above.

Posterior Surface of Petrous Portion

This is a triangular bony surface surrounded by the superior petrosal sinus above, inferior petrosal sinus below, and sigmoid sinus posteriorly. It forms the anterior border of the posterior cranial fossa and is also called its cerebellar surface. From the medial to lateral, the main anatomical landmarks are as follows: the porus of the internal auditory canal (IAC), subarcuate fossa, and fissure of the endolymphatic sac.

1. The middle part of the posterior surface of the petrous portion is the oblique positioned opening of the intracranial end of the IAC, with a sharp posterior rim and a flattened anterior rim.
2. The IAC is approximately 1 cm in length and sits in the petrous part of the temporal bone between the posterior cranial fossa and the inner ear. It provides a passage for the vestibulocochlear nerve, the facial nerve, and the labyrinthine artery between the posterior cranial fossa and the inner ear and the face. It also contains the vestibular ganglion. The fundus of the canal is divided into a smaller superior and larger inferior section by the transverse crest. Its upper lateral end is divided by a vertical bony plate, Bill's bar, into anterior and posterior sections.
3. There is a depression in the space between the IAC porus and the fissure of the endolymphatic sac for the passage of a small dural vein.
4. The fissure for the endolymphatic sac is a small slit located approximately 1 cm posterior and lateral to the porus of the IAC which accommodates the endolymphatic sac and the external aperture of the vestibular aqueduct.

Inferior Surface of Petrous Portion

This is an irregular surface that forms part of the skull base. The main bony landmarks are as follows:

1. The carotid canal is a bony opening located in the middle of the inferior surface of the petrosal part, anterior to the jugular foramen, where the internal carotid artery passes forwards and intracranially.
2. Postero-lateral to the opening of the carotid canal is the jugular fossa accommodating the jugular bulb and jugular foramen through which the bulb joins the internal jugular vein.

3. The jugulocarotid spine is a thin bony crest between the external aperture of the carotid artery and the jugular fossa. The inferior aperture of the tympanic canaliculus is seen in its external surface. The tympanic branch of the glossopharyngeal nerve (Jacobson's nerve) and the carotico-tympanic artery pass through the aperture into the tympanic cavity.
4. The external opening of the cochlear aqueduct, the cochlear canaliculus is at the anteromedial side of the jugular fossa through a triangular fossa medial to the carotid canal.
5. The jugular foramen sits between the posterior border of the petrous temporal bone and the anterior edge of the occipital bone. It is relatively large and positioned posterior to the carotid canal. The right foramen is usually larger than the left. The foramen gives passage to the IX, X, and XI cranial nerves, the inferior petrosal sinus, and is the site where the jugular bulb becomes the internal jugular vein.
6. The mastoid canaliculus sits in the lateral wall of the jugular fossa and transmits the auricular branch of the vagus nerve (Arnold's Nerve).
7. The rough anteromedial part of the inferior surface of the petrous portion gives attachment to the levator palati muscle, tensor veli palatini muscle, and the cartilaginous part of the Eustachian tube.

Three Margins of the Petrous Portion

1. The superior edge of the petrous portion is where the anterior and posterior surfaces of the pyramid meet. It is also called the petrous ridge. It contains a groove in its medial surface accommodating the superior petrosal sinus. There is a notch in the medial part of the superior border which contains the posterior part of the trigeminal nerve ganglion. The tip of the superior border connecting with the sphenoid bone by the petro sphenoidal (petroclinoid) ligament forms a small tube, through which the abducent nerve and the inferior petrosal sinus pass.
2. The posterior margin of the petrous portion where the posterior and inferior surfaces meet. There is the groove located in the internal part of the posterior border of the petrous portion, which contains the inferior petrosal sinus. The lateral segment of the posterior margin of the petrous portion and the jugular notch of occipital bone form the jugular foramen.
3. The anterior margin of the petrous portion. The internal part relates to the greater wing of the sphenoid bone to form sphenopetrosal fissure; the external part participates in forming the petrosquamous fissure and petrotympanic fissure; there are two bony tubes entering the tympanic cavity between the petrous portion and squamous portion, the upper one is the semicanal for the tensor tympani muscle and the lower is the Eustachian tube.

Styloid Process

The temporal styloid process is a process of bone that extends down from the temporal bone of the skull, just below the ear. The average length is approximately 25 mm. Its distal part gives attachment to the following structures: stylohyoid ligament, stylomandibular ligament, styloglossus muscle, stylohyoid muscle, and stylopharyngeus muscle. The stylomastoid foramen is between the styloid process and the mastoid. It is the external aperture of the facial nerve canal where the facial nerve passes out toward the parotid gland.

Bony Structures of the Temporal Bone

Ming-yu Han and Xue Gao

The temporal bones (are a pair of irregular bones, situated on each side of the skull. The squamous, tympanic, mastoid, petrous, and styloid process parts are its major components. The temporal, parietal, sphenoid, and occipital bones are connected at named fissures. Detailed knowledge of the bony structure and three-dimensional position of the temporal bone are the foundation and prerequisite for performing surgery on the ear.

The squamous portion of the temporal bone has four major landmarks: temporal line, zygomatic process, sulcus for the middle temporal artery, sulcus for the middle meningeal artery.

The mastoid portion of the temporal bone has six major features: external suprameatal spine (Spine of Henle), suprameatal triangle, parietal incisura, mastoid foramen, ridge of the digastric muscle and groove of the sigmoid sinus.

The major bony landmark of the anterior part of the tympanic portion is the endomeatal spine.

The vertical component of the squamous portion is irregular and complex. The major components of the three surfaces of the temporal bone are (1) superior surface: tegmen tympani, cupula of the tympanic antrum, mastoid roof, arcuate eminence, sulcus of GSPN, sulcus of LSPN, trigeminal impression; (2) posterior surface: ridge of petrous bone, superior petrosal sulcus, inferior petrosal sulcus, IAC porus, subarcuate fossa, fissure of endolymphatic sac; (3) Inferior surface: internal and external canals of the internal carotid artery, jugular fossa, jugular foramen, semicanal for the tensor tympani muscle, bony portion of the Eustachian tube and stylomastoid foramen.

The temporal bone is made up of a number of smaller irregular bones, and thus there are many fissures, including: tympanomastoid, occipitomastoid, petrotympanic, and petrosquamous fissures.

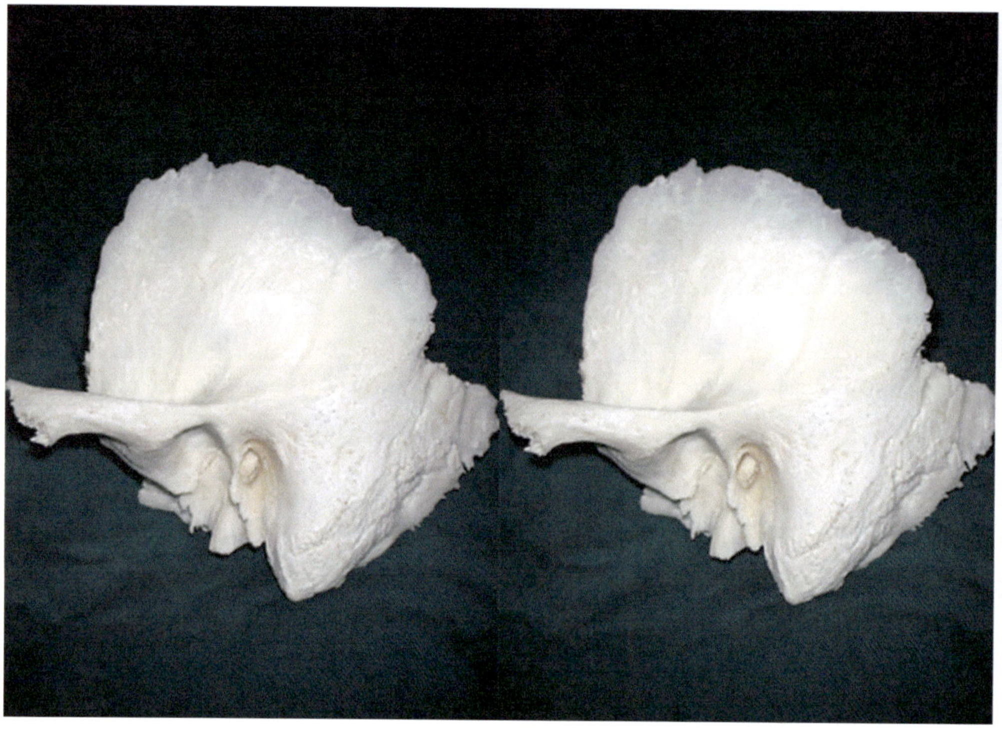

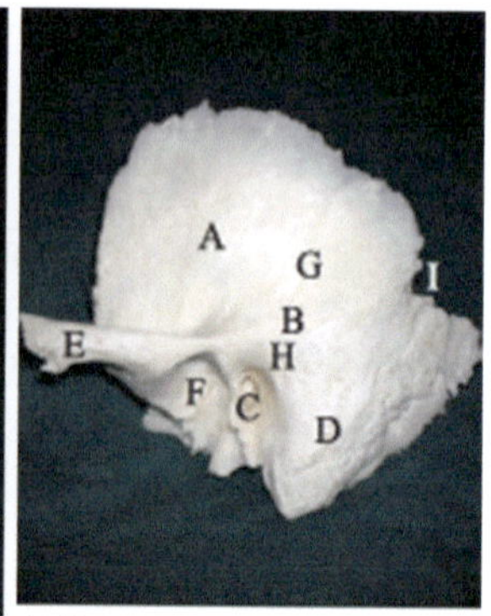

A. Squamous portion
B. Temporal line
C. Tympanic portion
D. Mastoid portion
E. Zygomatic process
F. Mandibular fossa
G. Sulcus for middle temporal artery
H. Suprameatal triangle
I. Parietal incisura

Fig. 2.1 Bony landmarks of the lateral side of the temporal bone (left) The outer surface of the squamous portion is relatively smooth. There is a sulcus for the middle temporal artery in its posterior half. A prominence on the inferior surface of the zygomatic process forms the anterior border of the mandibular fossa, and the bony part of EAC forms its posterior wall. The posterior expansion of the zygomatic process forms the temporal line. The surface of the mastoid process is rough and serves as the attachment for the sternocleidomastoid, trapezius, and splenius capitis muscles. The outside surface of the temporal bone provides approximate landmarks for the floor of the middle cranial fossa, facial nerve, and sigmoid sinus

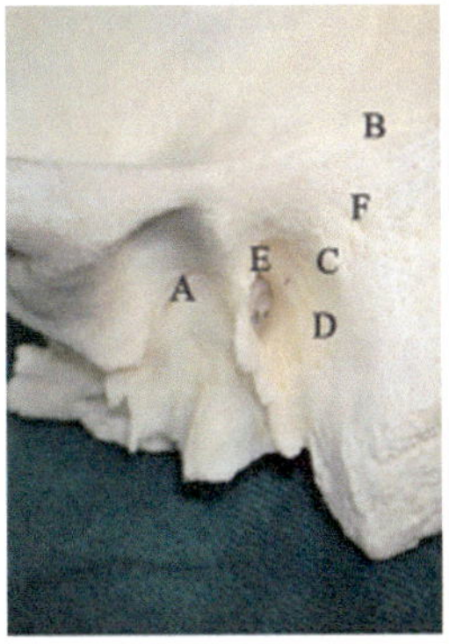

A. Petrotympanic fissure
B. Temporal line
C. Suprameatal spine
D. Tympanomastoid fissure
E. Endomeatal spine
F. Cribriform area

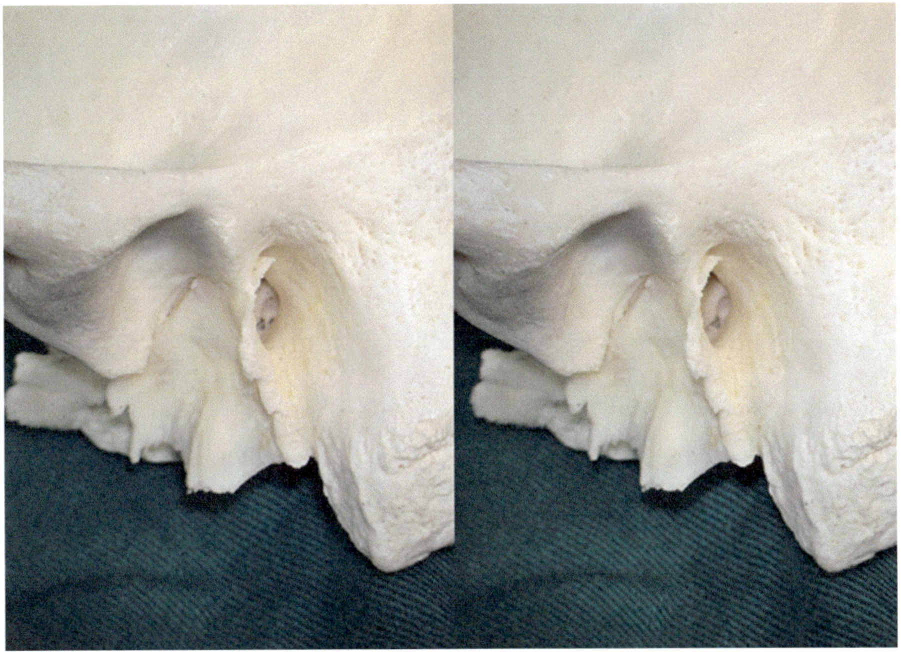

Fig. 2.2 Tympanic portion and bony EAC (left)
There are a little bony ridge and fissure in the anterior-superior wall of the EAC known as the endomeatal spine and fissure. It is usually necessary to remove the endomeatal spine to fully elevate EAC skin flaps by a trans-canal approach. The EAC branch of the auriculotemporal nerve passes through the endomeatal spine, making this a preferred site for infiltration of local anesthetic. In the posterior suprameatal region, there are the suprameatal spine and suprameatal triangle. Deep to this triangle is the mastoid antrum. The posterior fissure of the EAC is the tympanomastoid fissure, and deep to this is the vertical segment of the facial nerve. The petro-tympanic fissure lies between the tympanic bone and the petrous portion and at its anteromedial ends lies the canaliculus for the chorda tympani passing from the tympanic cavity to the infratemporal fossa

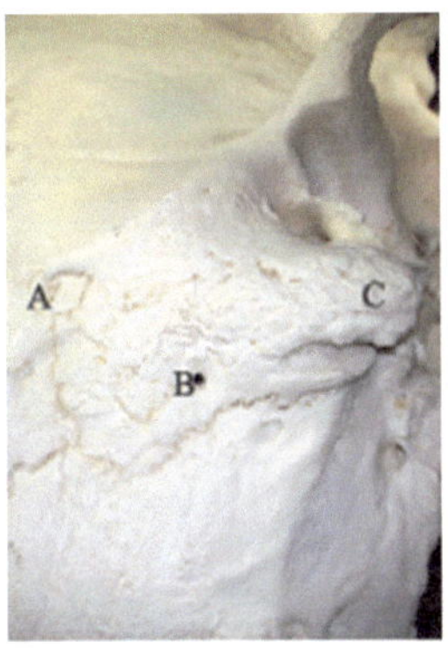

A. Parietal incisura
B. Mastoid foramen
C. Mastoid tip

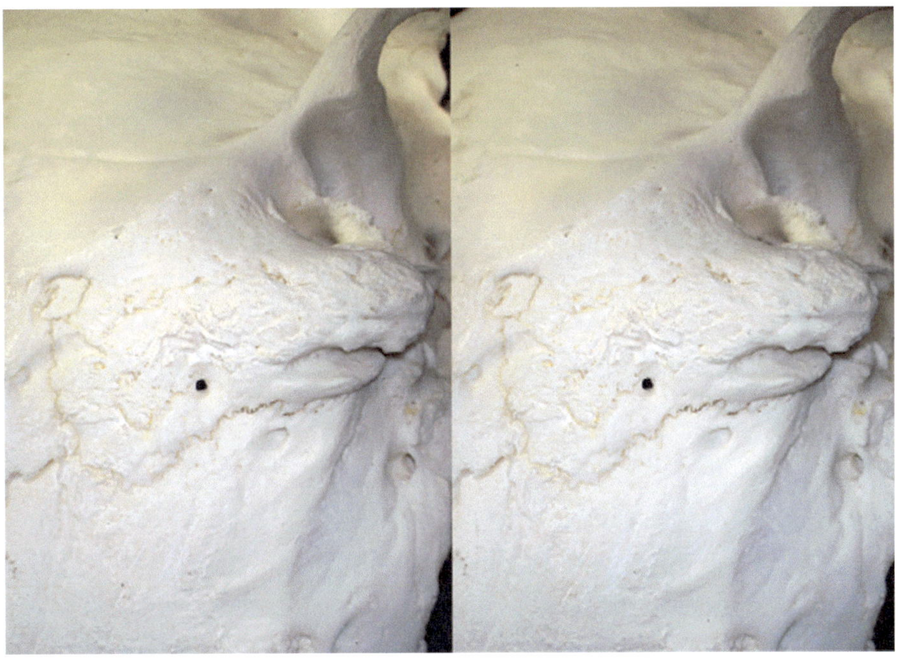

Fig. 2.3 Lateral surface of the mastoid and mastoid foramen (right)
The outer surface of the mastoid portion of the temporal bone is coarse. The sternocleidomastoid, trapezius, and splenius capitis muscles attach to the mastoid process infero-laterally. In the middle part of the posterior border of the mastoid portion, there are multiple foramina for the mastoid emissary veins joining the sigmoid sinus. On the medial surface of the mastoid tip is the mastoid notch (or digastric groove) where the posterior belly of the digastric muscle attaches. Corresponding to the notch inside the mastoid is the digastric ridge which is only seen when the mastoid cavity has been created surgically. The anterior end of the ridge abuts the line of the vertical segment of the facial nerve. It is safe to dissect in surgery outside the line of the ridge. There is a sulcus near the mastoid notch for the occipital artery

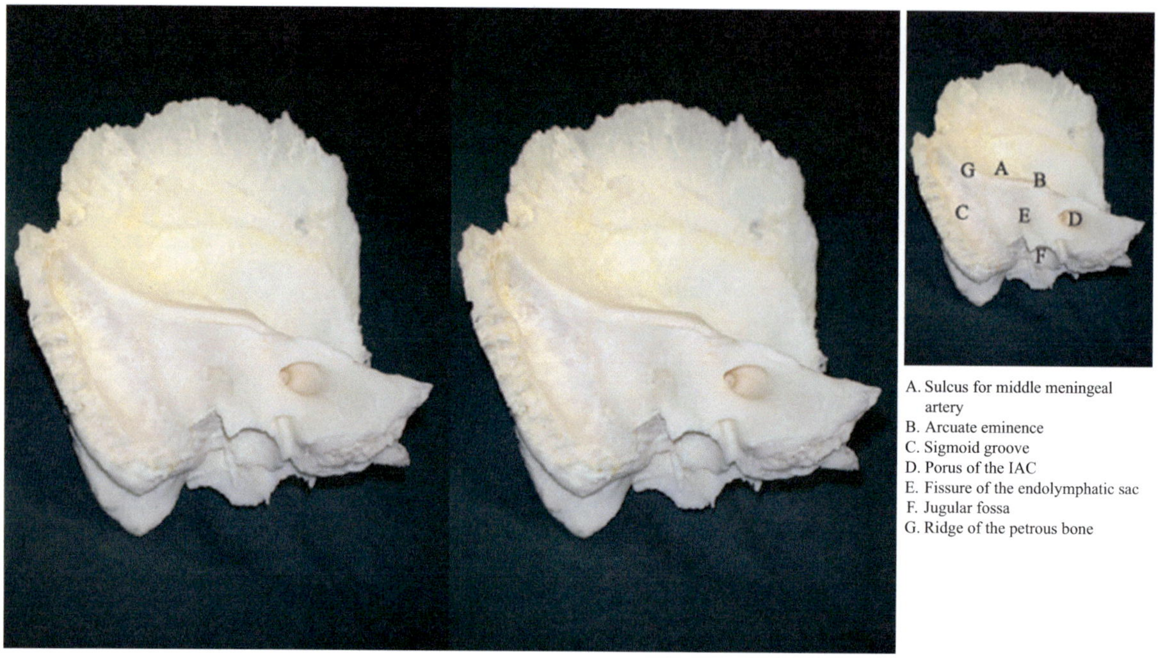

Fig. 2.4 Medial surface of squamous portion and posterior aspect of petrous bone (left)
On the inner face of the squamous portion of the temporal bone, there are depressions for the gyri of the temporal lobe and a sulcus for the middle meningeal artery. Along the ridge of the petrous bone is the sulcus for the superior petrosal sinus. The tentorium cerebellae also attaches to the petrous ridge. Inferiorly the petrous bone has a sulcus for the inferior petrosal sinus. The posterior-lateral portion of the petrous bone has an S-shaped sulcus for the sigmoid sinus. In the middle of the posterior surface of the petrous bone is the porus at the medial end of the IAC. Posterior to the IAC is a depression for the endolymphatic sac over the external aperture of the vestibular aqueduct which contains the endolymphatic duct

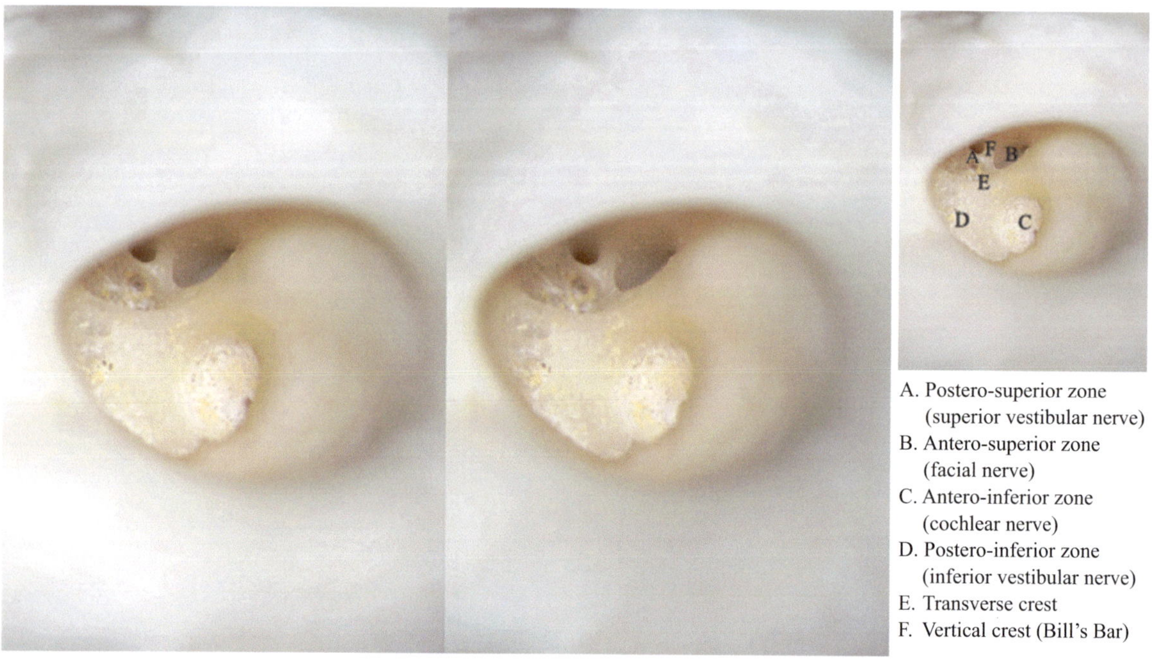

Fig. 2.5 Fundus of IAC (left)
(Viewed from inside to outside) The lateral end or fundus of IAC has a common wall with the medial part of the inner ear. The fundus is divided into two parts by the transverse crest (which also extends along the posterior wall of the canal). The superior part is further divided into anterior and posterior zones by a vertical crest also called Bill's Bar. The IAC fundus thus has four zones: anterosuperior zone (facial nerve passing through), anteroinferior zone (cochlea nerve passing through), posterosuperior zone (superior vestibular nerve passing through), and posteroinferior zone (inferior vestibular nerve passing through). Sometimes, the posteroinferior zone also has a foramen for the posterior ampullary nerve

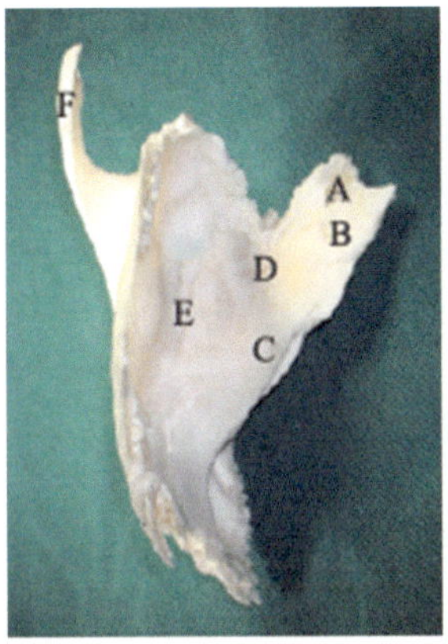

A. Internal aperture of the internal carotid canal
B. Trigeminal impression
C. Arcuate eminence
D. Sulcus of the GSPN
E. Tegmen tympani
F. Zygomatic process

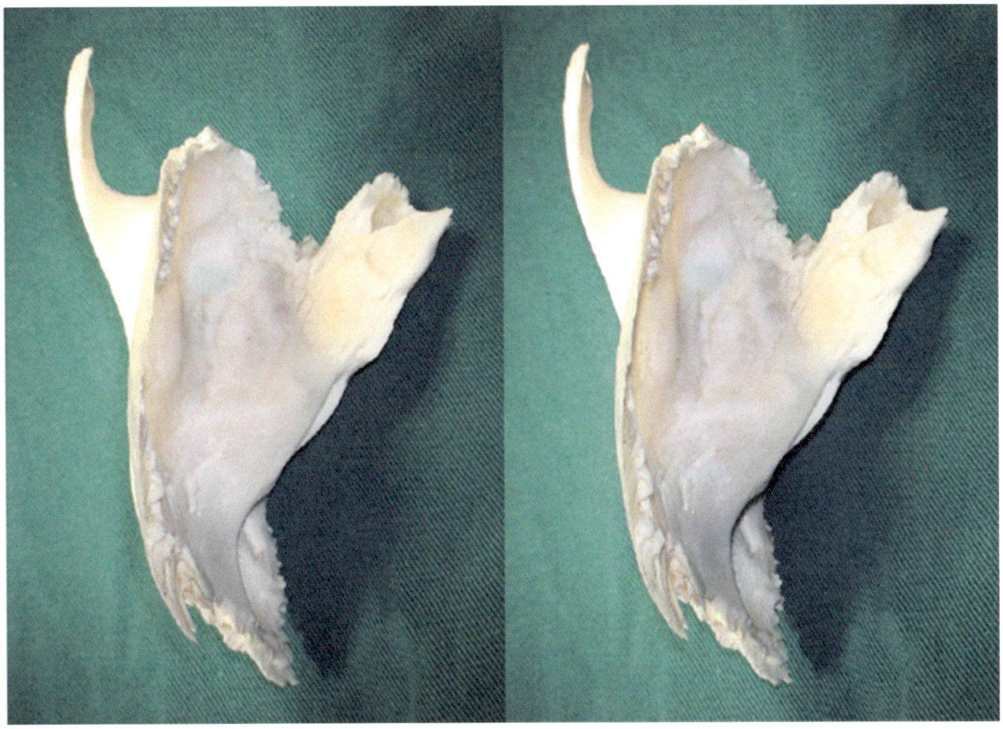

Fig. 2.6 View of the temporal bone from above (left)
In the middle of the superior surface of the petrous bone is the arcuate eminence of the superior semicircular canal. Laterally, is a slightly concave portion of the petrous bone formed by the tegmen tympani and tegmen mastoideum. The trigeminal semilunar ganglionic impression is close to the apex of the petrous bone. Antero-inferior to the apex of the petrous bone is the internal aperture of the internal carotid canal

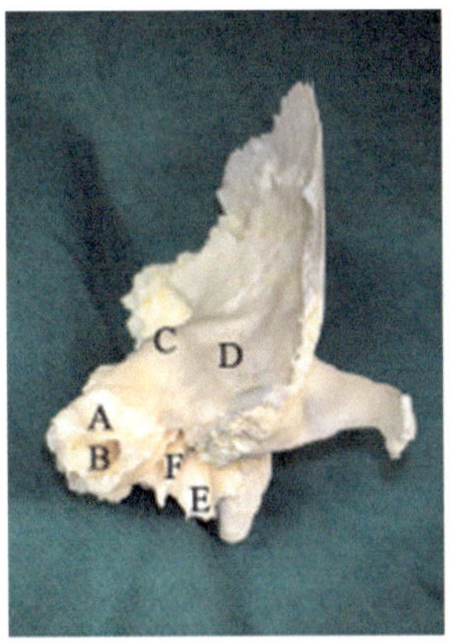

A. Trigeminal impression
B. Internal aperture of the internal carotid canal
C. Arcuate eminence
D. Tegmen tympani
E. Tympanic bone
F. The bony part of the Eustachian tube

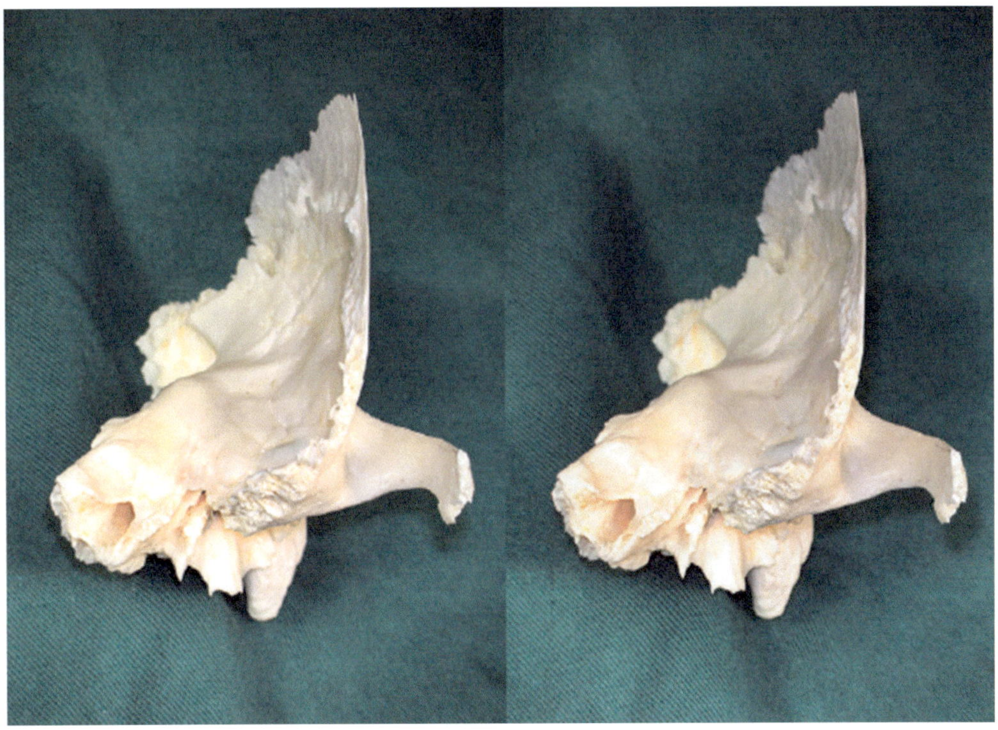

Fig. 2.7 Anterior view of the temporal bone (left)
The foramen lacerum is bounded by the apex of the petrous bone, the greater wing of the sphenoid bone, and the basal part of the occipital bone. It is closed in life by dense fibrous tissue. Postero-lateral to the trigeminal impression there are two parallel fissures. The lateral one is the sulcus of the LSPN and the medial one is the sulcus of the GSPN. At the lateral end of the GSPN sulcus is the hiatus of the facial nerve canal connecting the GSPN with the geniculate ganglion. The bony part of the Eustachian tube is located at the junction of the petrous and squamous parts of the temporal bone

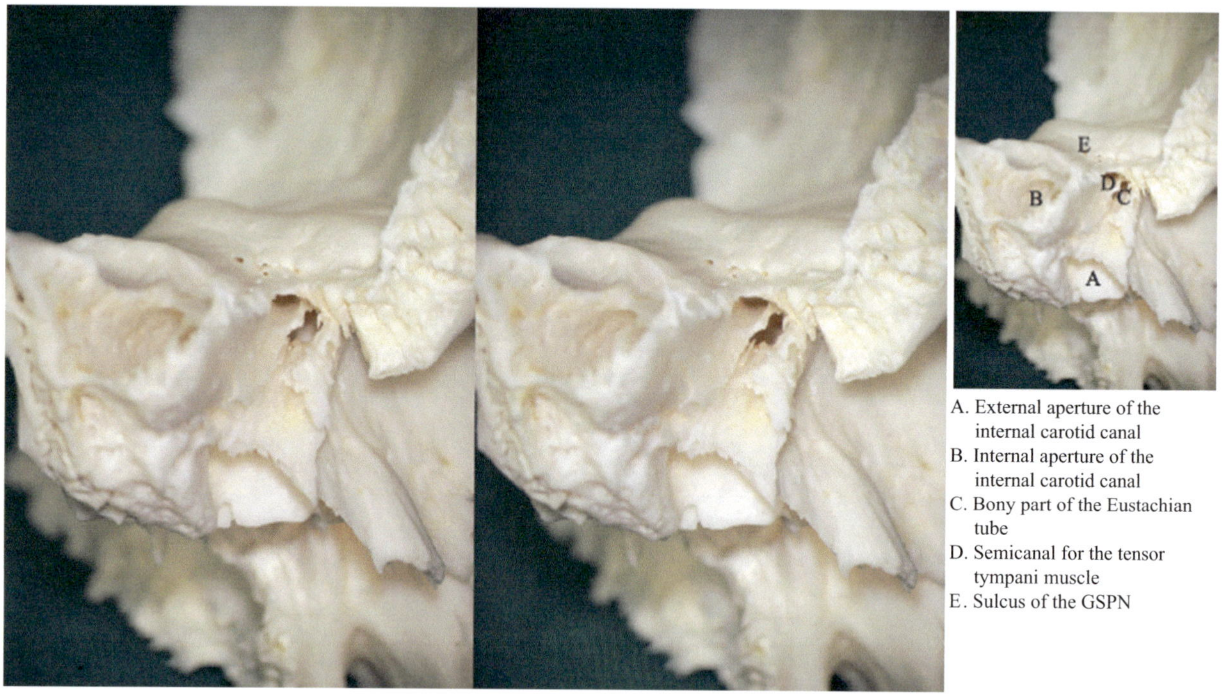

A. External aperture of the internal carotid canal
B. Internal aperture of the internal carotid canal
C. Bony part of the Eustachian tube
D. Semicanal for the tensor tympani muscle
E. Sulcus of the GSPN

Fig. 2.8 Anterior view of the temporal bone (left)
The external aperture of the internal carotid canal is located at the inferior aspect of the petrous bone, and the internal aperture of the internal carotid canal at the anteroinferior part of the petrous apex. Close to the horizontal segment of the internal carotid canal, there are two parallel bony canals. The superomedial one is the semicanal for the tensor tympani muscle and the inferolateral canal is the bony part of the Eustachian tube

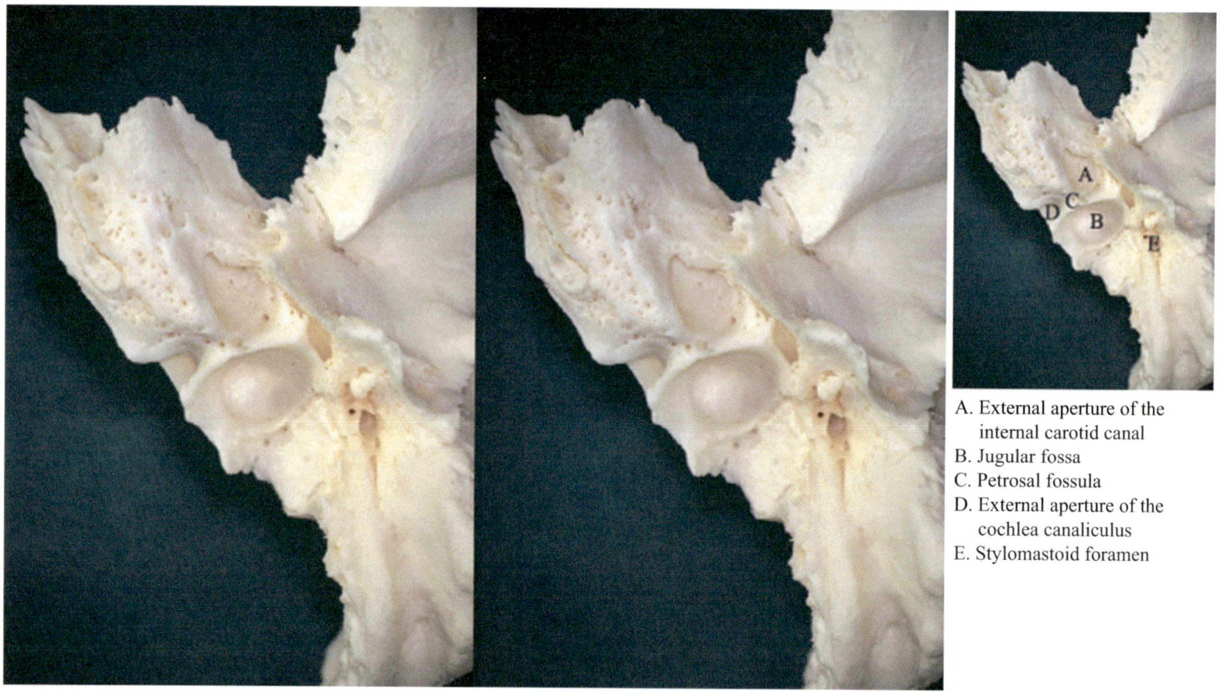

A. External aperture of the internal carotid canal
B. Jugular fossa
C. Petrosal fossula
D. External aperture of the cochlea canaliculus
E. Stylomastoid foramen

Fig. 2.9 Inferior surface of the temporal bone (left)
The inferior surface of the temporal bone is rough and complex. Close to the apex of the petrous bone are the attachments of the tensor veli palatini and levator veli palatini muscles and the cartilaginous part of the Eustachian tube. Postero-lateral to the petrous apex is the external aperture of the internal carotid canal and the jugular fossa. Between these two structures is the site of the ganglion derived from the glossopharyngeal nerve externally, sitting in a bony depression (the petrosal fossula). In the ridge between the internal carotid artery and jugular fossa is the aperture of the tympanic canaliculus containing Jacobson's nerve and the tympanic branch of the ascending pharyngeal artery. Postero-medial to the petrosal fossula is the external aperture of the cochlea canaliculus. The facial nerve exits the skull through the stylomastoid foramen

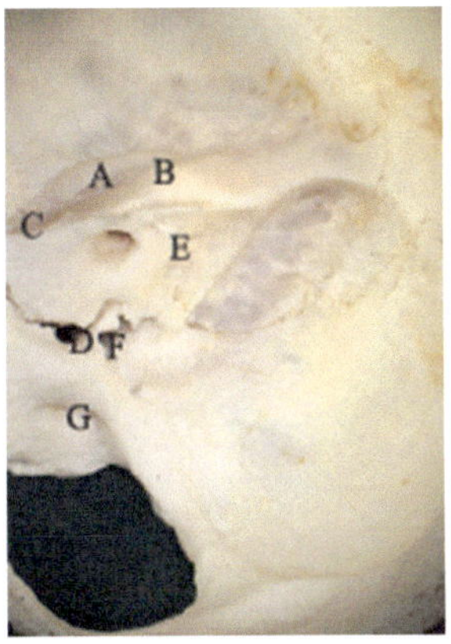

A. Tegmen tympani
B. Arcuate eminence
C. Trigeminal impression
D. Jugular foramen petrosal part
E. Fissure of the endolymphatic sac
F. Jugular foramen sigmoid part
G. Internal aperture of the hypoglossal canal

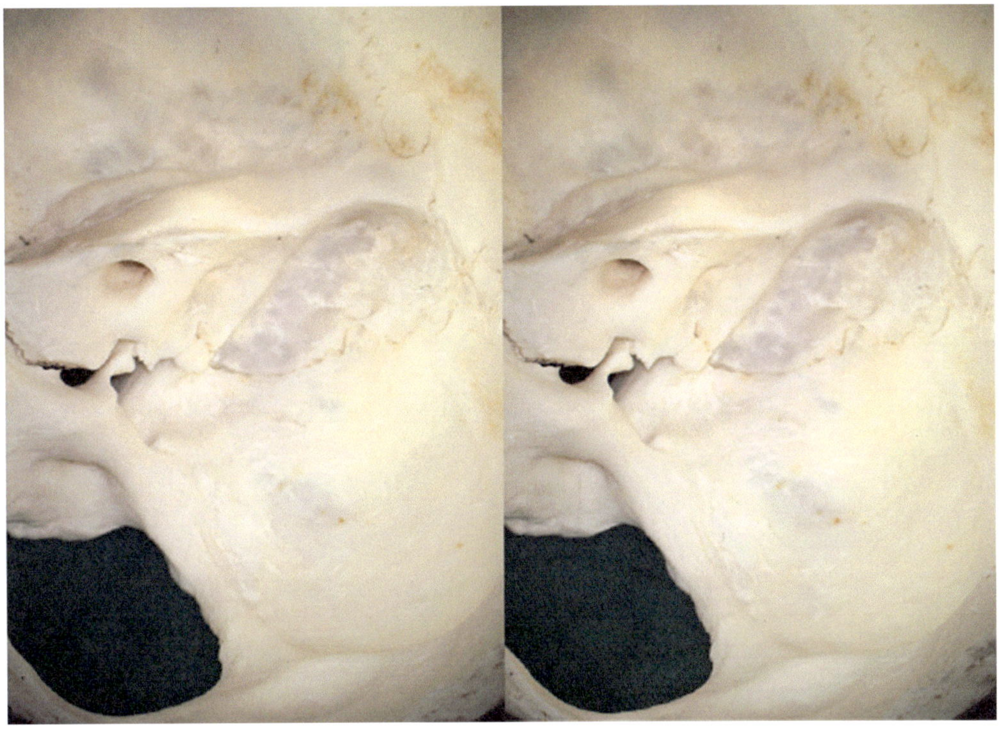

Fig. 2.10 Internal surface of the temporal bone and skull base (right)
The external aperture of the endolymphatic duct is within the fissure of the endolymphatic sac. The distance between the external aperture of the endolymphatic duct and porus of the IAC is 1 cm. Superior to the IAC porus and fissure of the endolymphatic sac is the subarcuate fossa through which passes the subarcuate artery. The sigmoid sinus sits in its groove and joins the internal jugular vein via the jugular bulb. The jugular foramen is divided into an anterior petrosal part and posterior sigmoid part containing the inferior petrosal sinus and sigmoid sinus, respectively

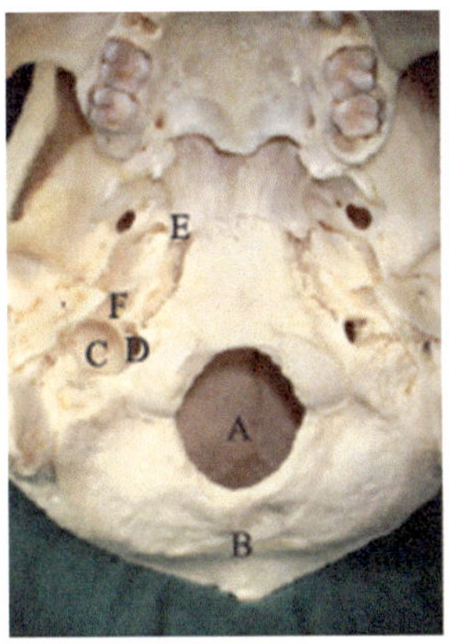

A. Foramen magnum
B. Occipital bone
C. Jugular fossa
D. Jugular foramen
E. Pterygoid process of the sphenoid bone
F. External aperture of the internal carotid artery

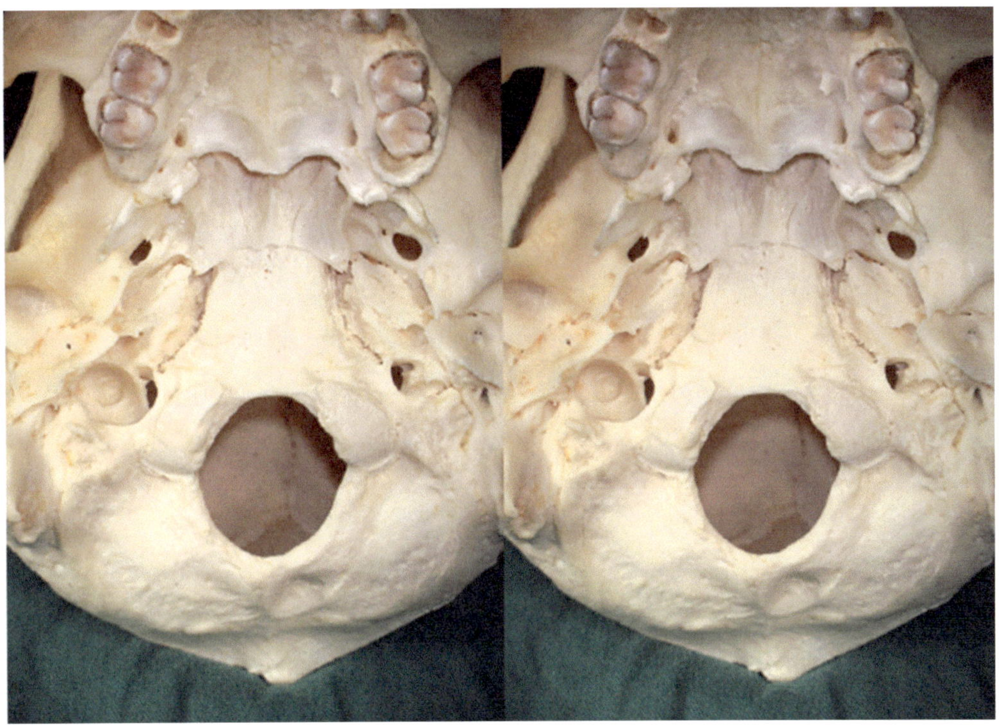

Fig. 2.11 Inferior surface of the skull
Corresponding to the internal surface of the cranial base (anterior, middle, and posterior cranial fossa), the inferior surface of the skull base can be divided into three parts, which are anterior, middle, and posterior skull base. The petrous apex and lateral skull base are mainly located in the middle and posterior zones. The important structures in the middle and posterior skull base include: petrous apex, sphenoid body, sella turcica, clivus, hypoglossal canal, temporal bone, and pterygoid process of the sphenoid bone

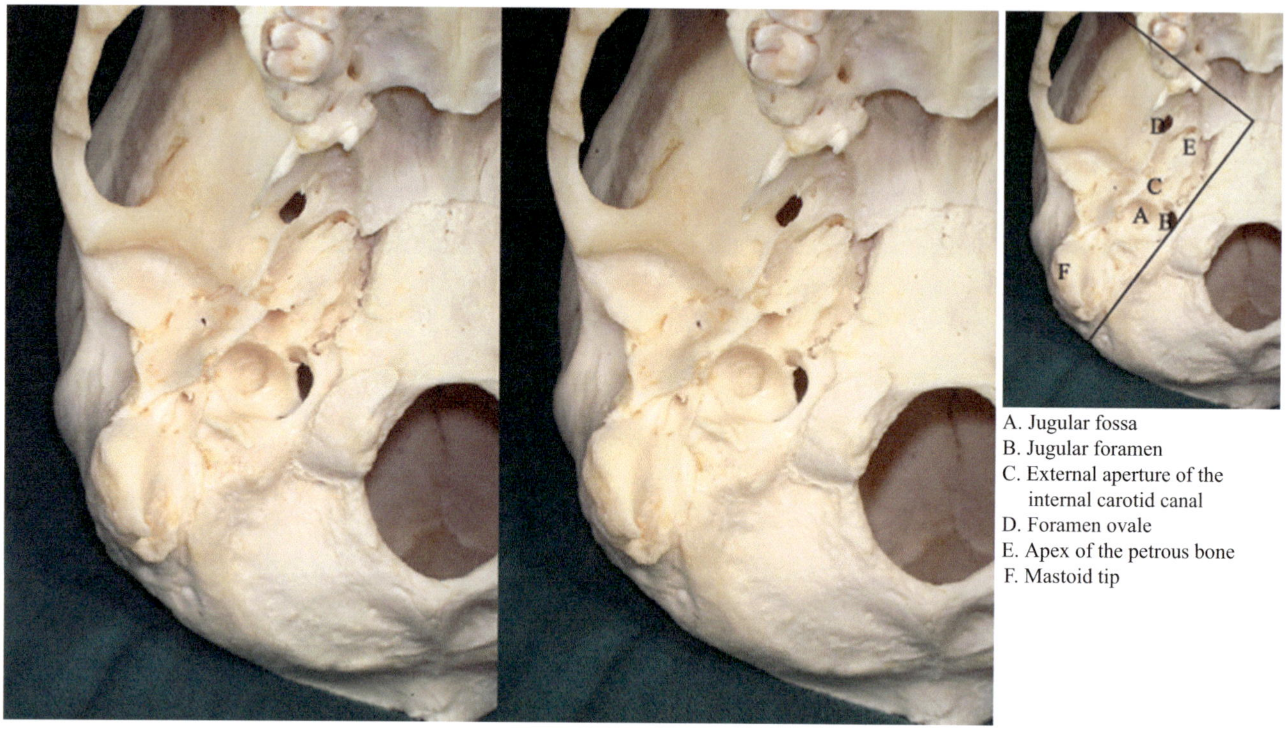

Fig. 2.12 Lateral skull base and its constituent parts (right)
Draw an imaginary line from the center of the nasopharynx roof medially, anterolaterally across the pterygopalatine fossa to the inferior orbital fissure and a second line from the mid-nasopharynx posterolaterally across the jugular fossa to the posterior margin of the mastoid, the triangular area between them is the lateral skull base region. In 1984, Van Huijzer divided the lateral skull base as follows: nasopharyngeal portion, Eustachian tube portion, neurovascular portion, acoustic portion, joint portion, and the inferior temporal portion

Bony Structures of Middle Ear

Meng-hang Wang and Pu Dai

The middle ear cleft is an air-filled, irregular space located within the temporal bone, which comprises the Eustachian tube, tympanic cavity, tympanic antrum, and mastoid cells. The middle ear is a crucial component in the transmission of sound from the air of the EAC to the fluids of the inner ear.

The tympanic cavity is irregular and the biggest air-filled space of the temporal bone. It is surrounded by squamous, tympanic, and petrous portions of the bone and the tympanic membrane. The tympanic cavity is connected to the nasopharynx anteriorly and medially by the Eustachian tube. Posteriorly and superiorly it connects via the aditus ad antrum to the mastoid antrum, a cavity in the mastoid process of the temporal bone. The tympanic cavity is 2–4 mm in depth, ~15 mm in vertical height, ~13 mm anteroposteriorly. It is ~2 mm deep in the mesotympanum, ~4 mm deep in the epitympanum, and ~6 mm deep in the hypotympanum. Its volume is 1–2 ml.

The tympanic cavity has six walls:

- Lateral wall: The lateral wall is formed mostly by the tympanic membrane and the bony wall of the epitympanum.
- Superior wall (Tegmental wall): The roof is formed by the tegmen tympani, which is part of the temporal bone.
- Inferior wall (Jugular wall): The floor is formed by a bone that separates the middle ear from the jugular bulb and internal jugular vein.
- Anterior wall (Carotid wall): The anterior wall separates the tympanic cavity from the carotid canal and artery. It has the opening for the Eustachian tube and the semicanal for the tensor tympani muscle.
- Posterior wall (Mastoid wall): The posterior wall has an opening called the aditus ad antrum that connects the tympanic cavity (epitympanum) to the mastoid air cells.
- Medial wall (Labyrinthine wall): The medial wall separates the middle ear from the inner ear. It includes the promontory of the labyrinthine wall and the oval and round windows.

The other related structures of middle ear:

- Eustachian tube: It consists of a bony part and a cartilaginous part. The bony part (1/3) is nearest to the middle ear and begins in the anterior wall of the tympanic cavity, ends at the angle of junction of the squamous and the petrous portions of the temporal bone, it is below the septum separating it from the semi-canal of the tensor tympani muscle and medial to the internal carotid artery. The cartilaginous portion (2/3) is nearest to the nasopharynx and is formed of a triangular plate of elastic fibrocartilage.
- Tympanic antrum: It is a large air space communicating posteriorly with the mastoid cells and anteriorly with the epitympanum above the middle ear space. The tympanic antrum is a very important anatomical landmark in middle ear surgery.
- Mastoid cells: Positioned in the lower part of the squamous portion of the temporal bone there are many air-filled cells, which exhibit great variety in their size and number.

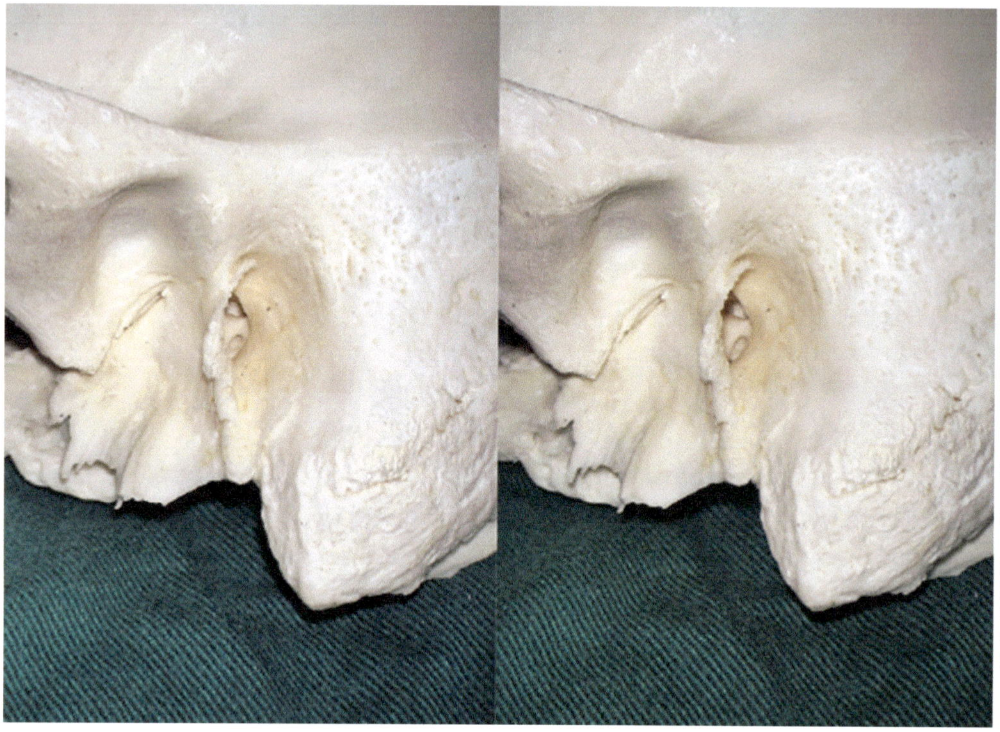

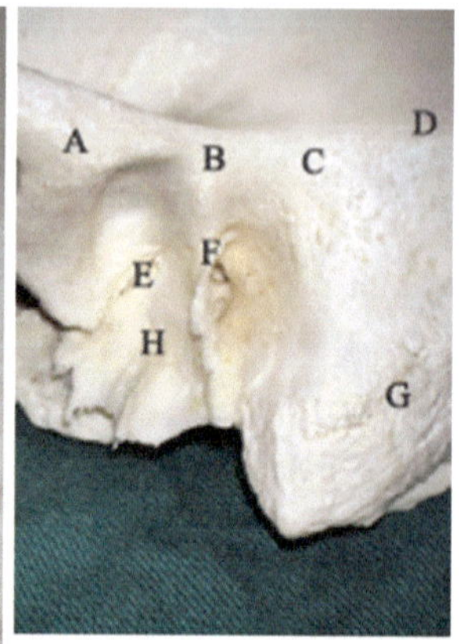

A. Anterior root of zygomatic process
B. Middle root of zygomatic process
C. Posterior root of zygomatic process
D. Temporal ridge (temporal line)
E. Petrotympanic fissure
F. Squamotympanic fissure
G. Mastoid
H. Tympanic bone

Fig. 2.13 Outer surface of the temporal bone (left vertical)
The outer surface of the temporal bone centers on the EAC and consists of three portions, the squamous, mastoid, and tympanic portions. The tympanic portion lies below the squamous portion, in front of the mastoid portion, and forms the front, inferior, and part of the posterior walls of the bony EAC. The superior wall of the bony EAC is the middle and posterior root of the zygomatic process. The line between the posterior root of the zygomatic process and parietal notch is named the temporal ridge (or temporal line) and is the surface projection of the bottom of the middle cranial fossa. Middle ear surgery should be undertaken below the level of the temporal ridge, which corresponds to the level of the dura

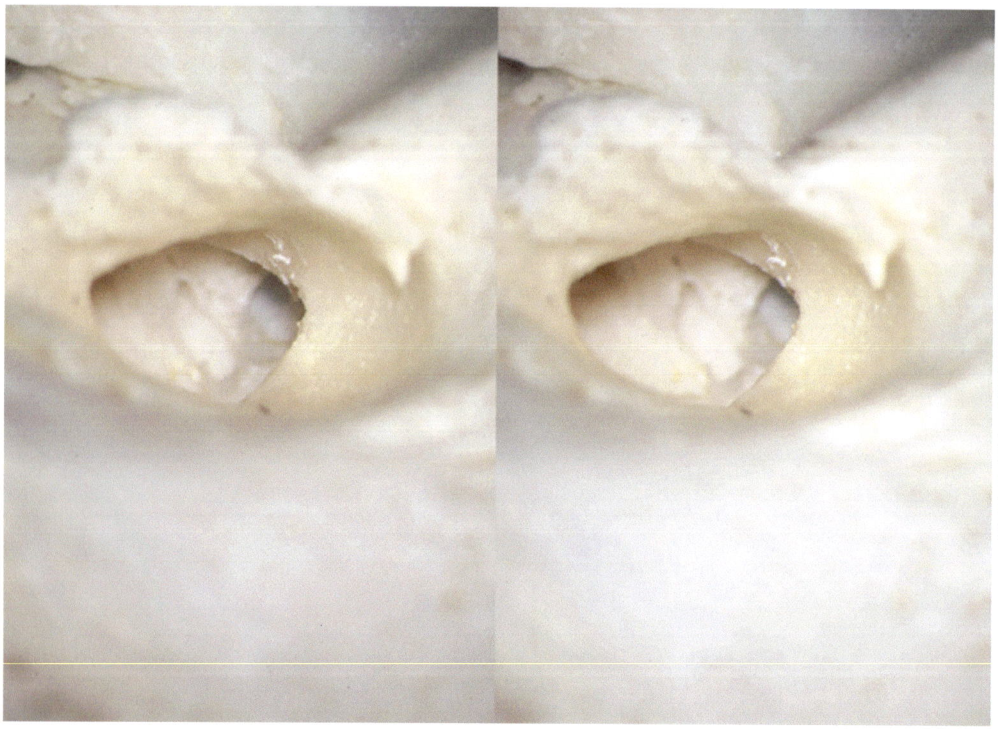

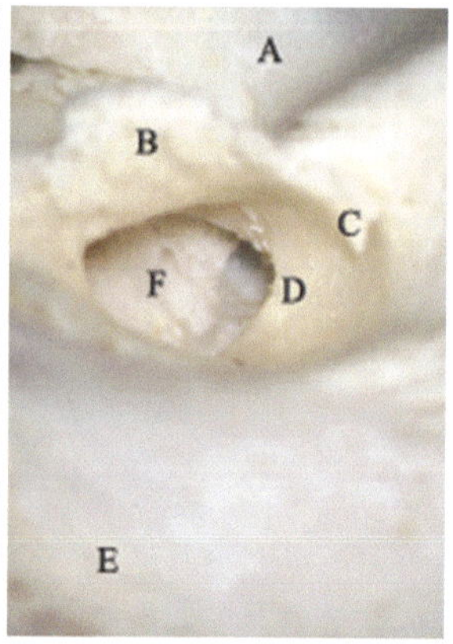

A. Mandibular fossa
B. Tympanic portion
C. Endomeatal spine
D. Scutum of the epitympanum
E. Mastoid portion
F. Mesotympanum

Fig. 2.14 Bony EAC and scutum of the epitympanum (left recumbent)
The anterior, inferior, and part of the posterior wall of bony EAC are formed by the tympanic portion, while the posterior-superior wall is formed by the squamous portion. The lateral bony wall (scutum) of the epitympanum is formed by the squamous portion, making up part of the lateral wall of the tympanic cavity and separating the epitympanum from the bony EAC

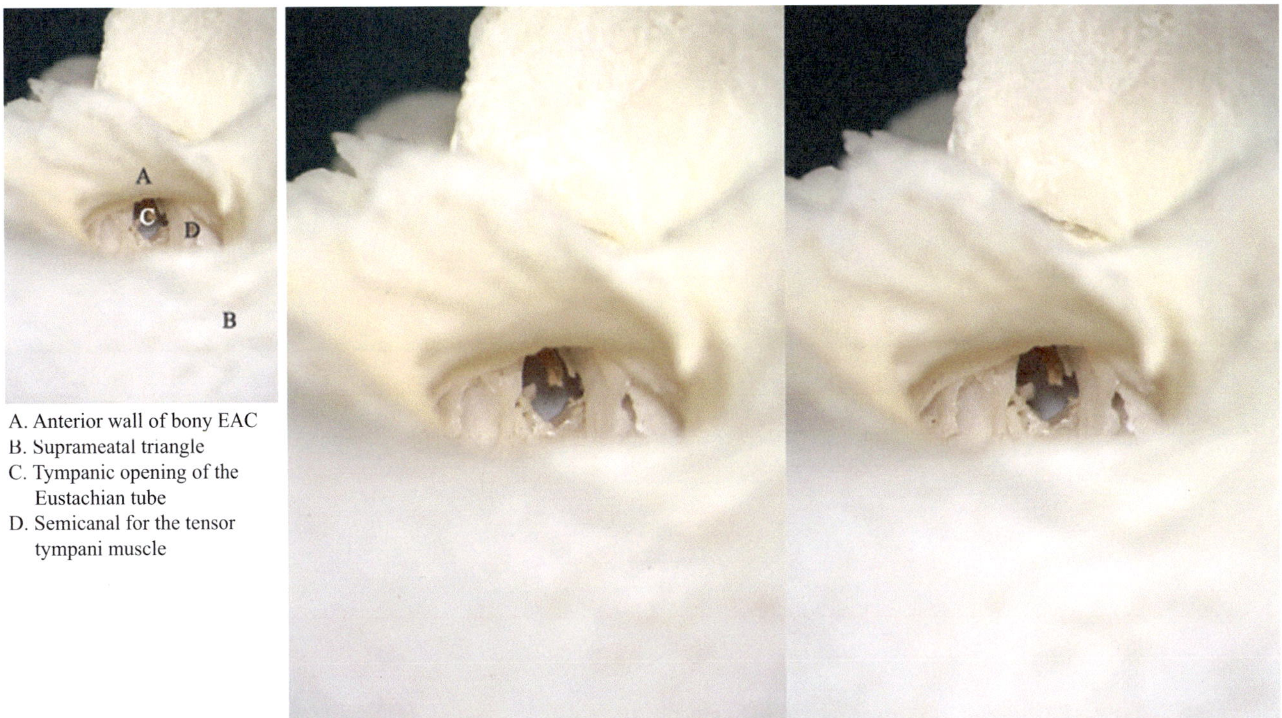

A. Anterior wall of bony EAC
B. Suprameatal triangle
C. Tympanic opening of the Eustachian tube
D. Semicanal for the tensor tympani muscle

Fig. 2.15 Tympanic part of the Eustachian tube (left)
The anterior wall of the tympanic cavity has the opening for the Eustachian tube just inferior to the semicanal for the tensor tympani muscle. A thin bony wall separates the tympanic cavity anteriorly from the internal carotid artery. Care should be taken when dissecting in the Eustachian tube, as the bony septum is sometimes dehiscent and the risk of injuring the artery exists

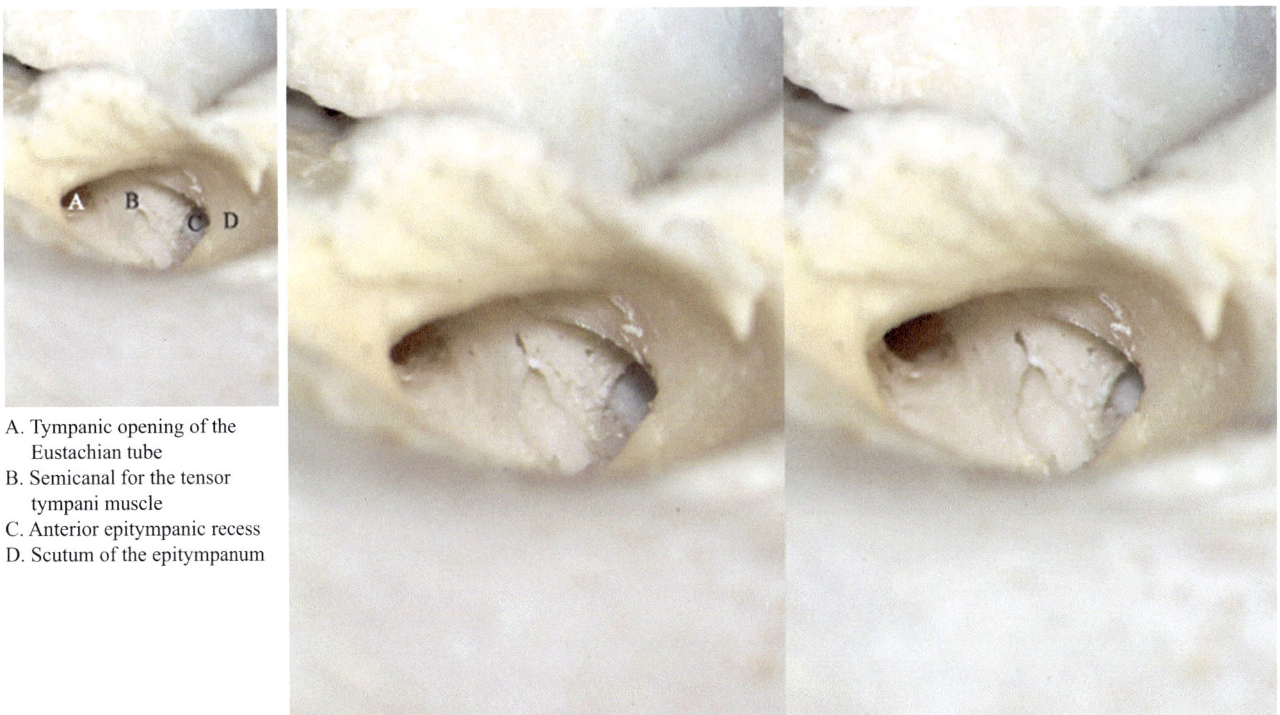

A. Tympanic opening of the Eustachian tube
B. Semicanal for the tensor tympani muscle
C. Anterior epitympanic recess
D. Scutum of the epitympanum

Fig. 2.16 Semicanal for the tensor tympani muscle (left)
The semicanal for the tensor tympani muscle lies superior to the tympanic opening for the Eustachian tube and contains the tensor tympani muscle which arises from the cartilaginous portion of the Eustachian tube and the adjoining part of the greater wing of the sphenoid. Passing backward through the canal, it ends in a slender tendon that enters the tympanic cavity, makes a sharp bend laterally around the posterior extremity of the septum, known as the cochleariform process, and is inserted into the neck of the malleus. The tympanic (horizontal) segment of the facial nerve lies from posterior to the cochleariform process and turns anteriorly and medial to reach the geniculate ganglion

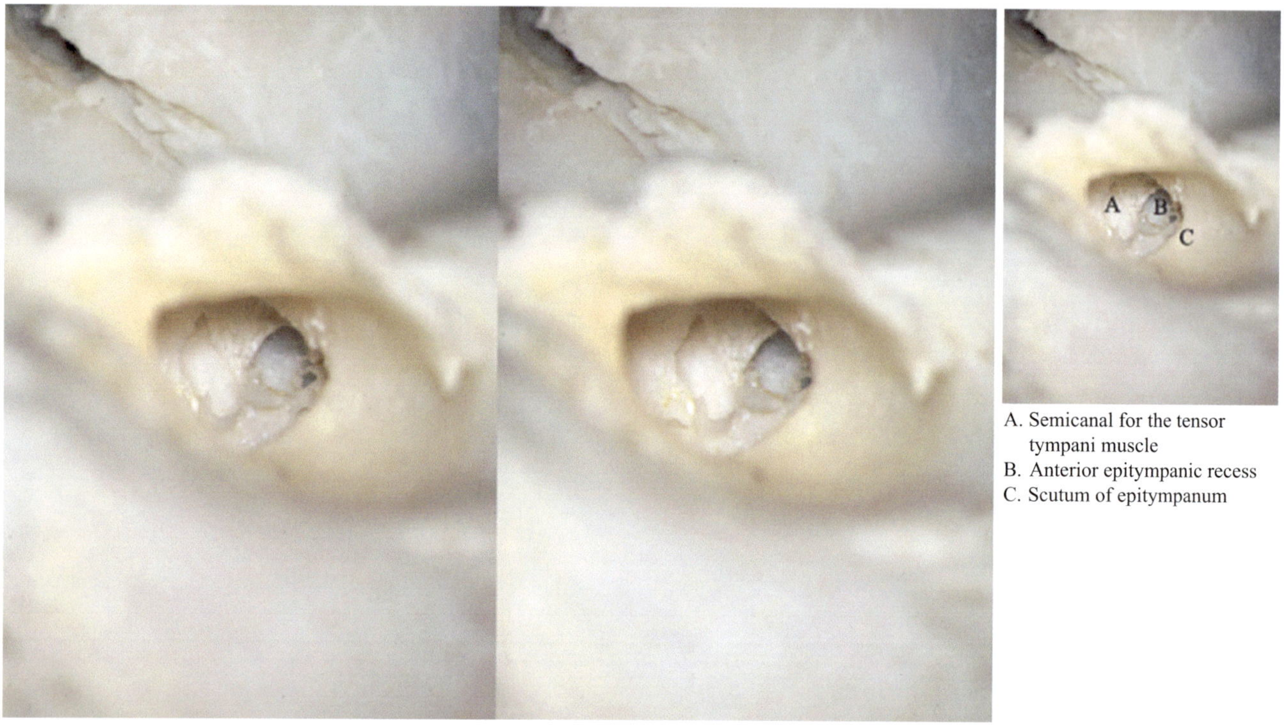

A. Semicanal for the tensor tympani muscle
B. Anterior epitympanic recess
C. Scutum of epitympanum

Fig. 2.17 Semicanal for the tensor tympani muscle and anterior epitympanic recess (left)
The epitympanum is that portion of the middle ear cleft located superior to the tympanic membrane. The anterior epitympanic recess is the anterior part of the epitympanum and is superior to the semicanal for the tensor tympani muscle. Medial to the anterior epitympanic recess are several sinuses called epitympanic sinuses which indicate the lateral surface of the geniculate ganglion

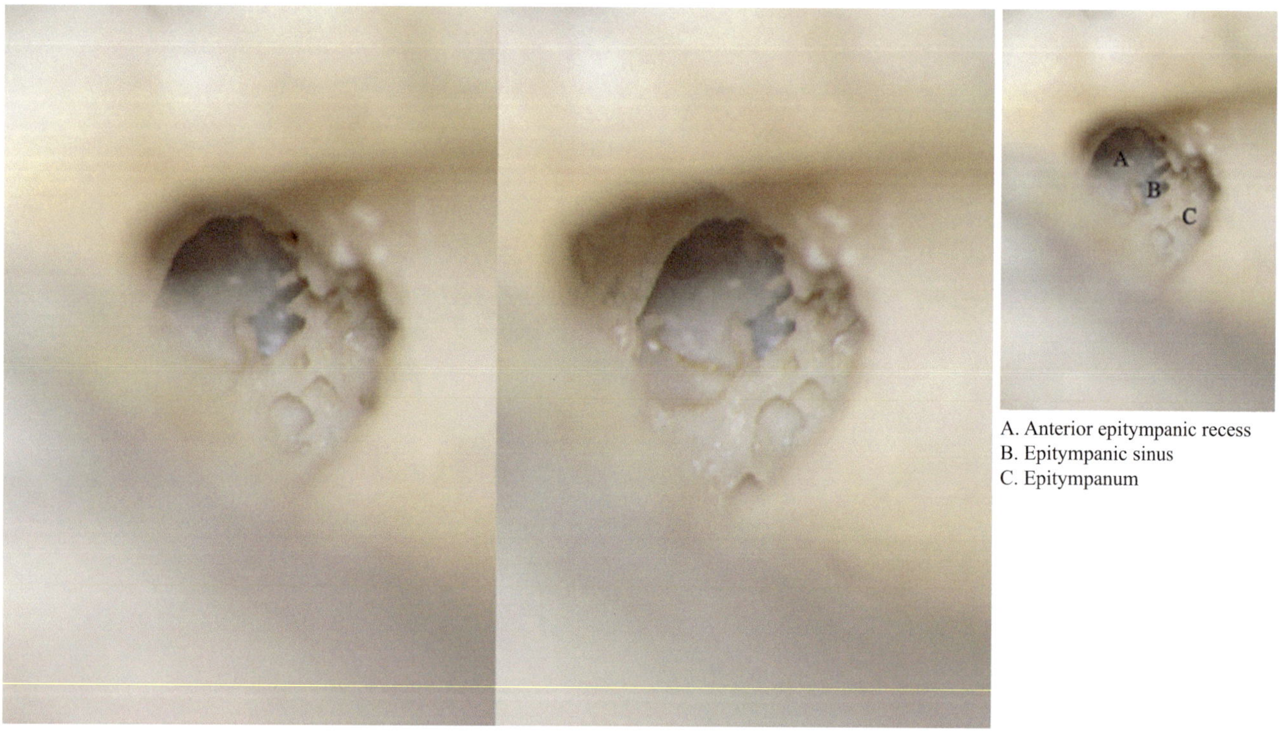

A. Anterior epitympanic recess
B. Epitympanic sinus
C. Epitympanum

Fig. 2.18 Epitympanum and anterior epitympanic recess (left)
Anterior epitympanic recess is the anterior part of the epitympanum. The epitympanic sinus is located in the medial wall of the epitympanum

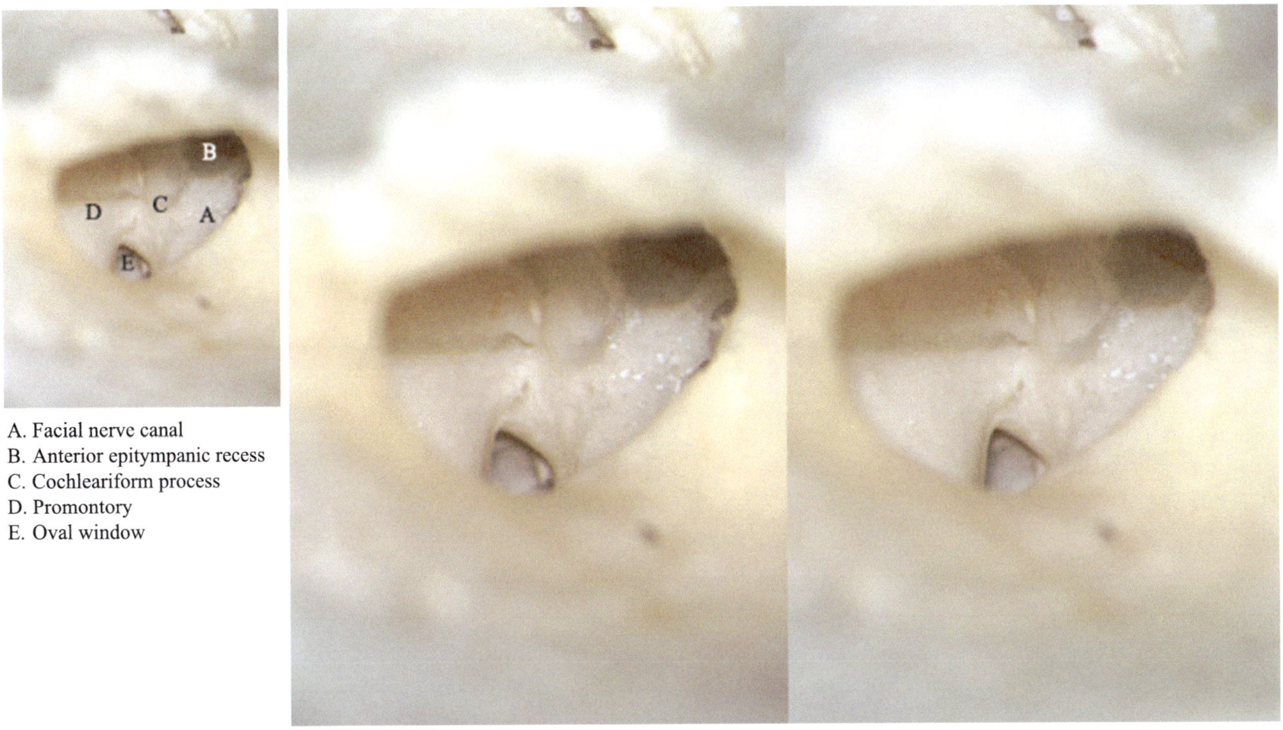

A. Facial nerve canal
B. Anterior epitympanic recess
C. Cochleariform process
D. Promontory
E. Oval window

Fig. 2.19 Upper part of medial wall of tympanic cavity (left)
In the medial wall of the tympanic cavity, the facial nerve canal is located postero-superiorly to the cochleariform process and contains the horizontal segment of the facial nerve. The oval window lies inferior to the facial nerve canal. The promontory is a prominent eminence located anteroinferior to the oval window and corresponds to the basal turn of the cochlea

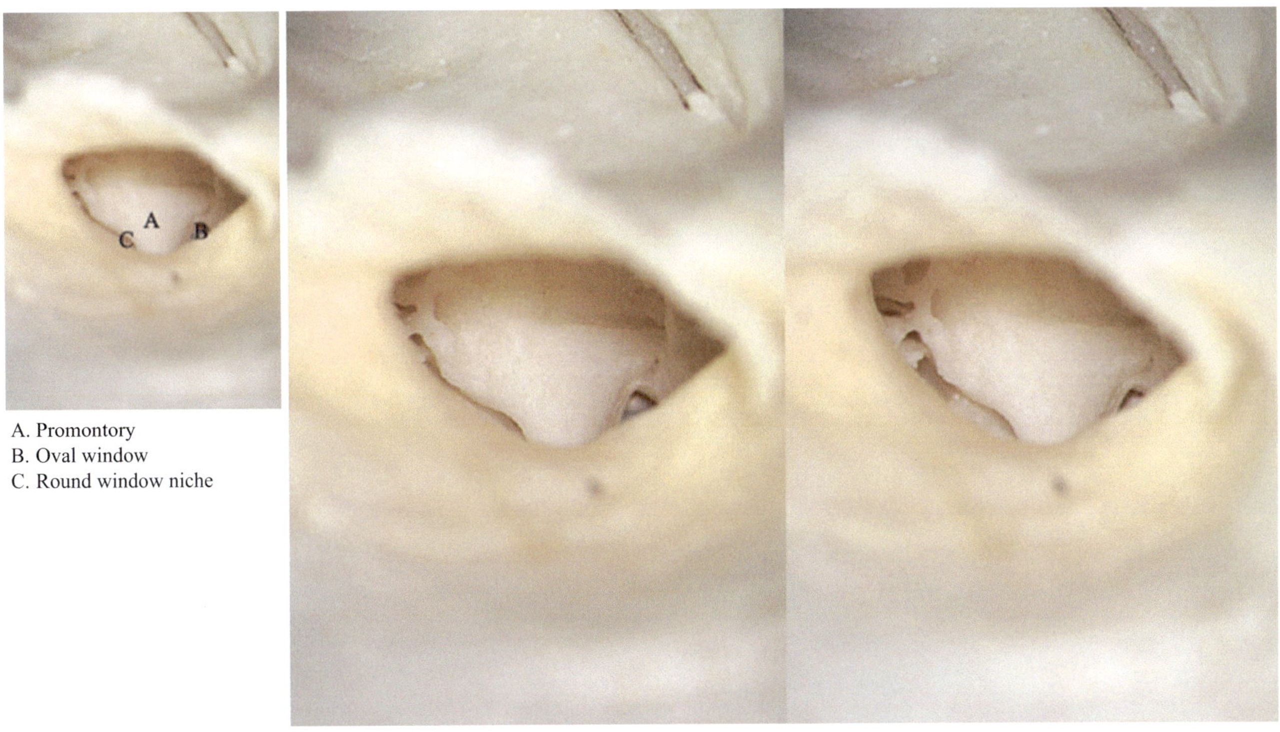

A. Promontory
B. Oval window
C. Round window niche

Fig. 2.20 Middle part of medial wall of tympanic cavity (left)
The promontory and the round window niche, which sits posteroinferior to it, form the middle section of the tympanic cavity's medial wall. The oval window is positioned above the round window niche at the depths of which lies the round window membrane. Surgical exposure of the membrane requires removing some of the superior and anterior bony overhang of the niche. The bone infero-posterior to the round window niche is rough and a branch of the inferior vestibular nerve (posterior ampullary nerve) runs beneath it

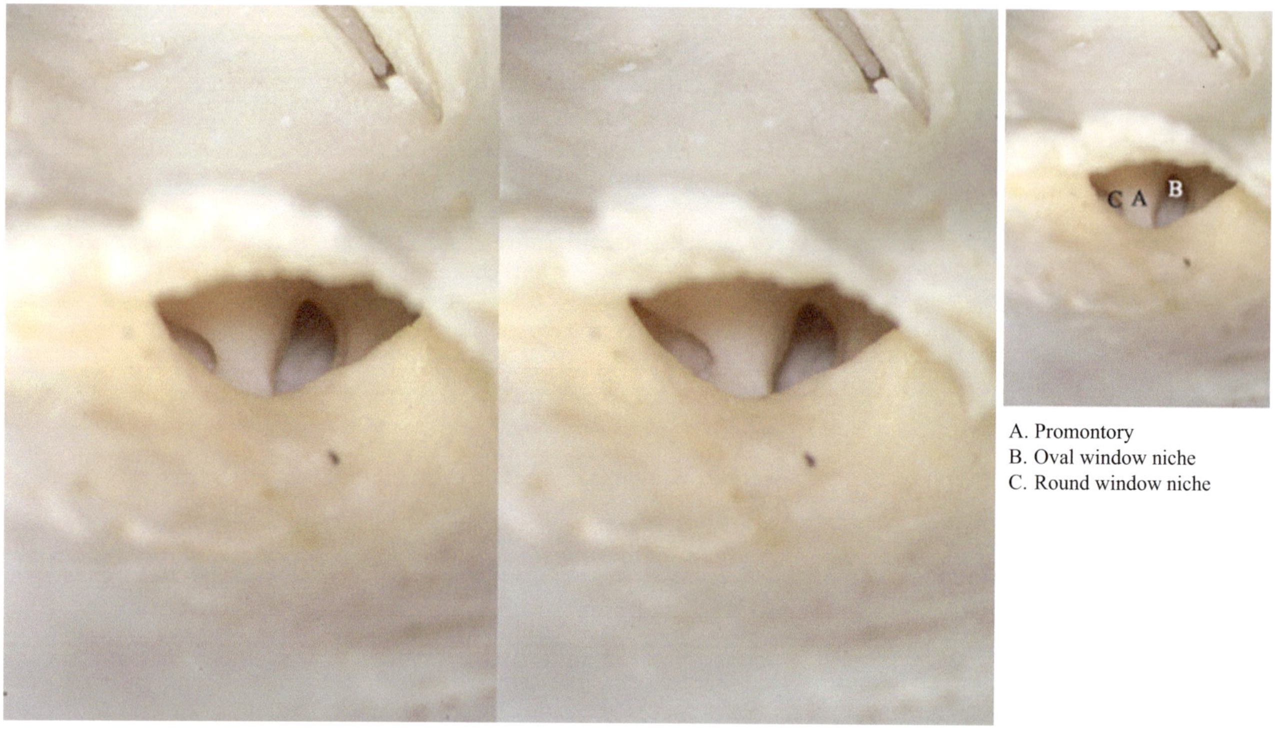

A. Promontory
B. Oval window niche
C. Round window niche

Fig. 2.21 Oval window niche and round window niche (left)
The oval window is in the vestibular window niche, superior to the round window. The round window is mostly sheltered by the round window niche in this case

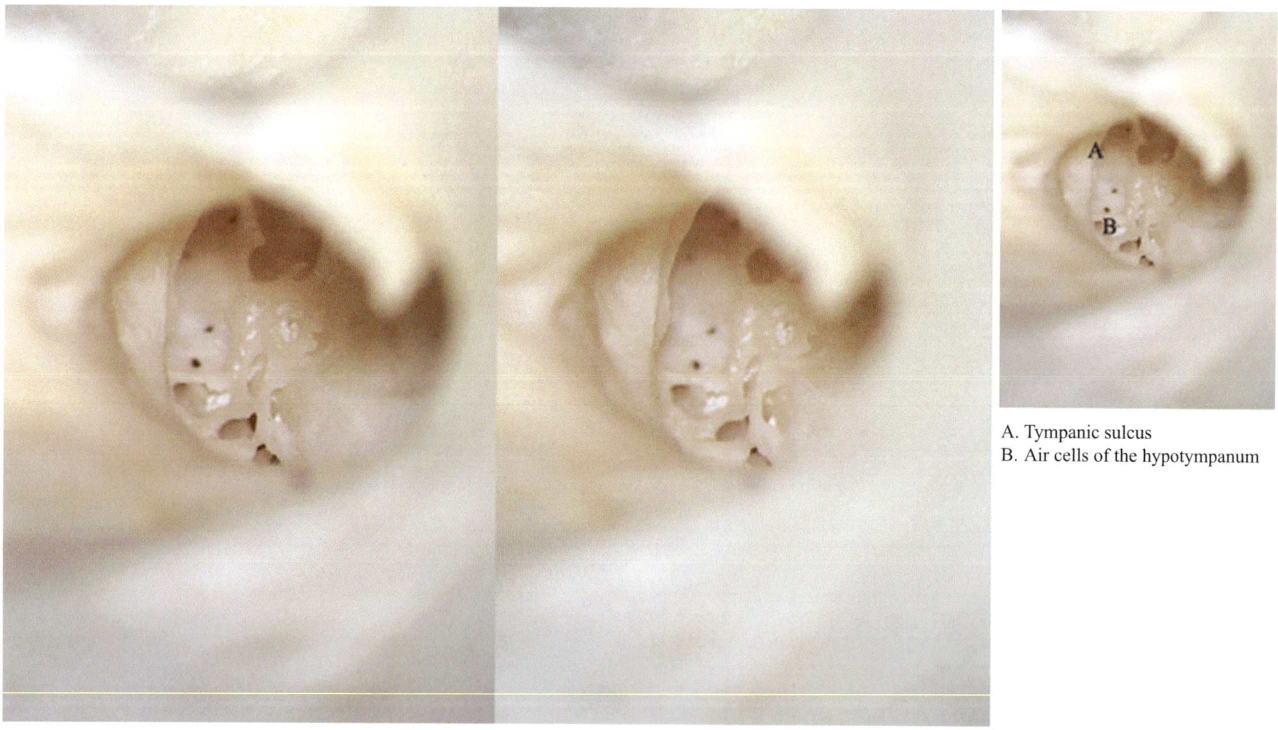

A. Tympanic sulcus
B. Air cells of the hypotympanum

Fig. 2.22 Inferior wall of tympanic cavity (left)
The tympanic membrane annulus is attached to a groove on the bony canal, called the tympanic sulcus, located at the medial end of the EAC. The inferior tympanic recess lies in the corner between the inferior and anterior walls of the tympanic cavity. The inferior wall of the tympanic cavity starts at the inferior tympanic recess and ends at the styloid apophysis. The inferior wall of the tympanic cavity is also called the Jugular wall: this floor is formed by bone that separates the middle ear from the internal jugular vein

Suggested Reading

Bai S-l. Systematic anatomy. Beijing: People's Medical Publishing House; 2001.

Dai P, Cousins V-C, Han D-y, Song Y-s. Stereo operative atlas of micro ear surgery. Singapore: Springer Nature; 2017.

Han D-y. Neuro-otology and lateral skull base surgery. Beijing: Science Press; 2008.

Huang X-z, Wang J-b, Kong W-j. Practical otolaryngology-head and neck surgery. 2nd ed. Beijing: People's Medical Publishing House; 2008.

Jiang S-c. Ear anatomy and temporal bone histopathology. Beijing: People's Military Medical Press; 1999.

Jiang S-c. Complete works of surgery – Volume of Otorhinolaryngology. Beijing: People's Military Medical Press; 1994.

3 Transcanal Approach

Guo-jian Wang, Bao-chun Sun, Jia-nan Li, Sen-yao Shao, Yun-juan Lin, Fei Yu, Qing-ling Bi, Sha-sha Huang, Li-li Ren, Yu-hua Zhu, and Pu Dai

Surgical Procedures Using the Transcanal Approach

The transcanal approach is an operative approach commonly used in otomicrosurgery. This approach is minimally invasive but provides limited exposure for some disease processes. Operations that can be performed via the transcanal approach include:

1. Incision of tympanic membrane and insertion of a ventilation tube
2. Resection of external auditory canal (EAC) cholesteatoma
3. Resection of EAC osteoma (exostoses)
4. Resection of cancer of the EAC in early stage
5. Myringoplasty
6. Tympanotomy
7. Tympanoplasty
8. Stapes surgery
9. Removal of middle ear cholesteatoma, glomus tympanicum tumor, and similar conditions with limited extent of disease

Related Anatomical Structures

1. Helix: slightly curled outer edge of the auricle.
2. Antihelix: this is a curving ridge that sits anterior to the helix and roughly parallel to it. At its upper end, it divides into upper and lower crura between which is an area called the triangular fossa
3. Triangular fossa: depression between upper and lower crura of the antihelix.
4. Scaphoid fossa: groove between the helix and antihelix; also known as the scapha.
5. Concha: deep pit anterior to antihelix, also divided by the crus (or root) of the helix into cymba conchae above and cavum conchae below; the outer ear canal lies in front of the cavity of the auricular concha.
6. Tragus: the protuberance containing cartilage that lies in front of the outer ear canal; the prominent lower end of the antihelix is the antitragus.
7. Anterior incisura: groove between the tragus and the crus of the helix.
8. Intertragic notch: hollow area between the tragus and antitragus.
9. External Auditory Canal (EAC): the passage leading from the opening of the external ear to the tympanic membrane.
10. Isthmus: narrowest part of the EAC, lying approximately 5 mm from the tympanic membrane.
11. Suprameatal spine: osseous spine in the posterosuperior edge of the osseous EAC; also known as spine of Henle.
12. Endomeatal spine: small and single osseous spine in the external end of the EAC behind the tympanosquamous fissure; this osseous spine must be negotiated when elevating a meatal flap.
13. Tympanic membrane: membrane closing the external sidewall of the tympanum; it is divided into pars tensa and pars flaccida.
14. Tympanic ring: inner edge of tympanic bone to which the tympanic membrane attaches; it is an incomplete ring, deficient superiorly.
15. Tympanic sulcus: the shallow groove in the tympanic ring; the edge of the pars tensa (i.e., the annulus) is embedded in the tympanic sulcus.
16. Tympanic notch: 5 mm gap in upper part of tympanic sulcus; the flaccid part of the tympanic membrane is

G.-j. Wang (✉) · J.-n. Li · F. Yu · S.-s. Huang · L.-l. Ren
Y.-h. Zhu · P. Dai
College of Otolaryngology Head and Neck Surgery, Chinese PLA General Hospital, Beijing, China

B.-c. Sun
Department of Otolaryngology Head and Neck Surgery, The Fourth Medical Center of PLA General Hospital, Beijing, China

S.-y. Shao · Y.-j. Lin
Department of Otolaryngology Head and Neck Surgery, Peking University International Hospital, Beijing, China

Q.-l. Bi
Department of Otolaryngology Head and Neck Surgery, China-Japan Friendship Hospital, Beijing, China

P. Dai et al. (eds.), *Stereoscopic Anatomical Atlas of Ear Surgery*, https://doi.org/10.1007/978-981-16-0927-5_3

attached to squamous bone in this notch; also known as the notch of Rivinus.
17. Tympanic scutum: posterosuperior wall of the medial end of the osseous EAC, forming part of the external wall of the epitympanum; it has a shield-like shape.
18. Tympanic cavity: an air-filled space in the temporal bone that is interposed between the tympanic membrane and the inner ear (otic capsule).
19. Malleus: the first of three ossicles, which lies between the incus and tympanic membrane; it is divided into the head, neck, lateral process, handle, and tip of handle.
20. Incus: the second of three ossicles, which lies between the malleus and stapes; it is divided into the body, long process, and short process. The end of the long process slightly expands on the inner side, forming the lenticular process.
21. Stapes: the smallest and most medial of the three ossicles, which lies in a horizontal plane and exhibits a stirrup shape; it is divided into the head, neck, arch with anterior and posterior crura, and footplate.
22. Superior recess of tympanic membrane: also known as Prussak's space. Its medial wall is the neck of the malleus and the lateral malleal fold; from superior to inferior, its lateral wall is formed by the scutum and the pars flaccida of the tympanic membrane. Its floor is formed by the lateral process of the malleus. This recess is the preferred site of formation of primary cholesteatoma.
23. Chorda tympani: branch of the facial nerve, which includes sympathetic and taste nerve fibers. It enters the tympanum through the posterior middle part of the tympanic ring; passes between the long process of the incus and malleus handle; then exits the tympanum and enters the infratemporal fossa through the anterior chorda tympani tubular opening in the inner end of the petrotympanic fissure.
24. Prominence of facial nerve canal: bony canal that passes above the oval window, which contains the horizontal segment of the facial nerve.
25. Promontory: protruding central part of the medial wall of the tympanum, which is formed by the basal turn of the cochlea that bulges into the tympanic cavity.
26. Promontory ponticulus: sharp ridge of bone that extends from the rear upper part of the promontory to the pyramidal process.
27. Promontory subiculum: extends from the rear of the promontory near the posterior edge of the round window and passes posteriorly, to join the styloid prominence. The ponticulus and subiculum are constant ridges at the back of the promontory, which form the upper and lower boundaries of the sinus tympani, respectively.
28. Round (cochlear) window niche: bony hollow in the lower part of the promontory that leads to the round window.
29. Oval (vestibular) window niche: oval window that lies below the prominence of the facial nerve and above the promontory and ponticulus.
30. Cochleariform process: lies anterior and superior to the upper part of the oval window and houses the tensor tympani tendon as it passes laterally to the neck of the malleus.
31. Eustachian tube: tube connecting the tympanum and nasopharynx; the medial two-thirds is composed of cartilage, while the outer one-third is bony. Its inner end opens in the lateral wall of the nasopharynx, while its outer end opens in the front wall of the tympanum.

Anatomy Overview

The main feature of the transcanal approach is that it involves minimal disruption of bony structures. The handling of the EAC tympanomeatal flap is the main aspect of the approach, allowing a gentle and minimally invasive procedure. Flap injury must be avoided. Anatomical training can provide familiarity with the key points of ear canal incisions and flap elevation.

1. Endaural incision (Lempert's approach). The first incision made in the transcanal approach begins longitudinally from the 12 o'clock position in the isthmus onto the bone surface, and extends 1.0–1.5 cm laterally into the anterior incisura; the skin, subcutaneous tissue, and temporal muscle surface are separated down to bone. The second incision begins from the 6 o'clock point, 6 mm lateral to the tympanic ring, and curves around superiorly to meet the first incision; the second incision is also deepened to the bone surface. After all incisions are completed, the EAC flap is elevated from lateral to medial along the bone surface. *Hints: (1) Because the endomeatal spine is typically closely bound to the skin, sharp dissection with a scalpel is necessary to separate the flap from it. Medial to the endomeatal spine, flap elevation can continue with a micro elevator. (2) Flap incisions should be deepened to bone along their full length prior to elevation, to avoid tearing the flap. (3) During the separation process, the micro elevator should always remain on the bone surface of the EAC; separation should be evenly completed to the deep part of the EAC.*
2. Intercartilaginous incision. The auricular cartilage should be pulled backward to expose the sulcus between the external meatal cartilage and auricular cartilage. The skin and subcutaneous tissue should be cut from 6 o'clock to 12 o'clock in an arc along the intercartilaginous sulcus. The anterior incisura should then be cut in an outward manner. Incision to the bone surface should be made backward and inward along the entire incision; the external meatal flap should be separated on the bony surface of

the mastoid process and EAC. *Hints: (1) The flap should be cut through to bone and continuity of the incisions should be ensured to avoid tearing the flap. (2) The flap should be thinned on the rear upper wall to expose the mastoid cortex; during flap separation, the endomeatal spine may need to be isolated and removed. (3) To enter the middle ear, the skin of the EAC should be cut 5–6 mm lateral to the fibrous annular tympanic ring then elevated medially.*

3. Ear canal incision. The flap is easily damaged because it is very thin; thus, the incision is typically completed with the assistance of an endoscope. The skin of the EAC should be cut from 6 o'clock to 12 o'clock, about 6 mm lateral to the fibrous tympanic ring. The EAC flap and tympanic ring should then be elevated. *Hints: The skin of the EAC flap should be cut through its full thickness and dissection must be gentle to avoid tearing the flap.*
4. The fibrous tympanic ring should be elevated and the tympanic cavity is then exposed. A middle ear elevator should be used to separate the tympanic ring from the tympanic sulcus; the chorda tympani should be separated with a hook to expose the middle ear cavity. *Hints: (1) The fibrous tympanic ring forms the posterior part of the pars tensa and can be separated intact from the tympanic sulcus. (2) Elevation of the ring should be performed carefully to avoid tearing the EAC flap and tympanic membrane. (3) To avoid damaging the chorda tympani and facial nerve, traction should not be excessive while using the hook to separate the chorda tympani.*

Purpose and Requirements of Anatomical Dissection

1. Mastery of the structures of the external ear.
2. Mastery of morphology and spatial relationships of the contents of the tympanic cavity.
3. Mastery of the methods for endaural incision.
4. Mastery of the methods for intercartilaginous incision.
5. Mastery of dissection of the endomeatal spine.
6. Mastery of techniques for elevation of EAC flap.
7. Mastery of methods for separation of fibrous tympanic ring from tympanic sulcus.
8. Mastery of the use of middle ear dissection instruments.

Anatomy of the External Ear

Jia-nan Li and Bao-chun Sun

The external ear is composed of two parts: the auricle and EAC. The auricle, with an angle of approximately 30°, is attached to the side of the skull by muscles, cartilage, ligaments, and skin. The rolled outer edge of the auricle is known as the helix. The upper end of the helix curves down to the rear of the EAC opening and is known as the crus of the helix. The lower end extends down to the ear lobule. The auricular tubercle is the small nodule on the posterosuperior surface of the helix. The antihelix is the curved prominence that lies anterior to and parallel to the helix. A hollow area in front of the antihelix is known as the concha. The cymba conchae is located above the crus of the helix, while the cavum conchae is located below the crus of the helix. The EAC opening is located anterior to the cavum conchae and posterior to the tragus. The EAC is 2.5–3.5 cm in length from its opening (meatus) to the tympanic membrane, with the lateral one-third cartilaginous and the medial two-thirds osseous. There are two narrow areas in the EAC: (1) the junction of the osseous and cartilage parts; and (2) the osseous part 0.5 cm lateral to the tympanic membrane, also known as the isthmus of the EAC.

The upper part of the bony EAC is composed of the temporal bone's squamous portion; the anterior, inferior, and posterior walls are composed of the tympanic portion. The lateral one-third of the EAC is lined with thicker skin that has hair follicles, sebaceous and ceruminous glands. The medial two-thirds is lined with simple thin skin that lies directly on the bone (unlike anywhere else in the human body) and does not contain hairs, glands, or a subcutaneous layer. This arrangement makes the medial skin very sensitive to pain.

The tympanic membrane is located at the medial end of the EAC; it is 9 mm in height, 8 mm in width, and 0.1 mm in thickness. It comprises three layers from lateral to medial: squamous epithelium, a combined radiating and circular fibrous layer, and an inner mucosal layer. The outer edge of the anterior, inferior, and posterior pars tensa presents the fibrous annulus which is a thickened component of the well-organized middle fibrous layer of that part of the tympanic membrane. The annulus sits in the circumferential bony tympanic sulcus which does not extend to the level of the epitympanum. The upper part of the membrane is the thinner pars flaccida which attaches peripherally to the notch of Rivinus.

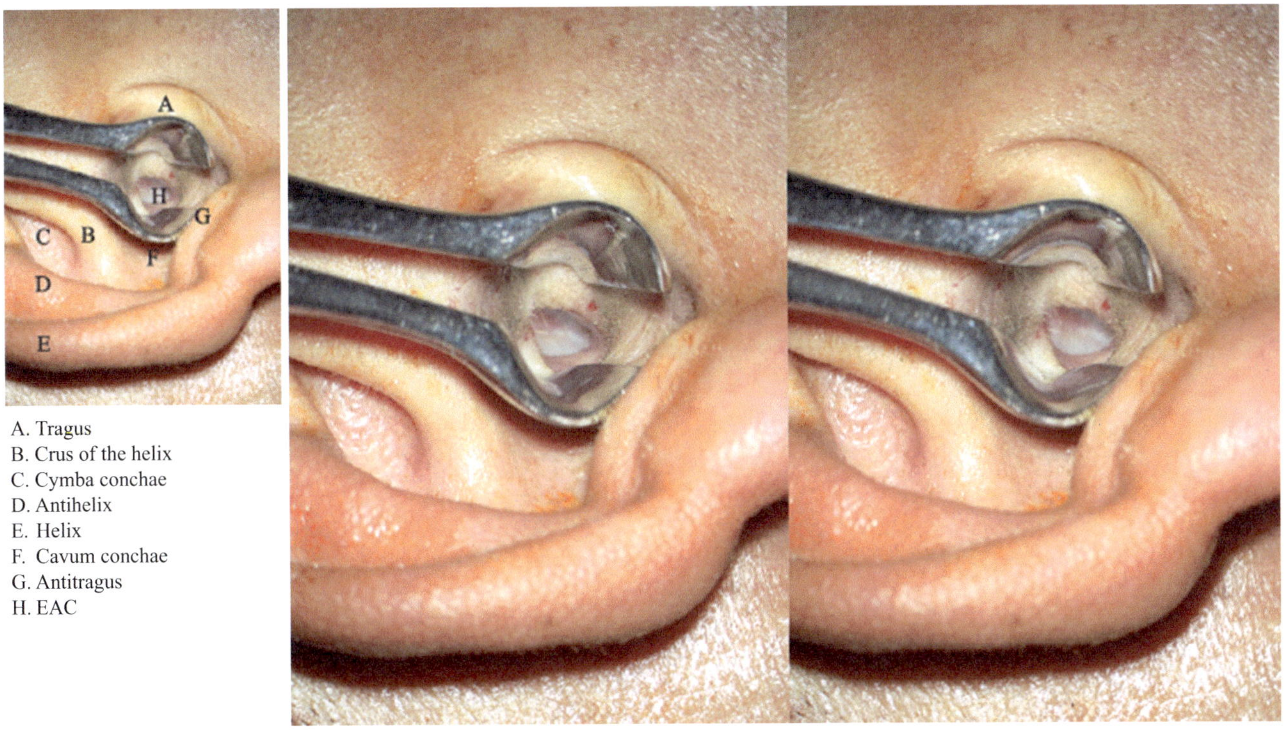

Fig. 3.1 Auricle and EAC (right)
The auricle is attached to the side of the skull by muscles, cartilage, ligaments, and skin. The incisura between the tragus and antitragus is known as the intertragic notch. The depression between the tragus and the crus of the helix is known as the anterior incisura. There is no cartilage in the anterior incisura; thus, an incision can be made through the anterior incisura directly to the cortex of bone without damaging the cartilage
Instruments: nasal speculum, scalpel

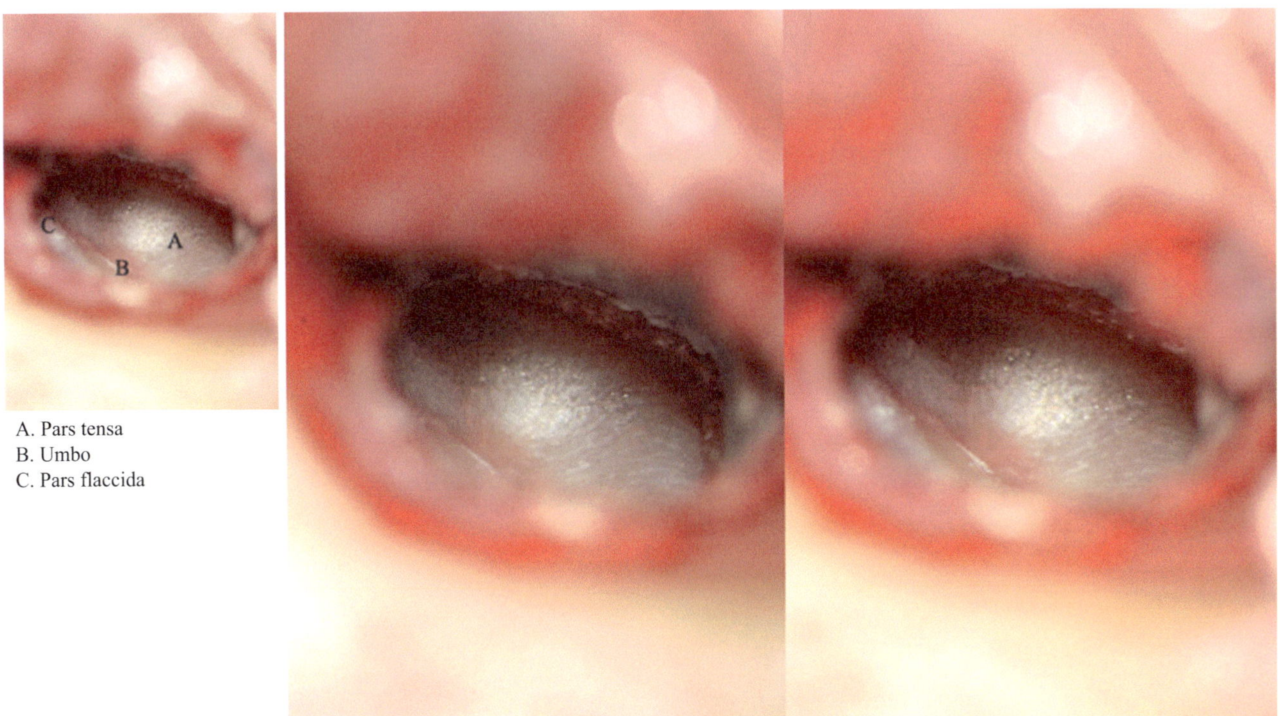

Fig. 3.2 Observation of tympanic membrane morphology (right)
The opening of the EAC can be enlarged with a retractor to observe the morphology of the EAC and tympanic membrane. The tympanic membrane is located at the medial end of the EAC; it is composed of the pars tensa and pars flaccida. Anatomic landmarks on the tympanic membrane surface are as follows: umbo, cone of light, malleal prominence, malleal stria, anterior malleal fold, and posterior malleal fold
Instruments: retractor, middle ear elevator

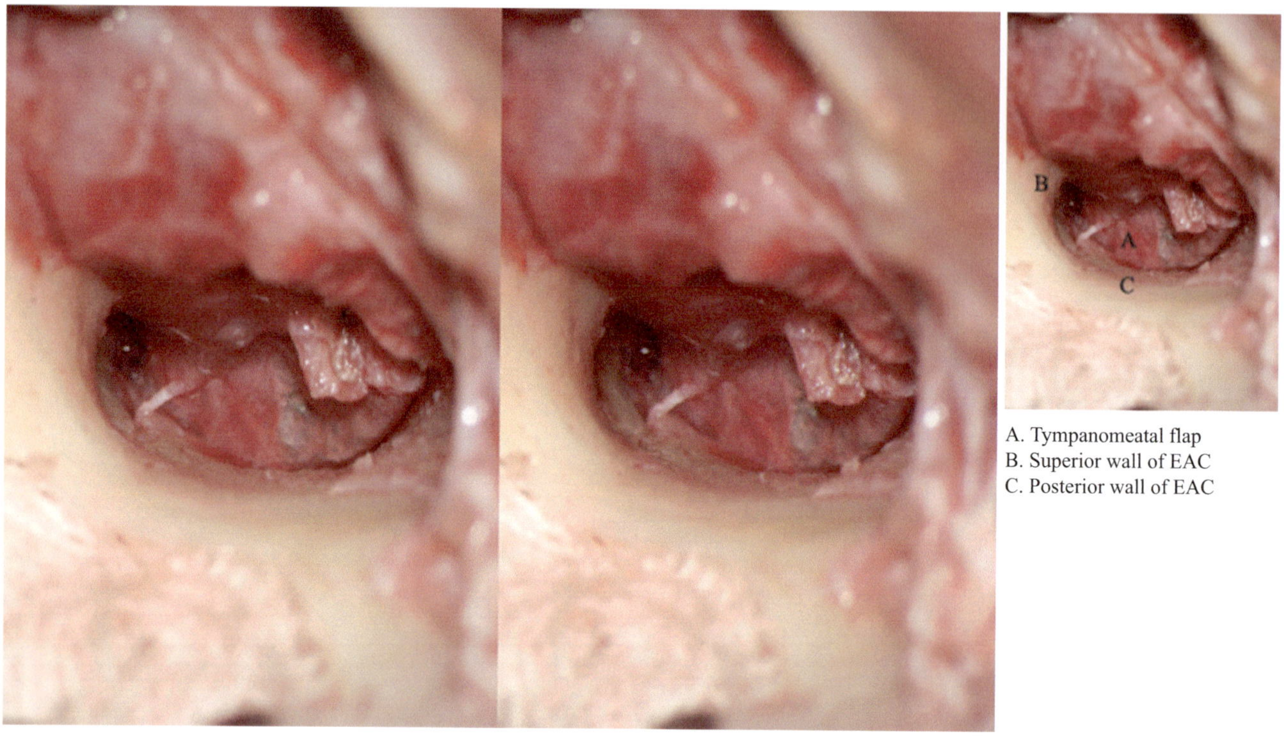

A. Tympanomeatal flap
B. Superior wall of EAC
C. Posterior wall of EAC

Fig. 3.3 Elevation of the tympanomeatal flap (right)
Using a middle ear elevator, elevate the tympanomeatal flap to the fibrous annulus. Note: the medial skin of the osseous EAC is very thin and delicate, without any adnexal structures or subcutaneous tissue, and can be easily torn. *Hints: (1) keep the elevator on the bone surface; (2) keep the surgical field clear; (3) avoid sucking on the tympanomeatal flap directly; and (4) use the side of the elevator, rather than the tip, to avoid tearing the flap*
Instruments: middle ear elevator, sucker

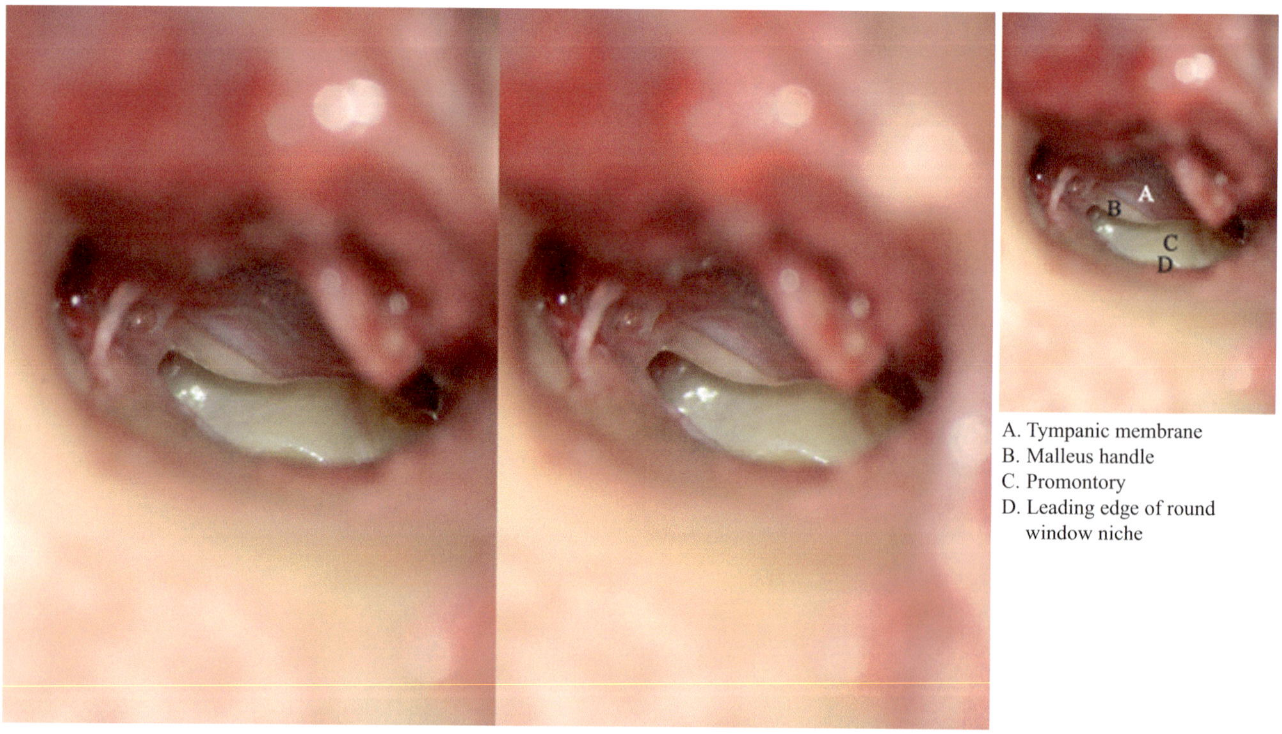

A. Tympanic membrane
B. Malleus handle
C. Promontory
D. Leading edge of round window niche

Fig. 3.4 Exposure of the mesotympanum (right)
Elevate the tympanomeatal flap to the fibrous annulus; along the pars tensa, the fibrous annulus can be separated from the tympanic sulcus using a middle ear elevator. The pars flaccida is attached to the notch of Rivinus. Using a middle ear elevator, probe into the epitympanum from the superior bone surface of the EAC; then, lift and elevate the pars flaccida along with the tympanomeatal flap to expose the epitympanum and mesotympanum
Instruments: middle ear elevator, sucker

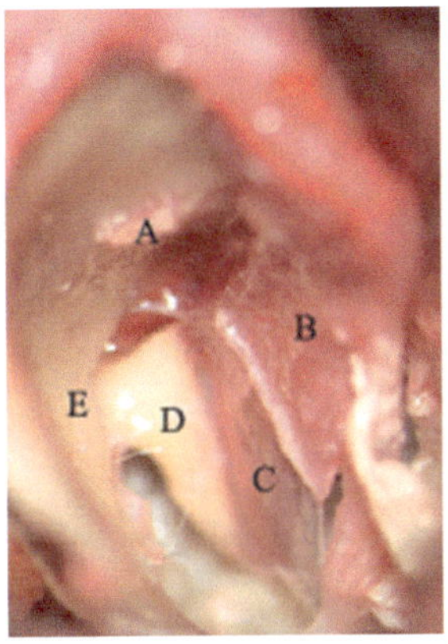

A. Endomeatal spine
B. Tympanomeatal flap
C. Tympanic membrane
D. Malleus
E. Lateral bony wall of the epitympanum

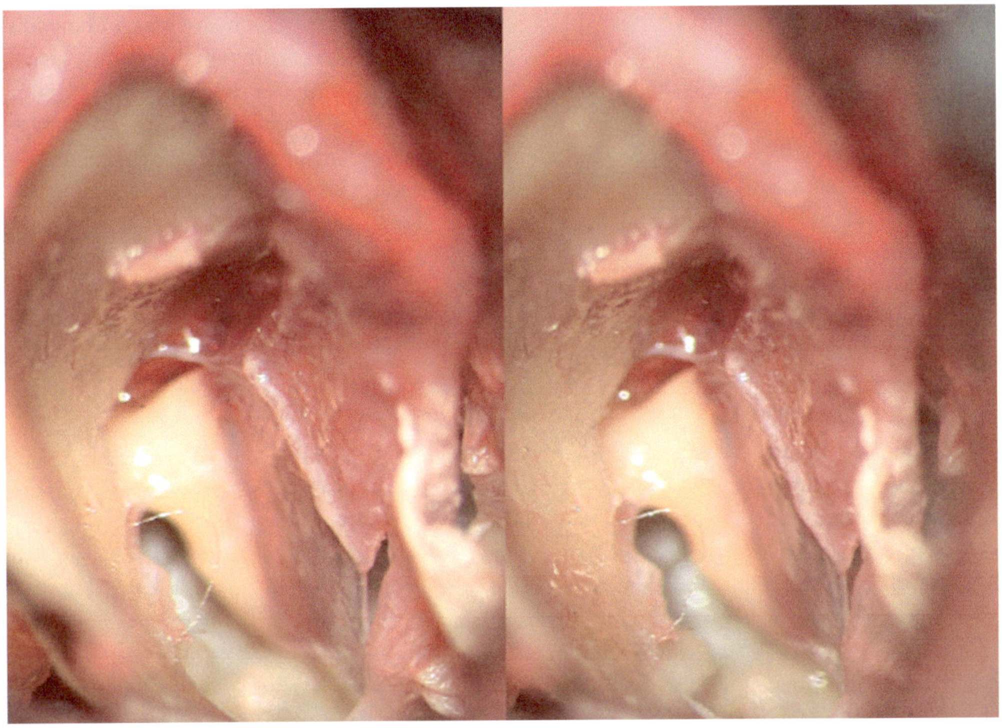

Fig. 3.5 Endomeatal spine (right)
There is a prominent bony spine on the anterosuperior wall of the EAC, known as the endomeatal spine. The endomeatal spine must be chiseled away, following separation of the meatal flap if it affects the exposure of the surgical field. *Hints: (1) the soft tissue around the spine can be separated with a #15 scalpel; (2) use blunt dissection along the bone surface to elevate the flap; (3) the endomeatal spine can be removed with an osteotome*
Instruments: middle ear elevator, scalpel, hammer, round chisel

Anatomy of the Middle Ear

Sen-yao Shao and Guo-jian Wang

The middle ear is located between the external and inner ears; its main function is to conduct external sound into the inner ear. The middle ear is generally regarded as the tympanic cavity and its contents.

The tympanic cavity is formed by the petrous, squamous, and tympanic portions of the temporal bone and the tympanic membrane; this cavity is the largest irregular pneumatic space in the temporal bone. There are many important structures surrounding the tympanic cavity. Laterally, the EAC is separated by the tympanic membrane. The medial wall features the promontory, oval and round windows of the inner ear. Anteriorly, the opening of the Eustachian tube passes down to the nasopharynx. Posteriorly, the aditus ad antrum joins to the antrum and pneumatic cells of the mastoid process. Horizontal planes passing through the upper and lower edges of the pars tensa of the tympanic membrane subdivide the tympanic cavity into epitympanum (attic), mesotympanum, and hypotympanum. The epitympanum is located above the upper plane; the mesotympanum is between the upper and lower planes, as well as between the tympanic membrane and medial wall of the tympanic cavity; and the hypotympanum is below the lower plane. The superoinferior dimension of the tympanic cavity is approximately 15 mm, while the anteroposterior dimension is approximately 13 mm. The distance between the lateral and medial walls varies: approximately 6 mm at the epitympanum, approximately 4 mm at the hypotympanum, and approximately 2 mm between the promontory and the umbo of the tympanic membrane. The tympanic cavity contains the auditory ossicles, muscles, and ligaments; it is covered by various types of mucous membranes. The tympanic membrane, posterior part of the promontory, auditory ossicles, epitympanum, tympanic antrum, and mastoid cells are covered by ciliated and nonciliated columnar epithelium; the remaining portion of the cavity (its anterior part) is covered by ciliated columnar epithelium.

The outer wall of the tympanum, also known as the tympanic membrane wall, is composed of membranous and bony portions. The membranous portion consists of the tympanic membrane, which is the main part of the wall; the smaller bony portion (i.e., the scutum) is the outer wall of the epitympanum. The scutum is a bony plate of the temporal squama, which forms the boundary between the upper medial bony external ear canal and epitympanum.

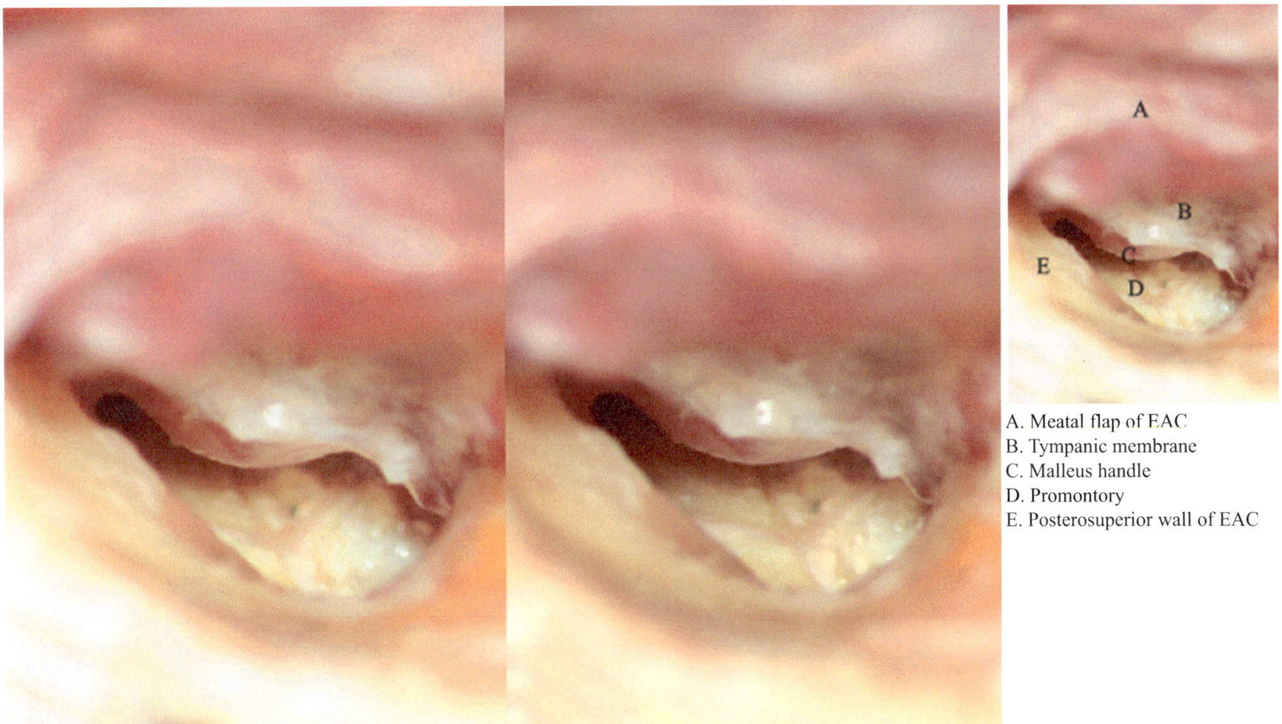

A. Meatal flap of EAC
B. Tympanic membrane
C. Malleus handle
D. Promontory
E. Posterosuperior wall of EAC

Fig. 3.6 Elevation of the tympanic membrane and exposure of the mesotympanum (right)
First, elevate the flap of the posterior wall of the EAC. Then, roll the flap forward and elevate the tympanic annulus from the tympanic sulcus, thereby raising the tympanic membrane forward and exposing the mesotympanum. The malleus handle and the promontory of the medial wall of the tympanic cavity can now be observed
Instruments: middle ear elevator

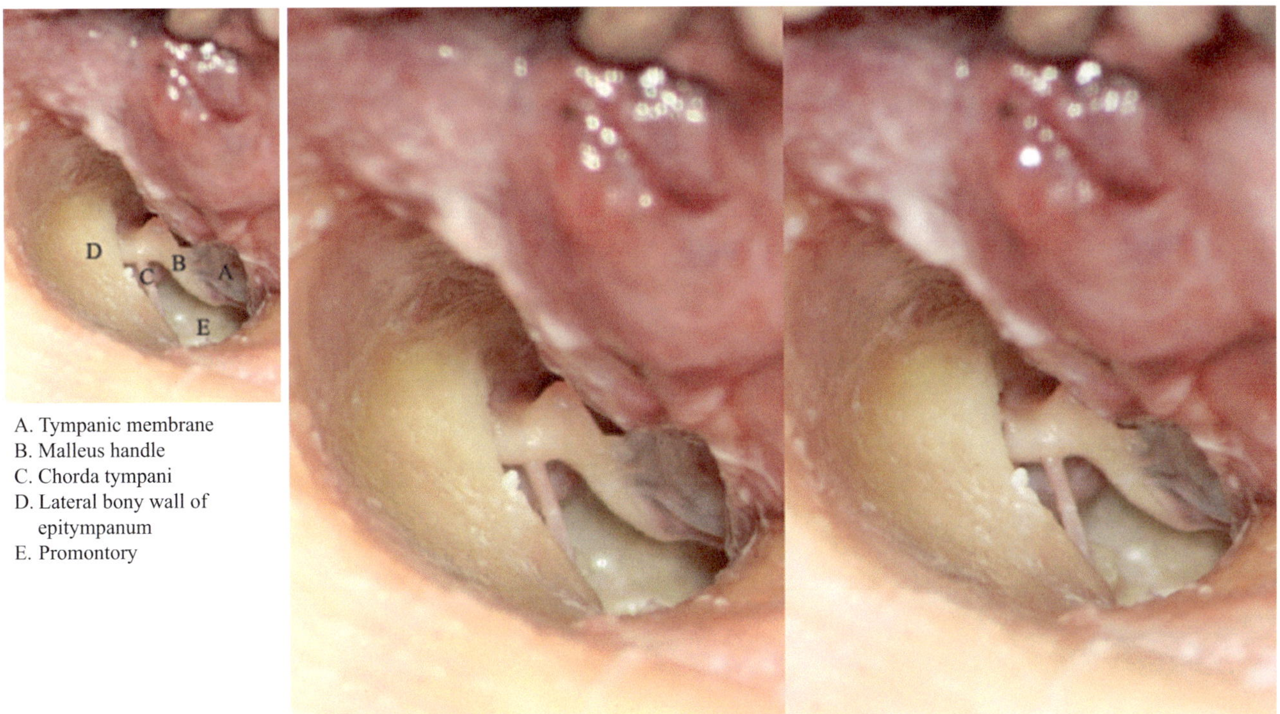

A. Tympanic membrane
B. Malleus handle
C. Chorda tympani
D. Lateral bony wall of epitympanum
E. Promontory

Fig. 3.7 Exposure of the epitympanum entrance (right)
Elevate the pars flaccida and expose the malleus neck, malleus lateral process, and chorda tympani. Then, identify the lateral wall of the epitympanum (scutum), locate the epitympanum, and probe the chorda tympani
Instruments: middle ear elevator, right-angle hook

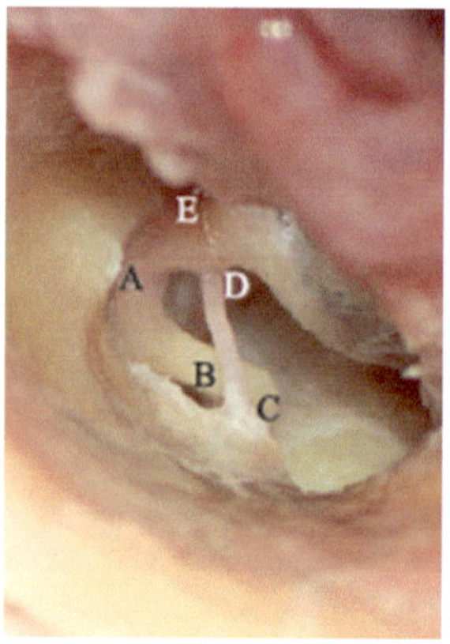

A. Incudomalleal joint
B. Long process of incus
C. Incudostapedial joint
D. Cochleariform process
E. Superior recess of tympanic membrane (Prussak's space)

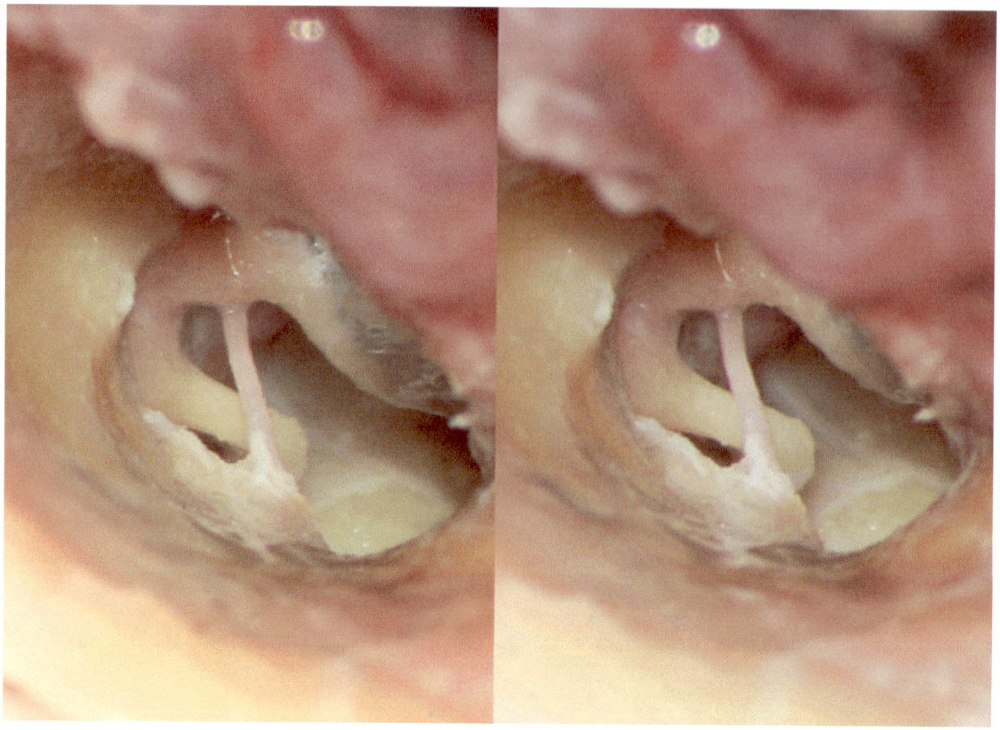

Fig. 3.8 Exposure of the incudostapedial joint (right)
Curette away part of the lateral wall of the epitympanum and reveal the inferior part of the epitympanum. Now, the following structures should be visible: complete malleus handle, lateral process of the malleus, neck of the malleus, and the superior recess of tympanic membrane (i.e., Prussak's space: the space between the neck and lateral process of the malleus, pars flaccida, and lateral ligament of the malleus), which is a common site of cholesteatoma formation. There are two methods for removing the bone: use of an electric drill (enables removal of bone progressively but is more likely to damage the flap) and use of an osteotome (avoids flap damage, but potentially risks damage to deeper structures)
Instruments: hammer, round chisel, right-angle hook

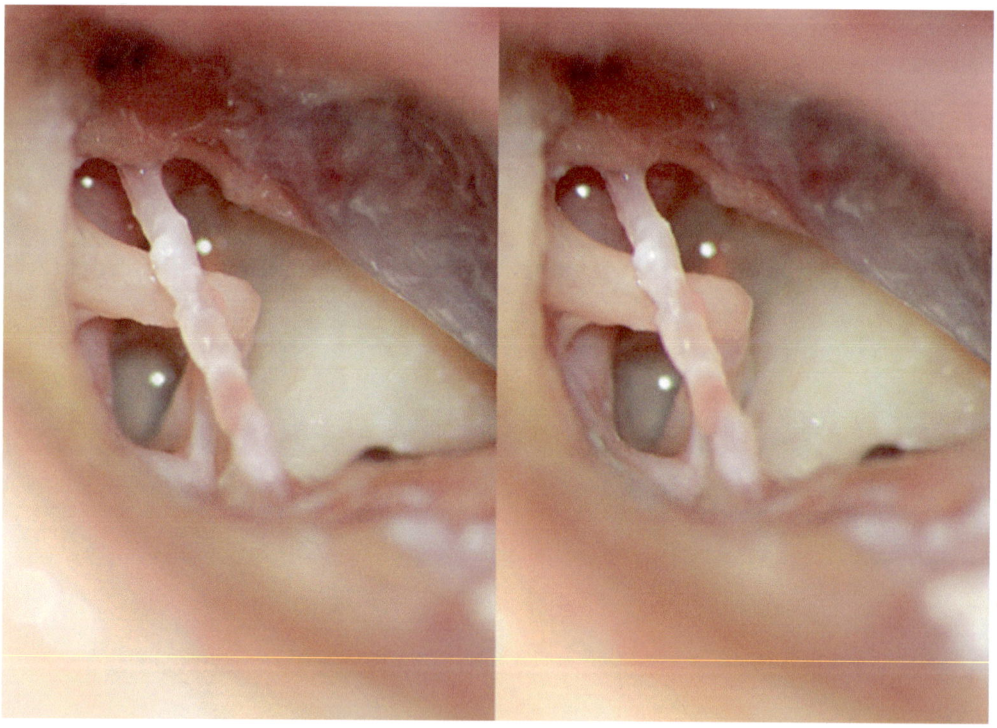

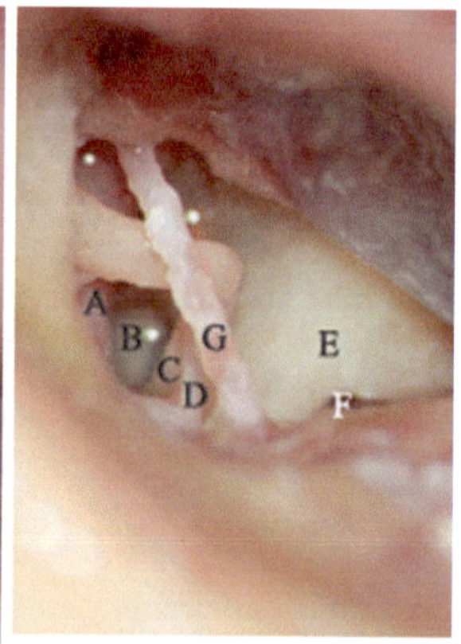

A. Prominence of the facial canal
B. Footplate of the stapes
C. Posterior crus of the stapes
D. Stapedius tendon
E. Promontory
F. Round window niche
G. Chorda tympani

Fig. 3.9 Exposure of the mesotympanum and lower region of epitympanum (right)
Probe the mesotympanum and lower region of the epitympanum, thereby enabling examination of the cochleariform process and the prominence of the facial canal. This procedure is useful for exploratory surgery of the ossicular chain and stapes
Instruments: hammer, round chisel

Hearing Reconstruction: Interposition of Reshaped Autogenous Incus

Yun-juan Lin and Pu Dai

Tympanoplasty is defined as surgical reconstruction of the sound transformer system and consists of ossiculoplasty and/or myringoplasty. It is a routine procedure in otomicrosurgery. Reconstruction of the ossicular chain is essential for the restoration of middle ear sound transmission function. Based on prognosis, Fisch et al. classified defects of the ossicular chain into three types: *type I* (remnant malleus and intact stapes), with intact and mobile stapes, malleus handle, and front part of tympanic membrane—the mean air–bone gap after ossiculoplasty may recover within 10 dB HL; *type II* (remnant malleus and intact footplate of the stapes), with an intact and mobile footplate but absent stapedial arch (superstructure), or with an intact but fixed footplate—aspects of the malleus handle and front part of the tympanic membrane resemble type I; *type III* (only the stapes present), only stapes without other ossicles—*type III (1)* involves an intact and mobile stapes, *type III (2)* involves an intact and mobile footplate, and *type III (3)* involves an intact but fixed footplate.

In the early 1950s, Wüllstein and Zöllner used a polyethylene columella as the first replacement prosthesis in otology; they inserted it between the mobile footplate and the grafted eardrum, thus initiating the practice of using ossicular replacement prostheses to reconstruct the conducting mechanism. In 1957, Hall et al. first attempted to use autogenous incus to rebuild hearing, thereby introducing autogenous ossicles into the options for ossicular-chain reconstruction. Subsequently, autogenous ossicular-chain prostheses (shaped autogenous incus) were found to exhibit many advantages in clinical practice, such as good biocompatibility and long-term stability, straightforward manipulation, low cost, and good sound transmission. The reshaped autogenous incus is therefore considered a safe and effective ossicular graft.

In general, the incus exhibits sufficient length to bridge the gap between the head of the stapes and the tympanic membrane; it can also be fashioned into different shapes and sizes as required. Currently, autogenous incus interposition is used mainly under the following circumstances: (1) Otitis media restricted to the ossicular chain: The most common ossicular-chain pathology is intact malleus and stapes, with resorption of the incus. Interposition of autogenous incus is the first operation considered when the ear is dry and exhibits no cholesteatoma invasion. (2) Abnormal connection of ossicular chain caused by trauma: Luxation of the incudostapedial joint and fracture of the long process of the incus are the most common ossicular defects; in such instances, the incus can be shaped to rebuild the ossicular chain. (3) Malformation of the incus or misconnection between the incus and the malleus or the stapes in the context of congenital ossicular chain malformation. (4) When the incus obstructs the view of the related ossicular chain or the horizontal segment of the facial nerve during surgery, the incus should be temporarily removed, then refashioned and reinserted at the end of the procedure.

Clinical practice has shown that ossiculoplasty using autogenous ossicles results in a good outcome, but there are also some limitations. Literature reports have primarily focused on the following aspects: (1) Bone absorption. Infection can lead to some dissolution and resorption of autogenous ossicles. Therefore, the use of an autogenous incus should only be considered in dry ears; the heat produced during shaping the incus by drilling can result in bone necrosis and increase the risk of bone resorption. Thus, a low drill speed and persistent irrigation with physiological saline solution are needed to reduce thermal damage during re-shaping. (2) Tiny latent disease nidus. Risks of osteitis and residual squamous epithelium are present in patients with cholesteatoma. Considering the relapse risk, these patients are not suitable candidates for procedures involving autogenous ossicles. (3) Adhesion and fusion of the autogenous incus with the surrounding bones. If these changes occur, a second operation to release and replace the shaped autogenous incus is inevitable. Thus, the autogenous incus must be accurately interposed, avoiding any connections to the surrounding bone; a gelatin sponge should be placed around the incus to prevent bony fixation. (4) Interposed ossicle shifting. An unstable connection between the interposed incus and the stapes may result in displacement. The groove in contact with the stapes should be deepened to prevent shifting.

In conclusion, when rigorous surgical indications and contraindications are observed, ossiculoplasty using autogenous ossicles can result in desired hearing restoration, if the autogenous incus is in good condition. Conditions that should be considered when choosing the interposition of the autogenous incus include: low disease relapse likelihood, infection-free middle ear, good Eustachian tube function, intact stapes, and fixed or misconnected incus.

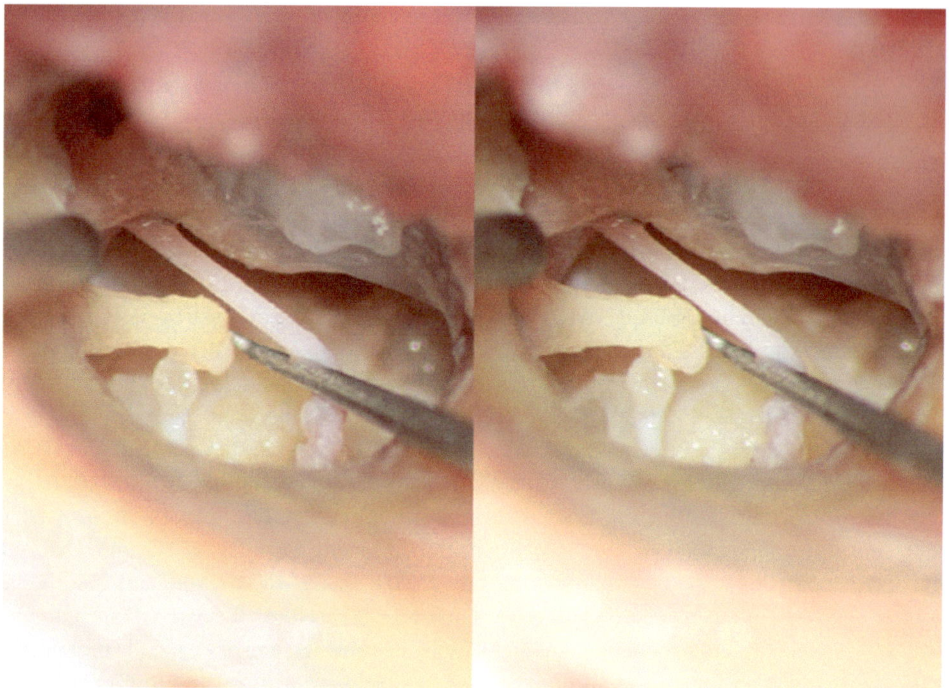

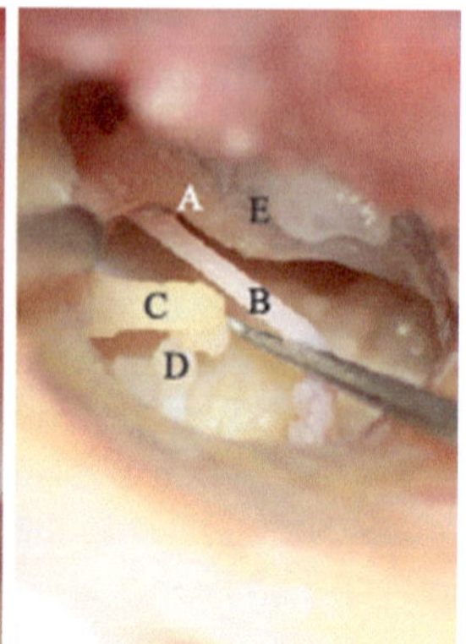

A. Handle of the malleus
B. Chorda tympani
C. Long process of the incus
D. Head of the stapes
E. Tympanic membrane

Fig. 3.10 Separation of the incudostapedial joint (right)
Elevate the tympanomeatal flap and expose the mesotympanum; locate the chorda tympani and gently move it in an anteroinferior direction to free it from the ossicular chain. Drill away the posterosuperior bone of the external canal (right ear from 9 o'clock to 12 o'clock; left ear from 12 o'clock to 3 o'clock) to sufficiently expose the incudostapedial joint. Use a right-angle hook to gently disrupt the incudostapedial joint and dislocate the incus, while ensuring that the chorda tympani remains protected
Instruments: middle ear elevator, round chisel, right-angle hook

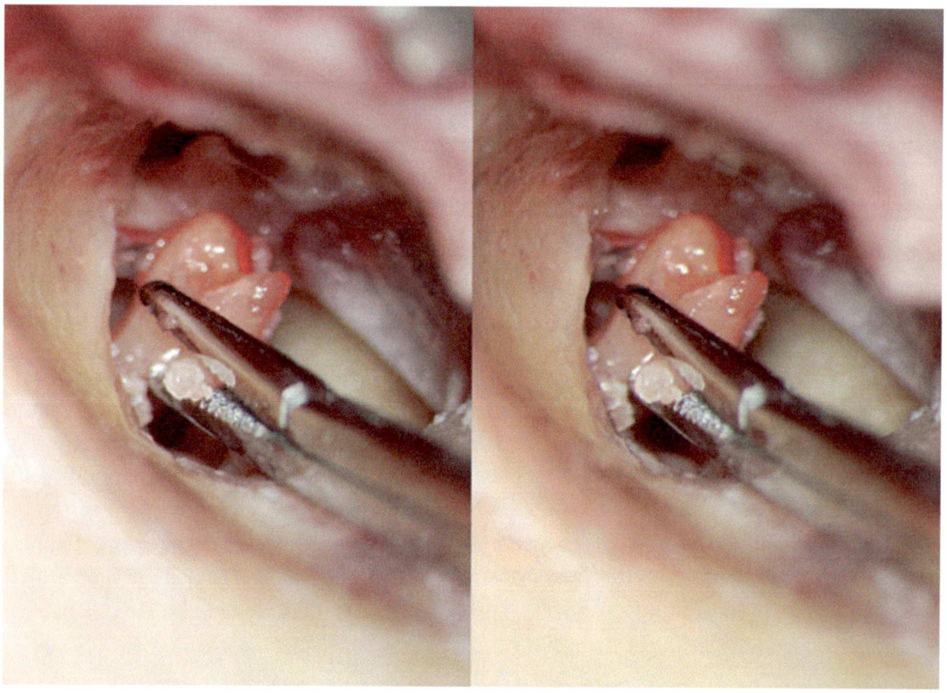

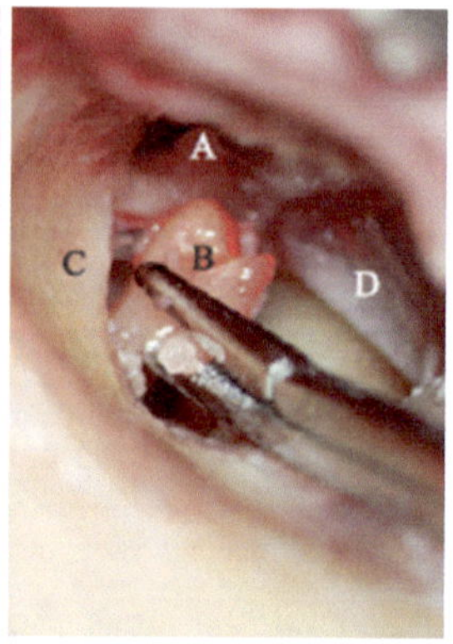

A. Lateral process of the malleus
B. Incus
C. Scutum
D. Tympanic membrane

Fig. 3.11 Removal of the incus (right)
Grasp the long process of the mobilized incus with alligator forceps (after ensuring it has been completely separated from the stapes); rotate it in a forward and lateral direction to disarticulate the incudomalleal joint. Then, detach the superior and posterior ligaments of the incus and remove the incus. Extraction of the incus must be performed carefully to protect the facial nerve, because the tympanic cavity is small and the bone shell covering the horizontal segment of the facial nerve (in the inner wall) is relatively thin; notably, the facial nerve may be naked of bone in the tympanic cavity in some instances. Attention should also be given to avoid injury or dislocation of the stapes when removing the incus
Instruments: alligator forceps

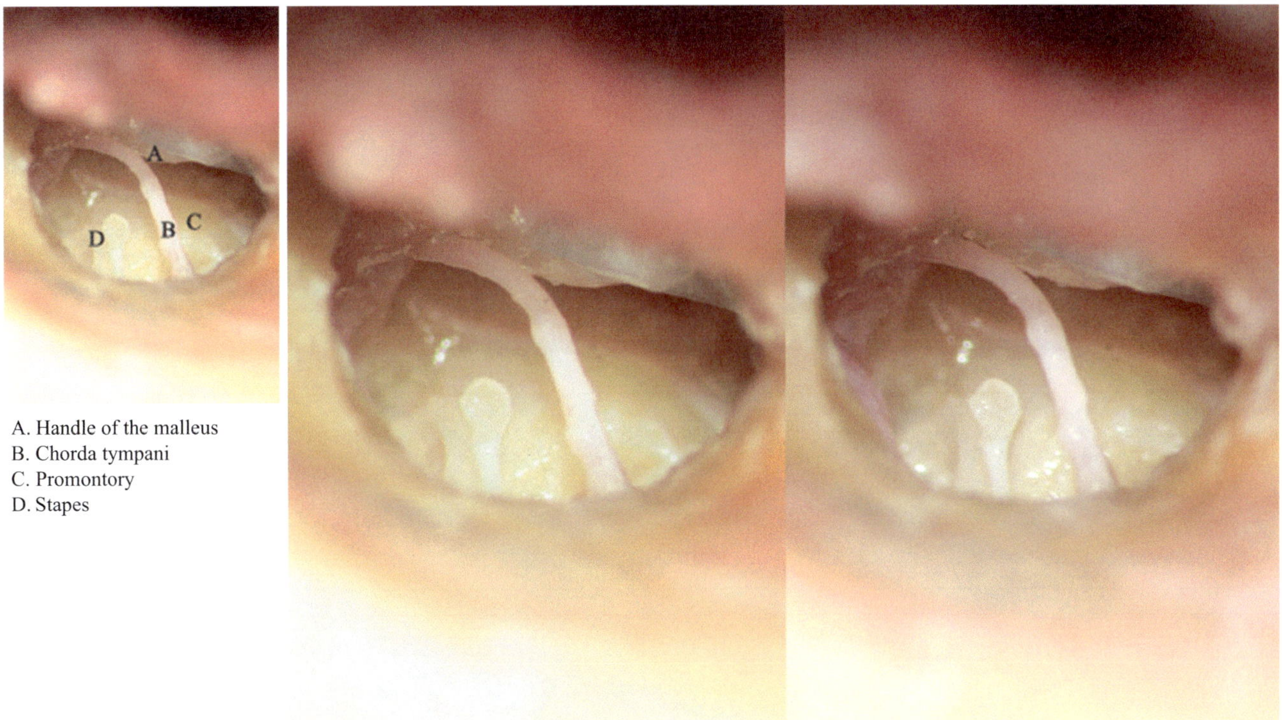

A. Handle of the malleus
B. Chorda tympani
C. Promontory
D. Stapes

Fig. 3.12 Measurement of distance and angle between the malleus and stapes (right)
View after extraction of the incus. Use a miniature measuring scale to assess the vertical distance between the head of the stapes and the malleus handle; this information can be used to determine the shape and size of the autogenous incus needed in ossiculoplasty
Instruments: miniature measuring scale

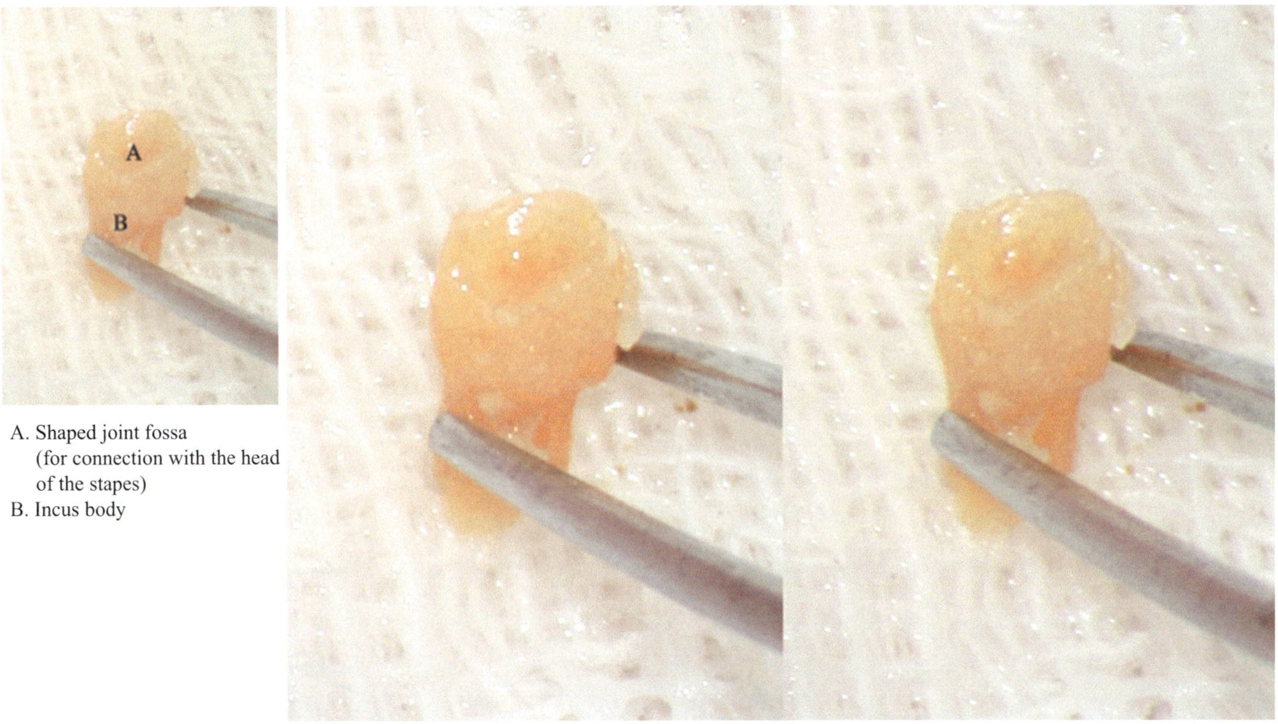

A. Shaped joint fossa (for connection with the head of the stapes)
B. Incus body

Fig. 3.13 Shaping of autogenous incus
Fasten the incus with toothed ophthalmic forceps, drill away the long process of the incus with a small diamond bur, and shape the incus into a columella. Drill a "joint fossa" at one end of the columella for placement on the head of the stapes; drill a groove to connect the malleus handle at the other end. Ensure low-speed drilling and continuous irrigation are used to prevent heat damage
Instruments: ophthalmic forceps, diamond burs

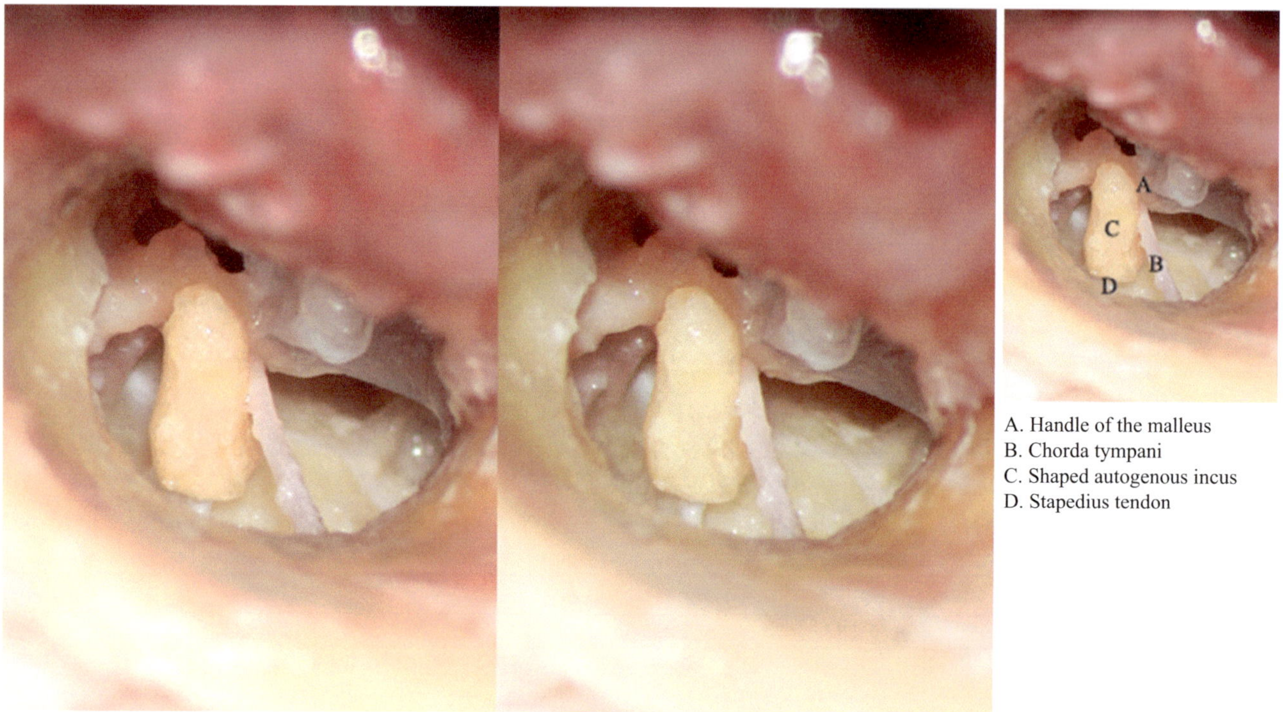

A. Handle of the malleus
B. Chorda tympani
C. Shaped autogenous incus
D. Stapedius tendon

Fig. 3.14 Interposition of the shaped incus and reconstruction of the ossicular chain (right)
Place the "joint fossa" end of the shaped incus onto the head of the stapes using a suction tip and a hook; place the groove end on the superior one-third of the malleus handle. The chorda tympani can be used to aid in the stabilization of the autogenous incus. Move the malleus handle gently to assess the mobility of the reconstructed ossicular chain. Tissue glue can be applied to the connections between the autogenous incus and the malleus, as well as the stapes. To protect the inner ear, avoid disturbing the stapes as much as possible
Instruments: suction cannulas, right-angle hook

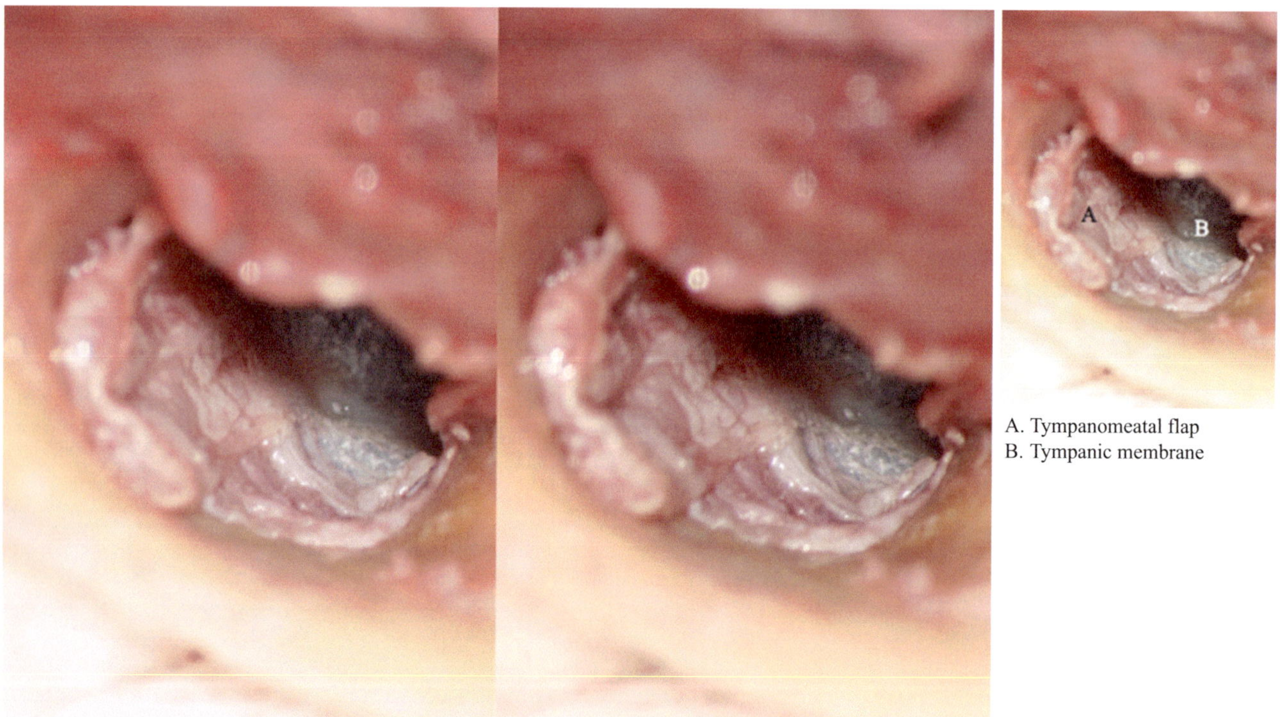

A. Tympanomeatal flap
B. Tympanic membrane

Fig. 3.15 Replacement of the tympanomeatal flap (right)
Replace the tympanomeatal flap; check repeatedly to confirm that the reconstructed ossicular chain is in a good position (not connected to surrounding bone) and the tympanic membrane is in an appropriate position
Instruments: middle ear elevator, alligator forceps

Hearing Reconstruction: PORP Implantation with Incus Removal

Fei Yu

When performing mastoidectomy, the main priority is to prevent the serious or fatal complications of otitis media. Since the 1950s, surgeons have been performing hearing reconstruction during the same surgical procedure, following resection and control of middle ear diseases, based on the understanding of the mechanism and transmission of middle ear diseases. Hearing reconstruction materials include autologous materials (autogenous ossicles, autogenous bone cortex, and autologous cartilage), allogenic materials (allogenic ossicles and allogenic cartilage), and artificial materials (high-molecular-weight polymer materials, hydroxyapatite, and titanium). The biocompatibility of autologous materials is ideal, while the use of autologous materials may result in reimplantation of residual disease. Allograft materials risk the spread of conditions such as human immunodeficiency virus infection, Creutzfeldt–Jakob disease, and various forms of hepatitis. The range of applications of the former two kinds of materials has therefore been gradually reduced. The compatibility, higher strength, and plasticity of titanium in biological artificial materials avoid the inherent disadvantages of autologous and allograft materials; these characteristics also reduce displacement and the need for removal with improved surgical technique and product design. In addition, titanium exhibits good compatibility for magnetic resonance imaging. In particular, titanium ossicular prostheses do not exhibit any obvious migration or heating in the high-intensity magnetic field of 3.0-tesla machines and are therefore promising middle ear implants.

With respect to form and purpose, titanium ossicular prostheses can be divided into partial ossicular replacement prostheses (PORPs), total ossicular replacement prostheses (TORPs), and pistons (artificial stapes). PORPs are used in patients who exhibit intact stapes, but lack a part of the lateral two ossicles; TORPs are used in patients who exhibit an intact footplate of the stapes but lack other ossicles. Pistons are used in patients with stapes fixation. PORPs and TORPs are made by different manufacturers and are available in different forms; they largely consist of a disk (tympanic membrane end), a stapes end, and a connecting rod. Artificial ossicles may exhibit adjustable or fixed length connecting rods.

The current design of artificial ossicles includes: (1) a perforated disk, which can expand the surgeon's field of view below the disk and reduce its weight as well; (2) an adjustable connecting rod, which enables customization of prosthesis height for each patient; (3) the medial frosted surface of the stapes end can improve the connection between the prosthesis and the head of the stapes; and (4) gaps in the stapes end, which can accommodate the tendon of the stapedius muscle and facilitate the installation.

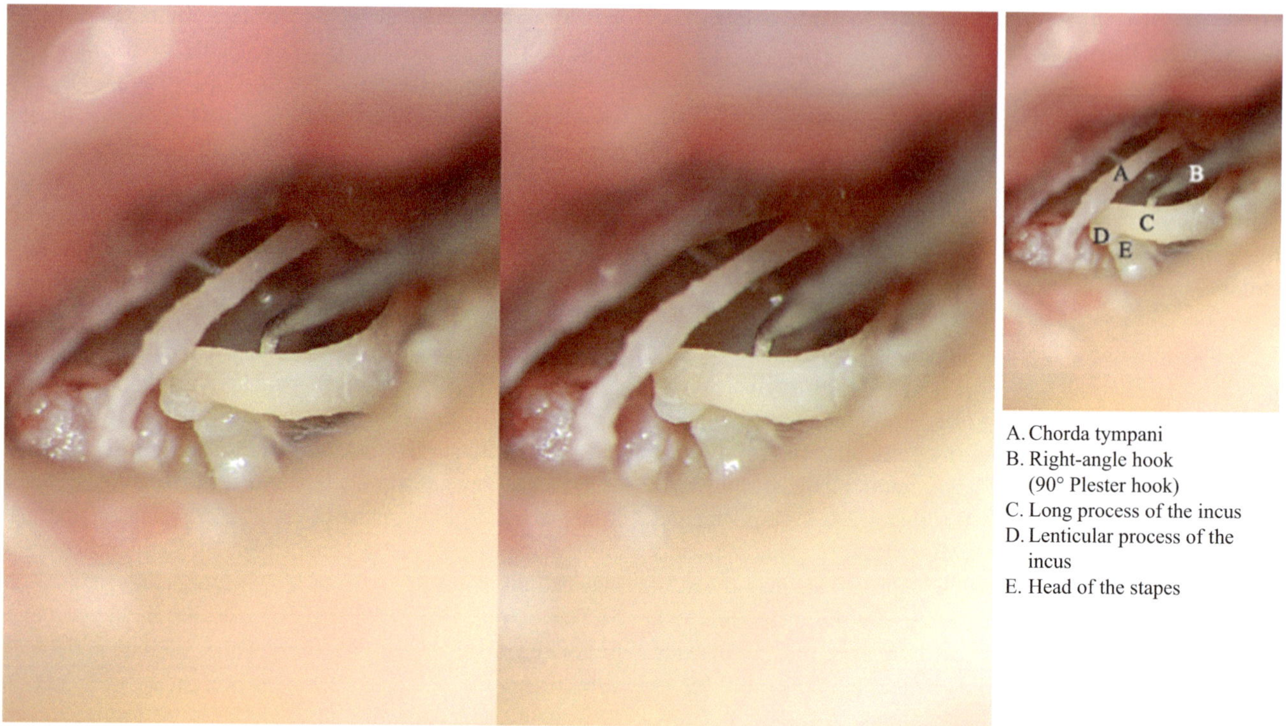

A. Chorda tympani
B. Right-angle hook (90° Plester hook)
C. Long process of the incus
D. Lenticular process of the incus
E. Head of the stapes

Fig. 3.16 Separation of the incudostapedial joint (left)
Elevate the tympanomeatal flap and enter the tympanic cavity; then, identify the chorda tympani, remove some of the scutum and expose part of the epitympanum; finally, explore the mobility of the ossicular chain and gently separate the incudostapedial joint between the lenticular process of the incus and the head of the stapes
Instruments: middle ear elevator, right-angle hook

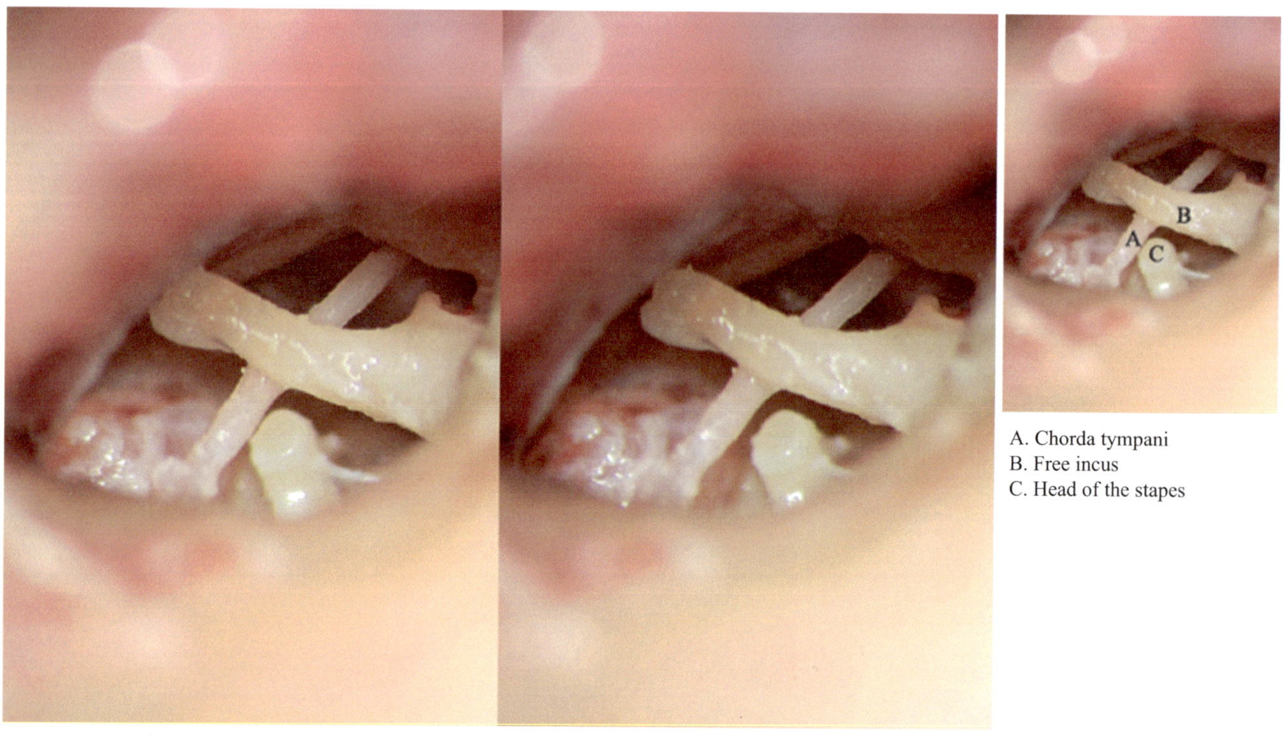

A. Chorda tympani
B. Free incus
C. Head of the stapes

Fig. 3.17 Separation of the incudomalleal joint and removal of the incus (left)
The shape of the incus is irregular. It lies in both the epitympanum and mesotympanum; the tympanic cavity is narrow, such that it can be difficult to remove. First, separate the incudostapedial joint using a right-angle hook, then displace the long process of the incus forward and backward. Dislocate the incudomalleal joint using a right-angle hook in the joint, then grasp the long process to remove the incus using ear forceps. During extraction, protect the chorda tympani, facial nerve, and stapes by using gentle dissection
Instruments: right-angle hook, ear forceps (serrated Hartmann ear forceps)

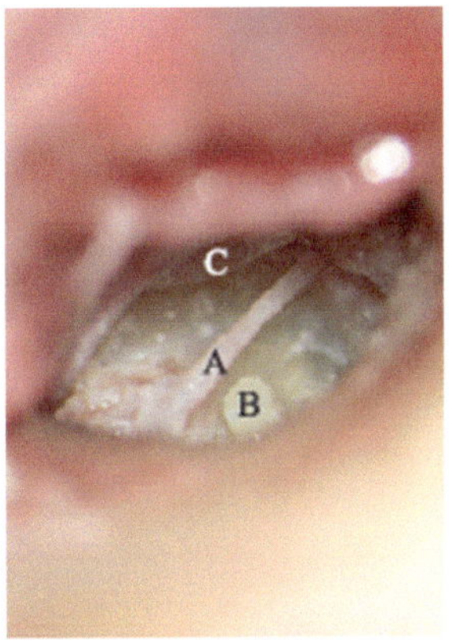

A. Chorda tympani
B. Head of the stapes
C. Handle of the malleus

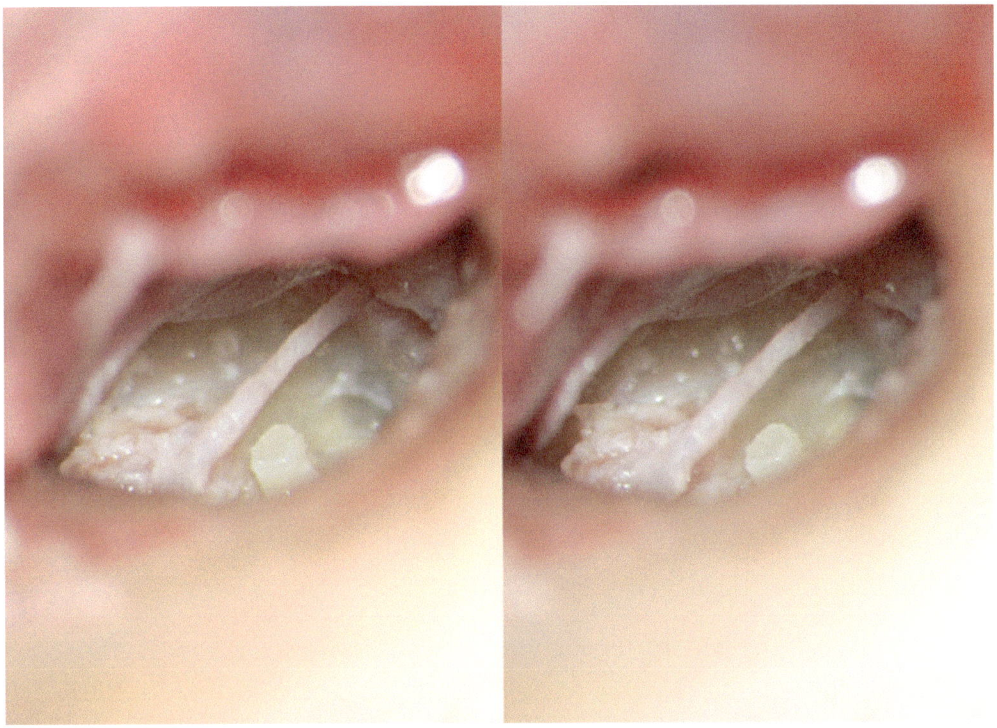

Fig. 3.18 Tympanic cavity after removal of the incus (left)
The stapes, handle of the malleus, and anteriorly folded tympanic membrane are visible after removal of the incus; in addition, the stapes exhibits good movement. In accordance with the Fisch type 1 classification, a PORP implant is feasible for repair of the ossicular chain
Instruments: #9 Suction cannulas, straight microneedle (0° microneedle)

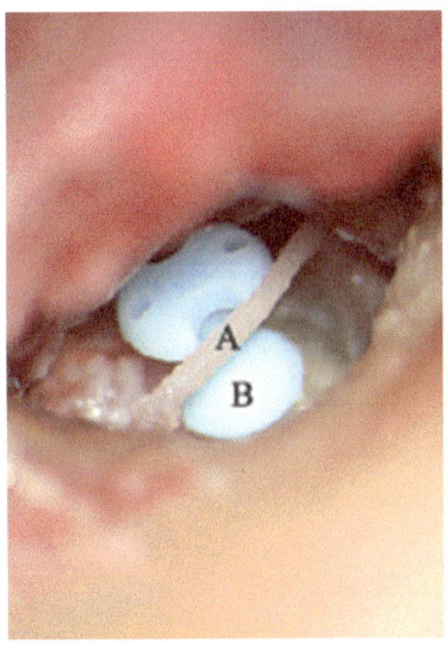

A. Chorda tympani
B. PORP model (Kurz)

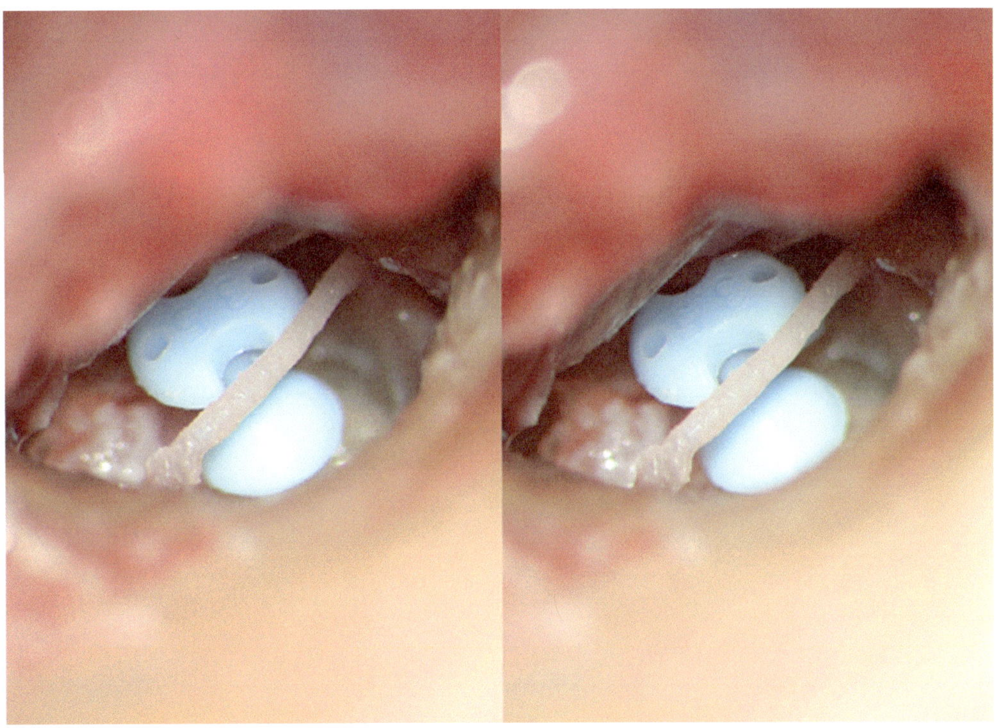

Fig. 3.19 Measurement of the distance between the handle of the malleus and the head of the stapes (left)
The distance between the head of the stapes and the tympanic membrane should be carefully assessed before PORP implantation. An appropriate PORP length is important for a suitable hearing outcome: a short PORP will cause disconnection of the ossicular chain, while a long PORP will risk tympanic membrane penetration. The implanted prosthesis should be slightly longer than the measurement taken to avoid disconnection of the ossicular chain caused by postoperative outward migration of the tympanic membrane. Measuring tools differ depending on the manufacturer. The image shown depicts a single-use PORP model from the Kurz company in Germany
Instruments: suction cannulas, right-angle hook

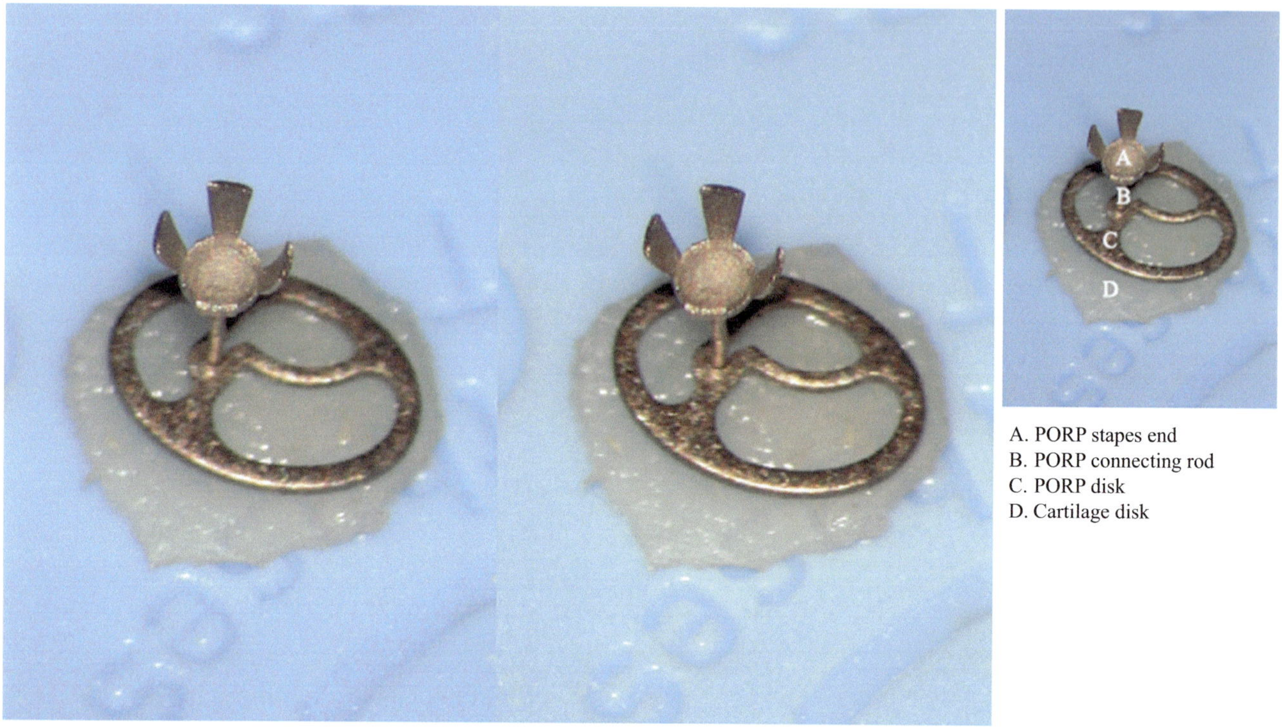

A. PORP stapes end
B. PORP connecting rod
C. PORP disk
D. Cartilage disk

Fig. 3.20 Assembly of the PORP and formation of the cartilage disk
A fixed-length PORP with suitable height or an adjustable PORP cut to the appropriate height should be selected in accordance with the measured distance between the head of the stapes and the tympanic membrane. A cartilage disk should be made in accordance with the size of the PORP disk end. The image shown depicts an adjustable titanium ossicle from Kurz. The stapes end is claw-shaped with the inner side surface dull polished, the disk is flat and perforated, and the length of the connecting rod is adjustable
Instruments: PORP assembly kit, scalpel

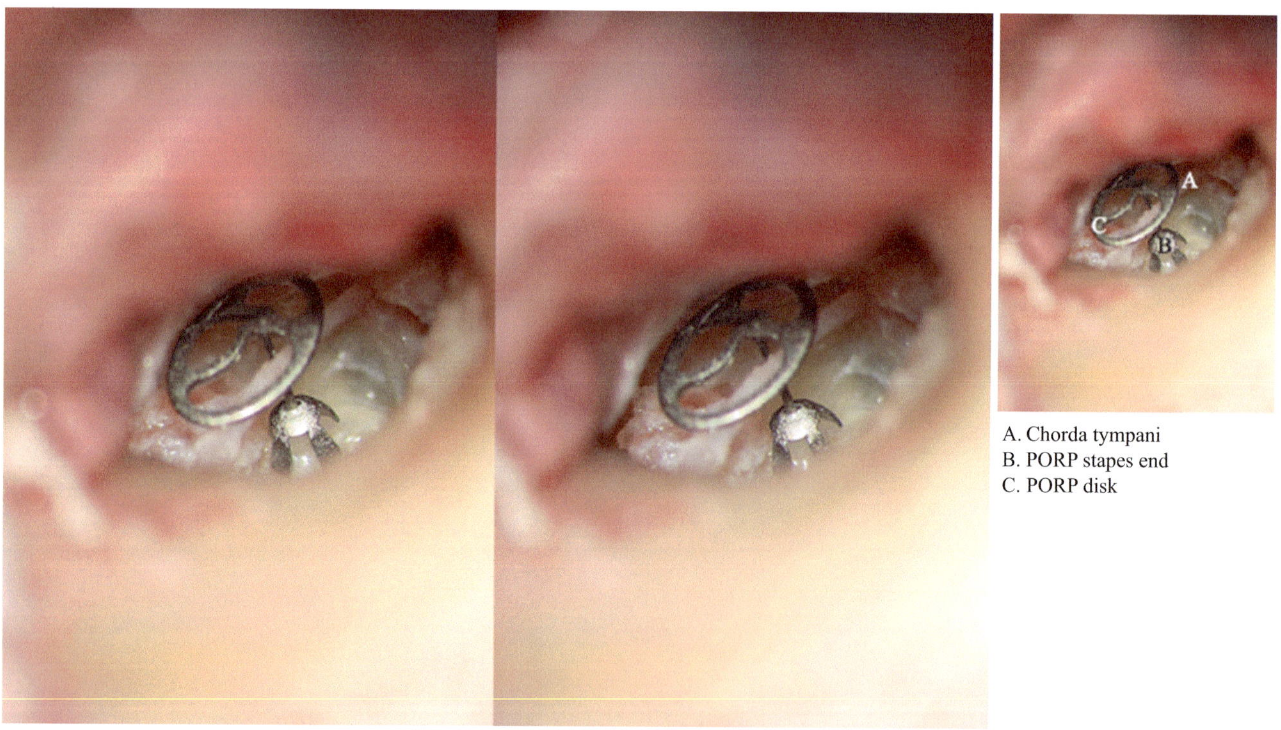

A. Chorda tympani
B. PORP stapes end
C. PORP disk

Fig. 3.21 Implantation of the PORP (left, Kurz)
Insert the selected PORP between the head of the stapes and the tympanic membrane. The deep part of the tympanic cavity can be observed through the perforated disk of the PORP
Instruments: right-angle hook, #9 suction cannulas

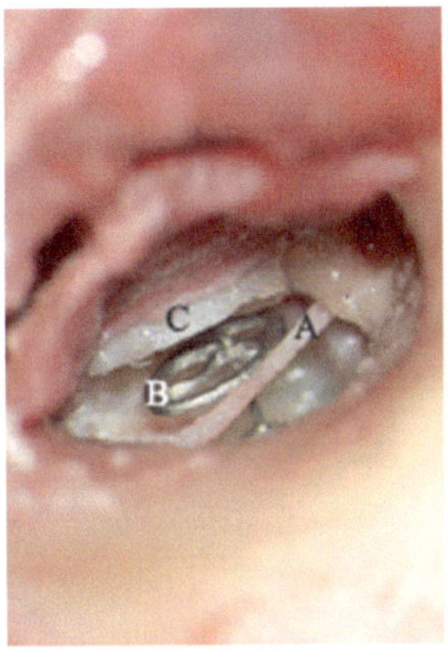

A. Chorda tympani
B. PORP disk
C. Cartilage disk

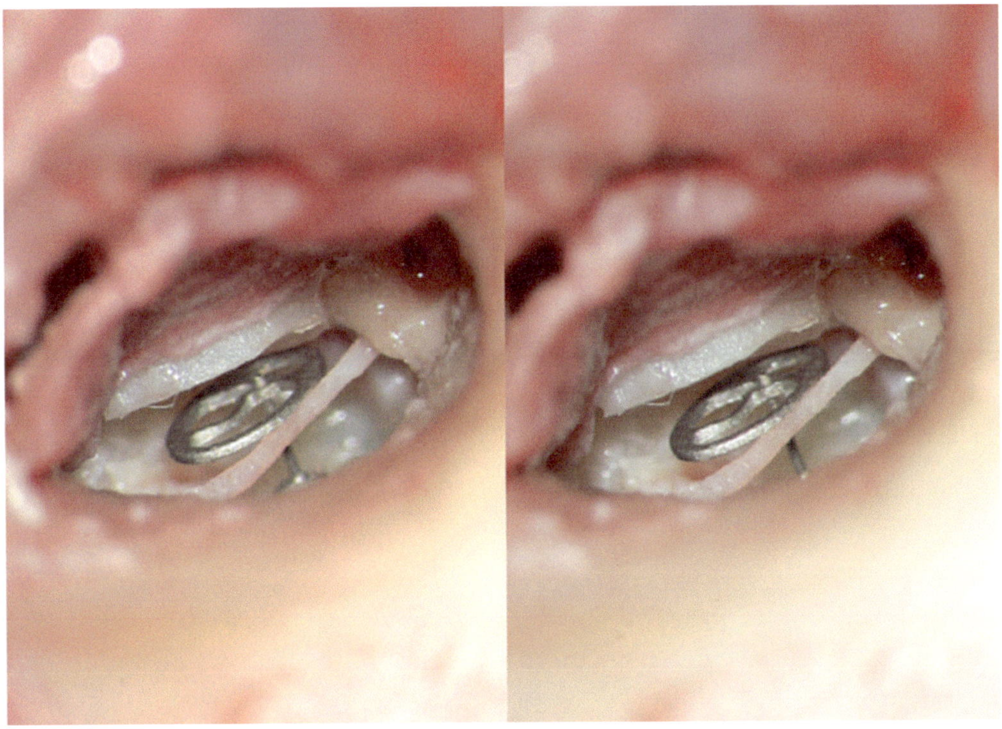

Fig. 3.22 Placement of the cartilage disk between the outer surface of the PORP and the tympanic membrane (left)
In all cases using metal ossicular replacement prostheses, a cartilage disk should be placed between the titanium surface of the PORP disk and the tympanic membrane. This avoids perforation of the tympanic membrane and extrusion of the artificial ossicle
Instruments: ear forceps, right-angle hook, #9 suction cannulas

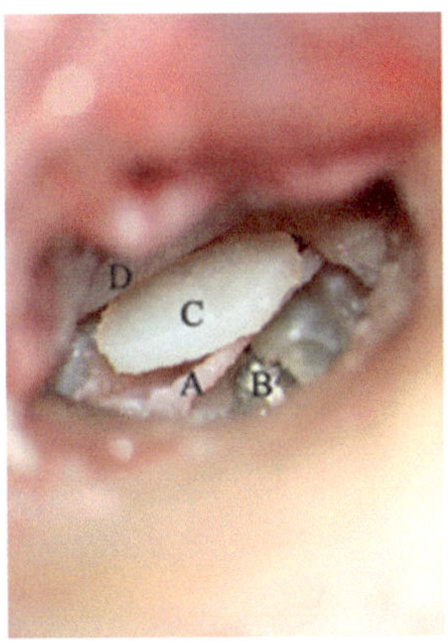

A. Chorda tympani
B. PORP stapes end
C. Cartilage disk
D. Tympanic membrane

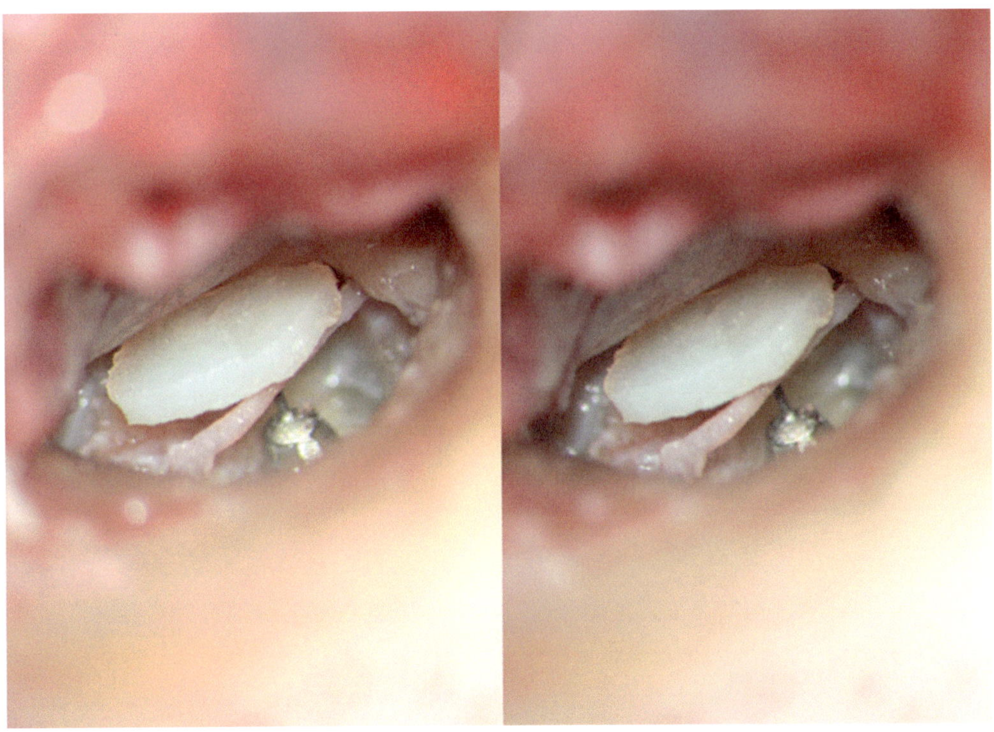

Fig. 3.23 Adjustment of the cartilage disk (left)
The trimmed cartilage disk should be inserted and adjusted to the right position. The disk covers the whole PORP disk and should make sufficient contact with the effective vibration area of the tympanic membrane. If necessary, the chorda tympani can be placed lateral to the cartilage disk to ensure it remains in place
Instruments: right-angle hook, #9 suction cannulas

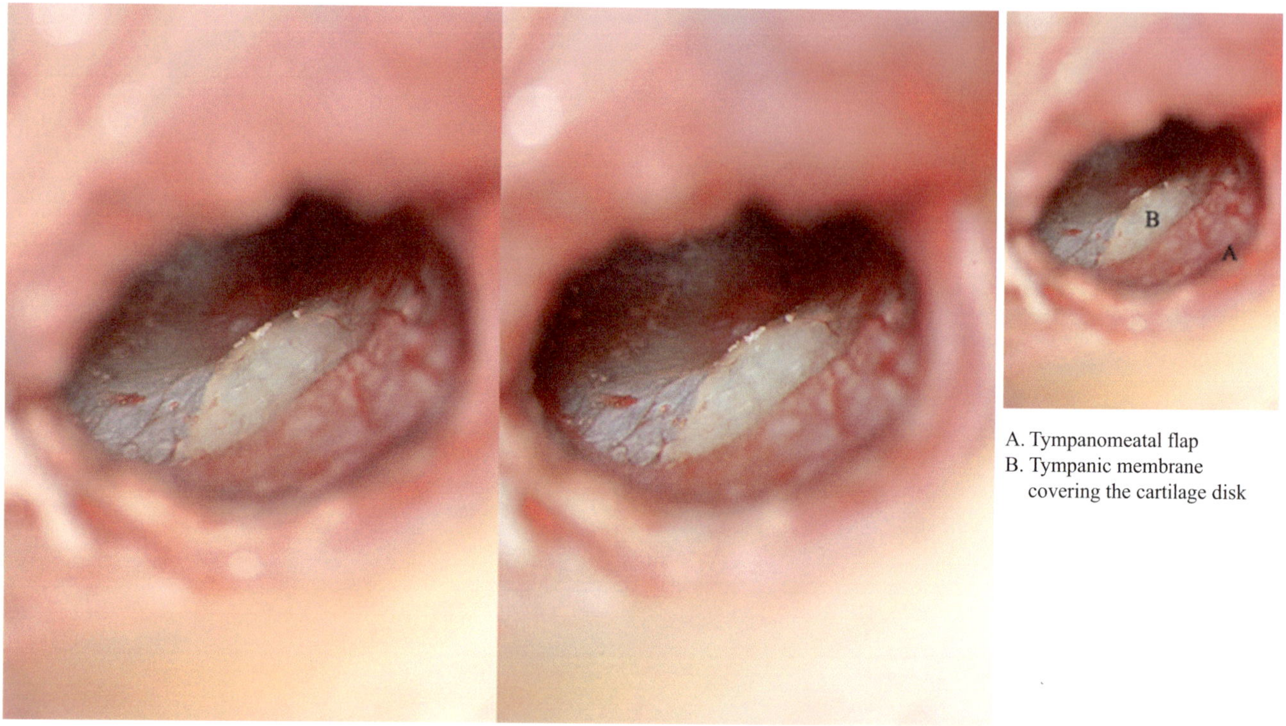

A. Tympanomeatal flap
B. Tympanic membrane covering the cartilage disk

Fig. 3.24 Reset of tympanomeatal flap (left)
Reset the tympanic membrane and tympanomeatal flap, confirm the length of the implanted PORP and the location of the cartilage disk, and ensure the absence of residual perforation of the tympanic membrane. Any abnormal finding should be corrected at this time

Instruments: middle ear elevator, eardrum flattening device (45° Rosen rounded knife)

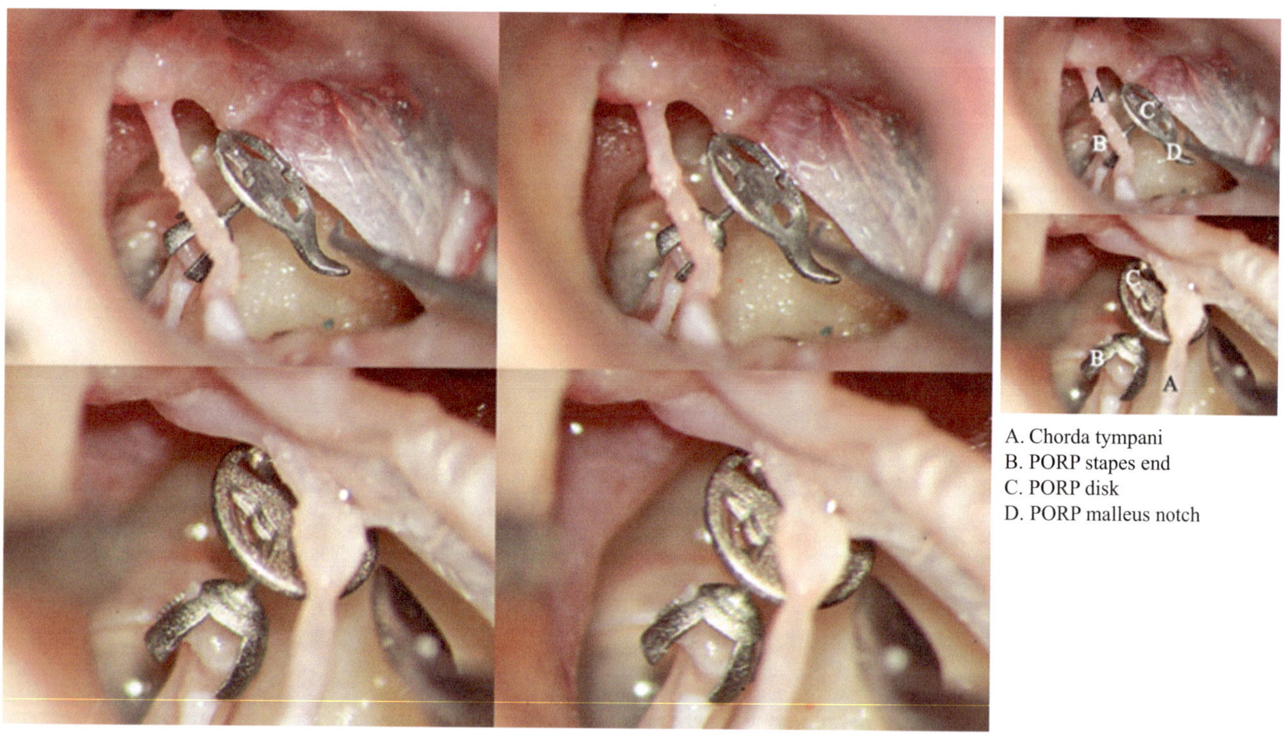

A. Chorda tympani
B. PORP stapes end
C. PORP disk
D. PORP malleus notch

Fig. 3.25 PORP (right, Kurz)
The malleus notch prosthesis (MNP, Kurz) exhibits a notched tail at the edge of the disk. The notch connects with the handle of the malleus to reinforce the reconstruction of the ossicular chain, reduce PORP compression on the tympanic membrane, and reduce the possibility of PORP extrusion. In addition, gaps in the stapes end of the PORP can be positioned over the tendon of the stapedius muscle, thereby allowing better connection between the PORP stapes end and the head of the stapes
Instruments: right-angle hook, #9 suction cannulas

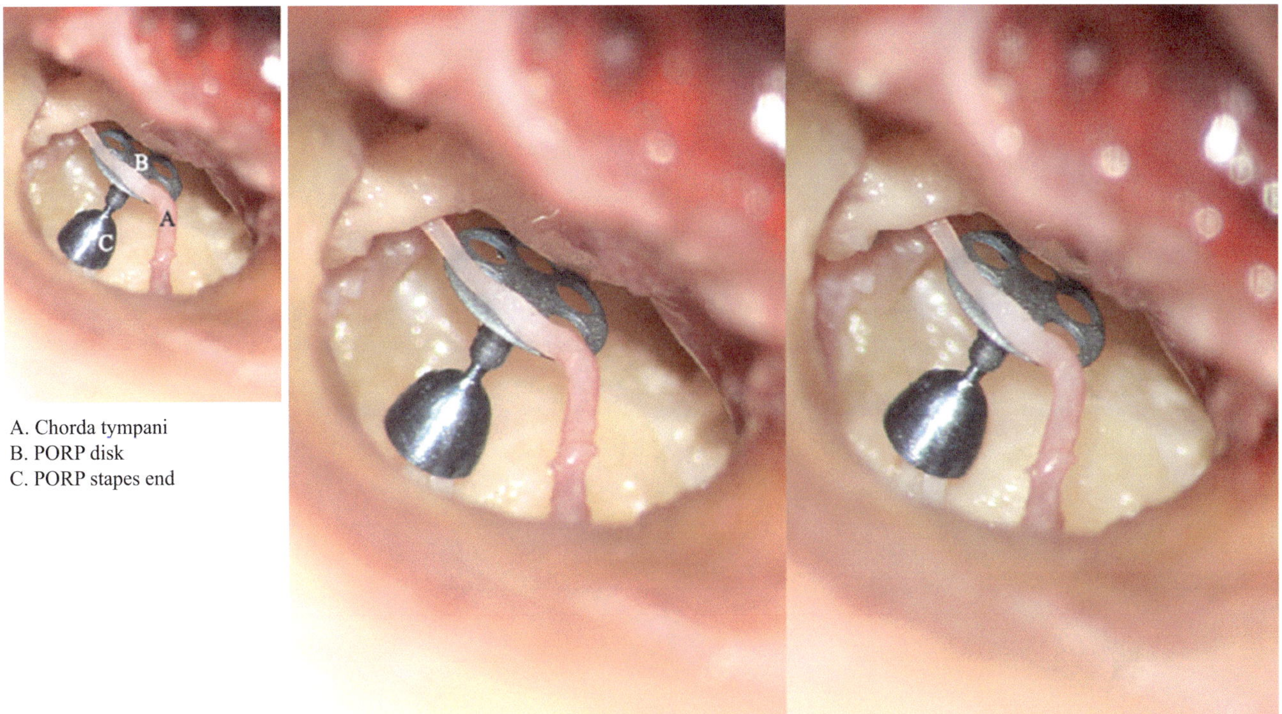

Fig. 3.26 PORP (right, Spiggle & Theis)
Based on the specific findings at surgery, PORPs of different shapes from different manufacturers can be used. The image depicts the all-titanium PORP disk with perforations (Spiggle & Theis), which can aid in the visualization of the deep cavity. The inside surface of the bell-shaped stapes end is already frosted to improve the connection between the prosthesis and the head of the stapes
Instruments: right-angle hook, #9 suction cannulas

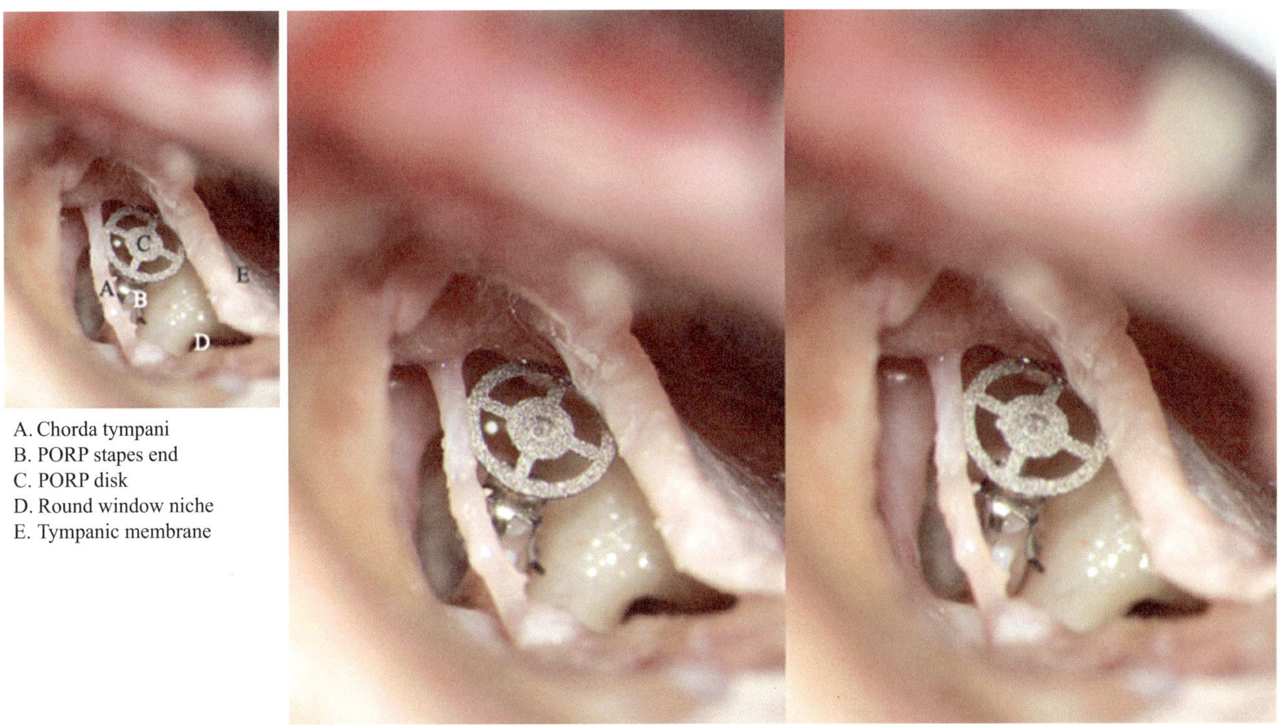

Fig. 3.27 PORP (right, Medtronic)
PORP from Medtronic, with fixed length, exhibits holes in the disk and a claw-shaped stapes end
Instruments: right-angle hook, #9 suction cannulas

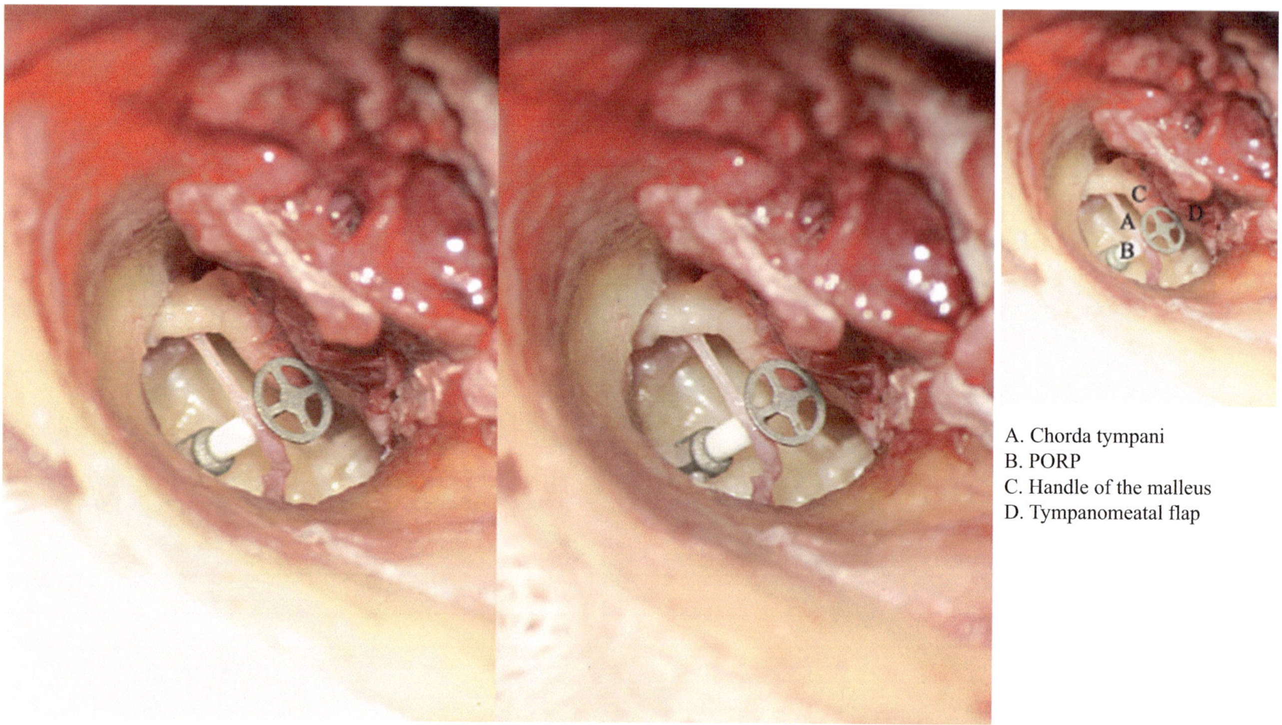

Fig. 3.28 PORP (right, Medtronic)
PORP from Medtronic, with adjustable length, exhibits holes in the disk and a claw-shaped stapes end

Instruments: right-angle hook, #9 suction cannulas

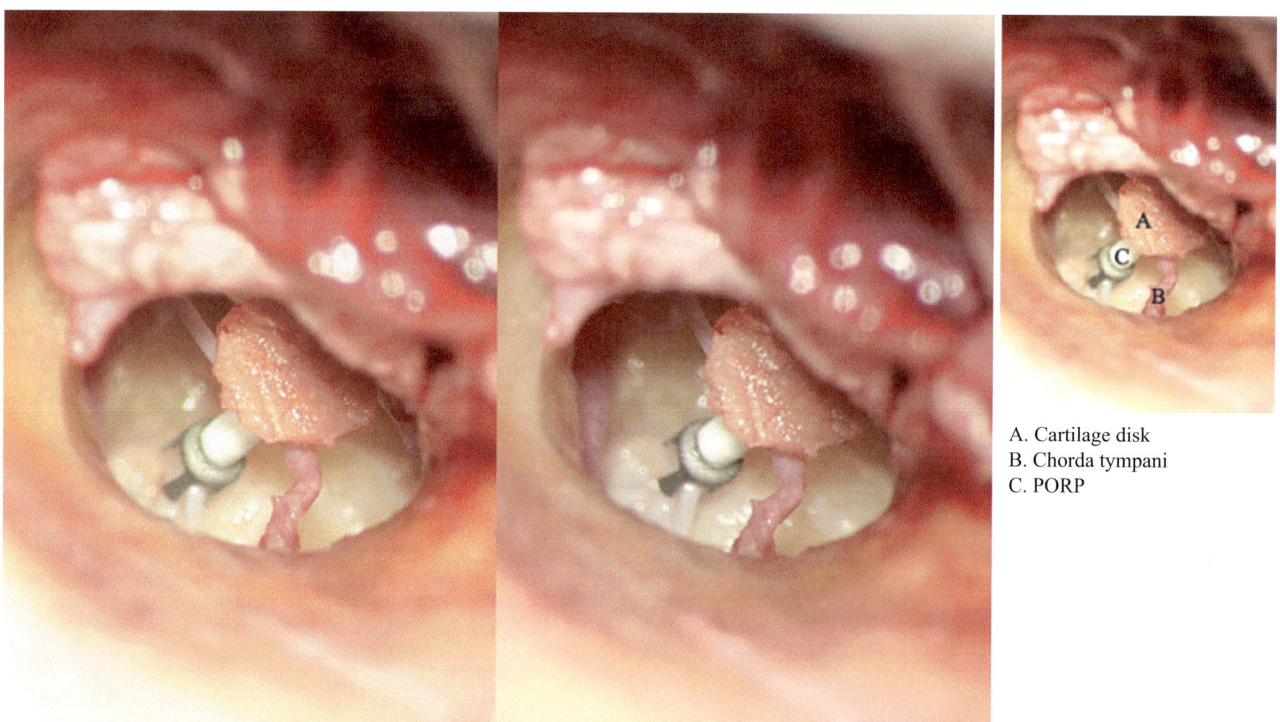

Fig. 3.29 Positioning of the cartilage disk (right)
To avoid perforation of the membrane and PORP extrusion, a cartilage disk must be placed over all types of metal PORPs under the tympanic membrane

Instruments: ear forceps, right-angle hook, #9 suction cannulas

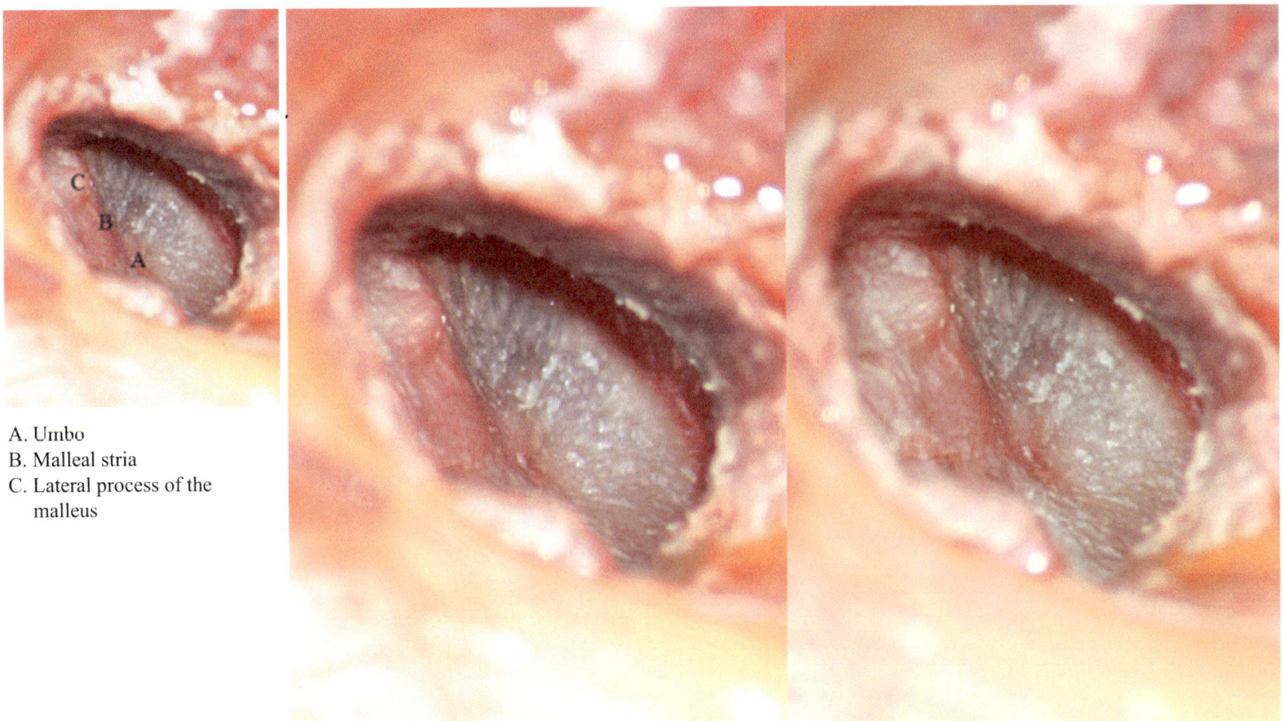

A. Umbo
B. Malleal stria
C. Lateral process of the malleus

Fig. 3.30 Reset of tympanomeatal flap (right)
Reset the tympanic membrane and tympanomeatal flap, then inspect repeatedly to ensure the ossicular chain and cartilage disk are stable and the tympanic membrane remains intact

Instruments: middle ear elevator, eardrum flattening device (45° Rosen rounded knife)

Hearing Reconstruction: PORP Implantation Without Incus Removal

Sha-sha Huang

There are many types of ossicular defects. If the remaining ossicular chain is normal apart from the incus, the abnormality is consistent with Fisch type I ossicular defect. With such a defect, the air–bone gap can be restored to within 10 dB HL by removal of the incus and implantation of a PORP to connect the malleus and stapes. It may be unnecessary to remove the incus if damage is limited to the end of the long process of the incus. In such instances, a special type of PORP can be used to preserve the lever function of the ossicular chain.

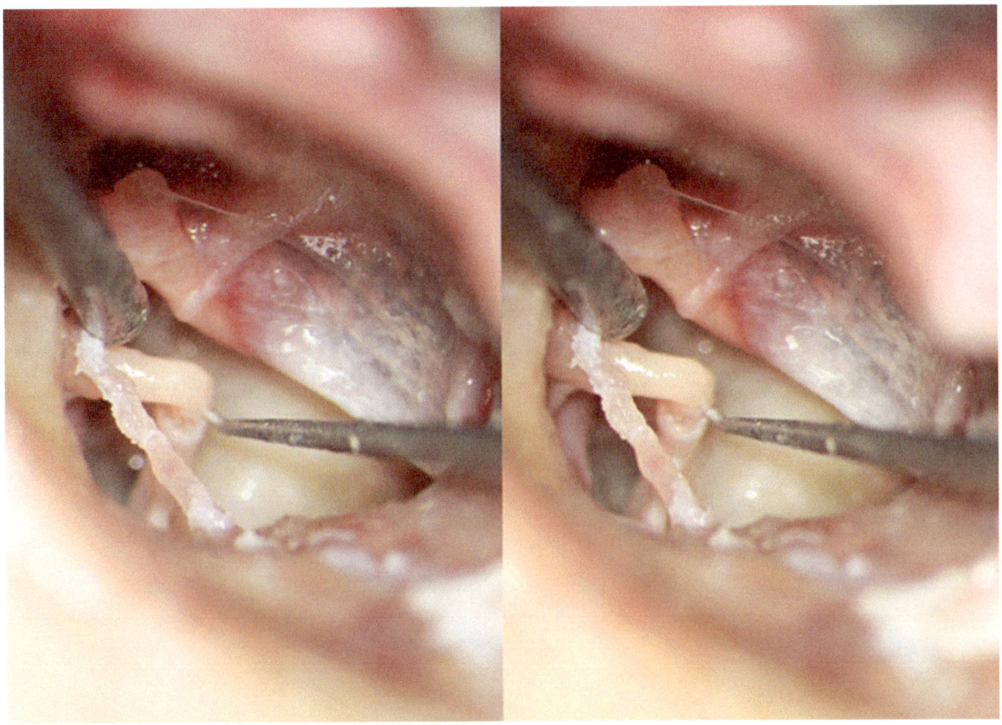

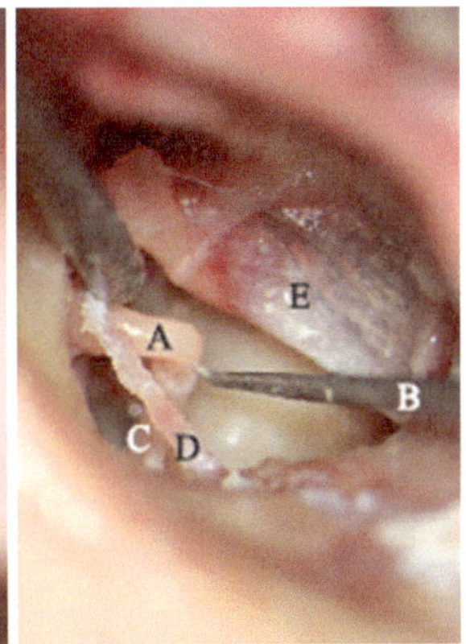

A. Long process of the incus
B. Right-angle hook
C. Posterior crus of the stapes
D. Chorda tympani
E. Elevated tympanic membrane

Fig. 3.31 Separation of the incudostapedial joint (right)
Elevate the tympanomeatal flap and tympanic membrane forward to explore the ossicular chain and chorda tympani. Then, remove the tympanic scutum, expose part of the epitympanum, and separate the incudostapedial joint with a right-angle hook

Instruments: scalpel, middle ear elevator, right-angle hook, suction cannulas

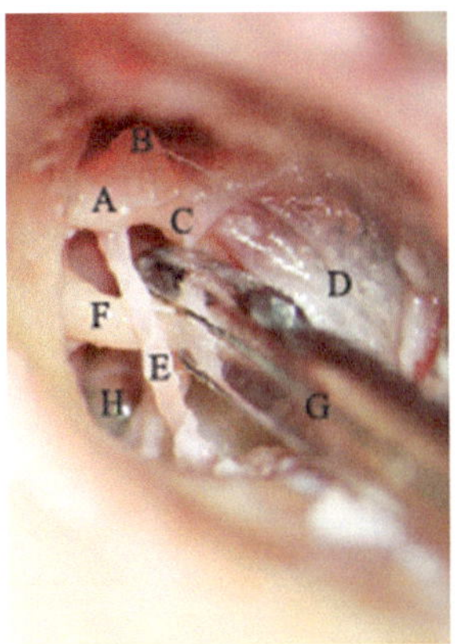

A. Neck of the malleus
B. Lateral process of the malleus
C. Malleus handle
D. Tympanic membrane
E. Chorda tympani
F. Long process of the incus
G. Malleus head scissors
H. Footplate of the stapes

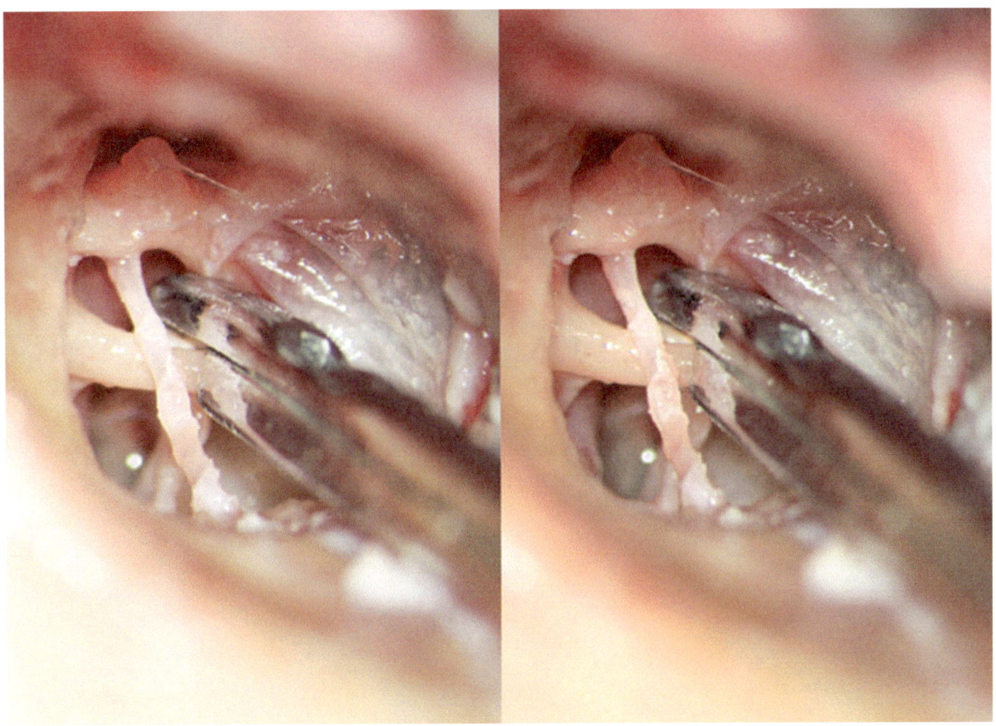

Fig. 3.32 Resection of the lenticular process of the incus (right)
Excise the end of the long process of the incus and its lenticular process using the malleus head scissors, following separation of the incudostapedial joint. This situation is to simulate a congenital incus deformity or incus long process erosion
Instruments: malleus head scissors, polyp forceps

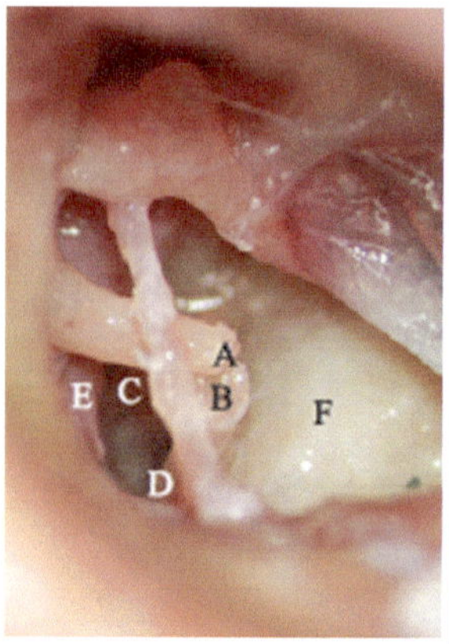

A. Deficient incus long process
B. Head of the stapes
C. Anterior stapes crus
D. Posterior stapes crus
E. Prominence of facial canal
F. Promontory

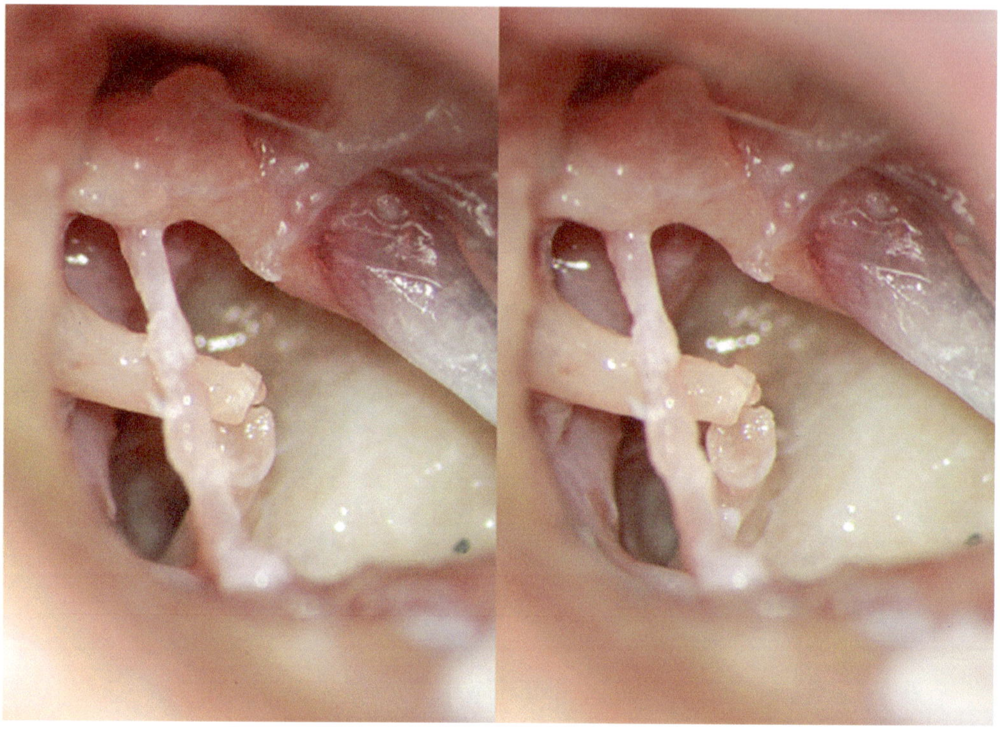

Fig. 3.33 Ossicular status after excision of the lenticular process of the incus (right)
Ossicular status: the malleus and stapes are both intact, while the mobile incus exhibits a deficient long process

Instruments: malleus head scissors, polyp forceps

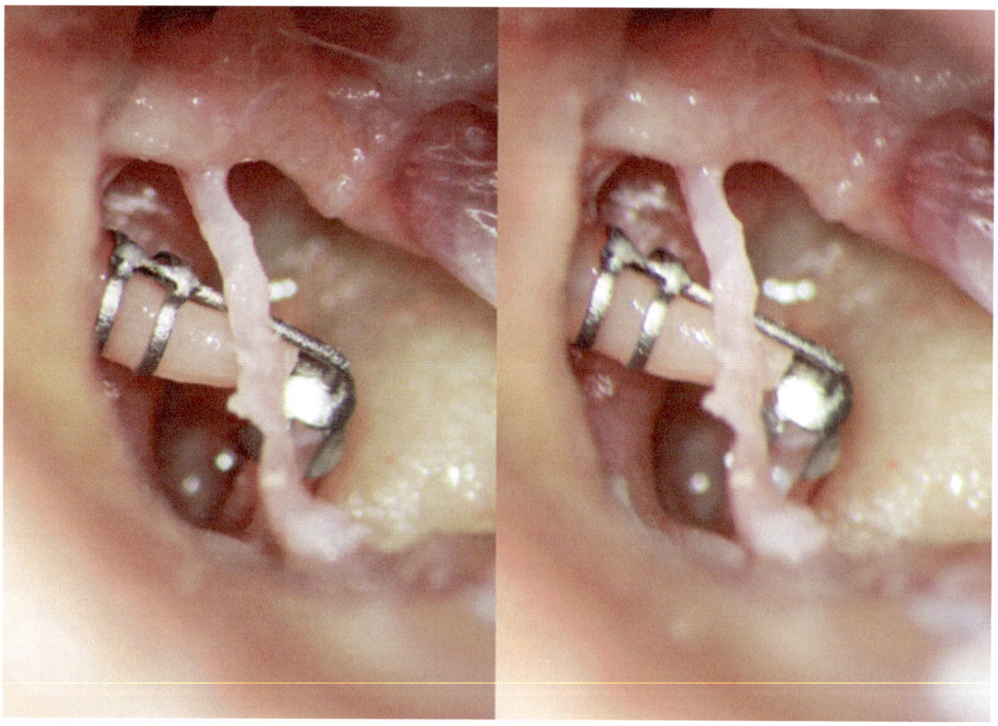

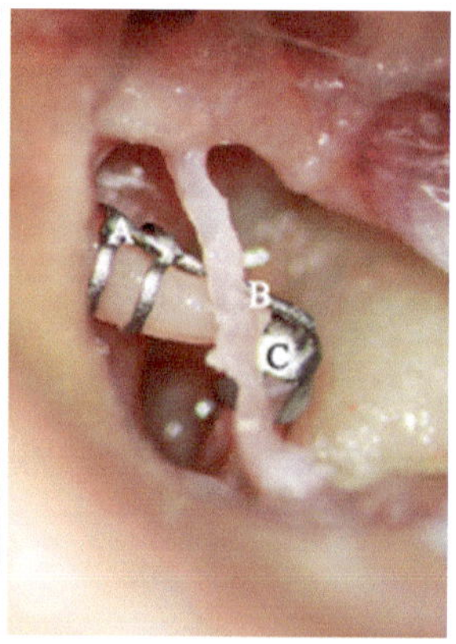

A. Incus end of the special PORP
B. Joint lever
C. Stapes end of the special PORP

Fig. 3.34 Implantation of a special PORP (right)
A special PORP is positioned between the long process of the incus and the head of the stapes; it consists of two claws for the long process of the incus, linked by a joint lever to a stapes head claw base. This type of PORP is used to reconnect the long process of the incus and the stapes and restore the normal function of the ossicular chain
Instruments: #9 suction cannulas, right-angle hook, polyp forceps

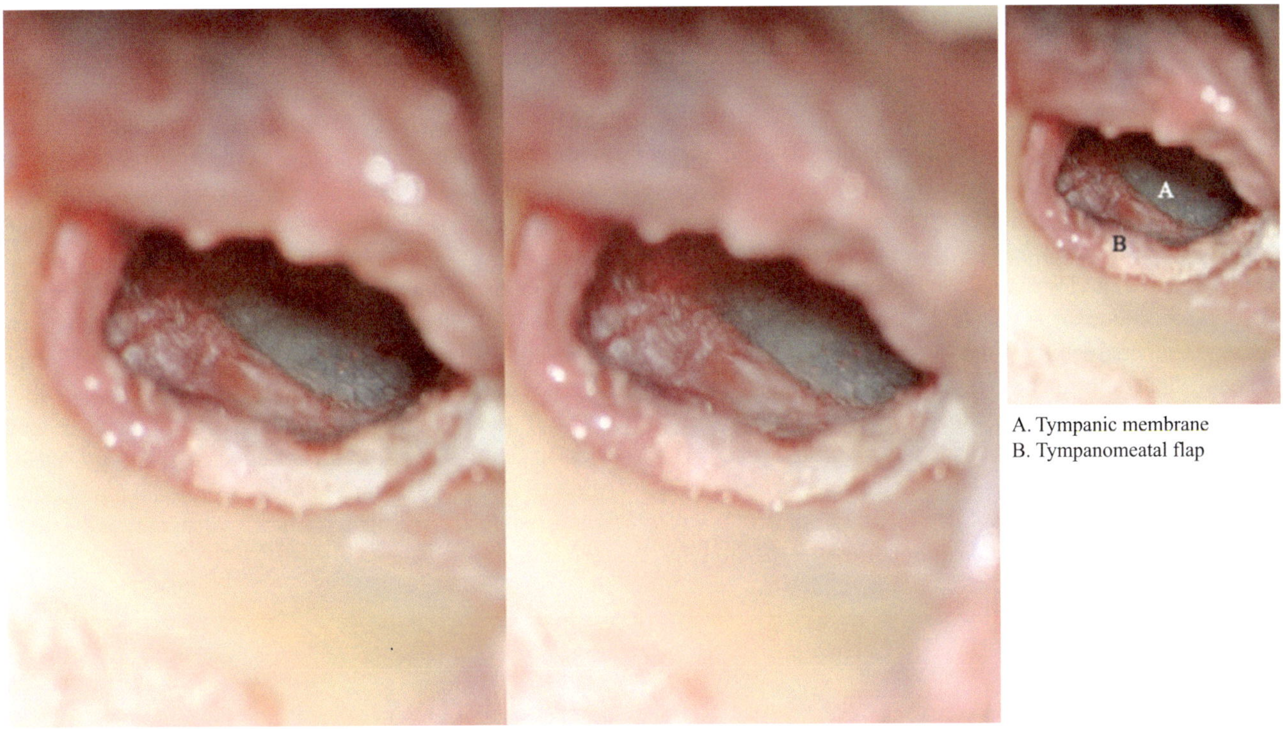

A. Tympanic membrane
B. Tympanomeatal flap

Fig. 3.35 Reset of the tympanomeatal flap (right)
Because the PORP exhibits no direct contact with the tympanic membrane, it is appropriate to reset the tympanomeatal flap without placement of a cartilage disk over the prosthesis

Instruments: middle ear elevator, eardrum flattening device (45° Rosen rounded knife), #12 suction cannulas

Hearing Reconstruction: TORP Implantation

Li-li Ren

The ossicular chain is an essential structure for the maintenance of normal acoustic transduction. Any lesion resulting in ossicular chain disruption or reduced mobility will inevitably cause hearing impairment. Similar to the PORP, the TORP is important for ossicular reconstruction.

The indications for TORP implantation are as follows: (1) damaged superstructure of the stapes by disease or trauma; (2) congenital deformity of the stapes superstructure; and (3) mobile stapes footplate, but autogenous ossicles cannot meet the demands for partial ossicular chain reconstruction.

Complications: (1) displacement of ossicles, which might be caused by an excessively short TORP or outward migration of the tympanic membrane; (2) perforation of the tympanic membrane, and extrusion of the TORP (potentially caused by an excessively long TORP, or by absorption or absence of the cartilage between the prosthesis and tympanic membrane); (3) fixation of ossicles, which might be caused by residual or recurrent pathology; and/or (4) fracture of the footplate, due to an excessively long TORP or an unsuitable prosthesis angle, which might cause sensorineural hearing loss.

Key points to improve TORP implantation: (1) the position of the TORP should guarantee vertical transduction of acoustic waves from the tympanic membrane; and (2) inappropriate contact between the TORP and surrounding structures will severely limit the mobility of the reconstructed ossicular chain. Therefore, avoid contact of the prosthesis with the following structures: the promontory, tympanic sulcus, horizontal bony canal of the facial nerve, and lateral wall of the epitympanum.

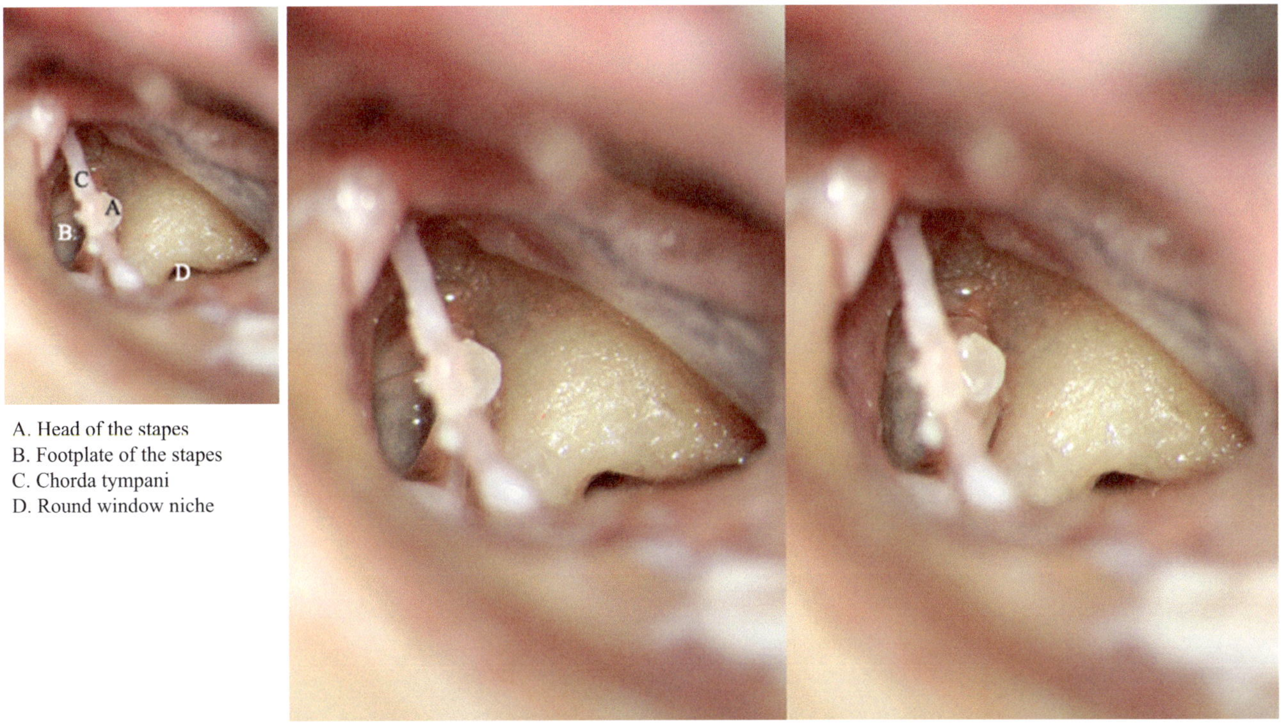

A. Head of the stapes
B. Footplate of the stapes
C. Chorda tympani
D. Round window niche

Fig. 3.36 Assessment of ossicular chain mobility and removal of the incus (right)
Endaural approach: perform an endaural incision and remove part of the tympanic scutum to expose the superior part of the upper tympanic cavity. Assess the mobility of the ossicular chain and remove the incus; then, measure the distance between the tympanic membrane and the footplate of the stapes to determine the proper TORP size
Instruments: middle ear elevator, right-angle hook, alligator forceps, miniature measuring scale, TORP assembly kit

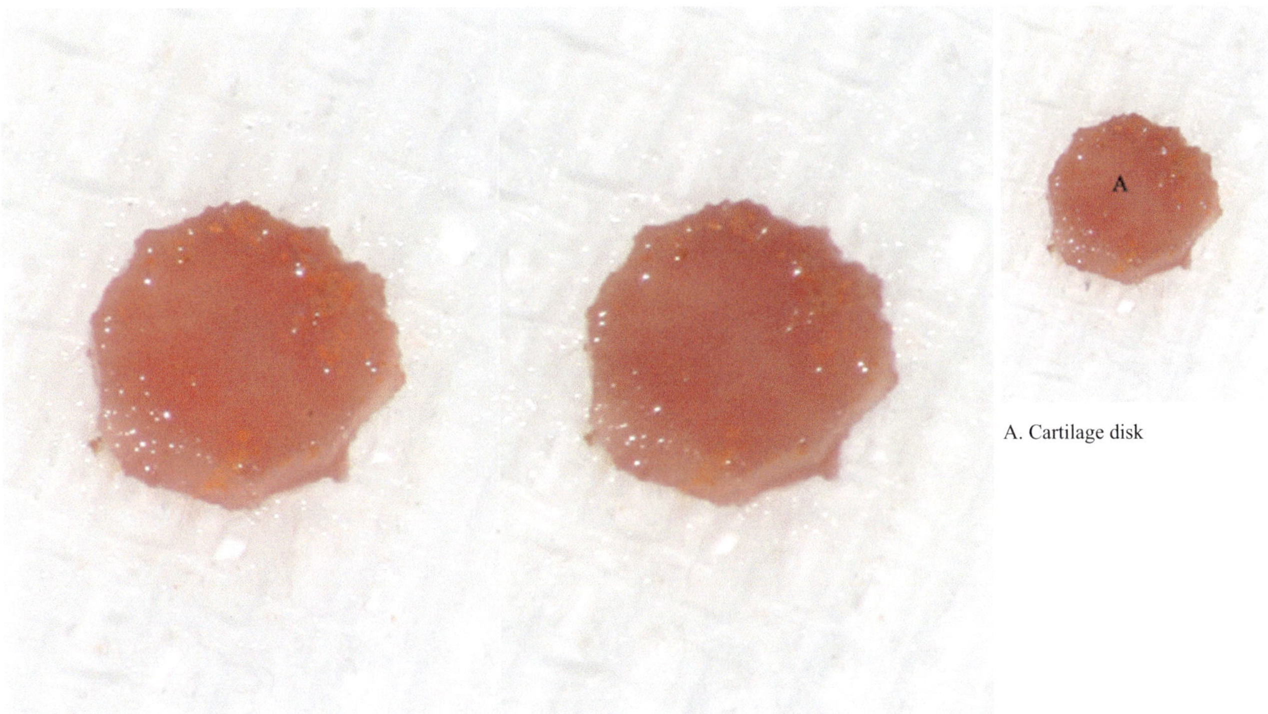

A. Cartilage disk

Fig. 3.37 Preparation of cartilage
Cut the appropriate size of the cartilage from the auricular concha or tragus, preserving the perichondrium. Trim the cartilage into a disk with a size equivalent to that of the tympanic membrane end of the TORP
Instruments: scalpel

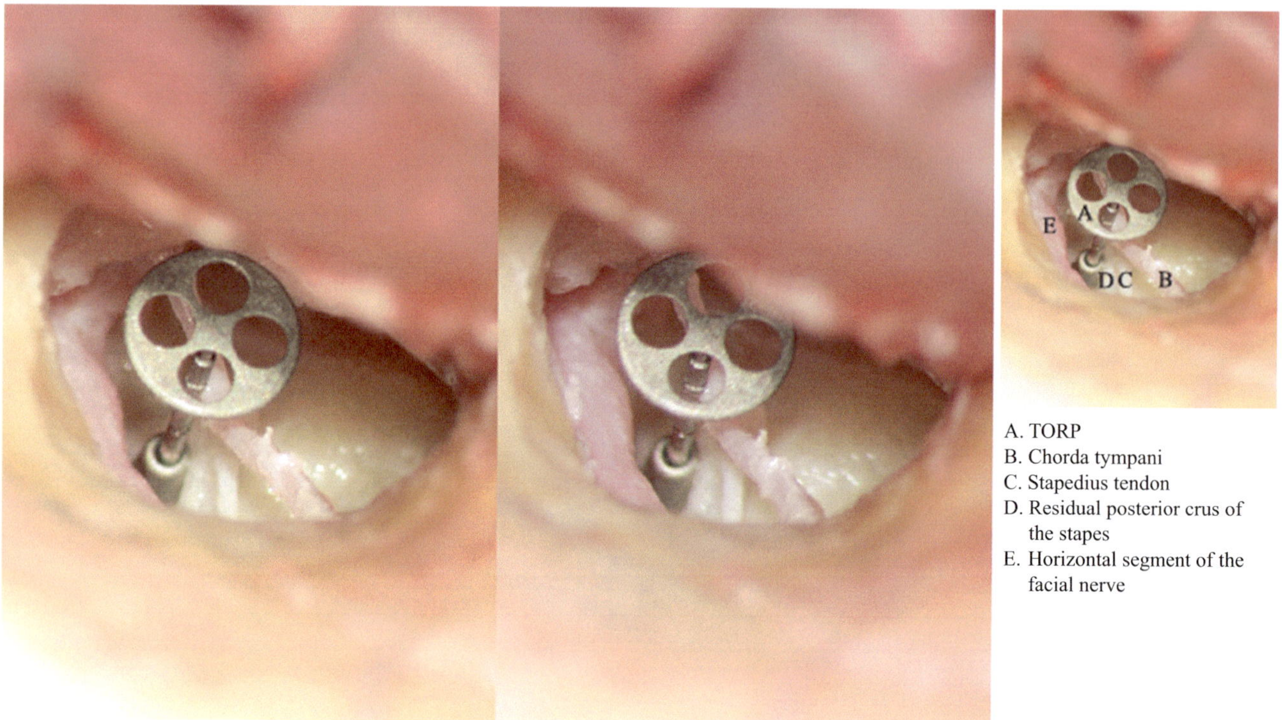

Fig. 3.38 Implantation of TORP (right, Spiggle & Theis)
Use a right-angle hook and size 9 sucker to implant the TORP. The stapes end of the TORP should be placed at the center of the stapes footplate, at right angles to the footplate. The tympanic membrane end of the TORP should be in contact with the umbo of the tympanic membrane. *Hints: (1) The presence of residual crura of the stapes can enhance the stability of the reconstructed ossicular chain by stabilizing the stapes end of the TORP. (2) If necessary, a piece of thin fascia can be placed between the footplate and TORP to protect the residual parts of the stapes*
Instruments: right-angle hook, suction cannulas

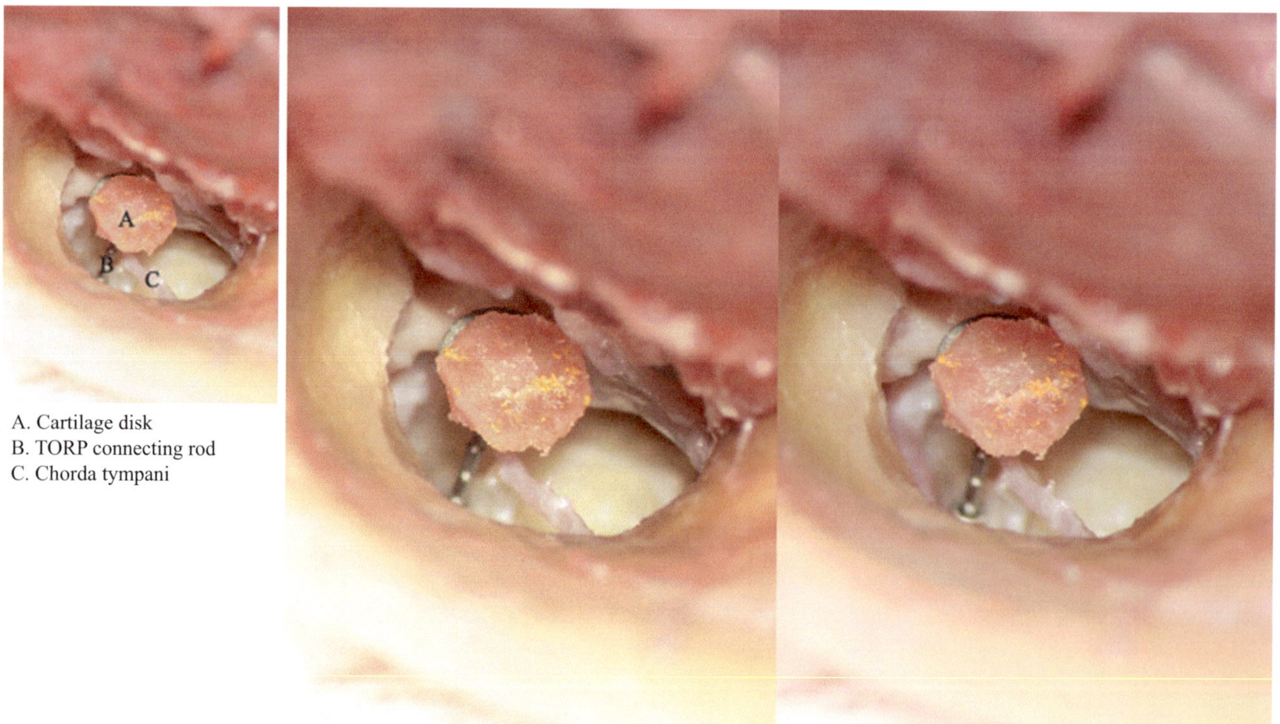

Fig. 3.39 Cartilage between the TORP and tympanic membrane (right)
Cartilage between the TORP and tympanic membrane will protect the TORP against extrusion from the middle ear; however, unnecessary contact between the cartilage or TORP and surrounding structures should be avoided
Instruments: right-angle hook, alligator forceps

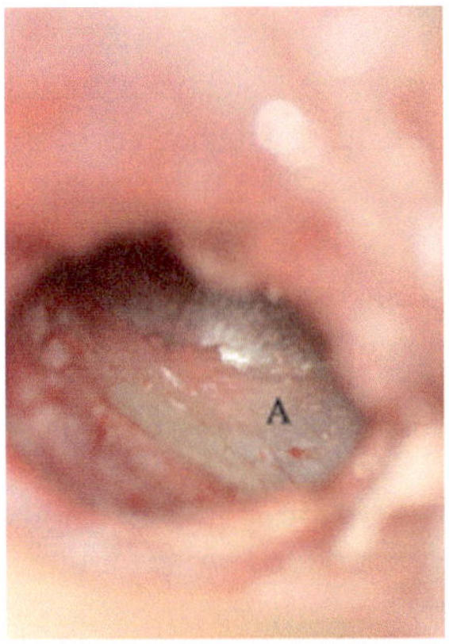

A. Tympanic membrane
(after reset)

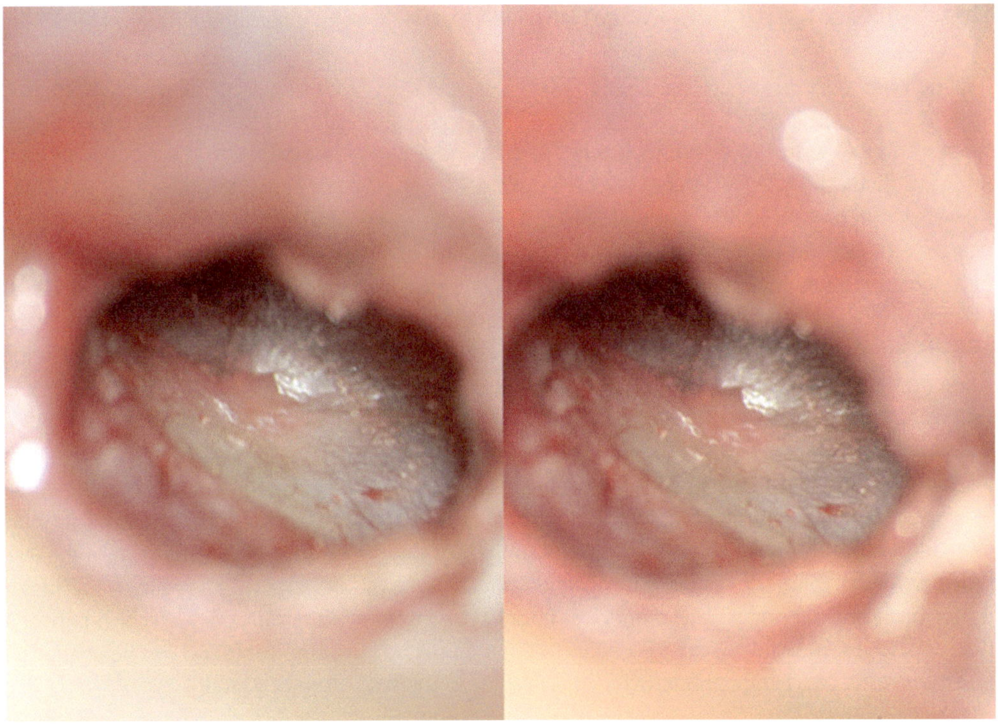

Fig. 3.40 Reset of the tympanomeatal flap (right)
Fill the tympanic cavity with a gelatin sponge; this can aid in the prevention of postoperative scarring and displacement of the ossicular chain. Then, reset the tympanomeatal flap

Instruments: middle ear elevator, suction cannulas

Hearing Reconstruction: Piston Implantation

Yu-hua Zhu

Stapes surgery with the piston technique is a considerably effective method for the treatment of conductive deafness or mixed deafness caused by stapes fixation. This technique was first introduced by Shea in 1956 and is now widely used in clinical practice.

Indications: (1) Otosclerosis: air conduction hearing loss >30 dB, air–bone gap >15 dB, speech recognition rate >60%. The ear with worse air conduction level should be treated first if both ears exhibit uniform bone conduction in patients with bilateral otosclerosis; the ear with better bone conduction level should be treated first if both ears exhibit the same loss of air conduction; if hearing loss is at the same level, the ear with worse tinnitus or semicircular canal function should be treated first. Surgery on the contralateral ear should be performed no sooner than 6–12 months and only after a continuing successful result of the first one. (2) Congenital stapes deformity. (3) Tympanosclerosis, adhesive otitis media accompanied by stapes fixation, with normal round window and Eustachian tube function.

Contraindications: (1) Severe sensorineural hearing loss with rapid development of the disease. (2) The patient's employment requires rapid rotation of the head, or high-altitude operations, and cannot be changed after operative intervention. (3) Active inflammatory disease in ear, nose, pharynx, and/or throat. (4) General health condition is poor and surgery cannot be tolerated.

Stapes footplate perforation can be performed with a miniature bur or triangular needle. In recent years, carbon dioxide and other types of laser technology for stapes footplate perforation have also been widely applied. The advantages of laser stapedotomy are its accuracy, safety, and speediness; it is especially suitable for patients in whom a floating stapes footplate may be caused by surgery. After piston installation, the reconstructed ossicular chain should be touched to observe its mobility and any necessary adjustments should be made. The diameter of the stapes footplate opening should be slightly larger than the piston. After implantation of the artificial stapes, the gap between the piston and the opening of the footplate can be sealed with a small fat graft and/or a drop of blood.

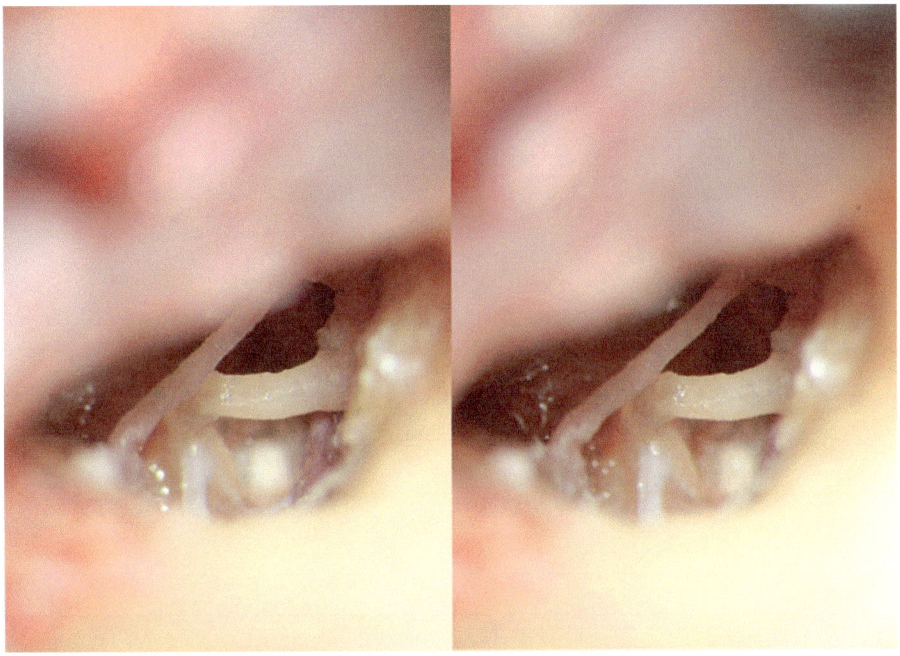

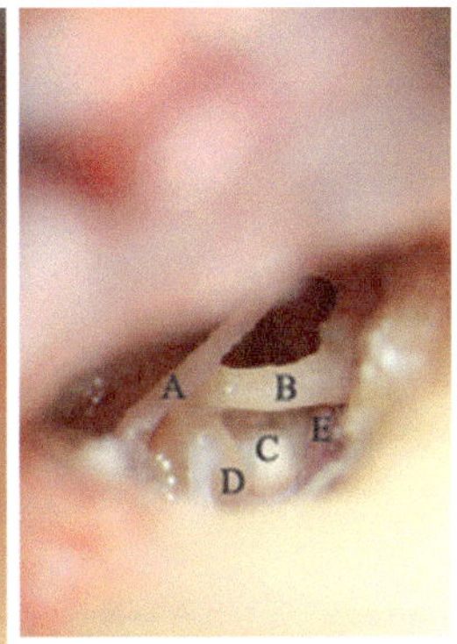

A. Chorda tympani
B. Long process of the incus
C. Stapes footplate
D. Posterior crus of the stapes
E. Horizontal segment of the facial nerve

Fig. 3.41 Elevation of the tympanomeatal flap and exposure of the mesotympanum (left)
Perform endaural incision and elevate the tympanomeatal flap; then, lift the tympanic membrane and expose the mesotympanum. Remove part of the scutum and expose the lower section of epitympanum until the incudostapedial joint, the stapes, stapedius tendon, and long process of the incus can be well observed. Looking upwards, the horizontal segment of the bony facial nerve can be observed, as well as whether the facial nerve is exposed or covers the oval window. Assess the mobility of each of the ossicles to confirm that the malleus and incus are mobile and only the stapes footplate is fixed. If the chorda tympani affects the exposed surgical field or interferes with the operation, it can be mobilized and displaced forward and downward
Instruments: scalpel, round chisel, hammer, middle ear elevator, right-angle hook

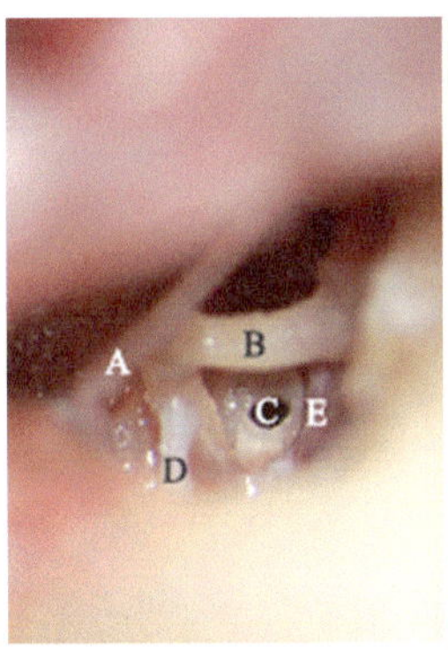

A. Chorda tympani
B. Long process of the incus
C. Stapes footplate perforation (stapedotomy)
D. Stapedius tendon
E. Horizontal segment of the facial nerve

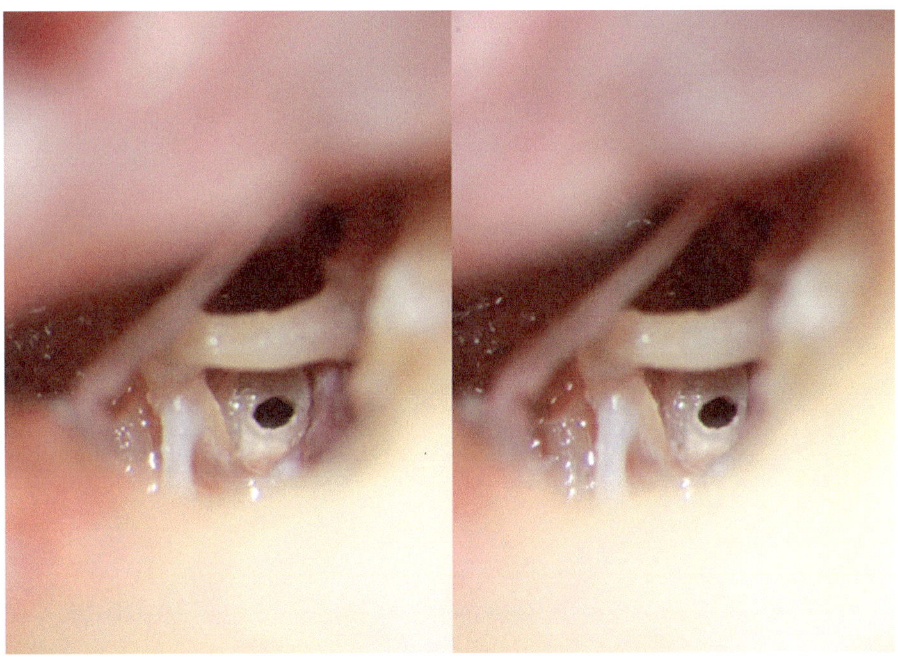

Fig. 3.42 Perforation of the stapes footplate (left)
Open the oval window by perforating the middle of the stapes footplate with a miniature bur, triangular needle, or laser (if the stapes footplate is floating, a carbon dioxide laser should be used for perforation). The operation of the stapedotomy must be gentle to avoid stapes footplate fragmentation. The inner ear must be protected as much as possible after stapes footplate perforation, as follows: (1) avoid direct suction against the hole in the footplate, which can lead to disturbance and loss of perilymph fluid; (2) avoid entry of foreign bodies and drugs into the vestibule (e.g., blood, bone fragments, or adrenaline); and (3) minimize the exposure duration of the inner ear
Instruments: miniature drill, triangular needle, laser equipment

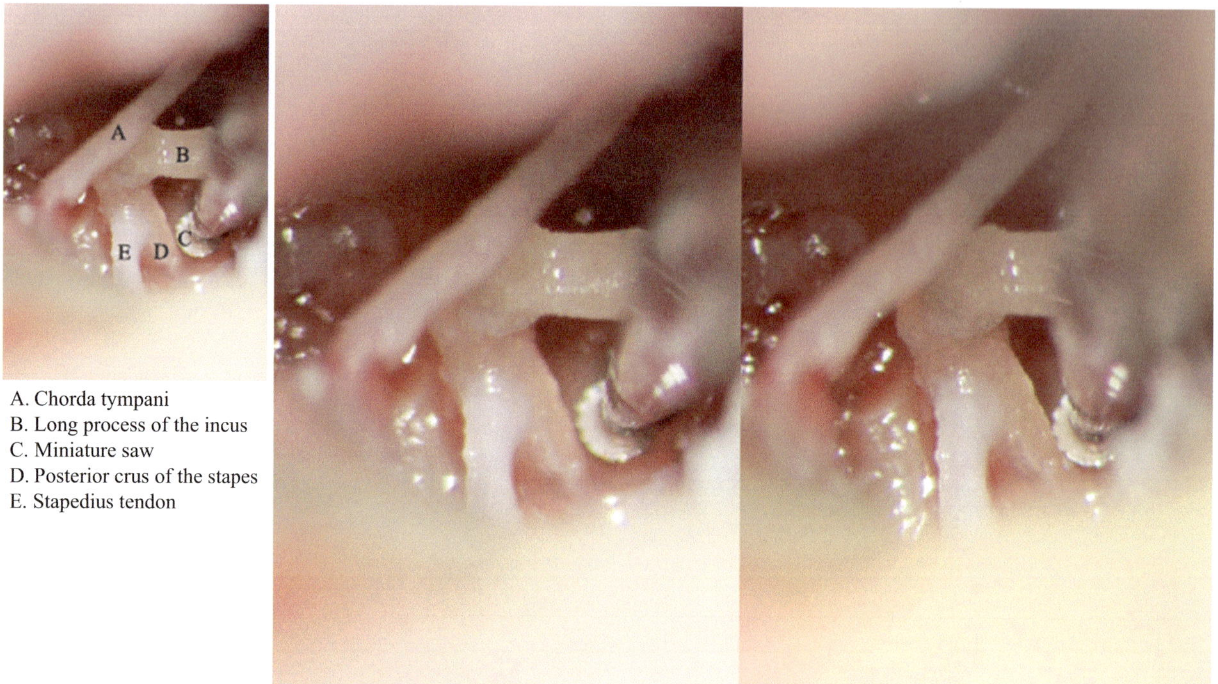

A. Chorda tympani
B. Long process of the incus
C. Miniature saw
D. Posterior crus of the stapes
E. Stapedius tendon

Fig. 3.43 Separation of the incudostapedial joint and resection of the superstructure of the stapes (left)
Following perforation of the stapes footplate, separate the incudostapedial joint, resect the anterior and posterior arches of the stapes with a miniature saw (or laser), and remove the arch and head of the stapes to prepare for artificial stapes implantation
Instruments: right-angle hook, miniature drill, middle ear micro scissors

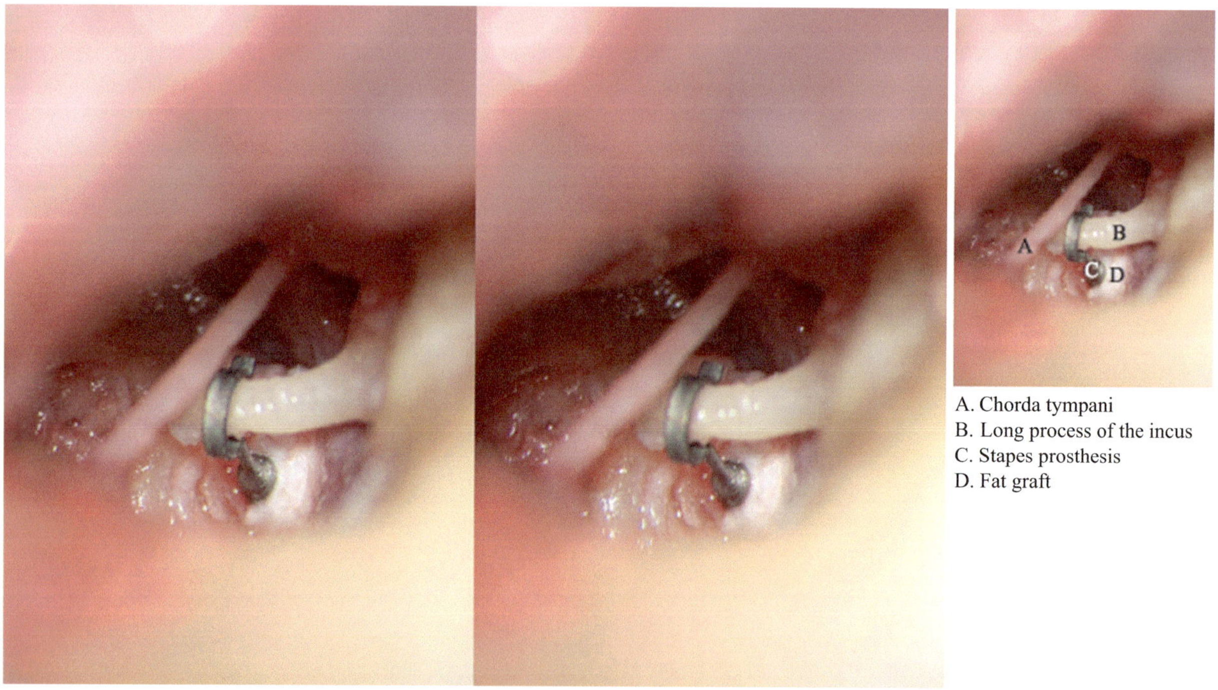

A. Chorda tympani
B. Long process of the incus
C. Stapes prosthesis
D. Fat graft

Fig. 3.44 Implantation of the artificial stapes (left, Piston)
Place the metal hook of the piston over the lower one-third of the long process of the incus; place the medial column end of the artificial stapes into the stapes footplate opening. Clamp the hook and fix the piston to the incus long process. Then, use a fat graft to seal the gap between the artificial stapes and the opening of the footplate. *Hints: (1) the length of the artificial stapes should be appropriate—it may become displaced if excessively short, whereas it may damage the membranous labyrinth if excessively long; (2) if the artificial stapes is placed at an improper angle, it will affect the transmission efficiency of sound; and (3) the clamping force of the hook on the incus should be moderate—the incus will become ischemic and may exhibit necrosis if excessively tight, whereas it may become detached if excessively loose*
Instruments: fine forceps, right-angle hook, artificial stapes installer

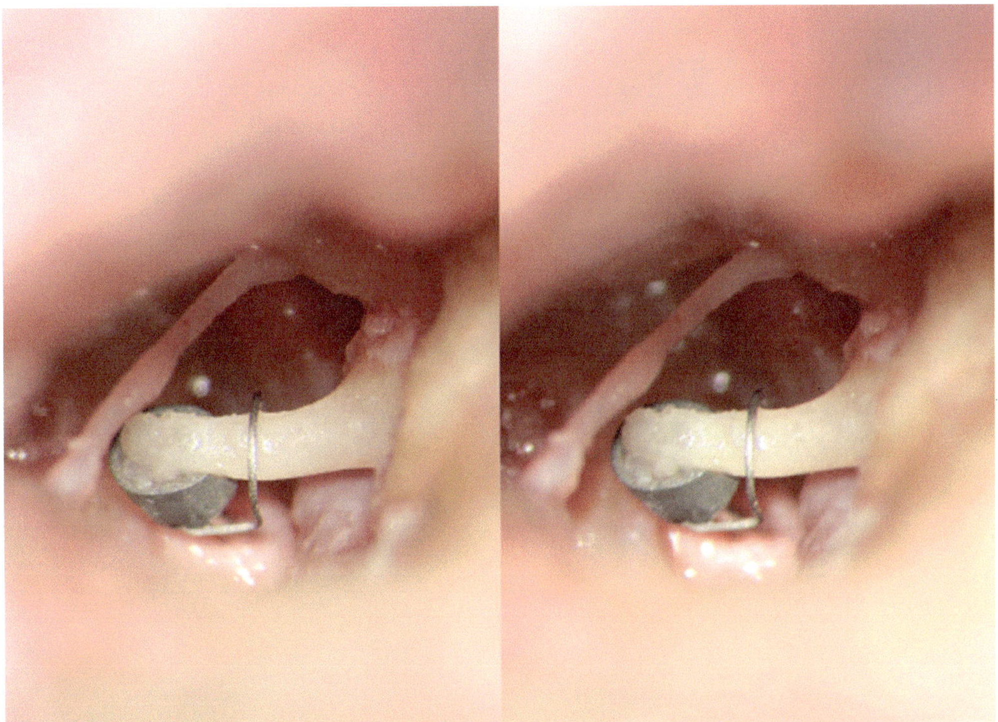

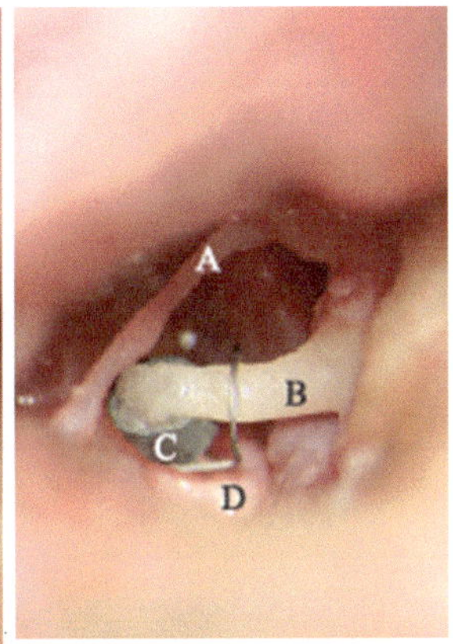

A. Chorda tympani
B. Long process of the incus
C. Artificial stapes prosthesis
D. Fat graft

Fig. 3.45 Artificial stapes with bucket handle (left, Medtronic Robinson Cupped Stapes Piston)
There are many variants of artificial stapes; the above figure depicts a representative type of artificial stapes that can ensure ossicular chain conduction efficiency while avoiding disruption to the incus blood supply. The artificial stapes is placed on the window edge of the footplate (not into the opening yet), then connect the bucket end of the prosthesis with the long process of the incus. The fixing ring (handle) of the bucket is rotated, such that it is placed over the long process of the incus; the artificial stapes is then eased into the opening of the stapes footplate
Instruments: right-angle hook, straight needle

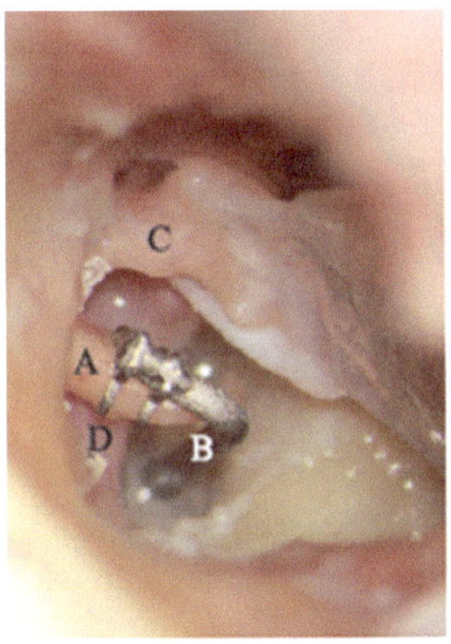

A. Long process of the incus with distal defect
B. Artificial stapes
C. Malleus
D. Horizontal segment of the facial nerve

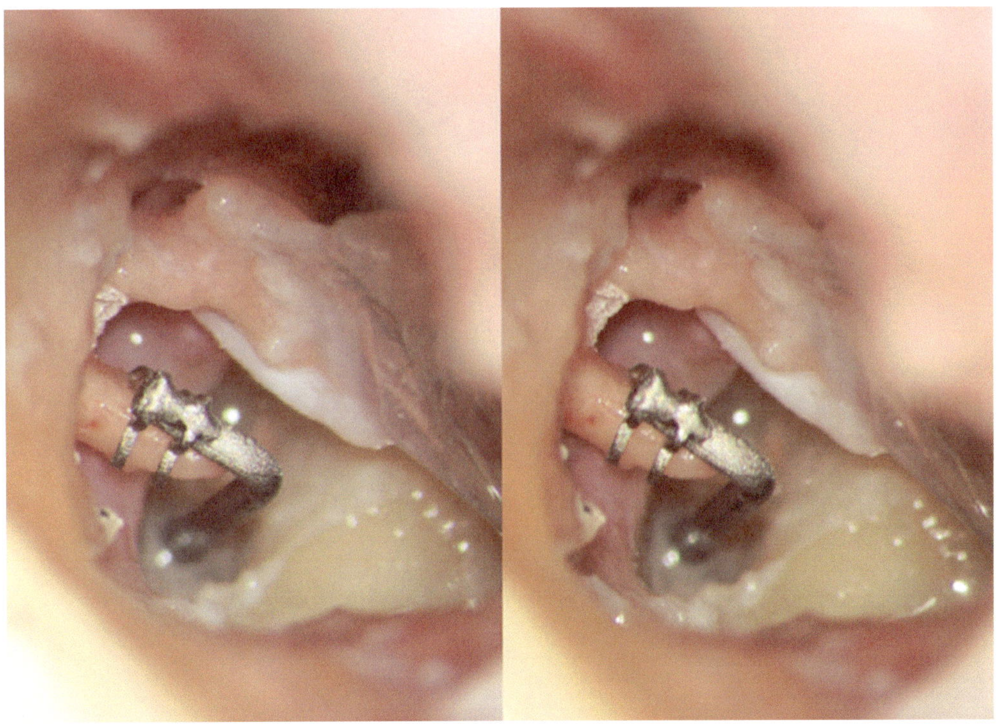

Fig. 3.46 Angular artificial stapes (right)
The tip of this artificial stapes is a claw-like structure that lies perpendicular to the major axis of the artificial stapes. This type is useful for patients with partial defects of the long process of the incus (i.e., middle ear deformity or pathologic erosion); it can replace the distal end defect of the long process and ensure that the inner end of the artificial stapes remains perpendicular to the oval window
Instruments: right-angle hook, fine forceps, artificial stapes installer

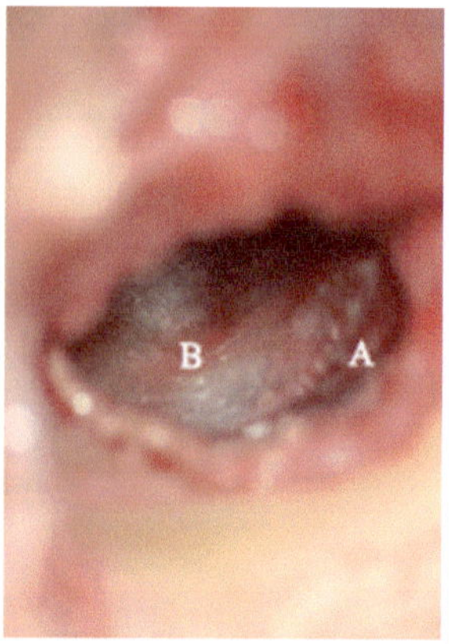

A. Reset tympanomeatal flap
B. Umbo region of the tympanic membrane

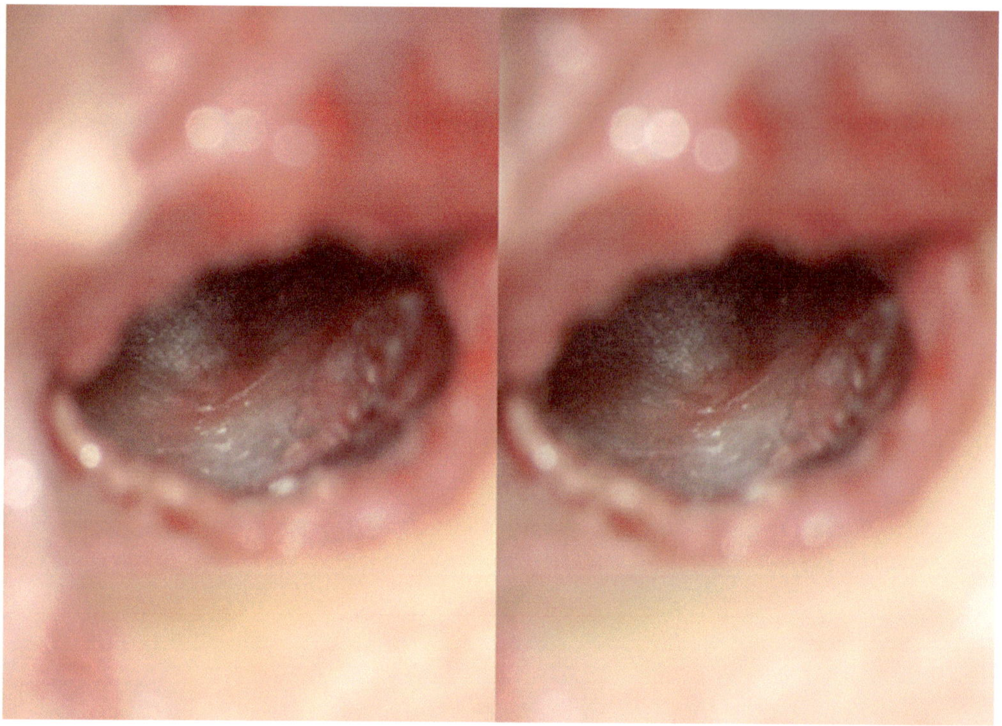

Fig. 3.47 Reset of the tympanomeatal flap (left)
After artificial stapes implantation, reset the tympanomeatal flap and check the integrity of the tympanic membrane. If a laceration of the tympanic membrane is present, it can be repaired with fat or fascia. The air and bone conduction hearing level can be roughly tested with a 256 Hz tuning fork in patients under local anesthesia. If necessary, the location of artificial stapes can be re-checked and adjusted
Instruments: middle ear elevator, eardrum flattening device

Suggested Reading

Dai P, Han D-y, Cousins VC, et al. Stereo operative atlas of micro ear surgery. Singapore: Springer; 2017.

Huang X-z, Wang J-b, Kong W-j. Practical otolaryngology-head and neck surgery. 2nd ed. Beijing: People's Medical Publishing House; 2008.

Jiang S-c, Yang W-y, Gu R. Otorhinolaryngology—head and neck surgery. 2nd ed. Beijing: People's Medical Publishing House; 2007.

Wang Q-h. Practical surgery anatomy of otolaryngology, head and neck. Beijing: People's Medical Publishing House; 2010.

Wüllstein H. The restoration of the function of the middle ear in chronic otitis media. Ann Otol Rhinol Laryngol. 1956;65:1020–41.

Zollner F. The principles of plastic surgery of the sound-conducting apparatus. J Laryngol Otol. 1955;69:637–52.

Postauricular Approach

4

Yu Su, Jian-hui Li, Su Jeong Lee, Hui-bing Wang, Bo Gao, Ya-qing Liu, Bing Han, Yi Sun, Bao-chun Sun, Song Gao, Chang Guo, Kun Ma, Zhan-guo Jin, Jun-fang Xue, Chao-chan Cai, Feng Xin, Xu-kun Yan, Xue Gao, and Vincent C Cousins

Surgical Options Using the Postauricular Approach

The postauricular approach is commonly used in ear microsurgery and is the routine surgical approach to the labyrinth and infratemporal fossa. It is key to temporal bone anatomical training. Surgical procedures that can be performed through the postauricular approach include the following:

1. Mastoidectomy
2. Endolymphatic sac decompression
3. Radical excision of endolymphatic sac carcinoma
4. Cerebrospinal fluid otorrhea repair/mastoid obliteration
5. Cochlear implantation
6. Vibrant Soundbridge implantation
7. Radical mastoidectomy (canal wall down technique)
8. Radical mastoidectomy (canal wall up technique)
9. Modified radical mastoidectomy
10. Semicircular canal obliteration
11. Facial nerve decompression
12. Sigmoid sinus reduction for sigmoid-sinus-related pulsatile tinnitus

Related Anatomical Structures

The temporal line (suprameatal crest): extends backward from the superior border of the zygomatic process, above the external auditory canal (EAC) and forms a slightly upwardly curved crest of bone, marking the inferior margin of the temporalis muscle, which attaches to it.

Mastoid air cells: cells with diverse shapes and sizes in the mastoid. Depending on the degree of development, they are classified into pneumatized, diploic, sclerotic, and mixed types.

Suprameatal spine, also called the Spine of Henle: a small bony spine located in the posterosuperior part of the osseous EAC.

Y. Su (✉)
Department of Otolaryngology Head and Neck Surgery, Chinese PLA General Hospital Affiliated Hainan Hospital, Sanya, China

J.-h. Li · B. Gao · B. Han · C. Guo · C.-c. Cai
College of Otolaryngology Head and Neck Surgery, Chinese PLA General Hospital, Beijing, China

S. J. Lee · K. Ma · J.-f. Xue
Department of Otolaryngology Head and Neck Surgery, Peking University International Hospital, Beijing, China

H.-b. Wang
Department of Otolaryngology Head and Neck Surgery, The Third Medical Center of PLA General Hospital, Beijing, China

Y.-q. Liu
Department of Otolaryngology Head and Neck Surgery, Children's Hospital of Nanjing Medical University, Nanjing, China

Y. Sun
Department of Otolaryngology Head and Neck Surgery, General Hospital of Central Theater Command, Wuhan, China

B.-c. Sun
Department of Otolaryngology Head and Neck Surgery, The Fourth Medical Center of PLA General Hospital, Beijing, China

S. Gao
Department of Otolaryngology Head and Neck Surgery, The 909th Hospital of PLA, South-East Hospital Affiliated to Xiamen University, Zhangzhou, China

Z.-g. Jin
Department of Otolaryngology Head and Neck Surgery, Air Force Medical Center, Beijing, China

F. Xin
Department of Otolaryngology Head and Neck Surgery, Second Hospital of Shanxi Medical University, Taiyuan, China

X.-k. Yan
Department of Otolaryngology Head and Neck Surgery, Beijing Tiantan Hospital, Capital Medical University, Beijing, China

X. Gao
Department of Otolaryngology Head and Neck Surgery, PLA Rocket Force Characteristic Medical Center, Beijing, China

V. C. Cousins
Department of Ear Nose and Throat Surgery, Alfred Hospital, Melbourne, Australia

Department of Surgery, Monash University, Melbourne, Australia

P. Dai et al. (eds.), *Stereoscopic Anatomical Atlas of Ear Surgery*, https://doi.org/10.1007/978-981-16-0927-5_4

Suprameatal triangle, also called MacEwen's triangle: area bordered by the temporal line, the Spine of Henle, and a vertical tangent through the posterior limit of the EAC.

Cribriform area: the bony surface in the suprameatal triangle, with numerous holes through which small blood vessels pass.

Parietal notch: the osseous incisura between the posterosuperior part of the squamous portion of the temporal bone and the superior border of the mastoid, in which is embedded the posteroinferior angle of the parietal bone.

Mastoid tip: the tip of the lower part of the mastoid. A line from the tip to the parietal notch is the surface marking of the sigmoid sinus.

Jugular bulb: a bulbous junction of the sigmoid sinus and internal jugular vein, located in the jugular fossa.

Stylomastoid foramen: the bony opening between the root of the styloid process and the mastoid tip, through which the facial nerve exits the skull.

Tympanomastoid fissure: between the posterior surface of the tympanic bone and the mastoid. It is the surface marking of the mastoid (vertical) segment of the facial nerve. In adults the fissure is closed, leaving only a shallow groove.

Körner's septum, also called the petro-squamous lamina: the thin bony plate between the superficial air cells of the mastoid and the antrum. It is formed by the growth of the squamous portion of the mastoid over the petrous portion during the development of the temporal bone.

Tegmen: a bony plate that separates the mastoid cavity and middle cranial fossa.

Sigmoid sinus: the meningeal venous sinus that sits in the sigmoid groove on the inner surface of the mastoid, connecting the transverse sinus and jugular bulb.

Sinodural angle: formed in the posterosuperior part of the mastoid cavity, it is the angle between the cerebral dura mater of the middle cranial fossa and the sigmoid sinus. The superior petrosal sinus is located deep to the sinodural angle.

Digastric ridge: a bony prominence lying in the sagittal plane inside the mastoid cavity. Its front end meets the stylomastoid foramen and lower mastoid segment of the facial nerve. On the external inferior surface of the skull is the digastric groove that corresponds to the digastric ridge and accommodates the posterior belly of the digastric muscle.

Superior petrosal sinus: lies along the petrosal ridge to which the tentorium cerebelli attaches. Its internal end joins the back of the cavernous sinus, and its posterior end connects to the junction of the transverse and sigmoid sinuses. The petrosal vein also drains into the superior petrosal sinus.

Trautmann's triangle: an area enclosed by the sigmoid sinus posteriorly, the superior petrosal sinus superiorly, and the bony labyrinth anteriorly. Deep to the bone of the triangle is the dura mater of the cerebellum.

Aditus ad antrum: the inverted triangular opening in the posterior wall of the upper part of the tympanic cavity. It is the connection point of the epitympanum and the mastoid antrum and air cells. Medial to the aditus is the anterior end of the lateral semicircular canal, above it is the posterior tegmen tympani and its lower angle points to the pyramidal segment of the facial nerve.

Mastoid (tympanic) antrum: the pneumatized space posterior to the epitympanum, and the main connection between the middle ear and mastoid air cells. Its surface marking is the suprameatal triangle.

Fossa incudis: a hollow in the posteroinferior part of the epitympanum that accommodates the short process of the incus. Medial to the fossa incudis is the second genu of the facial nerve.

Posterior tympanum: the part of the tympanic cavity medial to the posterior part of the pars tensa of the tympanic membrane.

Sinus tympani, also called the pyramidal recess: a bony fossa in the posterior part of the tympanic cavity, medial to the pyramid and the styloid eminence, bounded above by the ponticulus and below by the subiculum.

Facial recess: the triangular space with its base bounded above by bone lateral to the short process of the incus, the chorda tympani laterally and the vertical segment of the facial nerve medially.

Pyramidal eminence: a smaller osseous cone projecting from the middle of the posterior tympanic cavity wall, at the level of the oval window. The stapedius tendon passes forward from the tip of the pyramid to attach to the back of the stapes neck.

Promontory: the large bony prominence in the center of the inner wall of the tympanic cavity, formed by the basal turn of the cochlea. The tympanic nerve plexus grooves its surface as it passes from below upwards.

Incudostapedial joint: the articulation formed by the lenticular process of the incus and the head of the stapes. It can be seen from behind when the facial recess has been opened.

Prominence of the facial canal: the linear prominence lying horizontally above the oval window that contains the horizontal segment of the facial nerve.

Prominence of the semicircular canal: bony prominence formed by the lateral semicircular canal sitting posterosuperior to and 0.5–1.5 mm above the horizontal segment of the facial nerve. It is a good landmark for the nerve and a site of predilection for a labyrinthine fistula caused by chronic otitis media and/or cholesteatoma.

Round window niche, also called the cochlear window niche: the osseous cavity located in the posteroinferior part of the promontory, at the depths of which is the almost circular bony opening into the start of the scala tympani of the cochlea, which is closed by the round window membrane.

Oval window niche, also called the fossula fenestrae vestibuli: the hollow located in the posterosuperior part of the promontory. The elliptical bony window in the depths of the recess is called the vestibular or oval window.

Osseous semicircular canals: three mutually perpendicular bony tubes each forming 2/3 of a circle and constituting the posterosuperior part of the vestibular labyrinth. They are named the superior, posterior, and lateral semicircular canals according to their relationship with the vestibule. The lateral canal lies at an angle of 30° to the horizontal plane with its anterior end higher than its posterior end.

Vestibule: the other part of the bony labyrinth, which has a slightly elliptical shape and lies between the cochlea and the semicircular canals. It accommodates the saccule and utricle and has five openings, which communicate with the three semicircular canals.

Endolymphatic sac: an expanded part of the distal end of the endolymphatic duct. Its anterior half, the intraosseous part, lies in the vestibular aqueduct; the posterior half, the dural part, is located between two layers of the posterior fossa dura. The sac is involved with antigens, produces the immune response in the inner ear, and contains endolymph.

Cochlear aqueduct: a bony canal that connects the basal turn of the cochlear scala tympani and the subarachnoid space. Its internal aperture is near the round window and the external aperture is in the triangular fovea between the jugular foramen and the internal carotid artery. The internal aperture is closed by a membrane that separates perilymph and cerebrospinal fluid (CSF).

Anatomy Overview

Skin incision: parallel to the retroauricular groove, make a curving incision from the superior border of the root of the auricle to the mastoid tip. The distance from the middle of the incision to the retroauricular groove is 1.5 cm; the upper and lower ends are made 0.5 cm and 1.2 cm away from the root of the auricle, respectively. *Hints: (1) The tip of the retroauricular incision can be slightly extended to the site of attachment of the auricle by 0.3–0.5 cm to assist in reflecting the auricle forward; (2) The mastoid of children under 2 years of age is underdeveloped, the stylomastoid foramen is without a bony covering, and the facial nerve is shallow, so the lower end of the retroauricular incision should remain superficial and be located more posteriorly.*

Identification of osseous landmarks on the surface of the mastoid can help to locate the structures contained inside the temporal bone correctly. Surface landmarks to be identified in the postauricular approach include the temporal line, suprameatal spine, suprameatal triangle, cribriform area, parietal notch, and mastoid tip. The temporal line approximates to the level of the bottom of the middle cranial fossa, the dura of which is unlikely to be injured if drilling is performed only below this line when performing mastoidectomy. The suprameatal triangle is the surface marking of the mastoid antrum. When drilling out the triangle, take care not to injure the cerebral dura mater, ossicular chain, labyrinth, facial nerve, or other important structures. The line between the mastoid tip and the parietal notch marks the position of the sigmoid sinus and drilling only in front of the line can effectively protect the sigmoid sinus.

Mastoidectomy: the principle of anatomy when operating is "evidence-based progression"; the "evidence" refers to the anatomical landmarks, and "progression" emphasizes the order of operation. Identification of the bony landmarks on the surface of the mastoid is the initial guide in mastoidectomy, leading to accurate assessment and identification of the positions of the deep structures in the mastoid. With the temporal line as the upper boundary, the osseous posterior EAC wall as the anterior boundary, and the line connecting the mastoid tip and parietal notch as the posterior boundary, the three margins of the mastoidectomy are formulated. Remove the cortical bone of the mastoid with a coarse cutting bur to reveal the mastoid air cells and sigmoid sinus wall. Further resection of mastoid air cells allows the antrum to be opened and the bony labyrinth to be identified. Inferiorly the digastric ridge is exposed. Removal of the anterior antral wall with cutting and diamond burs will expose the aditus, fossa incudis, and short process of the incus. The posterior EAC wall is thinned further to expose the short process of the incus and lateral semicircular canal. The lower mastoid is opened more to expose the digastric ridge, whose anterior end is a good indicator of the stylomastoid foramen. Extend the drilling posteriorly to the antrum to expose the sinodural angle between the middle fossa dura and sigmoid sinus. The cavity is further developed by skeletonizing the sigmoid sinus, three semicircular canals, and the posterior cranial fossa bony plate. Locate the endolymphatic sac on or below a line through the lateral semicircular canal and behind the posterior semicircular canal. Open the facial recess to reveal the posterior tympanum. The margins of the facial recess are the incus buttress above, the chorda tympani anteriorly and the vertical facial nerve canal posteriorly. The order of steps performed in mastoidectomy varies with the surgeon's preference but must always follow the principle of "progression" based on "evidence". *Hints: (1) Cavity edges must not be left with overhanging bone; create an open cavity with smooth edges and without visual obstruction (an exception is in cochlear implantation, where the cavity edge should have overhanging bone, forming an "urn" shape to help to secure the electrode cable). (2) Anatomical landmarks are constantly reviewed when drilling the mastoid and deep drilling is not continued in any area if clear landmarks are not identified. (3) When smoothing the margins of the mastoid cavity, do not use a cutting bur which grinds away bone; use a larger diamond bur "floating" on the surface of the bone to "sweep" the bone away layer-by-layer, until the surface is smooth and internal structures are recognizable. (4) The internal structures of the mastoid cavity are numerous; their spatial arrangement is complex, and the use of a range of sizes and types of burs is necessary to reveal these structures.*

Purpose and Requirements of Anatomical Dissection

1. Master the corresponding relationship between the osseous landmarks on the surface of the mastoid and its deep structure.

2. Master the surface landmarks of the mastoid antrum, sigmoid sinus, and vertical segment of the facial nerve.
3. Master the method for locating every anatomical structure in the mastoid.
4. Master the technique of mastoidectomy.
5. Master the characteristics and scope of burs of different types and sizes, the choice of burs, and the appropriate use of drilling speed and pressure for each area in the mastoid.
6. Master the method of outlining the facial nerve and semicircular canals.
7. Master the method of identifying and opening the facial recess.

Mastoid Skeletonization

Su Jeong Lee

Skeletonization is a technical concept, referring to the removal of all the nonfunctional redundant bone of the mastoid cavity to expose the surfaces of the residual bony shell covering the important internal structures and bony margins. Extension of mastoid skeletonization may be required; superior to the base of the middle cranial fossa, posterosuperior to the sigmoid sinus anterior border, inferior to the mastoid tip, and anterior to the posterior canal wall. There are anatomical landmarks within the surgical cavity, such as the aditus ad antrum, short process of the incus, lateral semicircular canal, vertical and mastoid segments of the facial nerve, etc.

The recommended procedures to complete mastoid skeletonization quickly and safely are as follows:

1. Make an incision in the postauricular or intercartilaginous (between the root of the helix and tragus) region and expose the bony EAC and cortex of the mastoid.
2. Locate the suprameatal spine and suprameatal triangle. The aditus ad antrum is located in front of and deep to the suprameatal triangle.
3. Locate the anterior, superior, posterior, and inferior borders of the planned mastoid skeletonization.
4. Drill the superficial layer of mastoid air cells and find the sigmoid sinus located in the posterior wall of the mastoid cavity.
5. Drill out the suprameatal triangle to expose the aditus ad antrum and open the antrum.
6. The mastoid antrum and aditus ad antrum are anatomical landmarks; drill forward through the aditus ad antrum, then expose the short process of the incus (without touching it), the back of the epitympanum and the eminence of the lateral semicircular canal. Identify the back of the antrum as an anatomical landmark and drill posteriorly. Expose the mastoid roof (tegmen mastoideum) and continue drilling posteriorly until the sinodural angle is seen.
7. Expose the digastric ridge located inferiorly in the mastoid cavity.
8. Expose the whole length of the sigmoid sinus; drill the mastoid air cells to locate the internal edge of the sigmoid sinus and lateral part of the (pre-sigmoid) posterior cranial fossa dura.
9. Thin the posterior external canal wall and identify the line of the vertical segment of the facial nerve according to the anatomical landmarks, such as the front end of the digastric ridge, the eminence of the lateral semicircular canal, the short process of the incus, and the incudal fossa.
10. Lastly, remove the remaining air cells along each wall of the mastoid cavity with a diamond bur and polish the cavity walls well.

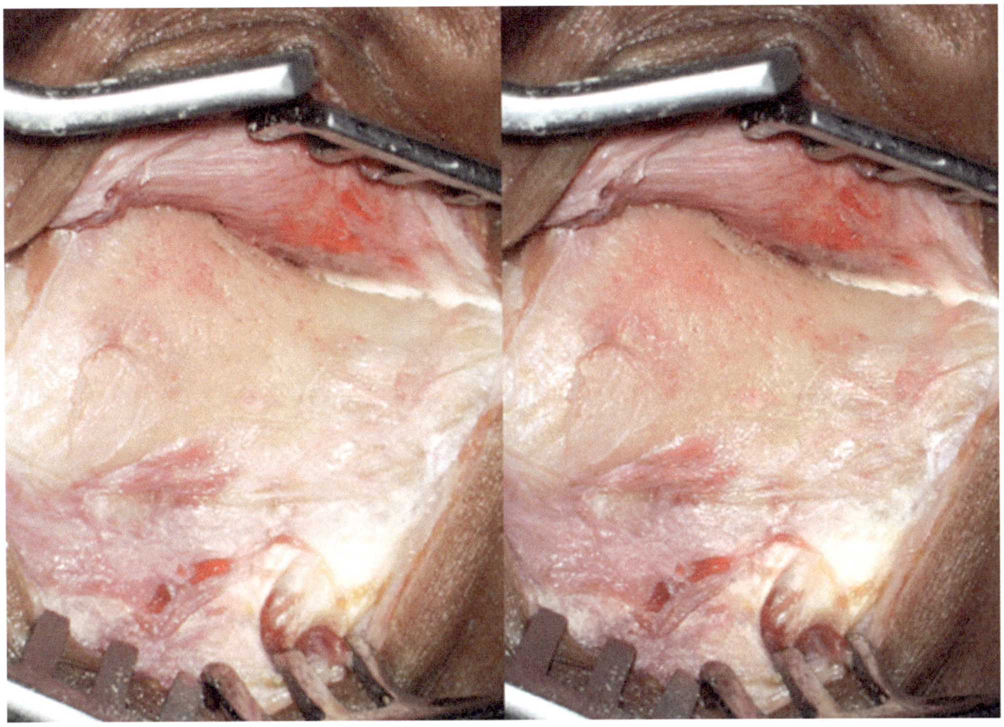

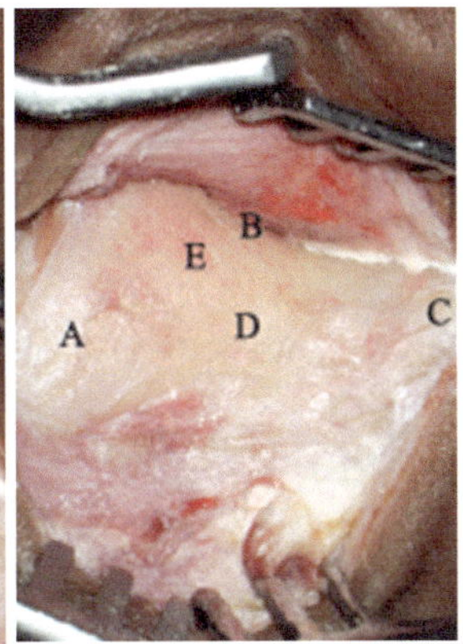

A. Temporal line
B. Suprameatal spine
C. Mastoid tip
D. Bony cortex of the mastoid
E. Cribriform area

Fig. 4.1 Expose the bony cortex of the mastoid (right)
Make the curved incision from the upper auricle root to the mastoid tip, parallel to the retroauricular groove. Cut through the skin and subcutaneous tissue; the maximal distance between the middle of the incision and the retroauricular groove is 1.5 cm, and the distances from the top and bottom of the incision to the retroauricular groove are 0.5 cm and 1.2 cm, respectively, which makes it easier to open the incision and roll the auricle forward. The flap is elevated off the bone surface to the posterior edge of the bony EAC with a periosteal elevator. Cut the sternocleidomastoid muscle attached to the mastoid. Hold the incision open with a self-retaining retractor and identify the anatomical landmarks; temporal line, suprameatal spine, suprameatal triangle and mastoid tip, etc.
Instruments: scalpel, periosteal elevator, retractor

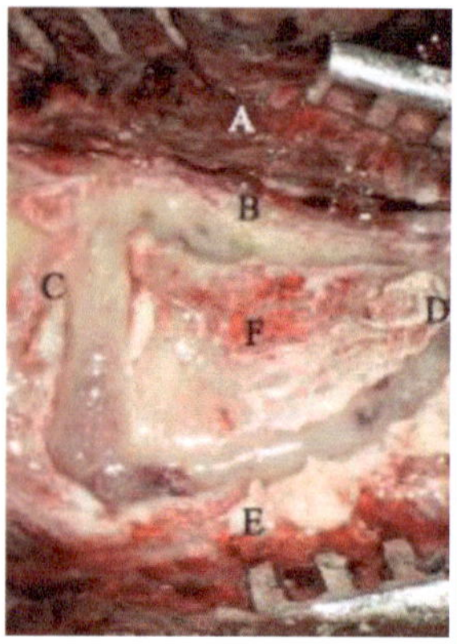

A. Post auricular flap
B. Anterior border of the mastoid
C. Temporal line
D. Mastoid tip
E. Posterior border of the mastoid
F. Mastoid cortex

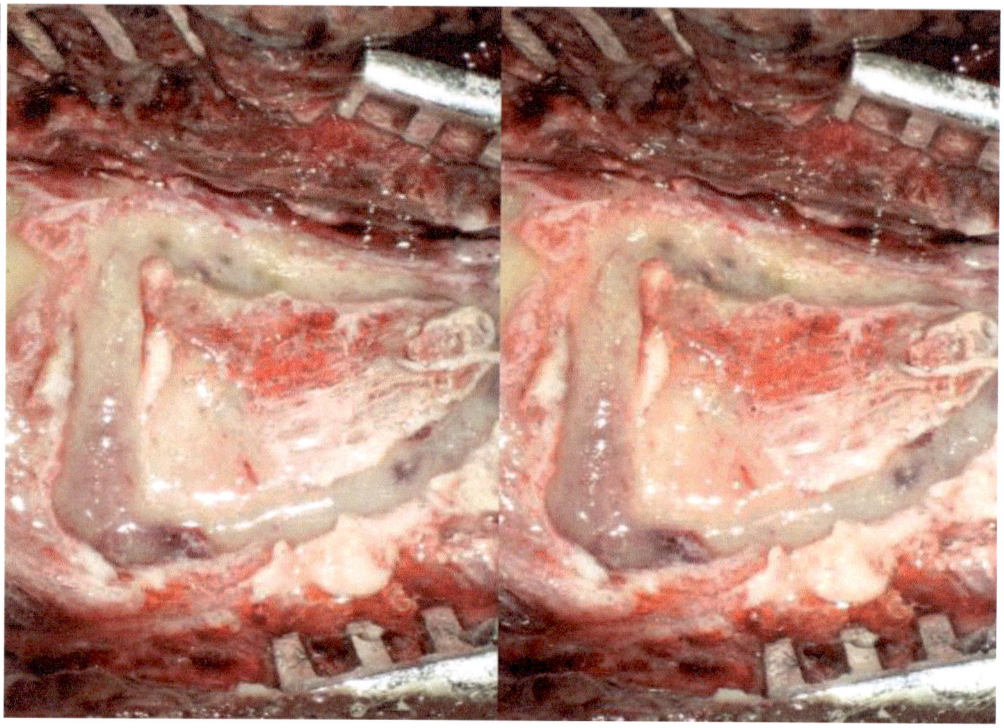

Fig. 4.2 Confirm the limits of mastoid skeletonization (right)
The mastoid cavity will be triangular in shape; its frontal margin is the posterior bone wall of the EAC. The superior border is the temporal line, and the posterior margin is the line connecting the mastoid tip to the parietal notch. Drill along the temporal line and the posterior wall of the EAC with a large cutting bur and drill out the anterior and superior borders of the intended mastoid cavity. Drill a groove in the bone along the three intended boundaries of the cavity to define the margins of the extent of mastoid skeletonization
Instruments: periosteal elevator, large-sized cutting burs

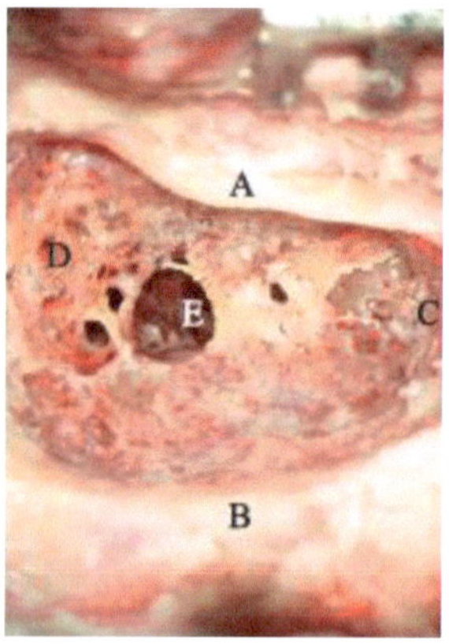

A. Posterior wall of the EAC
B. Posterior border of the mastoid
C. Mastoid tip
D. Mastoid air cells
E. Opened Körner's septum

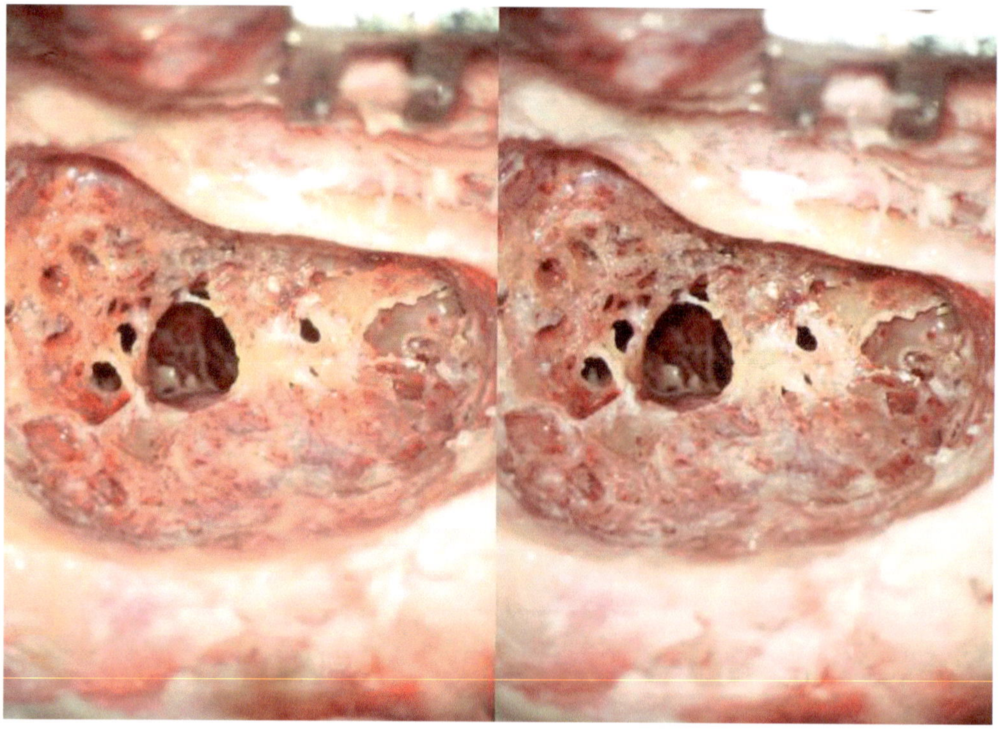

Fig. 4.3 Remove the mastoid air cells; open the Körner's septum (right)
After drilling away the mastoid cortex, the mastoid cavity with various size air cells is seen. The number and sizes of the air chambers are related to the pneumatization of the mastoid. The Körner's septum (petro-squamosal lamina) is visible in some temporal bones
Instruments: large- and medium-sized cutting burs

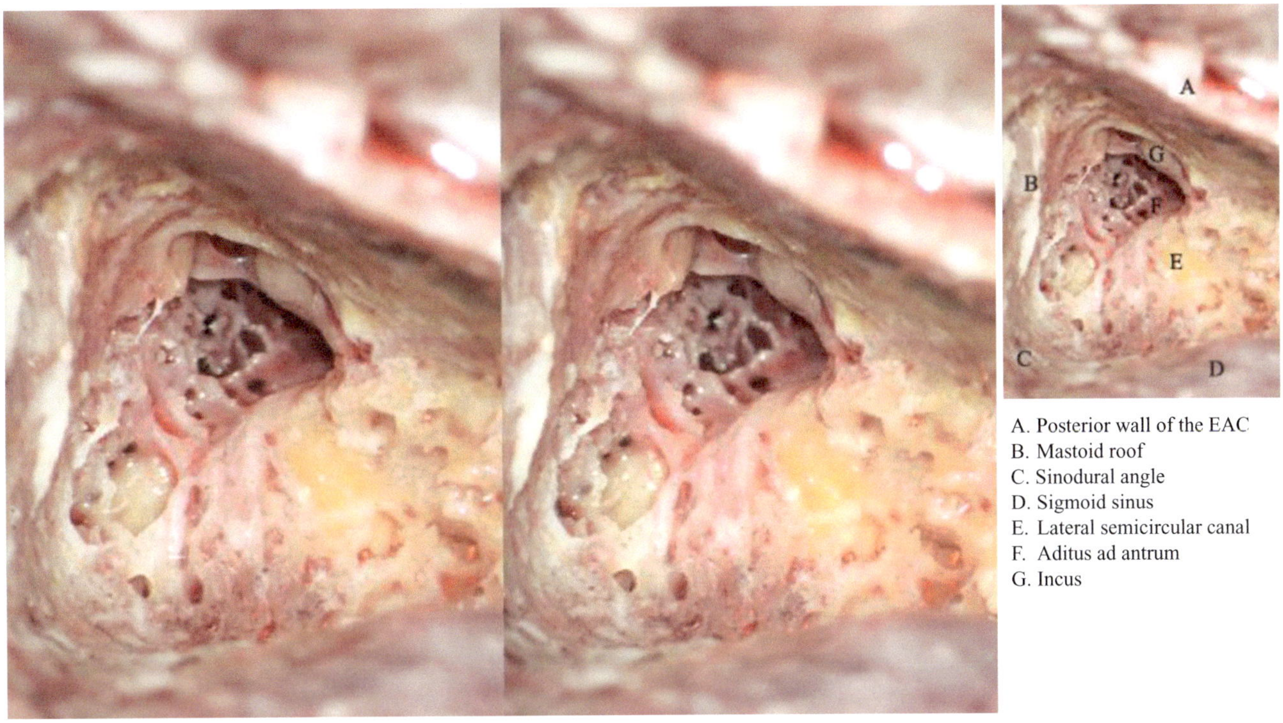

A. Posterior wall of the EAC
B. Mastoid roof
C. Sinodural angle
D. Sigmoid sinus
E. Lateral semicircular canal
F. Aditus ad antrum
G. Incus

Fig. 4.4 Fashion the upper part of the mastoid cavity (right)
To create the upper part of the mastoid cavity, thin the posterior wall of the EAC to enlarge the aditus ad antrum. The posterior epitympanum, short process of the incus, incudal fossa (located below the aditus ad antrum), and the eminence of the lateral semicircular canal (located medial to the aditus ad antrum) can be seen. The tegmen tympani (bone plate above the tympanic cavity) and mastoid roof (tegmen mastoideum) (bone plate above the mastoid) are also seen. The angle between the sigmoid sinus and mastoid roof is called the sinodural angle. The superior petrosal sinus is located deep and within the dura of the sinodural angle. The triangle formed by the sigmoid sinus, superior petrosal sinus, and the bony labyrinth is called Trautmann's triangle. The dura mater over the cerebellum is located deep to this triangular bony plate
Instruments: medium-sized diamond burs

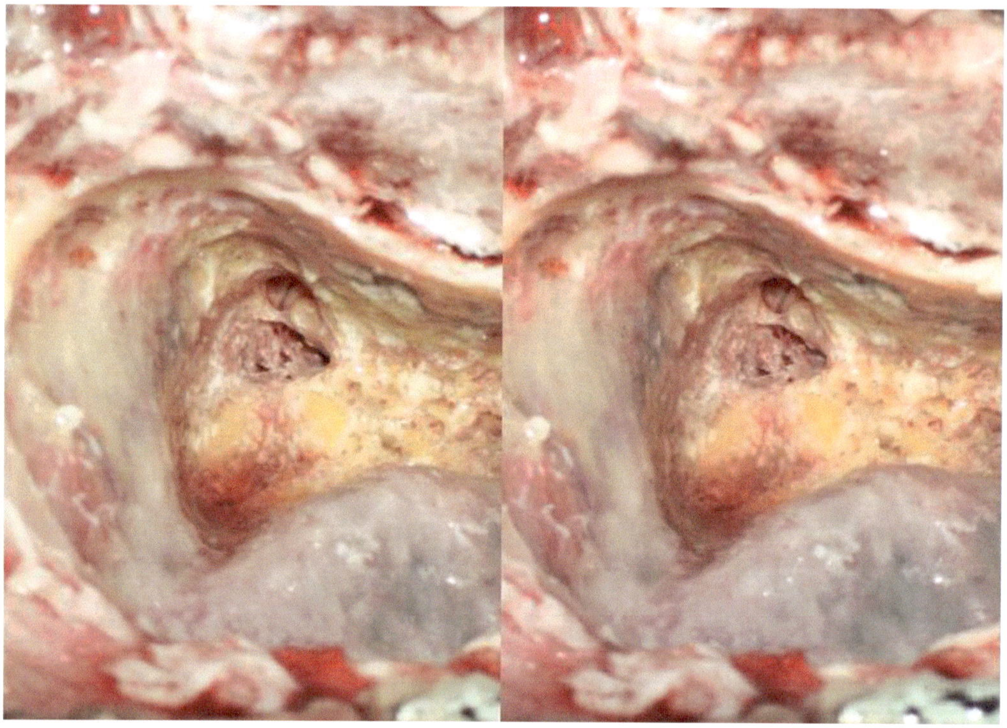

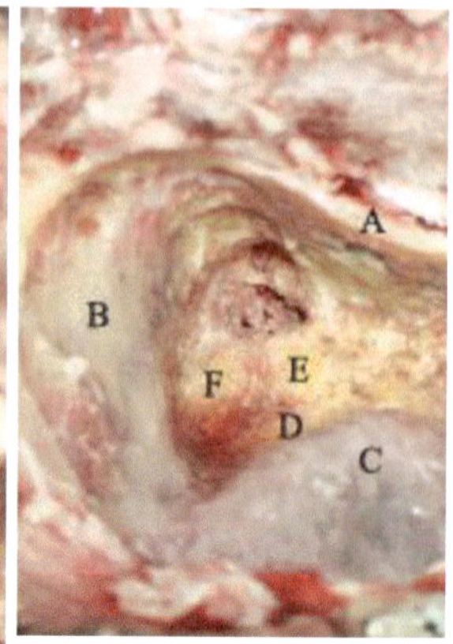

A. Posterior wall of the EAC
B. Mastoid roof
C. Sigmoid sinus
D. Posterior semicircular canal
E. Lateral semicircular canal
F. Superior semicircular canal

Fig. 4.5 Skeletonization of the upper part of the mastoid cavity (right) Thin the posterior wall of the EAC in the front of the cavity, and expose the mastoid roof (tegmen mastoideum), sinodural angle, sigmoid sinus, and posterior cranial fossa dura. Remove the air cells covering the bony labyrinth to expose its lateral surface. *Hint: A low-lying mastoid roof and anterior sigmoid sinus are common, so identification and drilling must be done carefully when close to the tegmen and sigmoid sinus*
Instruments: medium-sized diamond burs

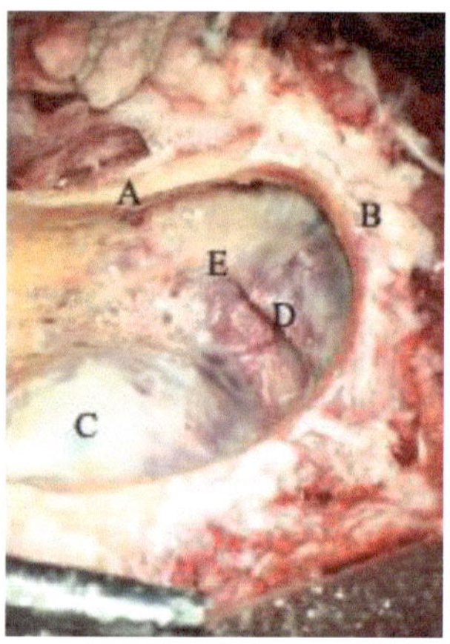

A. Posterior wall of the EAC
B. Mastoid tip
C. Sigmoid sinus
D. Digastric ridge
E. Junction of digastric ridge and facial nerve canal

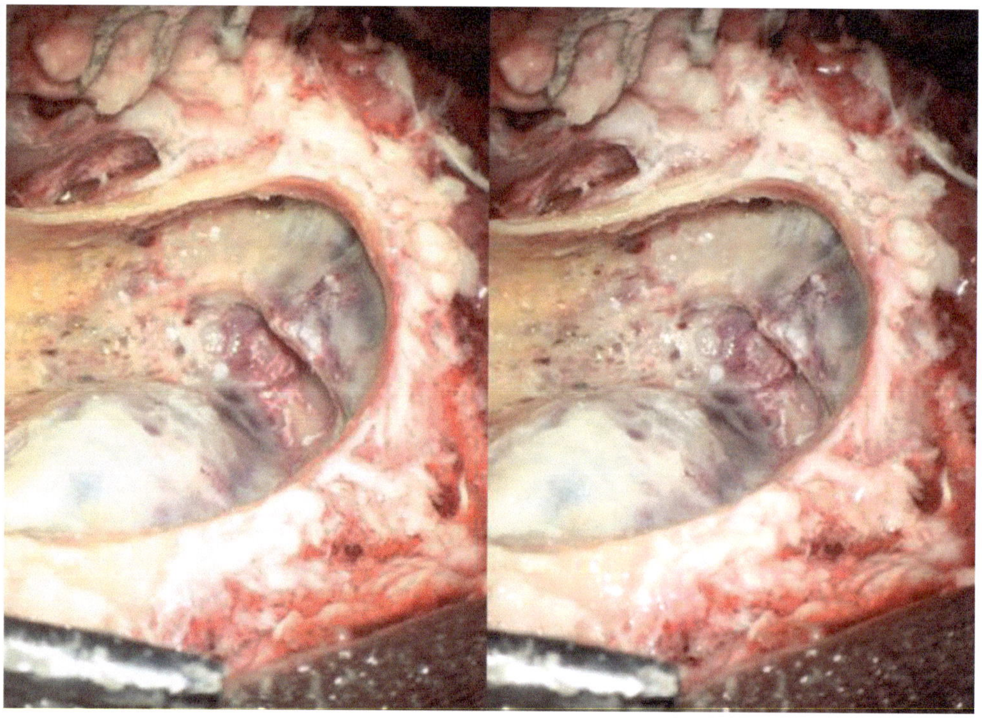

Fig. 4.6 Skeletonization of the lower part of the mastoid cavity (right) Develop the lower half of the mastoid cavity in the same way. The anterior wall of the cavity is the thinned-down posterior wall of the EAC; the bony canal of the vertical segment of the facial nerve can be seen at its inner edge. The digastric ridge can be seen inferiorly. The stylomastoid foramen is located at the junction of the anterior end of the digastric ridge and the vertical segment of the facial nerve canal. The posterior wall of the cavity is formed by the sigmoid sinus, which runs from above down to join the jugular bulb, medial to the mastoid tip, then continues on as the internal jugular vein
Instruments: large-sized cutting burs, medium-sized diamond burs

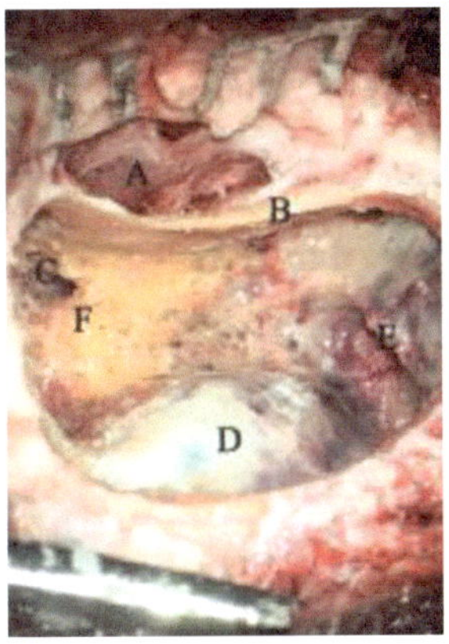

A. Skin flap of the EAC
B. Posterior wall of the EAC
C. Partly opened epitympanum
D. Sigmoid sinus
E. Digastric ridge
F. Lateral semicircular canal

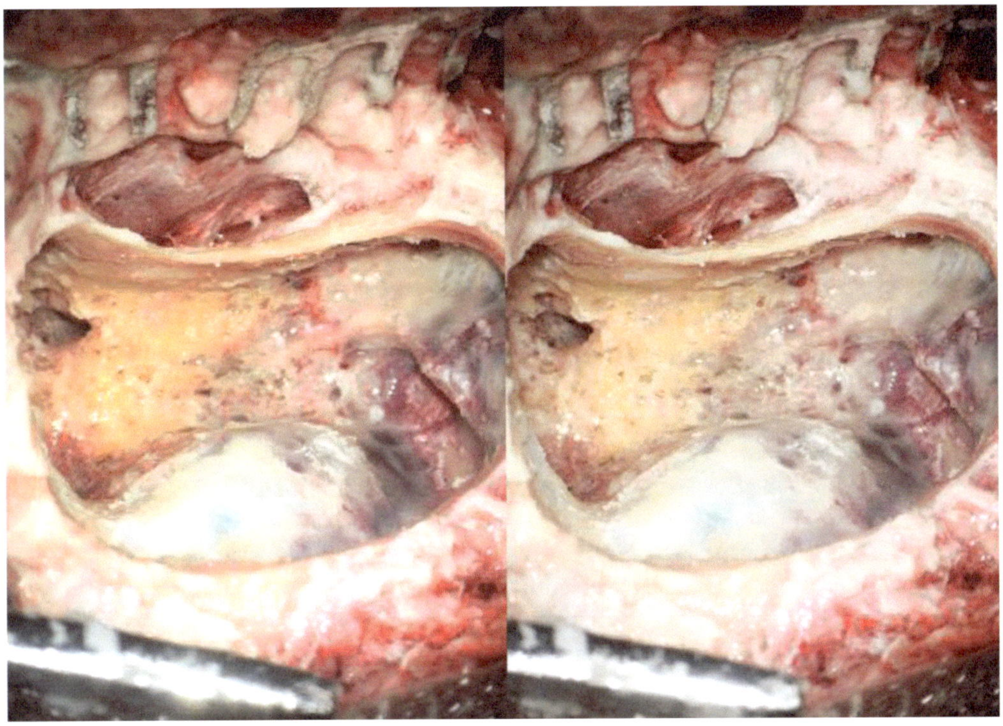

Fig. 4.7 The operative field after mastoid skeletonization (right)
The operative cavity after mastoid skeletonization should be smooth, with anatomical landmarks clearly visible. These include the thinned posterior wall of the EAC, contoured tegmen of the epitympanum, mastoid roof, sinodural angle, sigmoid sinus, vertical segment of the facial nerve canal, digastric ridge, epitympanum, incus, and bony labyrinth

Anatomy of the Facial Recess

Hui-bing Wang

The facial recess and the sinus tympani are located lateral and medial to the pyramidal eminence, respectively, in the posterior tympanum, and they are often hidden locations for cholesteatoma. The posterior tympanum can be revealed through the posterior tympanotomy approach; the mesotympanum and epitympanum junction area can be revealed if the incudal fossa is opened in continuity with the facial recess approach; and the hypotympanum can be better revealed if the lower part of the recess is enlarged.

The facial recess is shaped like an inverted triangle. The anterior boundary of the facial recess is the medial part of the posterior wall of the EAC and the chorda tympani (ca. 9.3 mm in length); the posterior boundary is the mastoid segment of the facial nerve (ca. 8.8 mm in length); and the upper boundary is the incudal fossa (ca. 2.9 mm wide). The transverse width of the middle of the facial recess is 2.65 mm.

The procedure to reveal the facial recess is to skeletonize the mastoid cavity, expose the aditus ad antrum and the prominence of the lateral semicircular canal, expand the aditus ad antrum to reveal the short process of the incus, and thin the lateral part of the posterior wall of the EAC in the plane of the mastoid segment of the facial nerve, while keeping these structures intact. At this point, the three boundaries of the facial recess can be approximately located.

Choose diamond burs of appropriate size (usually smaller than 2 mm) to open the facial recess according to the specific anatomy. Start to open the facial recess just below the short process of the incus where it is widest, then expand the recess gradually until the required exposure is achieved.

Hints: (1) The structure and function of the facial nerve must be protected when opening the facial recess. (2) The chorda tympani can be freed, displaced, or removed in special circumstances. (3) The incus buttress must be preserved to support the short process of the incus if the ossicular chain is to be kept intact. (4) The drill must not touch the incus.

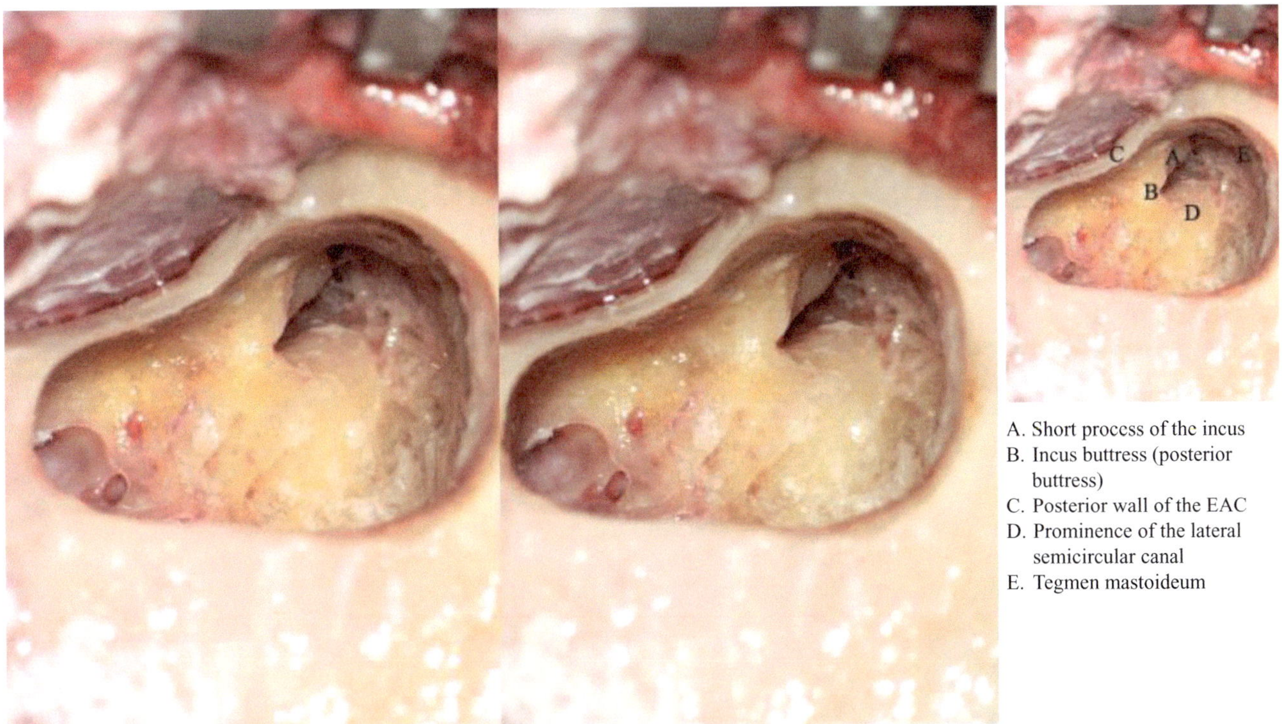

A. Short process of the incus
B. Incus buttress (posterior buttress)
C. Posterior wall of the EAC
D. Prominence of the lateral semicircular canal
E. Tegmen mastoideum

Fig. 4.8 Mastoid skeletonization (left)
Make a postauricular incision, open the mastoid cavity from the cribriform area, remove most of the mastoid cells, and mastoid skeletonization is completed. After determining the location of the mastoid antrum, widen the aditus ad antrum anteriorly to show the short process of the incus and the prominence of the lateral semicircular canal
Instruments: large- and medium-sized cutting burs, large- and medium-sized diamond burs

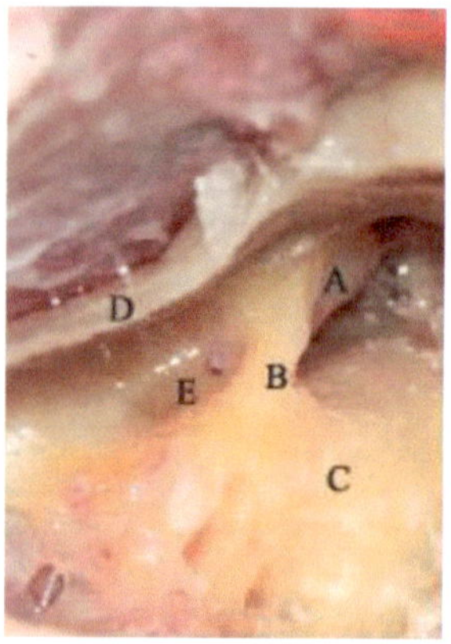

A. Short process of the incus
B. Incus buttress
C. Prominence of the lateral semicircular canal
D. Posterior wall of the EAC
E. Unopened facial recess

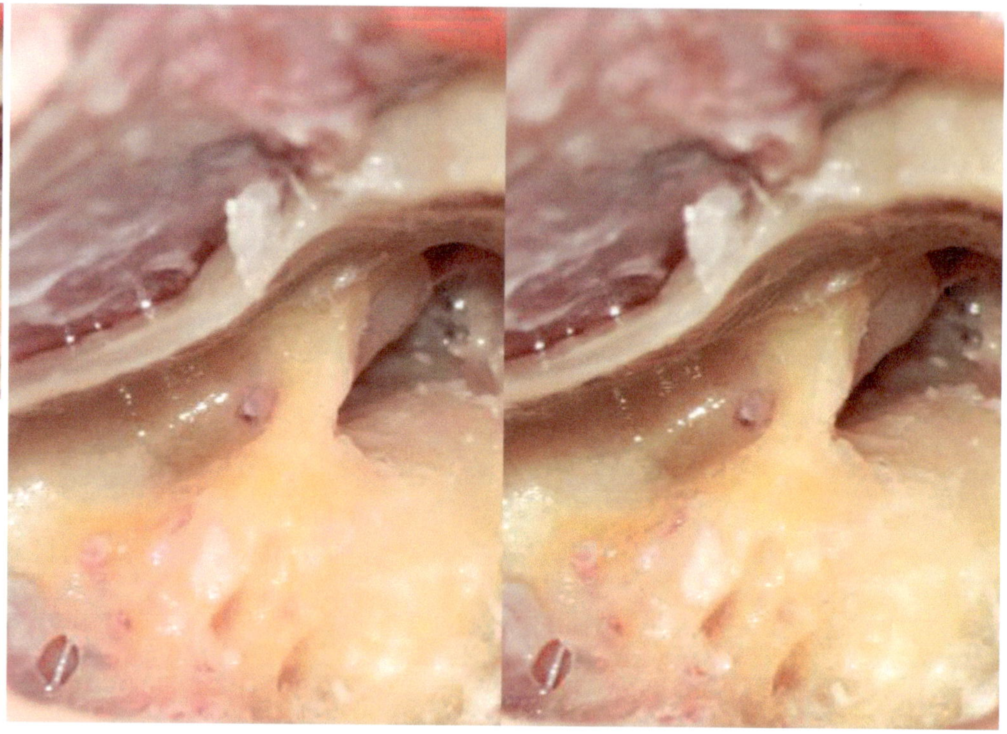

Fig. 4.9 Location of the facial recess (left)
Thin down the posterior wall of the EAC, and use the short process of the incus and the lateral semicircular canal as anatomical landmarks to locate the facial recess. The upper boundary of the facial recess is the incus buttress, the anterior boundary is the medial part of the posterior wall of the EAC and the chorda tympani, and the posterior boundary is the mastoid segment of the facial nerve. To open the facial recess safely, start to open it from just below the incus buttress, which is the widest part of the recess. In the course of removing the bone of the facial recess, note the following: (1) Remove the bone layer by layer to prevent injuring deeper structures. (2) Use liberal irrigation to clear bone chips, to prevent heating, and to better observe color changes of the bone surface. (3) The direction of movement of the drill must be along the long axis of the facial nerve, so as not to damage it
Instruments: small-sized diamond burs

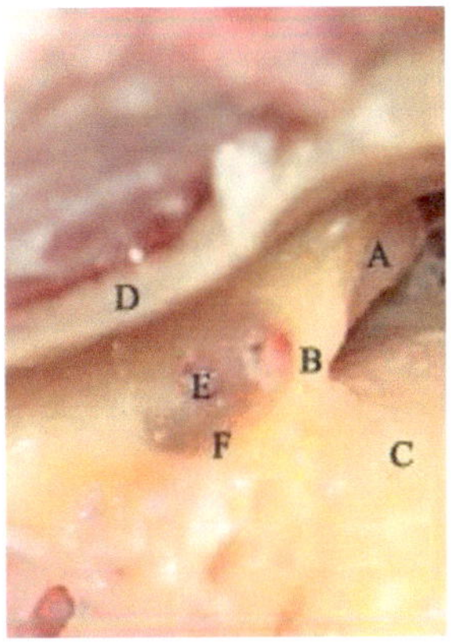

A. Short process of the incus
B. Incus buttress
C. Prominence of the lateral semicircular canal
D. Posterior wall of the EAC
E. Posterior tympanic mucosa
F. Posterior boundary of the facial recess (bony facial canal)

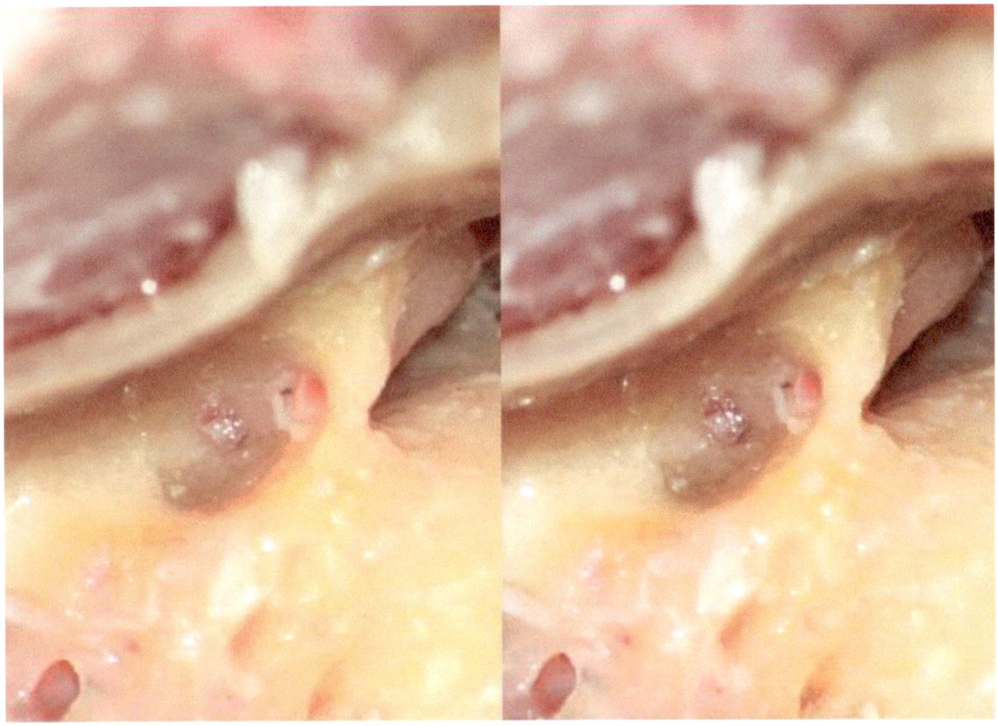

Fig. 4.10 Removal of bone of the facial recess (left)
After being located, open the facial recess layer by layer using small diamond burs. Any soft tissue in this area should be carefully dissected and the bone removed superiorly and inferiorly to identify whether it is the facial nerve. Mastoid air cells are occasionally seen anterior to the facial nerve and can be mistaken for the tympanum, so they must be explored using a hook and correctly identified
Instruments: small-sized diamond burs, right-angled hook

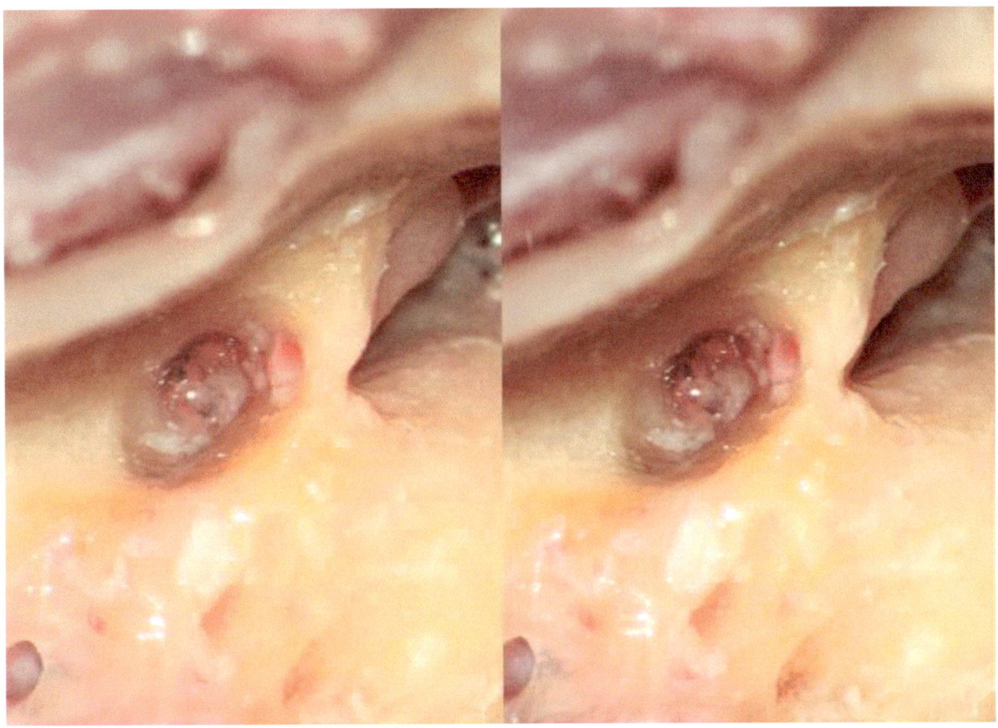

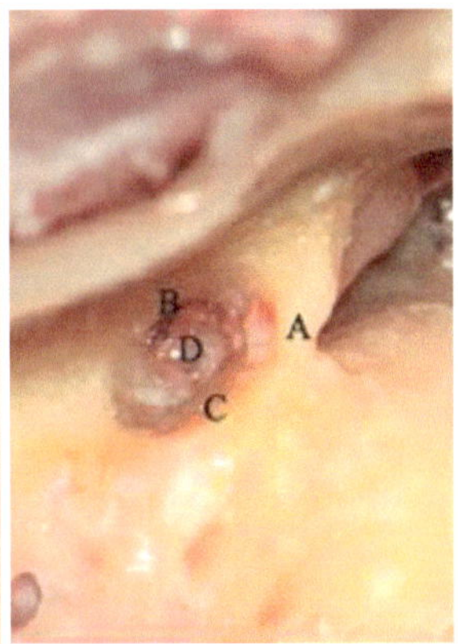

A. Incus buttress
B. Anterior boundary of the facial recess
C. Posterior boundary of the facial recess
D. Posterior tympanic mucosa

Fig. 4.11 Exposure of the posterior tympanic mucosa (left)
Gradually open the facial recess until the tympanic mucosa is exposed. The posterior tympanic mucosa is the last barrier to entering the posterior tympanum. The mucosa should be opened using a hook, not a bur, to prevent injury to the ossicular chain and inner ear
Instruments: small-sized diamond burs, right-angle hook

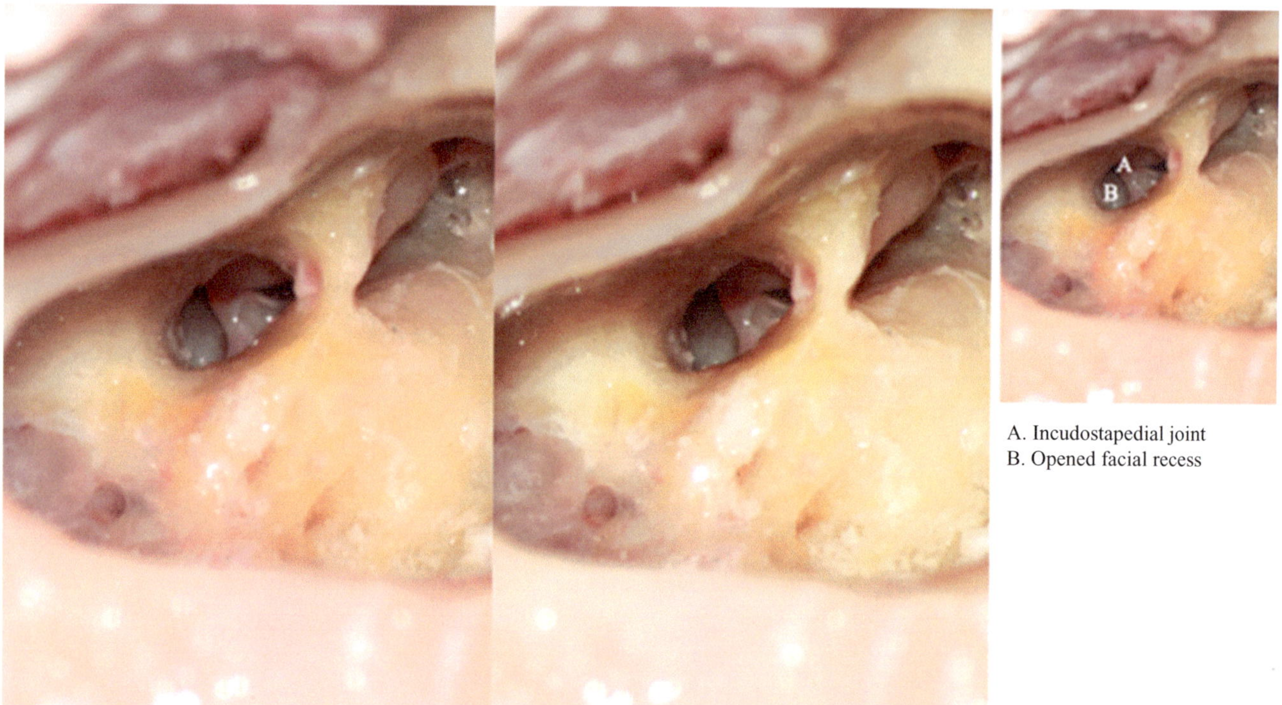

A. Incudostapedial joint
B. Opened facial recess

Fig. 4.12 Open facial recess to expose the posterior tympanum (left)
Remove the posterior tympanic mucosa, and the posterior tympanum is exposed. The incudostapedial joint and part of the tympanic medial wall can be observed through the facial recess. The posterior tympanum is explored using a hook, preparing to widen the recess exposure
Instruments: small-sized diamond burs, right-angle hook

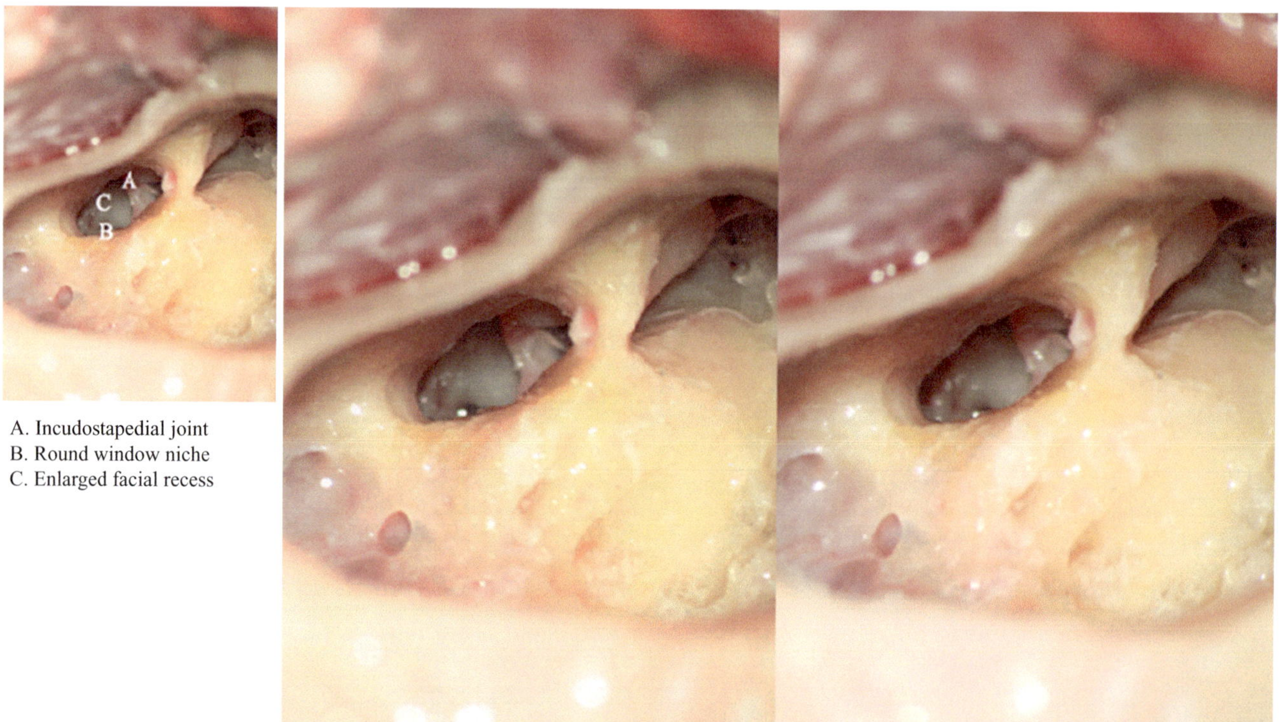

A. Incudostapedial joint
B. Round window niche
C. Enlarged facial recess

Fig. 4.13 Enlarge the facial recess to reveal the round window niche (left)
Enlarge the facial recess step by step, working parallel to the mastoid segment of the facial nerve and the chorda tympani. In the course of removing the bone of the facial recess, use a right-angle hook to keep exploring the scope of the posterior tympanum. Use copious irrigation and watch closely for any color change of the bone surface to distinguish any soft tissue early and identify whether the facial nerve sheath is exposed. In most cases, the round window niche can be fully revealed with adequate enlargement of the facial recess. To show the area of the round window niche better, the chorda tympani can be freed, displaced, or removed if the facial recess is extremely narrow
Instruments: small-sized diamond burs, right-angle hook

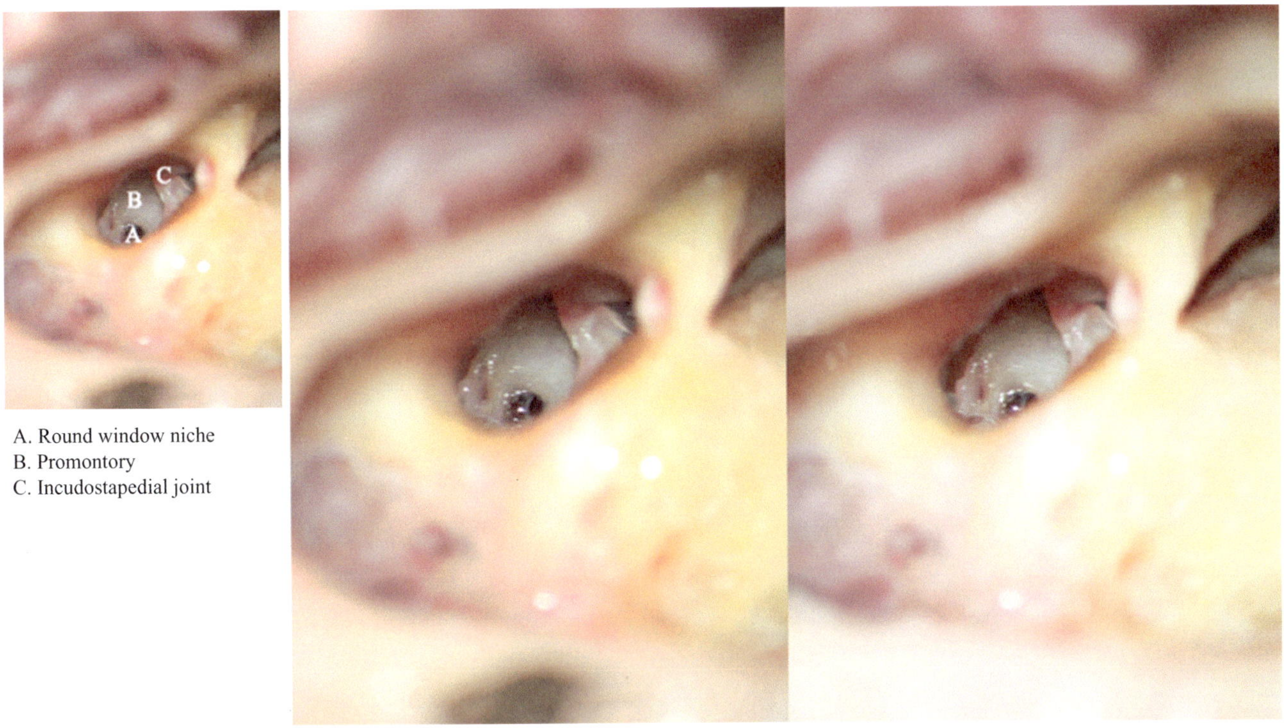

A. Round window niche
B. Promontory
C. Incudostapedial joint

Fig. 4.14 Expose the promontory and round window niche (left)
The promontory and round window niche can be observed under a microscope at high magnification. The window is located deep in the round window niche. Generally, one can observe only the aperture of the round window niche and the mucosal folds overlying it through the facial recess. When the bone anterior to and above the round window niche has been removed, the window and its closing membrane can be seen
Instruments: small-sized diamond burs

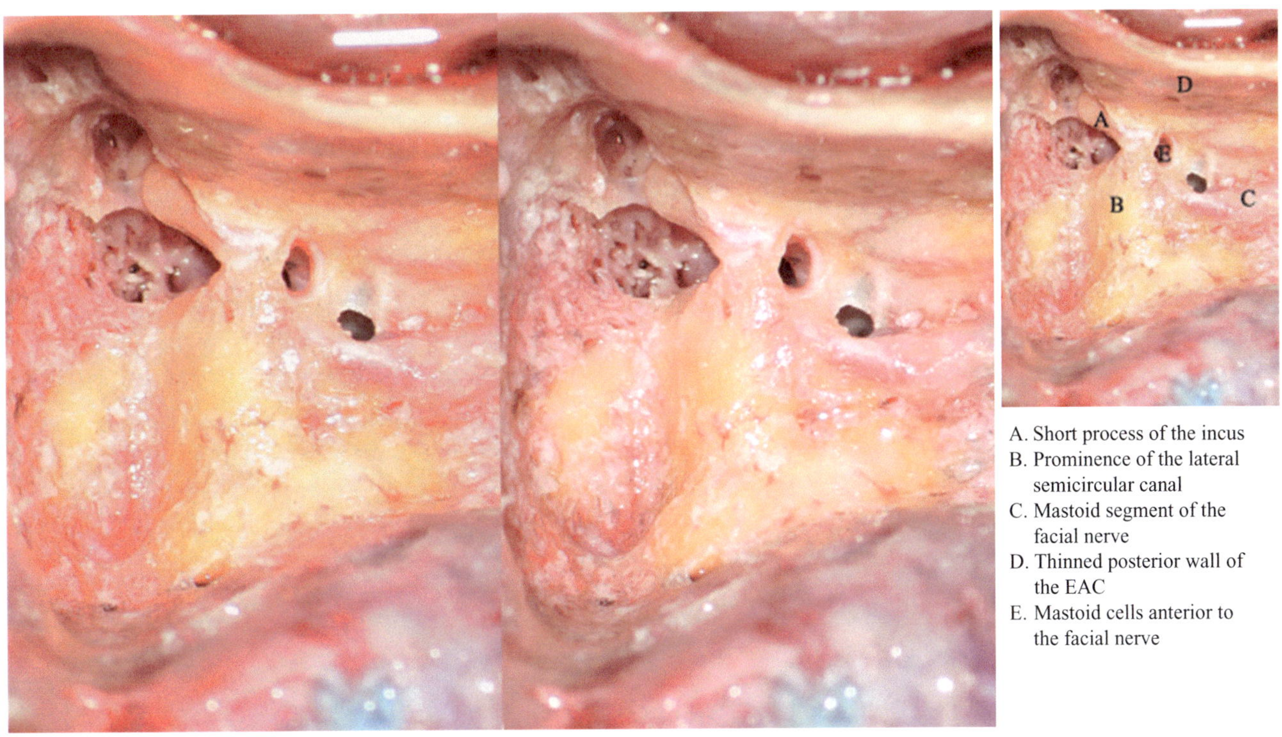

A. Short process of the incus
B. Prominence of the lateral semicircular canal
C. Mastoid segment of the facial nerve
D. Thinned posterior wall of the EAC
E. Mastoid cells anterior to the facial nerve

Fig. 4.15 Mastoid cells anterior to facial nerve (right)
Mastoid cells may be present anterior to the facial nerve below the incus buttress in some well-pneumatized cases. Generally, it is more convenient and safer to open the facial recess through these cells
Instruments: small-sized diamond burs

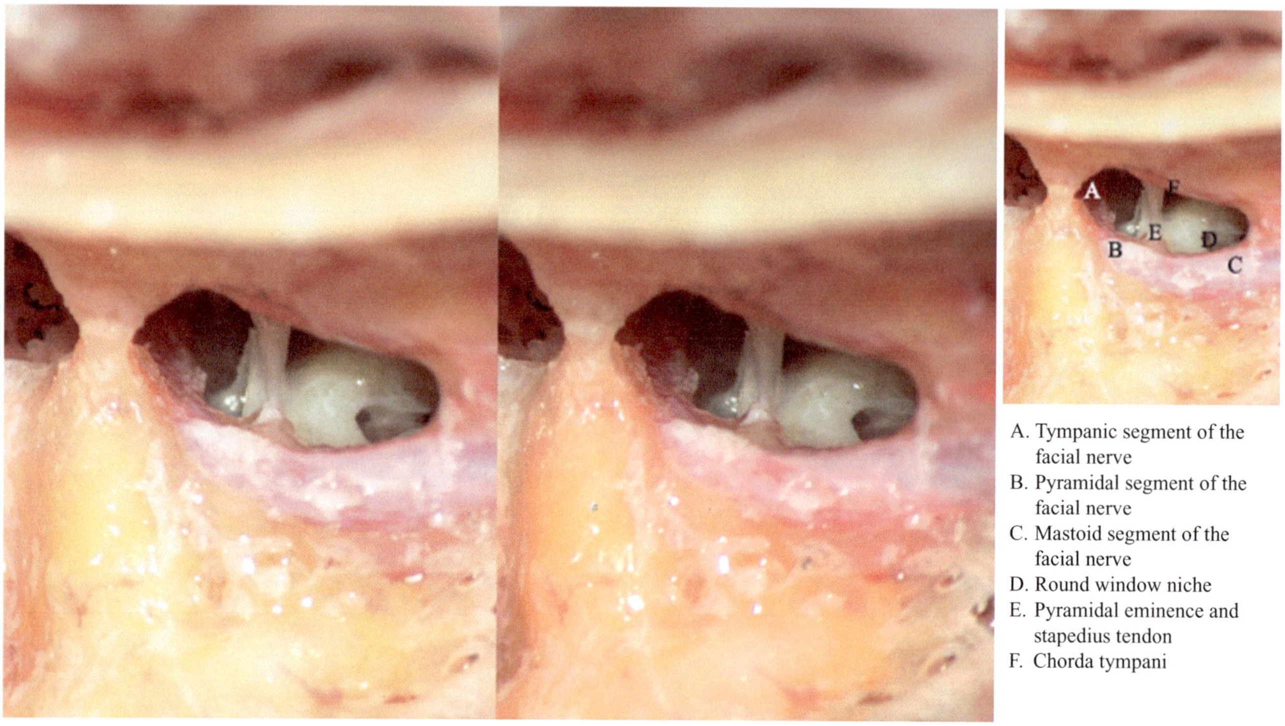

A. Tympanic segment of the facial nerve
B. Pyramidal segment of the facial nerve
C. Mastoid segment of the facial nerve
D. Round window niche
E. Pyramidal eminence and stapedius tendon
F. Chorda tympani

Fig. 4.16 Fully opened facial recess (right)
The pyramidal eminence is used as an anatomical marker for the position of the mastoid segment of the facial nerve. Many structures can be seen through the fully opened facial recess, such as the tympanic, pyramidal, and mastoid segments of the facial nerve, chorda tympani, pyramidal eminence, incudostapedial joint, oval window, promontory, and the round window niche
Instruments: small-sized diamond burs

Anatomy of the Facial Nerve

Yu Su and Bo Gao

The Course of the Facial Nerve

The anatomy of the facial nerve is one the most complex of the cranial nerves. It is categorized in terms of its relationship to the temporal bone of the skull (into three parts: intracranial, intra-temporal, and extra-temporal bone) and can be further divided into nine anatomical segments, or its four distinct neural components (branchial motor, visceral motor, general sensory, and special sensory).

The nine segments are as follows:

1. Supranuclear segment: the facial nerve is initiated within the brain by supranuclear inputs arising from the cerebral cortex, the precentral gyrus of the frontal lobe projecting to the facial nucleus.
2. Nuclear segment: The facial nerve leaving the facial nucleus courses dorsomedially toward the fourth ventricle to loop around the VIth (abducens) nerve nucleus and extend laterally to exit at the junction of the medulla and pons.
3. Cerebellopontine segment: the motor and sensory roots of the facial nerve exit the brainstem and cross the cerebellopontine angle (CPA) to leave the cranial cavity through the internal auditory canal (IAC). These nerves are devoid of epineurium but are covered in pia mater and bathed in cerebrospinal fluid. The branchial motor nerve and nervus intermedius complex travels about 10–14 mm through the CPA before beginning their combined course within the temporal bone by passing through the IAC porus.
4. Meatal segment: in the IAC, the facial nerve lies with the cochlear and vestibular nerves for 8–10 mm before it enters the fallopian canal.
5. Labyrinthine segment: the thinnest and shortest segment of the facial nerve, about 2–4 mm long. It passes from the fundus of the IAC to the geniculate ganglion. The first branch of the facial nerve, the greater superficial petrosal nerve (GSPN), leaves the anterior surface of the geniculate ganglion, runs through the facial hiatus and then the pterygoid canal and synapses at the pterygopalatine ganglion. Postsynaptic fibers of the GSPN innervate the lacrimal gland and mucosal glands of the nose, palate, and pharynx.
6. Tympanic (horizontal) segment: extends from the geniculate ganglion to the pyramidal segment (second genu). After curving posteriorly from the ganglion at an angle of 60–90°, the facial nerve continues as the tympanic segment, lying just under the bony surface of the medial wall of the tympanic cavity and forms a prominence above the oval window and promontory. This segment begins at the point between the bony crest called the cog above and the cochleariform process below. The nerve then passes posteriorly and inferiorly below the prominence of the lateral semicircular canal. The average length of the tympanic segment is 9–11 mm.
7. Pyramid segment: the second genu of the facial nerve, which lies below the inferiorly angled lateral semicircular canal as it curves to run downward as the mastoid segment.
8. Mastoid (vertical) segment: pyramidal process to stylomastoid foramen. The second genu marks the beginning of the mastoid segment which passes directly inferiorly into the stylomastoid foramen in the anterior part of the mastoid process. The mastoid segment is the longest one within the temporal bone and measures between 12 and 16 mm in length. The mastoid segment gives off three main branches: the nerve to stapedius muscle, the chorda tympani and a nerve that joins with the auricular branch of the vagus nerve. This auricular nerve arises from the superior vagal ganglion, passes through the jugular foramen, and joins the facial nerve inferior to the exit point of the nerve to the stapedius. The auricular nerve supplies sensation to the EAC including pain fibers. The chorda tympani is the terminal branch of the nervus intermedius and sits laterally in the middle ear on the medial surface of the tympanic membrane then passes forward between the handle of the malleus and the long process of the incus. It then exits the anterior part of the tympanic cavity via the petrotympanic fissure and joins the lingual nerve. Preganglionic parasympathetic secretory motor fibers to the submandibular and sublingual glands are carried in the chorda. Taste fibers, which are special sensory afferent from the ipsilateral anterior two-thirds of the tongue travel in the chorda as do some sensory fibers from the EAC posterior wall, subtending the senses of touch, pain, and temperature.
9. Extra-temporal facial nerve: stylomastoid foramen to the pes anserinus. The facial nerve leaves the skull through the stylomastoid foramen and passes lateral to the styloid process as a single structure to enter the posterior surface of the parotid gland. It generally separates into a superior and an inferior trunk between the superficial and deep lobes of the gland. The trunks then form a variable branching anastomosis, the pes anserinus, which gives off the five main motor branches, the temporal, zygomatic, buccal, marginal mandibular, and cervical, which exit the gland's anterior curving border to then innervate the muscles of facial expression. These branches may be single or multiple.

The Composition of the Facial Nerve

The facial nerve is complex and carries afferent fibers, general somatic afferent (GSA) and special afferent (SA) and efferent fibers, general visceral efferent (GVE) and branchial efferents (BE). It exits the brainstem laterally at the pontomedullary junction as a larger motor nerve containing BE fibers with the smaller nervus intermedius which has SA fibers for taste and the parasympathetic GVE and GSA fibers. The two components usually join to form one main nerve when passing through the fundus of the IAC.

BE fibers: cell bodies of the nerves that form the frontal branches have input from both sides of the cerebral cortex. Those to the lower four branches have cortical innervation from the contralateral side. Spontaneous facial movements are the result of input from multiple levels of the brain from the cortex down via the extrapyramidal system which also controls facial muscle tone and voluntary facial movement. Emotional responses are controlled by the hypothalamus. The facial nerve lower motor neurons' cell bodies sit in the facial nuclei which receive input from above from both the pyramidal and extrapyramidal systems. The lower motor neurons leave the facial nuclei, band together to pass around the sixth cranial nerve (abducens) nucleus to form the facial colliculus which sits on the floor of the fourth ventricle. The main (motor) facial nerve exits the brainstem at the pontomedullary junction where it is joined by the finer nervus intermedius. The nerves pass across the CPA bathed in cerebrospinal fluid (CSF). They are surrounded by pia mater but have no epineurium, similar to spinal nerve roots. The motor (BE) fibers innervate the muscles derived from the second branchial arch: the muscles of facial expression and scalp, the stapedius, the stylohyoid, and the posterior belly of the digastric.

Nervus intermedius: derives its name from the fact that it sits between the main facial nerve and the vestibulocochlear nerve as they pass across the CPA. It is a complex nerve that carries: taste fibers from the anterior two-third of the tongue brought by the chorda tympani, taste fibers from the soft palate brought by the GSP and palatine nerves and preganglionic parasympathetic fibers that innervate the lacrimal, sublingual, and submandibular glands. The facial nerve's parasympathetic visceral motor fibers have their cell bodies in the superior salivary nucleus which sits in the tegmentum of the pons. Involuntary activation is mediated via hypothalamic input. Lesions occurring above the nuclei including those in the internal capsule or motor cortex present with loss of voluntary control of facial movement below the eyebrows but preserved facial tone and spontaneous movement. The cell bodies in the facial nuclei that supply the forehead and scalp receive cortical input from both sides of the brain. In unilateral supranuclear lesions, upper facial movement is therefore preserved but voluntary movement below the brow is not. Reflexes, such as the blink reflex (trigeminal afferent and facial efferent), are not lost in lesions that occur above the facial nuclei. In view of the close relationship of the motor cortex and internal capsule control centers for facial, tongue, and hand movements, a central injury usually affects all three.

Sensory nerve fibers: a few sensory fibers in the facial nerve join the vagus nerve branch and innervate the EAC skin.

Anomalous Courses of the Facial Nerve

The facial nerve travels a long distance through the temporal bone and its pathway can be variable.

1. Dehiscence of the facial nerve: sites where the nerve is exposed due to absent bone covering, such as the horizontal segment, make it more susceptible to injury during otologic surgery.
2. Course anomalies: (1) the horizontal segment may run more inferiorly between the oval and round windows, vertically anterior to the lateral semicircular canal, superior to the lateral semicircular canal, make an extra bend (knuckle) at the pyramidal (second) turn, prolapse inferiorly to contact the stapes, bifurcate around the stapes, or deviate in various ways across the promontory; (2) the vertical segment may run backward, adjacent to the sigmoid sinus, or run more forward, adjacent to the posterior wall of the EAC; (3) the main nerve may run through the stapedius muscle; or (4) it may run through the anterior wall of the EAC.
3. Abnormal branching of the facial nerve: (1) the facial nerve may be divided into two branches, one running horizontally through the connective tissue while another tiny branch running through the normal bone canal; (2) the horizontal segment may run vertically with its branches passing through connective tissue to the tympanic opening of the Eustachian tube after leaving the geniculate ganglion, and then leave the temporal bone; (3) the horizontal segment may divide into two branches, running separately superior and inferior to the oval window; and (4) the mastoid segment may divide into two or three branches and traverse the temporal bone separately or merge together.
4. Facial nerve dysplasia: (1) narrow facial nerve; (2) the mastoid segment ends abruptly or only a slim branch passes through the stylomastoid foramen; (3) a thin flat facial nerve runs on the surface of the promontory on the medial wall of the tympanic cavity.

Causes of Facial Paralysis and Facial Nerve Decompression

Facial nerve paralysis is a common problem that affects any structure innervated by the nerve; it may be caused by supranuclear or infranuclear lesions. Facial palsy associated with ENT conditions manifests mainly as peripheral facial paralysis. The pathway of the facial nerve is long and relatively convoluted, and there are many causes of facial nerve paralysis, including Bell's palsy, trauma, infection, tumor, iatrogenic, etc. The most common is Bell's palsy, an idiopathic disease diagnosed by exclusion of all other causes.

When the facial nerve is permanently damaged due to infection, trauma, tumor, or other disorders, surgery including facial nerve decompression, direct repair, cross facial nerve grafting or masseteric facial nerve transfer may help to restore facial movement. Facial nerve decompression relieves pressure from the confining bony canal to allow recovery of facial nerve function, on the premise that continuity of facial nerve fibers is preserved. The surgical strategy is chosen according to the clinical presentation of the patient and includes transmastoid, middle cranial fossa (MCF), translabyrinthine, transcochlear and combined transmastoid-MCF approaches.

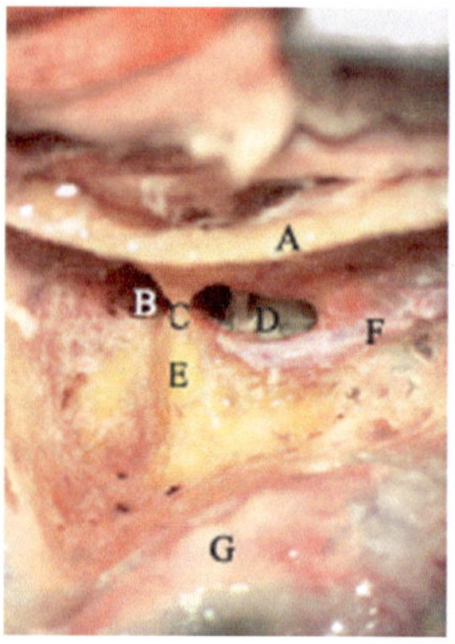

A. Posterior wall of the EAC
B. Aditus ad antrum
C. Incus buttress
D. Facial recess
E. Prominence of the lateral semicircular canal
F. Vertical segment of the facial nerve
G. Sigmoid sinus

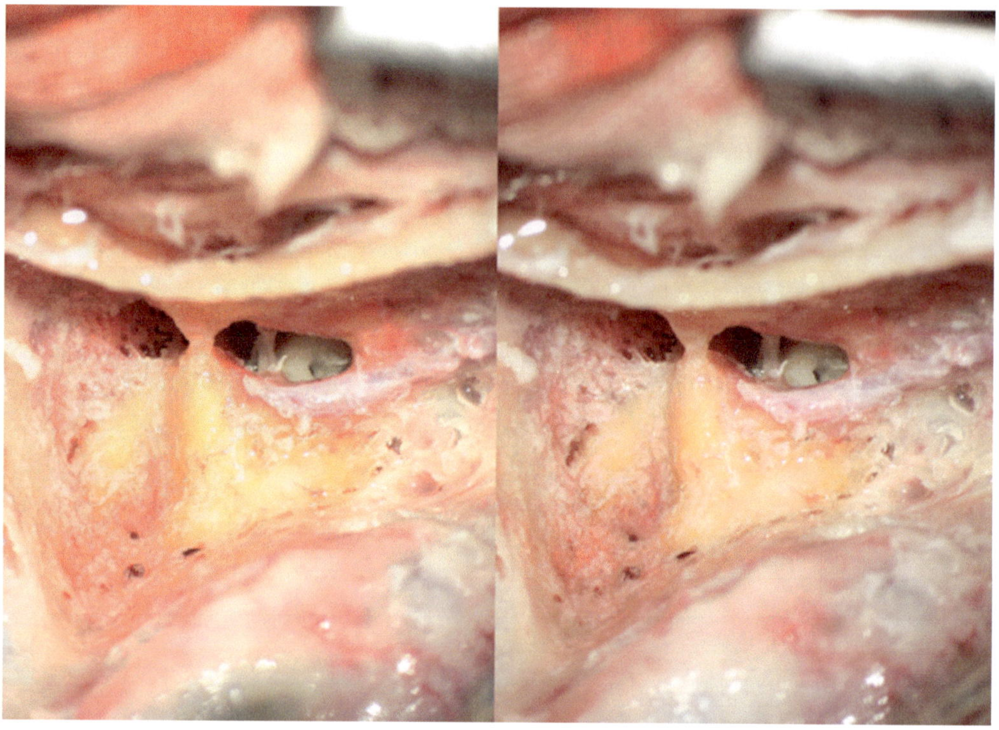

Fig. 4.17 Outline mastoid process and open facial recess (right)
The vertical segment of the facial nerve is located in the bone behind the posterior wall of the EAC, beginning below the prominence of the lateral semicircular canal, and intersects with the digastric ridge. First, outline the mastoid process, then open the facial recess, using the posterior wall of the EAC, short process of the incus, and prominence of the lateral semicircular canals as anatomical landmarks. Then expose the upper part of the vertical segment of the facial nerve. There are two anatomical landmarks of the facial nerve in the picture above; the pyramidal eminence and the prominence of the lateral semicircular canal. Through the facial recess, the incudostapedial joint, the stapes, and its tendon, the round window niche, and the promontory can be seen
Instruments: large- and medium-sized cutting burs, medium- and small-sized diamond burs

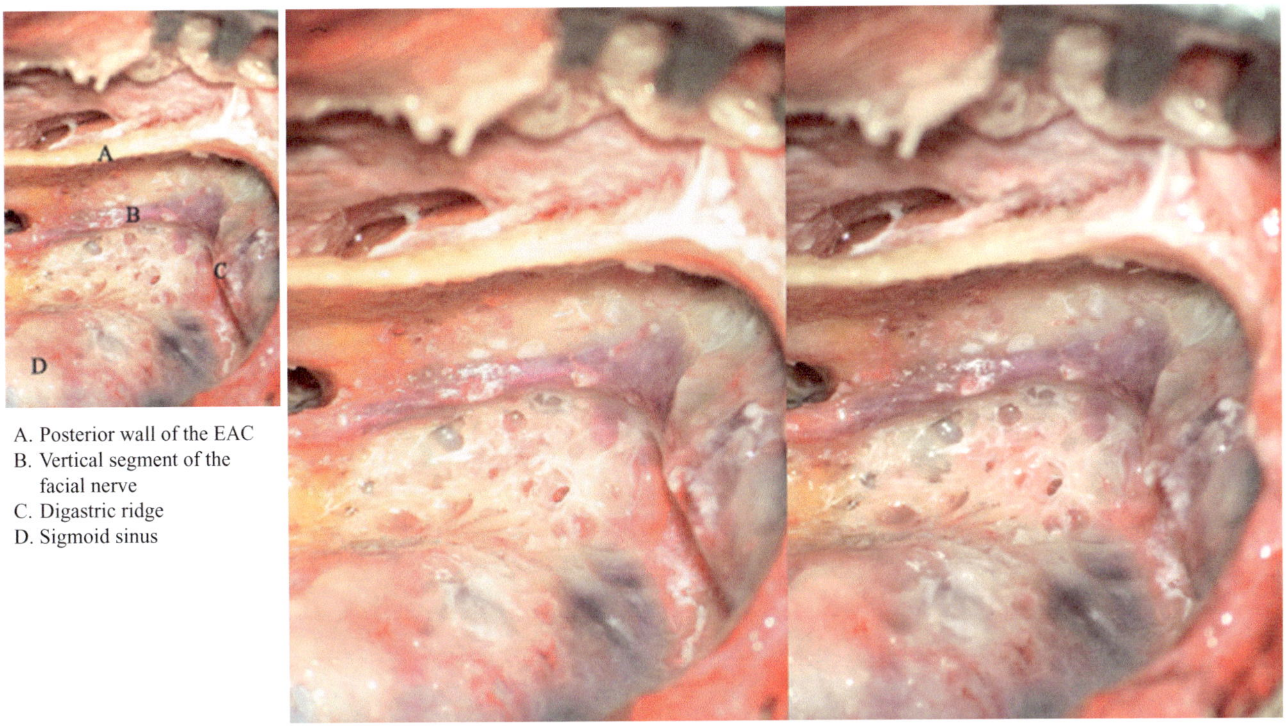

Fig. 4.18 Exposure of digastric ridge and vertical segment of facial nerve (right)
First, outline the digastric ridge and trace it forward until the stylomastoid foramen is found. After confirming the location of the vertical segment of the facial nerve, drill off the bone with medium-sized burs along the direction of the facial nerve until it is clearly exposed. *Hints: (1) the direction of movement of burs should be parallel to the course of the facial nerve; (2) drill the bone layer by layer, and notice the quality and color change of bone; (3) while outlining the vertical segment of the facial nerve, remember to drill the bone lateral and posterior to it*
Instruments: medium- and small-sized cutting burs

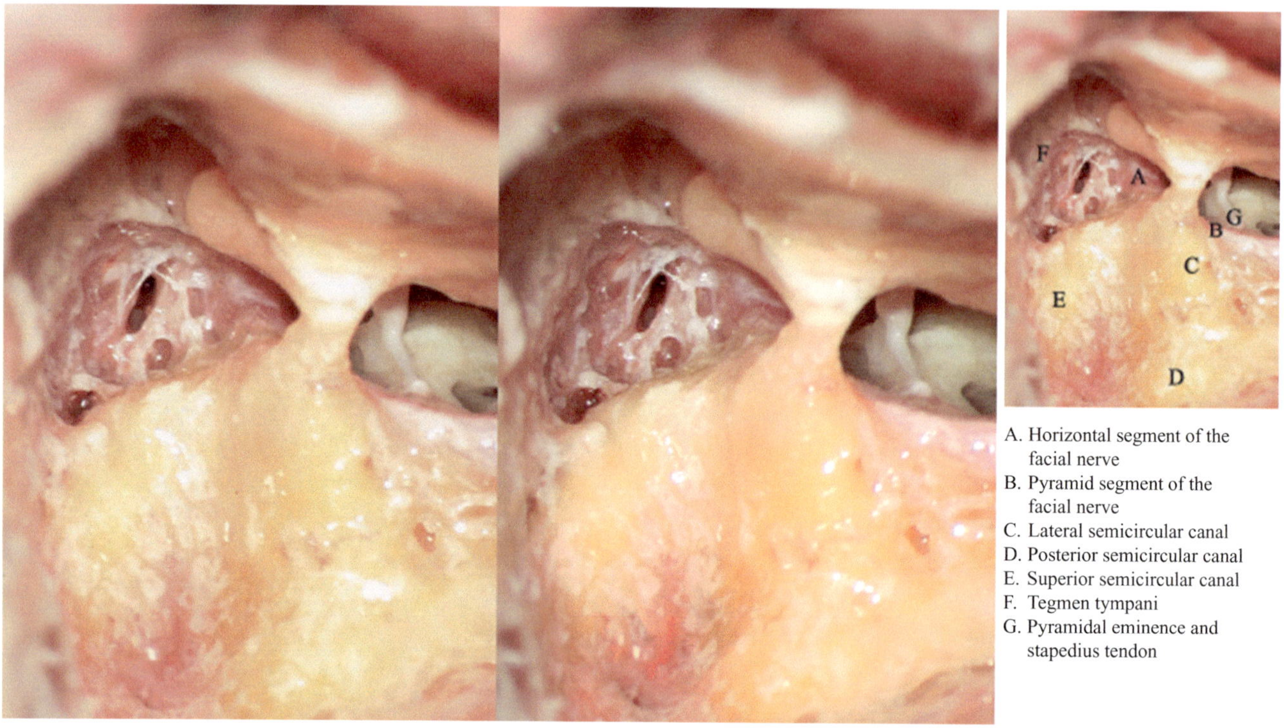

Fig. 4.19 Exposure of horizontal segment of facial nerve (right)
Note the prominence of the facial nerve canal though the expanded epitympanic approach, above the incus buttress in this image. Some cases have incomplete facial nerve canals with the nerve exposed to the tympanic cavity directly. Outline the superior and lateral semicircular canals, drill away the air cells to expose the tympanic antrum and epitympanum, and expose the first half of the horizontal segment of the facial nerve and geniculate ganglion. If the mastoid type is diploic or sclerotic, and it is difficult to expose the horizontal segment of the facial nerve and geniculate ganglion, the labyrinth or dura mater of the middle fossa may be used as landmarks
Instruments: small-sized diamond burs

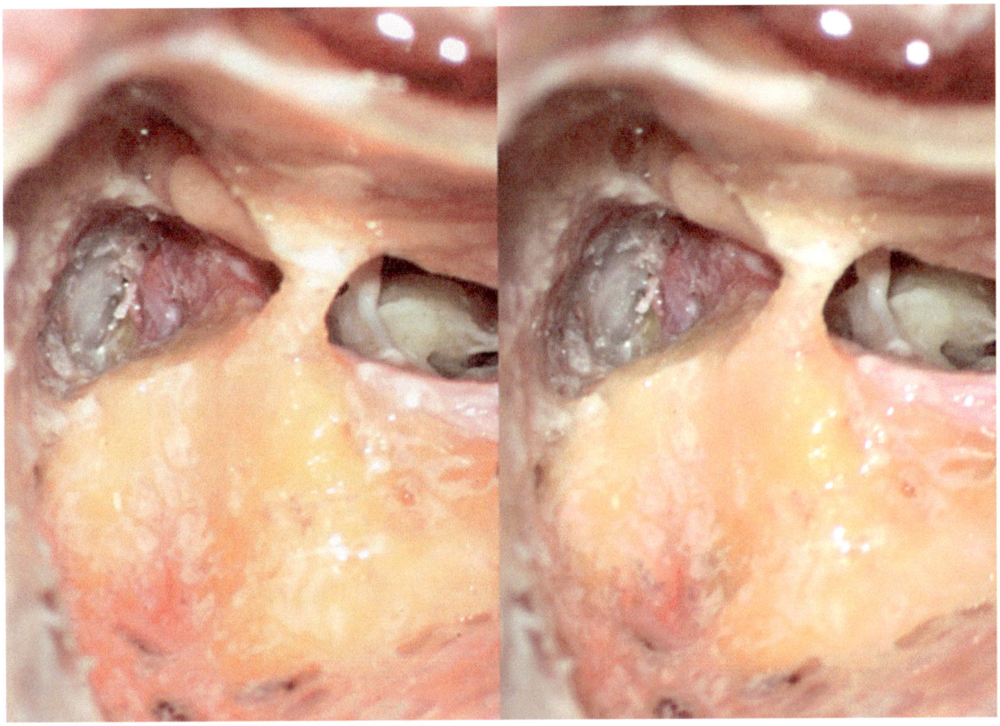

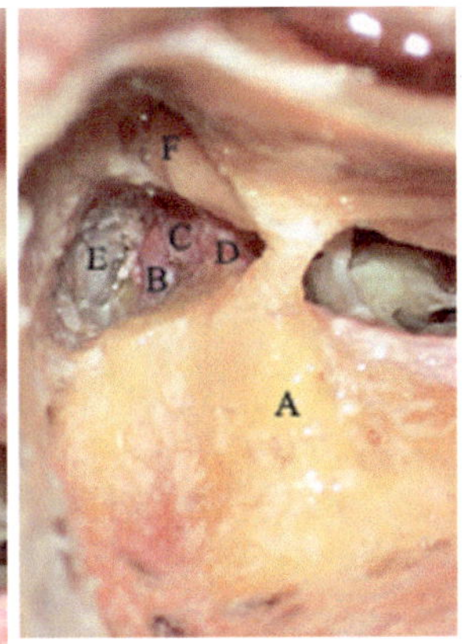

A. Lateral semicircular canal
B. Labyrinthine segment of the facial nerve
C. Geniculate ganglion
D. Horizontal segment of the facial nerve
E. Dura mater of the middle fossa
F. Incudomalleal joint

Fig. 4.20 Exposure of labyrinthine segment of the facial nerve and geniculate ganglion (right)
Carefully drill away the air cells above the horizontal segment of the facial nerve, to expose the horizontal segment, geniculate ganglion, and part of the labyrinthine segment of the facial nerve. Superior to this area is the dura mater of the middle fossa, posterior is the bony labyrinth, inferior is the horizontal segment of the facial nerve, anterior is the geniculate ganglion and lateral is the incudostapedial joint. The nerve in this area has the following features: (1) The horizontal segment of the facial nerve is almost parallel to the longitudinal axis of the petrous portion of the temporal bone. Longitudinal temporal bone fractures often involve this segment. (2) The geniculate ganglion forms the sharp angle between the horizontal and labyrinthine segments of the facial nerve. (3) The labyrinthine segment of the facial nerve is under the middle fossa and is the shortest segment of the facial nerve. (4) The narrowest part of the facial nerve canal is located in the entrance to this segment in the fundus of the IAC
Instruments: small-sized diamond burs, right-angle needle

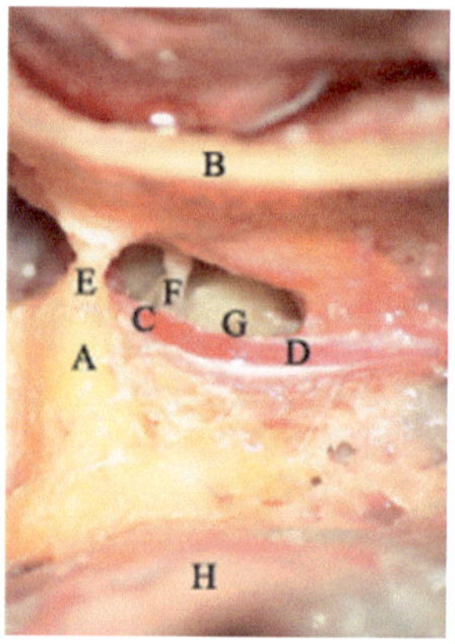

A. Lateral semicircular canal
B. Posterior wall of the EAC
C. Pyramid segment of the facial nerve
D. Vertical segment of the facial nerve
E. Incus buttress
F. Stapes
G. Round window niche
H. Sigmoid sinus

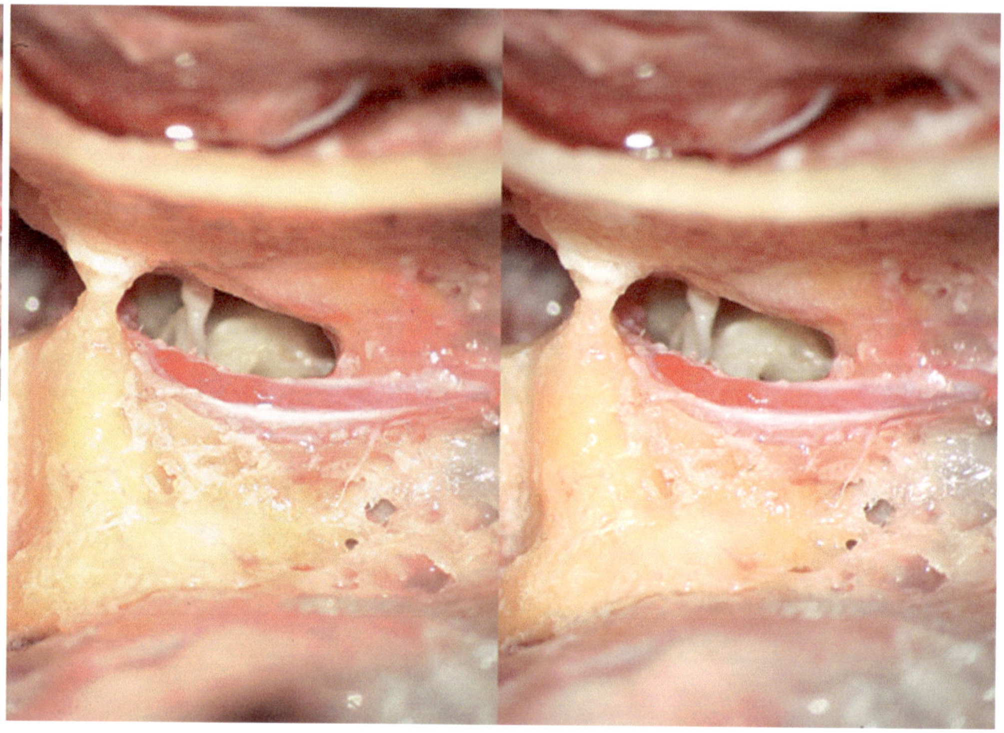

Fig. 4.21 Facial nerve decompression (pyramid and vertical segment, right)
Outline the facial nerve with spiral drilling, removing bone from the facial nerve canal, and expose the epineurium of the facial nerve. The spiral drilling technique is necessary as bone removal is safest posterior to the nerve in the lower vertical segment, lateral to the nerve at the second genu, and inferior to the nerve in the horizontal segment. Use a surgical sickle knife to open the epineurium to decompress the facial nerve; only the back of the knife should be in contact with the nerve. The incision should follow the spiral course, excising the epineurium along the length of the nerve from the bottom of the vertical segment to the labyrinthine segment, also removing it from the superior surface of the geniculate ganglion
Instruments: sickle knife, needle

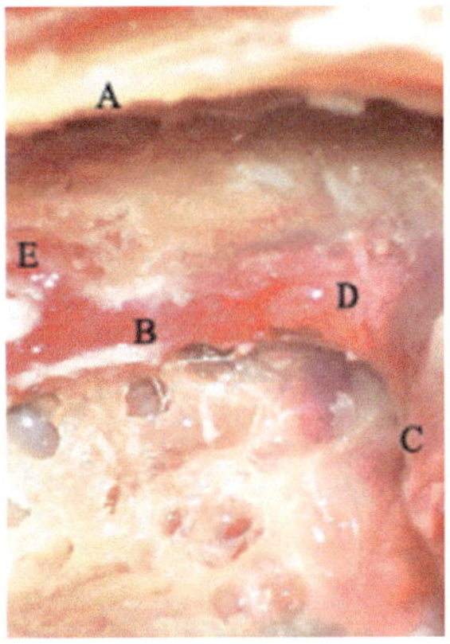

A. Posterior wall of the EAC
B. Neural fibers of the vertical segment of the facial nerve
C. Digastric ridge
D. Stylomastoid foramen
E. Chorda tympani

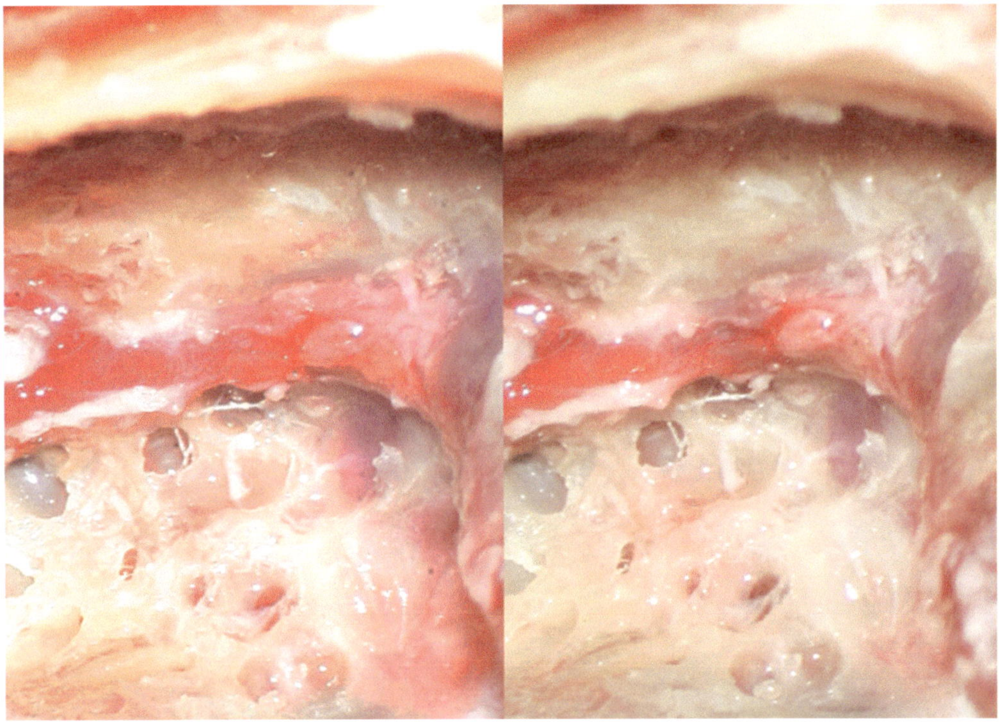

Fig. 4.22 Facial nerve decompression (pyramid and vertical segment, right)
Remove the posterolateral epineurium along the course of the vertical segment of the facial nerve to the stylomastoid foramen

Instruments: sickle knife, needle

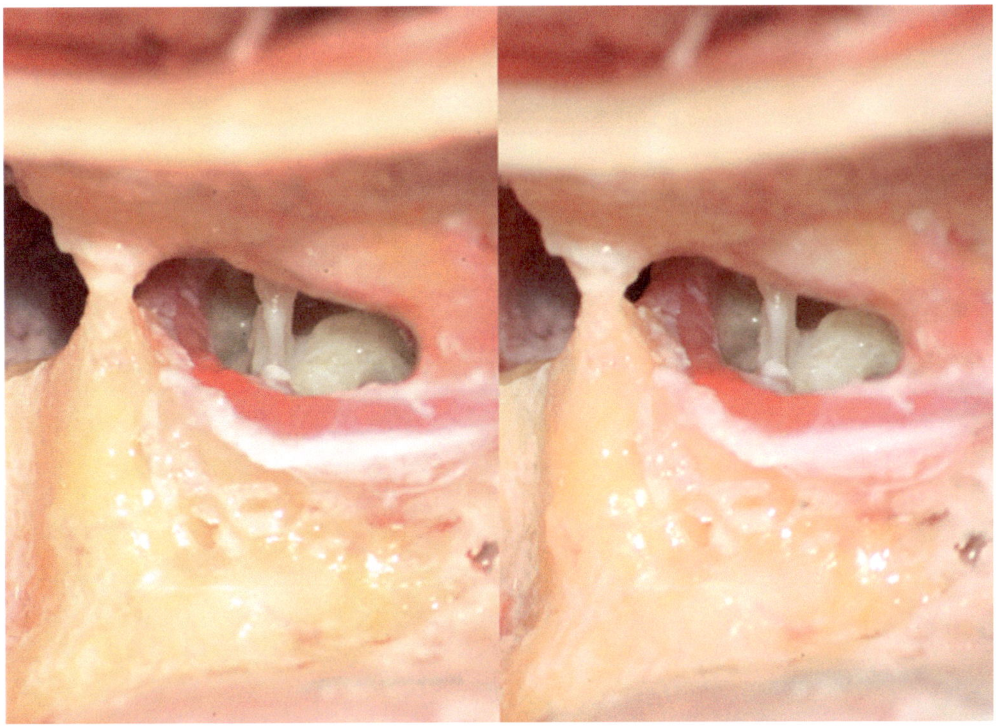

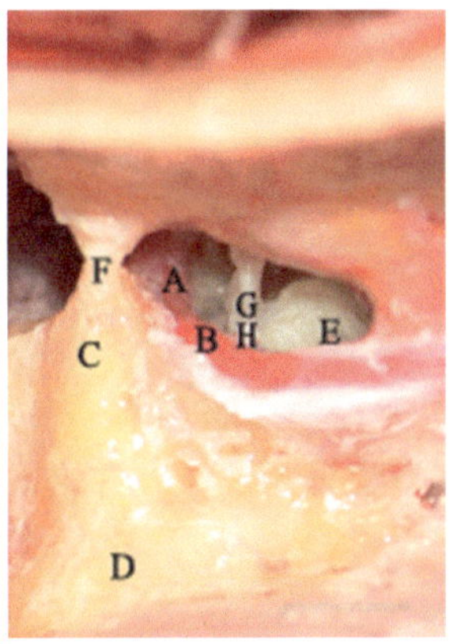

A. Horizontal segment of the facial nerve
B. Pyramid segment of the facial nerve
C. Lateral semicircular canal
D. Posterior semicircular canal
E. Round window niche
F. Incus buttress
G. stapedius tendon
H. pyramidal eminence

Fig. 4.23 Facial nerve decompression (pyramid and vertical segment, right)
Remove the lateral epineurium from the pyramidal segment of the facial nerve and inferior epineurium from the posterior horizontal segment of the facial nerve

Instruments: sickle knife, right-angled needle

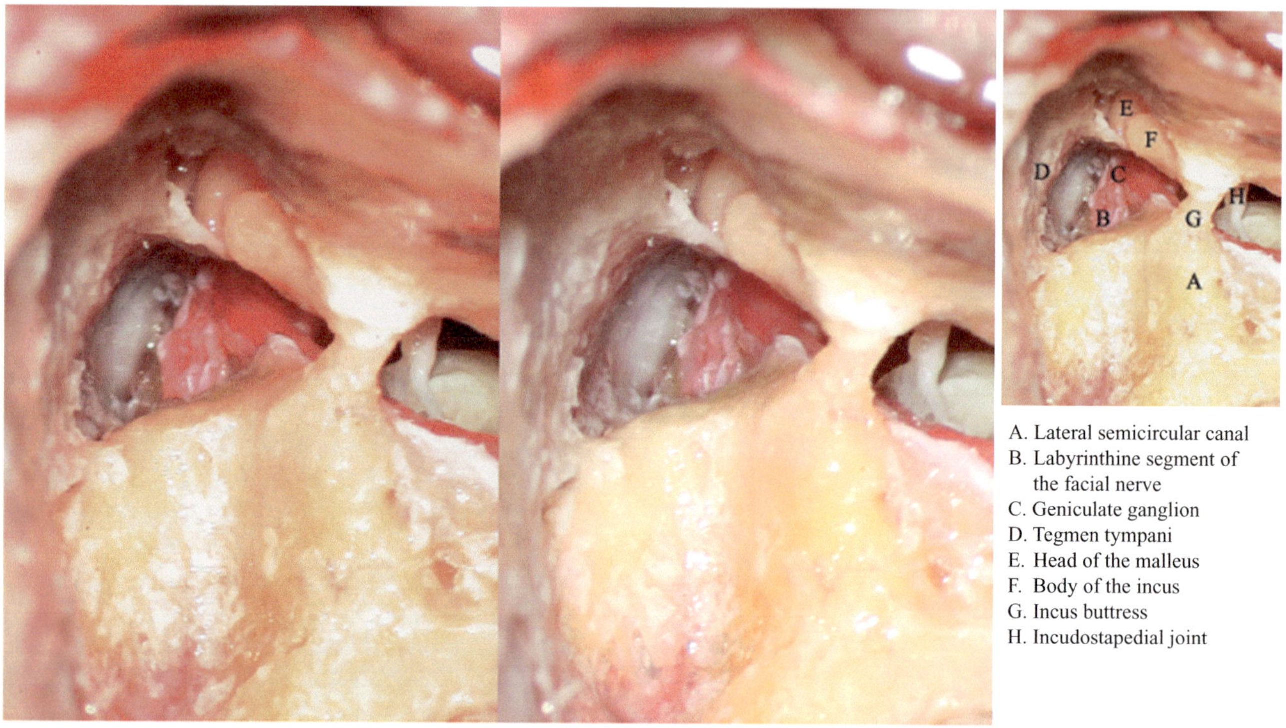

Fig. 4.24 Facial nerve decompression (horizontal segment, geniculate ganglion, and part of labyrinthine segment, right)
Remove the superior epineurium from the anterior horizontal segment, the superolateral epineurium off the geniculate ganglion, and the lateral epineurium from the labyrinthine segment to decompress the facial nerve. The labyrinthine segment is below the middle fossa, and part of it can be seen through the transmastoid approach
Instruments: right-angled needle

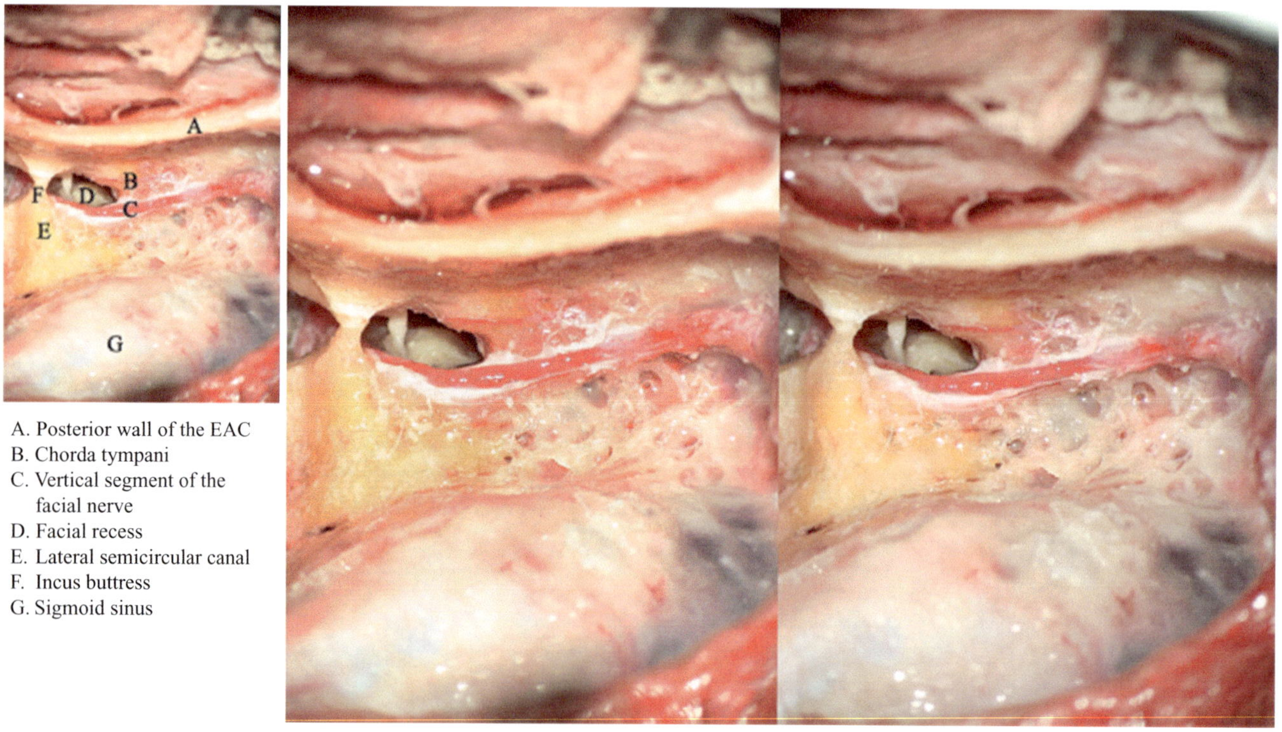

Fig. 4.25 Panorama of facial nerve decompression through transmastoid approach (right)
The transmastoid approach allows decompression of the facial nerve from the stylomastoid foramen to the labyrinthine segment, while keeping intact the posterior wall of the EAC, incus buttress, and ossicular chain

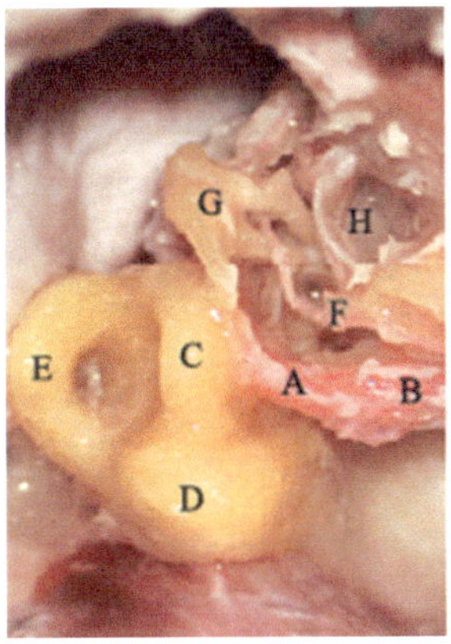

A. Pyramid segment of the facial nerve
B. Vertical segment of the facial nerve
C. Lateral semicircular canal
D. Posterior semicircular canal
E. Superior semicircular canal
F. Chorda tympani
G. Ossicles
H. Tympanic membrane

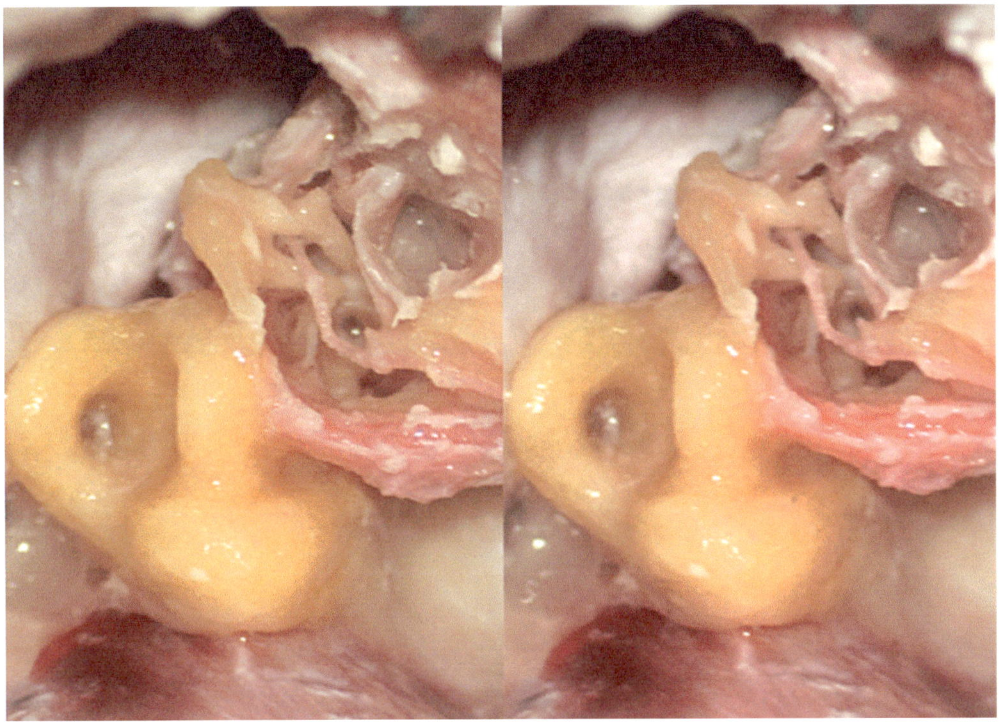

Fig. 4.26 Anatomic relationships of facial nerve (right)
Remove the bone of the middle and posterior fossa plates, and the lateral, anterior and superior walls of the epitympanum. The relationship of the tympanic membrane, ossicular chain, labyrinth, and facial nerve can be seen: (1) landmarks of the facial nerve; lateral semicircular canal, incudal fossa, pyramidal eminence, and cochleariform process (after removing the incus) (2) landmarks of the facial recess; short process of the incus, lateral semicircular canal, posterior wall of the EAC and chorda tympani; (3) the chorda tympani may arise from any part of the facial nerve, most commonly from the lower third of the vertical segment

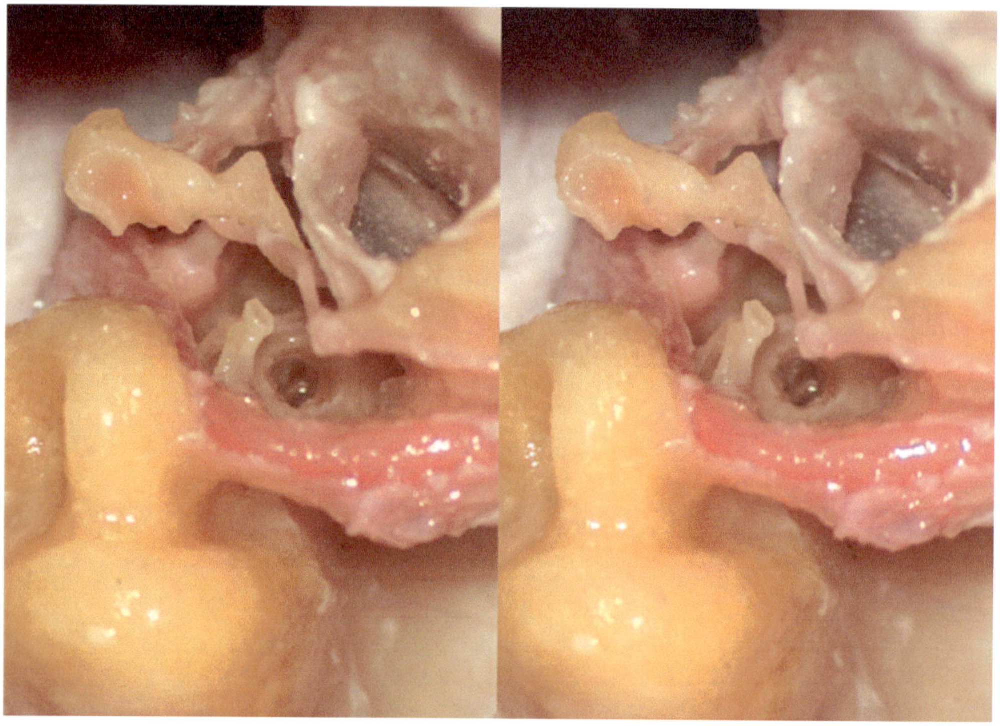

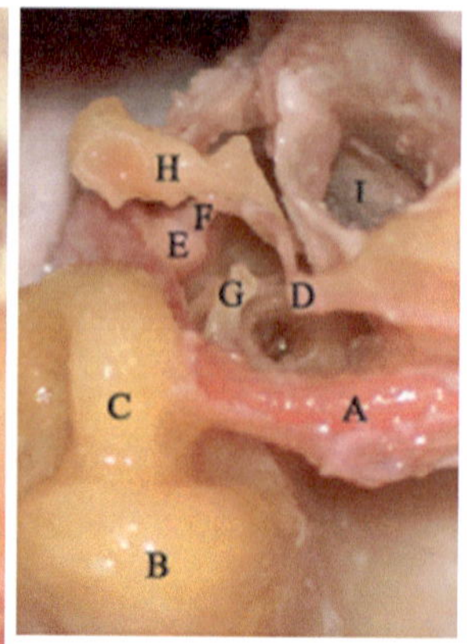

A. Vertical segment of the facial nerve
B. Posterior semicircular canal
C. Lateral semicircular canal
D. Chorda tympani
E. Cochleariform process
F. Tensor tympani tendon
G. Stapes
H. Malleus
I. Tympanic membrane

Fig. 4.27 Anatomic relationships of facial nerve after removing incus (right)
Remove the incus; the tensor tympani tendon comes from the cochleariform process almost at a right angle and inserts onto the medial surface of the neck of the malleus. The location of the cochleariform process is constant; it is superior to the oval window, inferior to the horizontal segment of the facial nerve, and it is an important landmark for the facial nerve. The bone of the canal of the horizontal segment is relatively thin and easily injured in surgery. Identification of the prominence of the lateral semicircular canal, cochleariform process, pyramidal eminence, and round window niche are beneficial in locating the facial nerve rapidly and safely (the round window is opened)
Instruments: right-angled needle

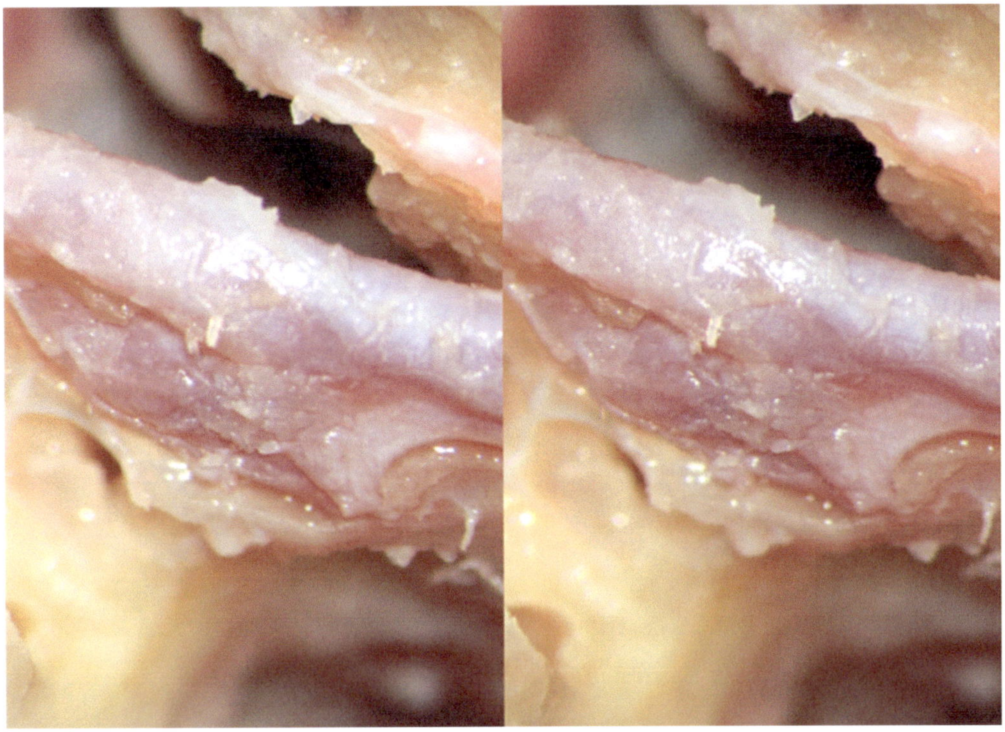

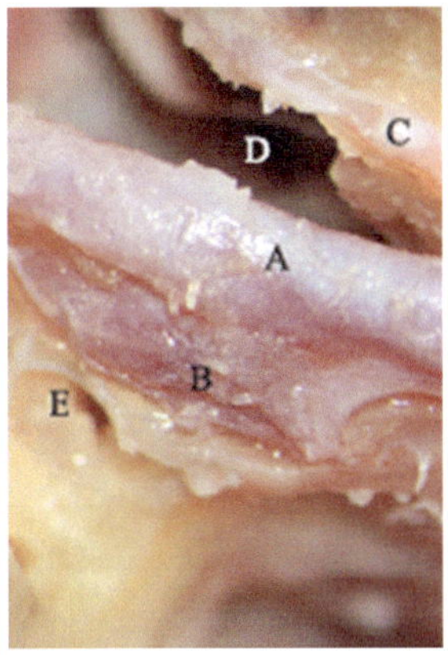

A. Facial nerve
B. Stapedius muscle
C. Chorda tympani
D. Facial recess
E. Opened posterior semicircular canal

Fig. 4.28 Facial nerve and stapedius muscle (right)
Remove the bone behind the vertical segment of the facial nerve, exposing the stapedius. Observe the surgical cavity from behind the facial nerve; the stapedius muscle is located in the bony canal medial to the vertical segment of the facial nerve. The facial nerve branch to the stapedius is at the level of the pyramidal eminence, and innervates the stapedius, serving the efferent arm of the stapedial reflex
Instruments: diamond burs, needle

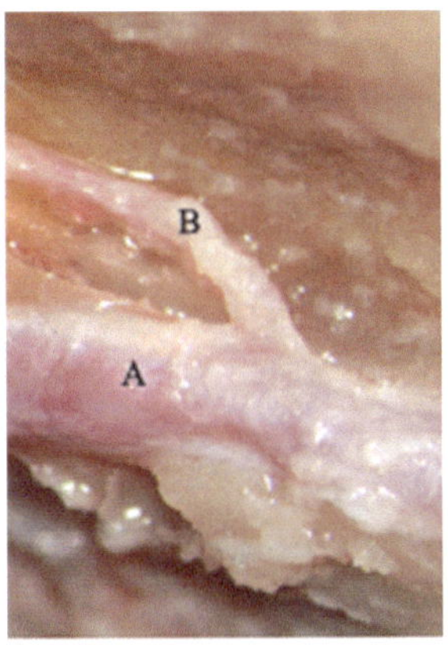

A. Facial nerve
B. Chorda tympani

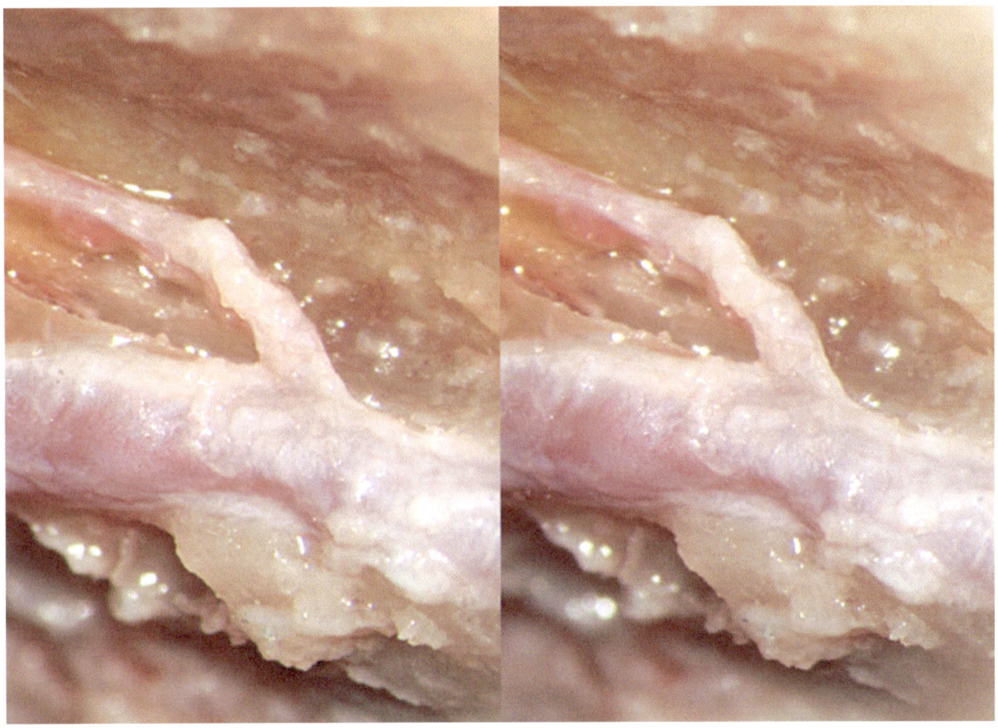

Fig. 4.29 Facial nerve and chorda tympani (right)
Thin the posterior wall of the EAC, then remove bone layer by layer 4–6 mm above the stylomastoid foramen and identify the origin of the chorda tympani. The majority of chorda tympani nerves arise from the medial side of the lower third of the vertical segment of the facial nerve; a minority come from the lateral side
Instruments: small-sized diamond burs

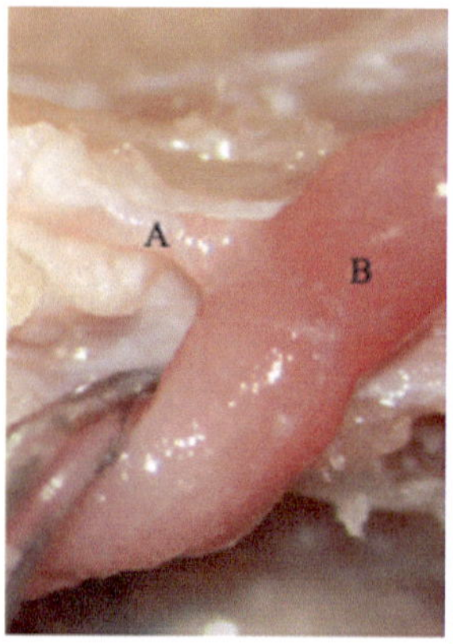

A. Neural fibers of the chorda tympani
B. Neural fibers of the vertical segment of the facial nerve

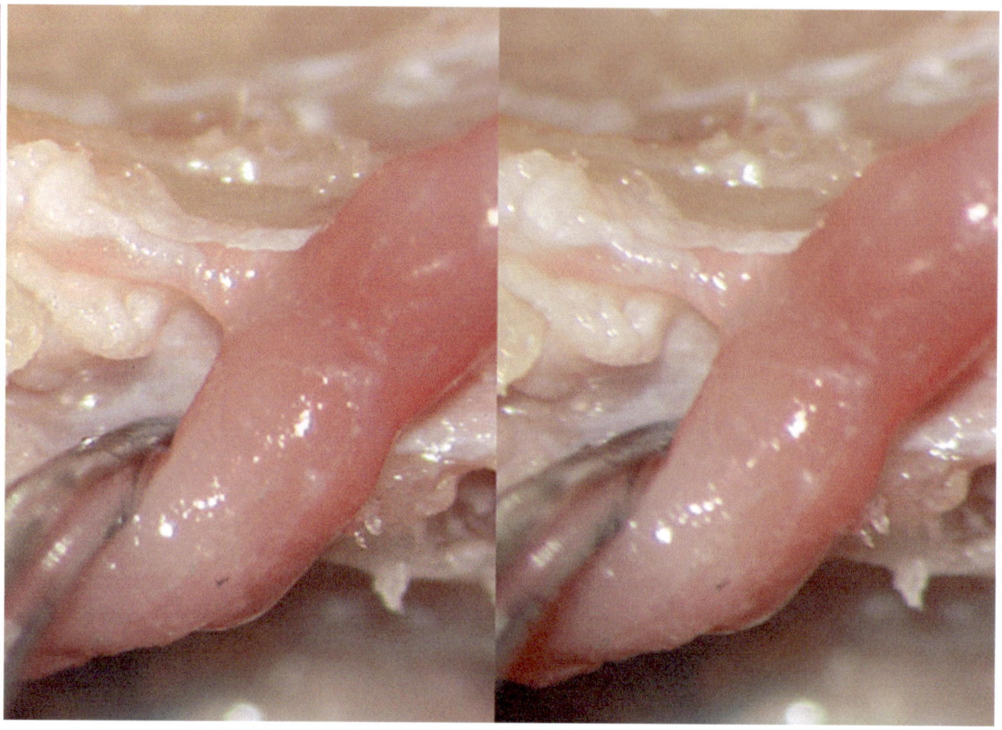

Fig. 4.30 Facial nerve and chorda tympani (right)
The chorda tympani is an important branch of the facial nerve. The majority of chorda tympani nerves come from the vertical segment. It lies in its own canal, passing from inferomedial to anterosuperior in the posterior wall of the EAC, and emerges near the top of the posterior part of the tympanic sulcus. It passes across the tympanic cavity between the long process of the incus and the handle of the malleus, then to the lateral infratemporal fossa through the petrotympanic fissure. The gustatory nerves of the chorda tympani then travel in the lingual nerve and parasympathetic fibers join the submandibular ganglion. The portion of the chorda tympani where it exits the facial nerve is seen in the picture above

Anatomy of the Endolymphatic Sac

Ya-qing Liu and Jian-hui Li

The endolymphatic sac is located in the endolymphatic fissure of the petrous bone, which is the expanded part of the distal end of the endolymphatic duct. The endolymphatic duct passes through the bony vestibular aqueduct, connecting the membranous labyrinth and endolymphatic sac, which is divided into two: the medial bony and lateral dural parts. The intraosseous part is located within the vestibular aqueduct and has walls with rich plications, also known as the rough endolymphatic sac. The dural part is located between the two layers of dura mater behind the petrous bone; it has smooth walls and is slightly flattened. The distal segment of the endolymphatic sac is 7–16 mm long and 5–10 mm wide.

There is a large variation in endolymphatic sac morphology due to different degrees of development. It can essentially be divided into three types: Type I endolymphatic sac, with the upper edge near Donaldson's line (extension line through the plane of the lateral semicircular canal). It is easy to identify due to the large external orifice of the vestibular aqueduct in a well-pneumatized temporal bone; Type II (medium) endolymphatic sac. Its superior border is not as high as Donaldson's line, and the external aperture of the vestibular aqueduct is of medium size; Type III (small) endolymphatic sac, located well below Donaldson's line, more anterior and even medial to the facial nerve. It is often in contact with the jugular bulb and associated with poor mastoid pneumatization and anterior displacement of the sigmoid sinus, which limits the exposure of the trailing edge of the sac.

Location: The endolymphatic sac is located below the plane of the lateral semicircular canal, below and posterior to the posterior semicircular canal, anteromedial to the sigmoid sinus, in the posterior fossa dura mater, behind the vertical segment of the facial nerve and above the jugular bulb. Take care not to damage surrounding structures, such as the semicircular canals, vertical segment of the facial nerve, and sigmoid sinus. Remove the bone over the dura in this region to expose the white, thicker, and nonvascular endolymphatic sac, which is usually a quite different color to the pale blue of the posterior fossa dura.

Endolymph is mainly absorbed by the endolymphatic sac, which plays an important role in the maintenance of vestibular function. Injury to the endolymphatic sac or scarring of local structures can cause disorders of the endolymph circulation, leading to endolymphatic hydrops, for which endolymphatic sac decompression or drainage may be performed. In some patients with Meniere's disease, intractable attacks of vertigo, and poor physical functioning, but with useful hearing still present, endolymphatic sac decompression may achieve good results.

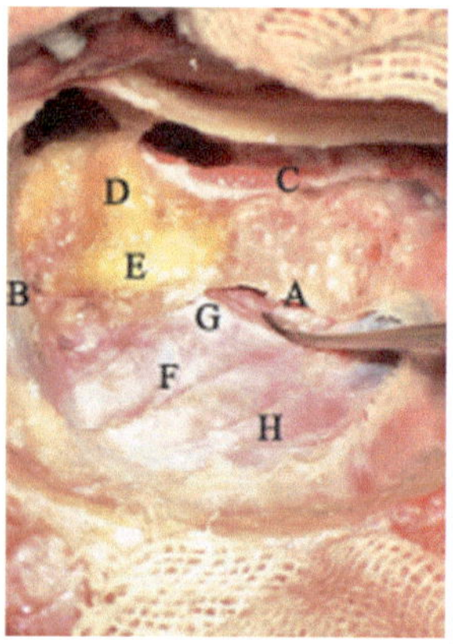

A. Posterior margin of the residual temporal bone
B. Tegmen mastoideum
C. Vertical segment of the facial nerve
D. Lateral semicircular canal
E. Posterior semicircular canal
F. Posterior fossa dura mater
G. Endolymphatic sac
H. Sigmoid sinus

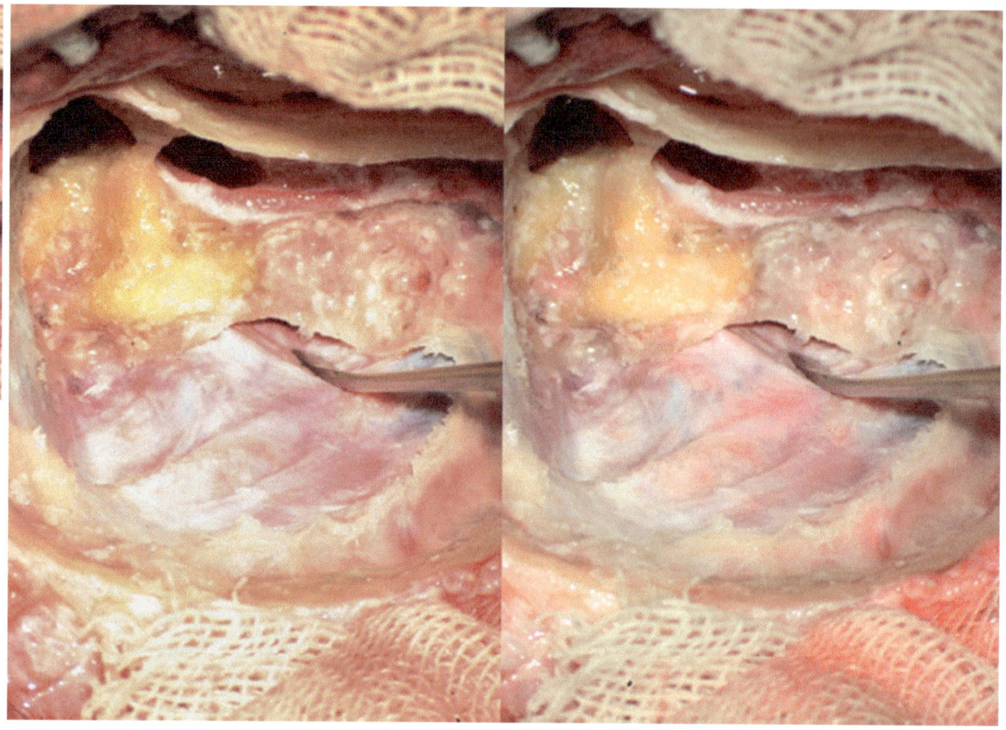

Fig. 4.31 Locate the endolymphatic sac (right)
After opening the mastoid antrum and outlining the mastoid cavity, the lateral and posterior semicircular canals, sigmoid sinus, and vertical segments of the facial nerve are used to locate the endolymphatic sac. Completely remove the bone over the posterior fossa dura. The outer wall of the endolymphatic sac is fan shaped and slightly thicker, and whiter than the surrounding dura mater. When the dura behind the petrous bone is compressed with an elevator, the narrow endolymphatic duct can be seen running in the vestibular aqueduct. Usually, the dura here is more tightly attached to the petrous bone at the bony eminence, which sits next to the opening of the endolymphatic duct. It is helpful to determine the location of the endolymphatic sac accurately by dissecting the endolymphatic duct
Instruments: large-sized cutting burs, large- and medium-sized diamond burs, middle ear elevator

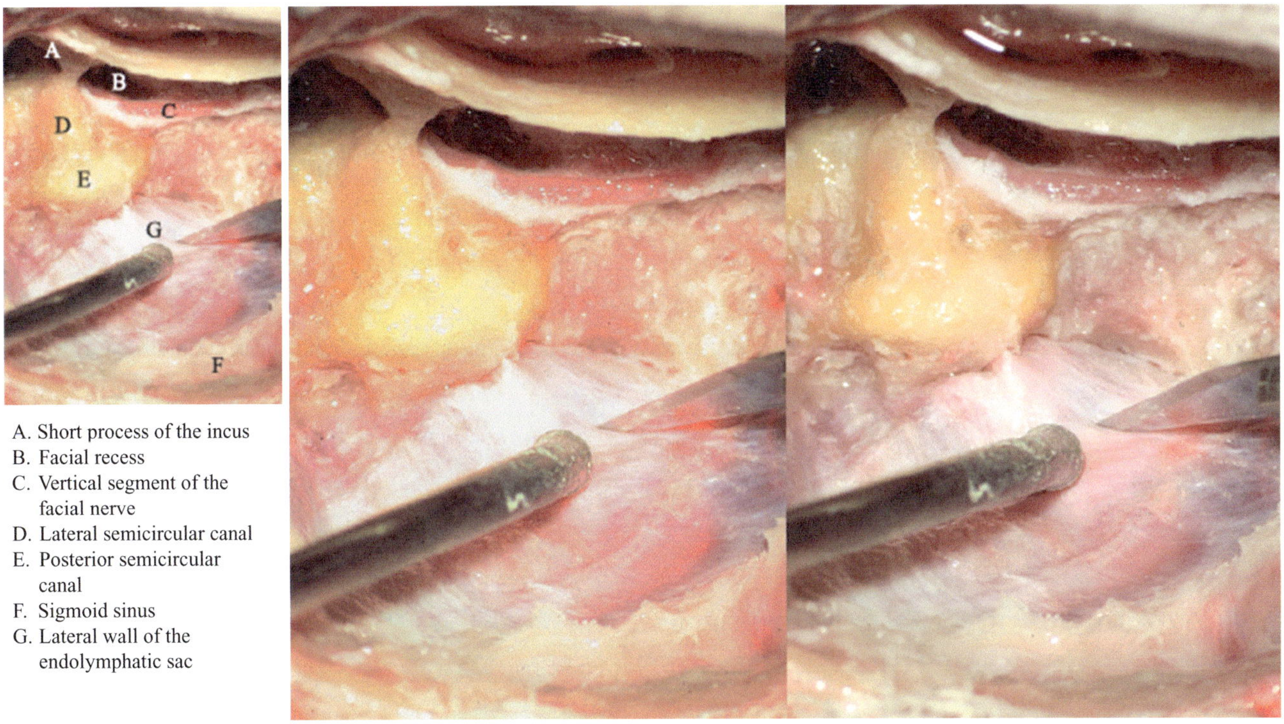

Fig. 4.32 Open lateral wall of endolymphatic sac (right)
After determining the position of the endolymphatic sac, use a #11 blade or sickle knife to open the endolymphatic sac through its lateral wall. Pay attention to the strength and depth of the lateral wall so as not to damage the medial wall of the endolymphatic sac, which can lead to cerebrospinal fluid leakage
Instruments: #11 surgical knife or sickle knife

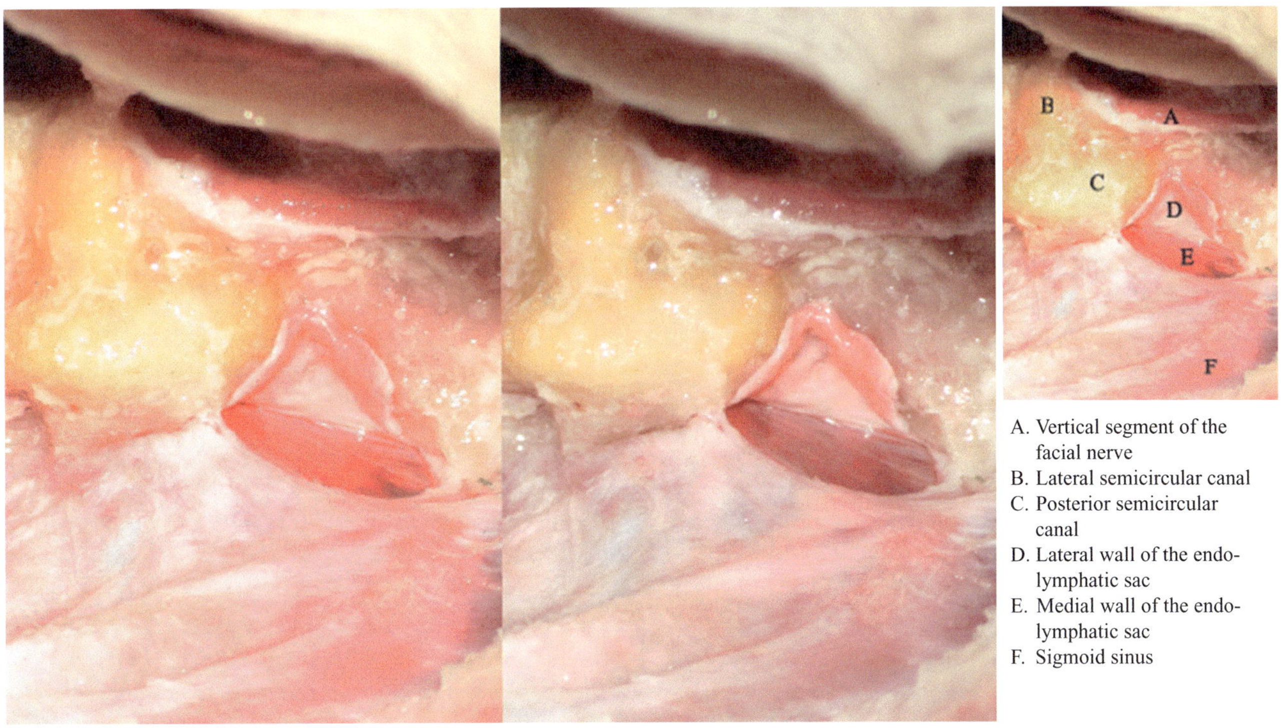

Fig. 4.33 Open endolymphatic sac (right)
Incise the outer wall of the endolymphatic sac to confirm its identity. During surgery, the smooth, slightly reflective inner wall of the sac can be seen. In the above image, the endolymphatic sac consists of inner and outer layers of dura mater, connected with lymphatic vessels
Instruments: middle ear elevator, middle ear scissors

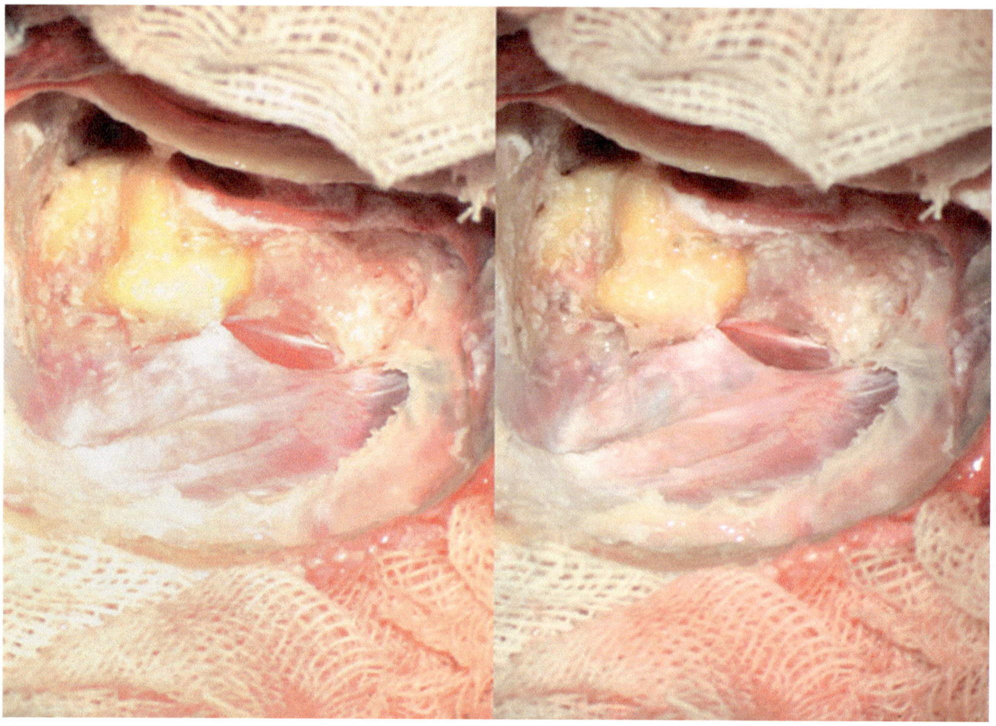

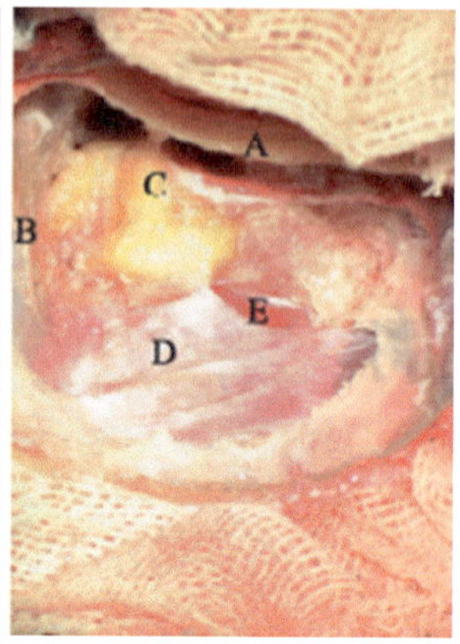

A. Thinned posterior wall of the EAC
B. Tegmen mastoideum
C. Lateral semicircular canal
D. Posterior fossa dura mater
E. Opened endolymphatic sac

Fig. 4.34 Complete endolymphatic sac decompression (right)
Reflect forward the lateral wall of the endolymphatic sac onto the posterior surface of the petrous bone (or excise it) to open the cavity of the sac and prevent closure from healing. This completes decompression of the endolymphatic sac
Instruments: middle ear elevator

Anatomy of the Vestibule and Semicircular Canals

Bing Han

Vestibule: it is a cavity in the bony inner ear that contains two important parts of the membranous labyrinth, the saccule, and utricle. It is situated between the IAC fundus medially and the oval window laterally with the semicircular canals posterior to it and the cochlea anteriorly. There are five openings of the semicircular canals in its posterior wall. It is connected to the scala vestibuli of the cochlea anteriorly by the ductus reuniens.

Semicircular Canals: the lateral semicircular canal forms a convex protrusion into the antrum, forming part of its medial wall. It sits at approximately 30° to the horizontal plane. The ampulla of the lateral semicircular canal forms its anterior end. It contains the ampullary sensory apparatus and is connected to the utricle. The three semicircular canals are positioned approximately perpendicular to each other. The posterior end of the lateral semicircular canal sits just in front of the middle of the posterior canal. The long axis of the posterior semicircular canal lies almost parallel with the plane of the posterior fossa dura behind it and its ampulla sits at its inferior end close to or medial to the vertical segment of the facial nerve. The non-ampullated ends of the superior and posterior canals join to form the common crus. The superior semicircular canal sits in or just below the mastoid tegmen with its ampulla forming its anterior end and sitting just above and medial to the ampulla of the lateral canal. These two ampullae form part of the medial wall of the epitympanum.

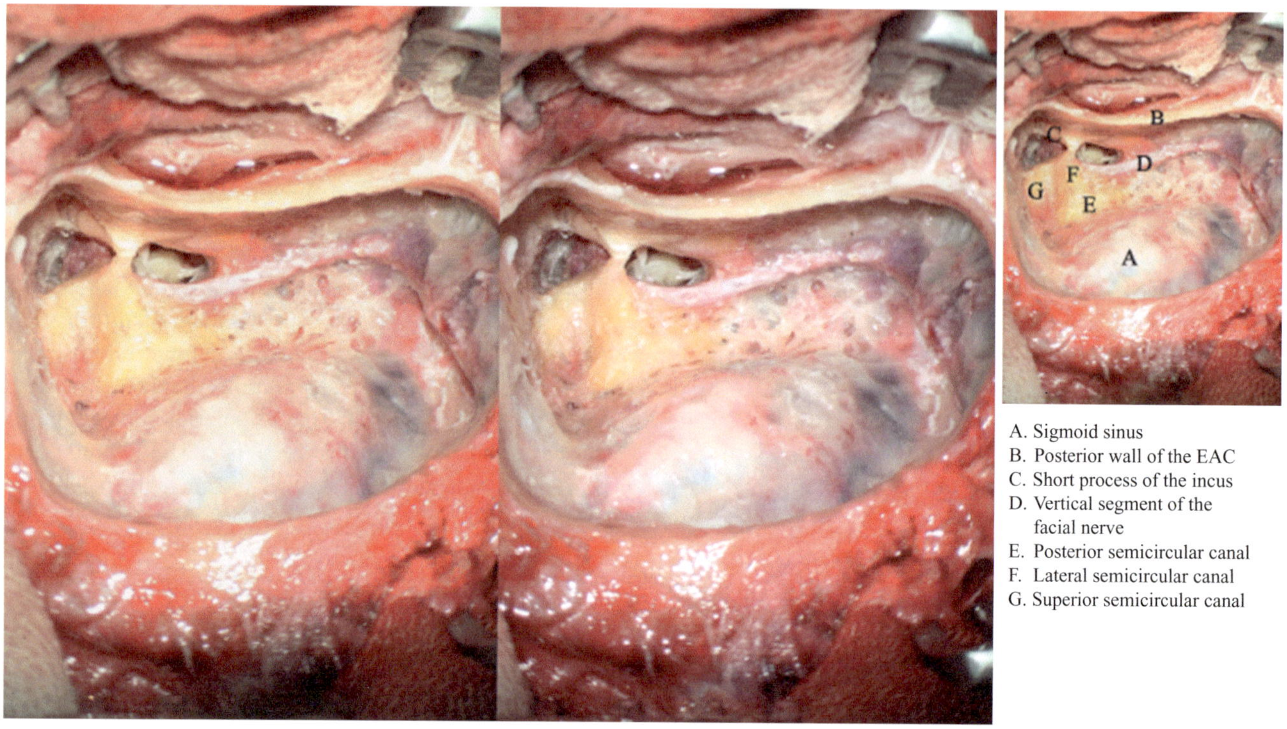

A. Sigmoid sinus
B. Posterior wall of the EAC
C. Short process of the incus
D. Vertical segment of the facial nerve
E. Posterior semicircular canal
F. Lateral semicircular canal
G. Superior semicircular canal

Fig. 4.35 Mastoid skeletonization (right)
As much as possible of the mastoid cavity bone should be removed. The bony capsule of the labyrinth is yellowish in color, compact and hard. The lateral semicircular canal is always located on the floor of the tympanic antrum, and based on the location of the lateral semicircular canal, the superior and posterior semicircular canals can be located. The canals are easier to identify in a well-pneumatized mastoid
Instruments: large-sized cutting burs; medium-sized diamond burs

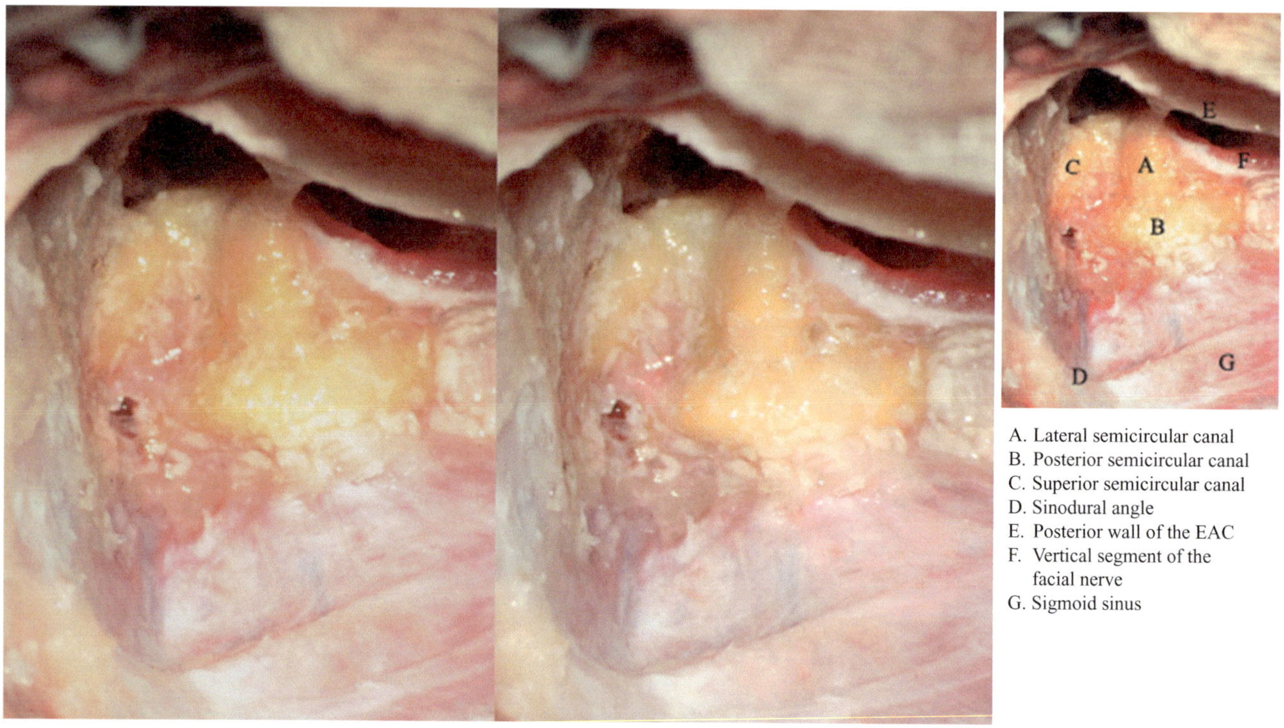

A. Lateral semicircular canal
B. Posterior semicircular canal
C. Superior semicircular canal
D. Sinodural angle
E. Posterior wall of the EAC
F. Vertical segment of the facial nerve
G. Sigmoid sinus

Fig. 4.36 Semicircular canal contouring (right)
Identify the position and configuration of the three semicircular canals. Remove the bone around the semicircular canals with different sized diamond burs to outline the shape of the three canals clearly. In this operative procedure, identify the anatomical landmarks of the incus short process, tegmen mastoideum, facial nerve, etc. Deep bone removal is not required in every procedure; proceed layer by layer, as necessary
Instruments: medium-sized cutting and diamond burs

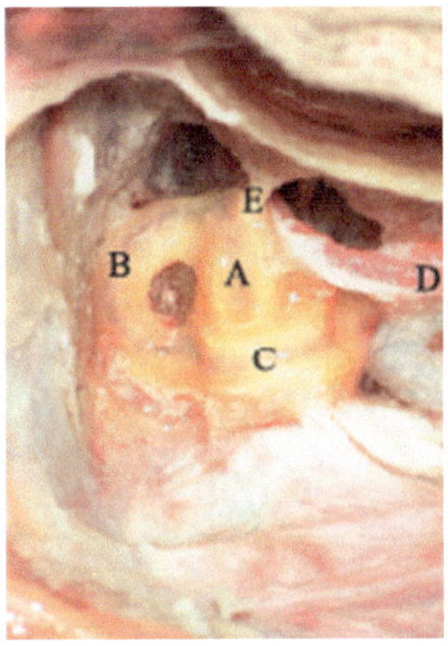

A. Blue line of the lateral semicircular canal
B. Blue line of the superior semicircular canal
C. Blue line of the posterior semicircular canal
D. Vertical segment of the facial nerve
E. Incus buttress

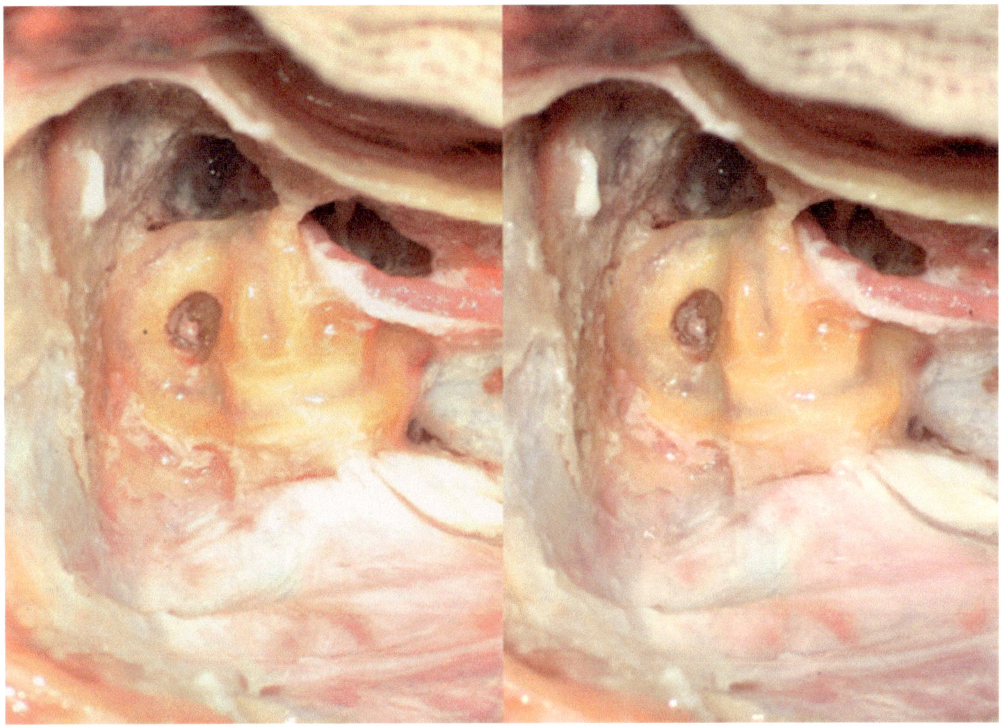

Fig. 4.37 Expose the blue lines of the semicircular canals (right)
After the shapes of the three canals have been clearly exposed, remove more bone from their lateral walls until the blue lines appear. Be careful to protect the membranous labyrinth

Instruments: medium-sized diamond burs

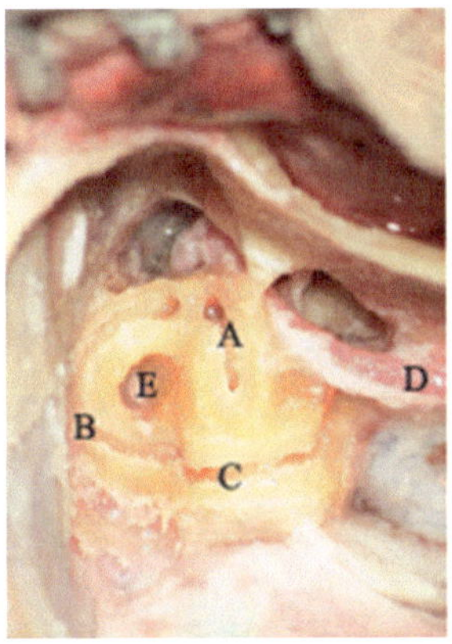

A. Opened lateral semicircular canal
B. Opened superior semicircular canal
C. Opened posterior semicircular canal
D. Mastoid segment of the facial nerve
E. Subarcuate artery

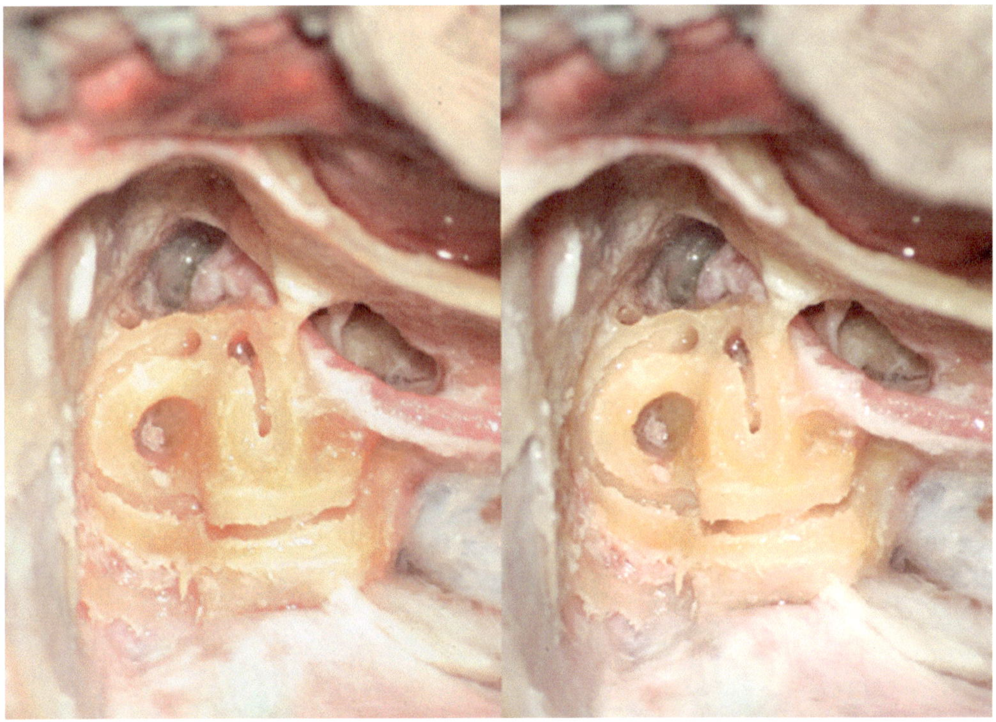

Fig. 4.38 Open semicircular canals (right)
Use a hook to remove the outer thinned bone of the three semicircular canals, then clearly identify their shapes. The superior and posterior semicircular canals are situated almost perpendicular to the lateral canal. The posterior end of the lateral canal sits just in front of the posterior canal level with its mid-point. The long axis of the posterior semicircular canal lies almost parallel with the plane of the posterior fossa dura behind it and its ampulla sits at its inferior end close to or medial to the vertical segment of the facial nerve. The superior end of the posterior semicircular canal joins the posterior end of the superior canal to form the common crus
Instruments: hooks

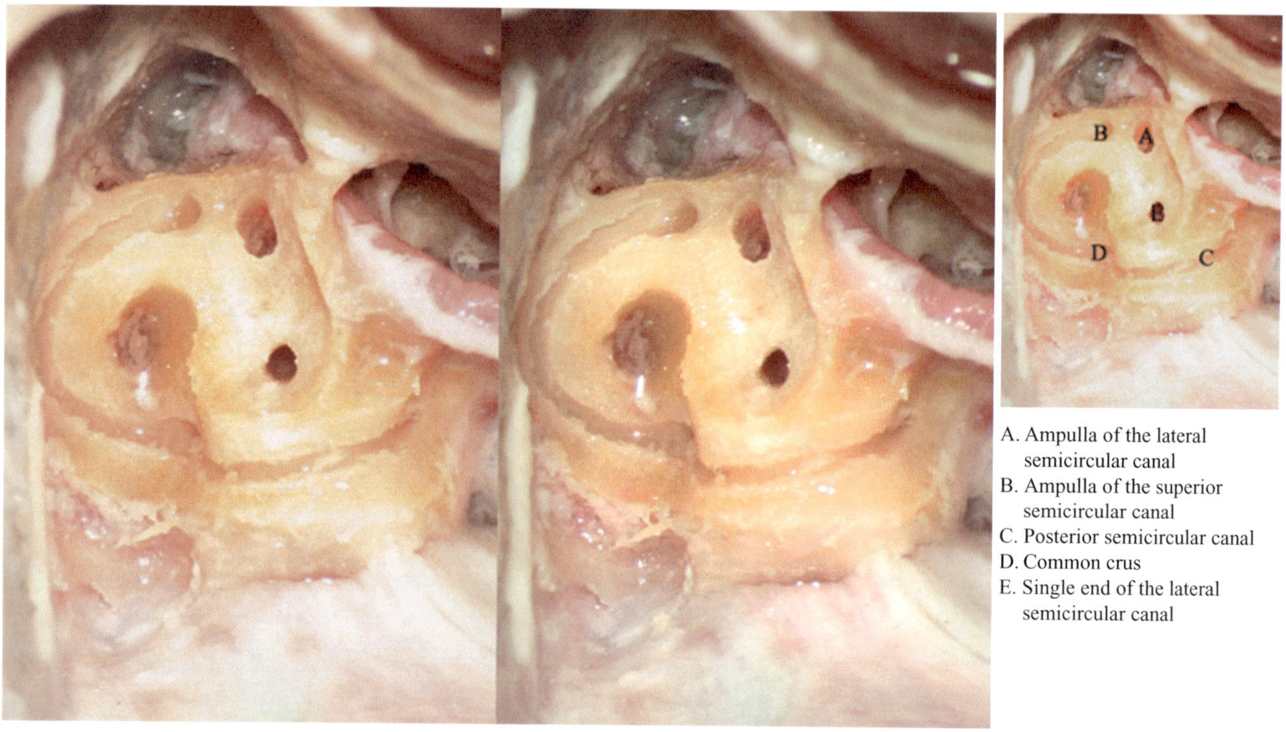

A. Ampulla of the lateral semicircular canal
B. Ampulla of the superior semicircular canal
C. Posterior semicircular canal
D. Common crus
E. Single end of the lateral semicircular canal

Fig. 4.39 Remove part of the lateral semicircular canal (right)
The three canals all connect with the vestibule. After drilling off more bone from the lateral semicircular canal, the vestibule can be clearly identified. The non-ampullated ends of the posterior and superior semicircular canals combine to form the common crus. The tympanic segment of the facial nerve is always close to the lateral semicircular canal
Instruments: medium-sized diamond burs

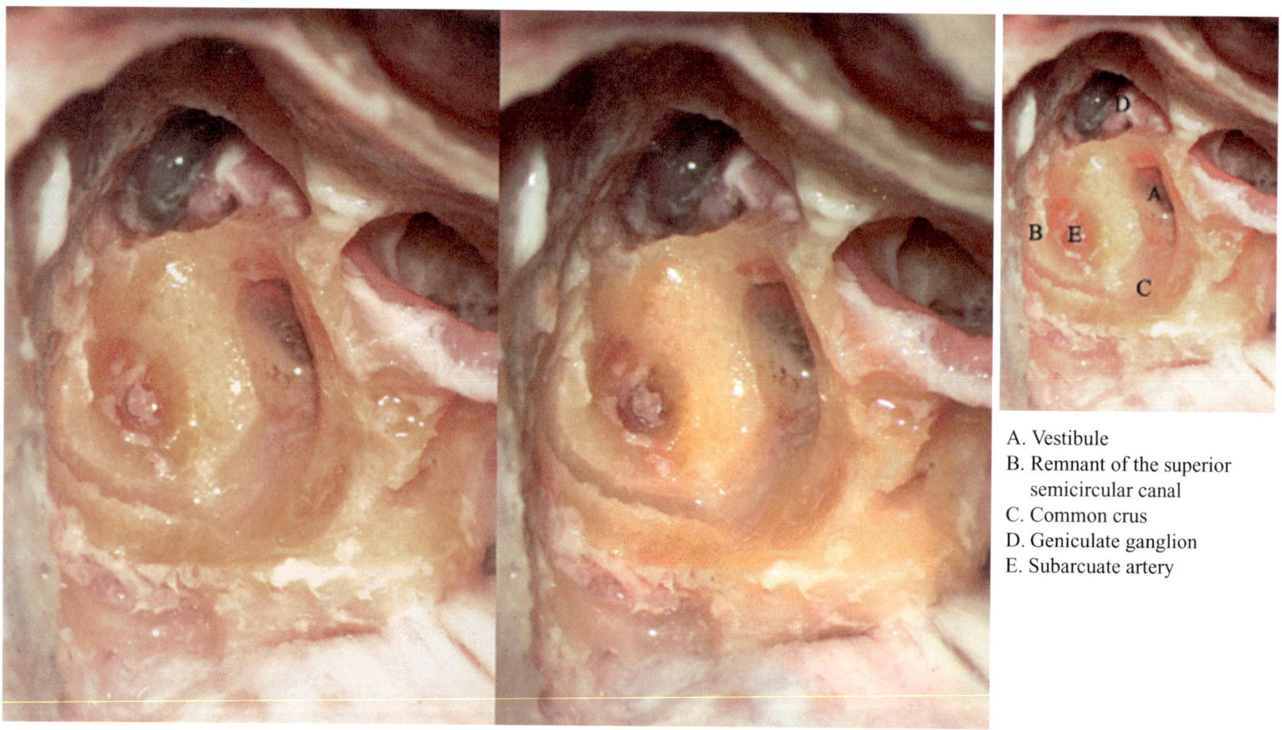

A. Vestibule
B. Remnant of the superior semicircular canal
C. Common crus
D. Geniculate ganglion
E. Subarcuate artery

Fig. 4.40 Open vestibule (right)
With the outer bony wall of the vestibule drilled away, its cavity is exposed. It lies between the IAC fundus medially and the oval window laterally. It is anterior to the semicircular canals whose five openings open into its posterior wall. The cochlea lies anterior to the vestibule with the ductus reuniens connecting the vestibule to the scala vestibuli of the cochlea
Instruments: medium-sized diamond burs

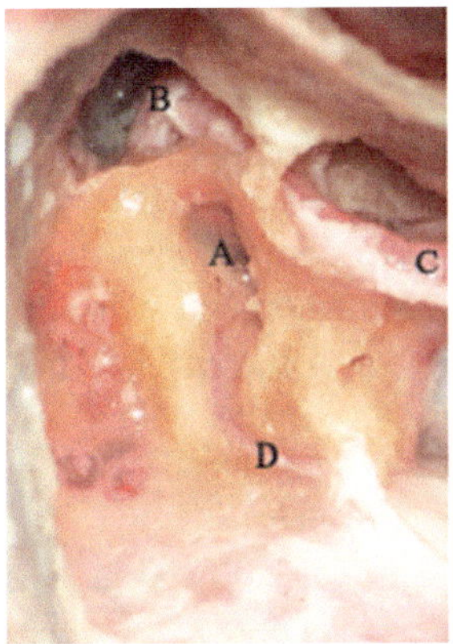

A. Opened vestibule
B. Geniculate ganglion
C. Mastoid segment of the facial nerve
D. Endolymphatic duct

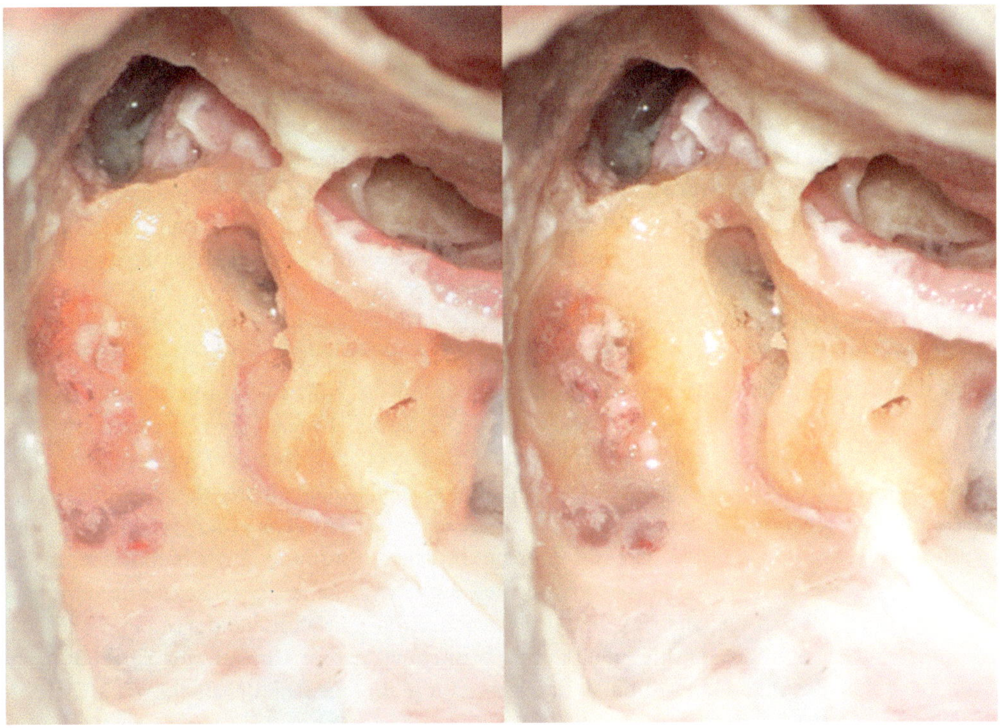

Fig. 4.41 Exposure of endolymphatic duct (right)
After drilling away the bone containing the common crus, the endolymphatic duct can be clearly identified. The endolymphatic duct connects the utricle and the saccule to the endolymphatic sac

Instruments: small-sized diamond burs

Anatomy of Sigmoid Sinus and Jugular Bulb

Yi Sun

The sigmoid sinus is located within a bony sulcus lying at the posterior edge of the mastoid segment of the temporal bone, starting at the end of the transverse sinus and ending at the jugular bulb. The sigmoid sinus is a space between the inner and outer layers of the dura, separated from the mastoid air cells by a thin layer of bone. The imaginary line connecting the parietal notch with the mastoid tip can be taken as the surface landmark of the sigmoid sinus. The average distance between the posterior wall of the EAC and the anterior wall of the sigmoid sinus is about 1.4 cm. The average distance between the cortex of the mastoid bone and the lateral wall of the sigmoid sinus is about 1 cm.

The position of the sigmoid sinus depends on the pneumatization of the mastoid. A posteriorly located sigmoid sinus is found in well-pneumatized mastoids, whereas an anteriorly located sigmoid sinus is found in poorly pneumatized mastoids. An anterior location is the most common anatomic variation of the sigmoid sinus. If the distance between the posterior wall of the EAC and the anterior wall of the sigmoid sinus is less than 1 cm, the sinus is said to be anterior. This distance can be accurately measured in axial sections of high-resolution computed tomography (HRCT). CT scanning is currently a very reliable tool in determining such anatomic variations.

The sigmoid sinus ends at the posterior margin of the jugular fossa, where it expands and arches upward to form the jugular bulb. The jugular bulb is located within the posterior compartment of the jugular fossa lying beneath the petrous bone and joins inferiorly with the internal jugular vein. Its width is about 15 mm and its height is about 14 mm. The position and size of the jugular bulb are variable. Pulsatile tinnitus is a common symptom in ENT practice and may be due to a dilated mastoid emissary vein or sigmoid sinus diverticulum. Their presence is suspected if the tinnitus is in time with the heart rate and can be relieved by soft compression of the lateral side of the internal jugular vein in the neck.

Anatomic variations in the jugular bulb include a high jugular bulb, jugular bulb diverticulum, and medially or laterally located jugular bulb. A high jugular bulb and jugular bulb diverticulum are the most common. A high jugular bulb is most commonly seen on the right side, which usually has the dominant sigmoid sinus-internal jugular vein complex, and is larger than the left. Anatomic variations in the jugular bulb can usually be identified using HRCT. The incidence of a high jugular bulb has been variously reported in different studies because of different diagnostic criteria. A high jugular bulb incidence is reported when the jugular bulb extends above the inferior aspect of the bony annulus—6%, the basal turn of the cochlea—20.3%, the level of the round window—24%, and the bottom portion of the IAC—9%, respectively.

A high jugular bulb is diagnosed if the jugular bulb dome reaches or extends over the level of the round window or the basal turn of the cochlea. Jugular bulb diverticulum is an irregular outpouching that may extend to the anterior, medial, or superior surface of the petrous bone, or to the IAC, and results in relative rarefaction of bone between the posterior fossa dura and the posterior semicircular canal. The incidence of a jugular bulb diverticulum is lower than that of a high jugular bulb, at less than 1%.

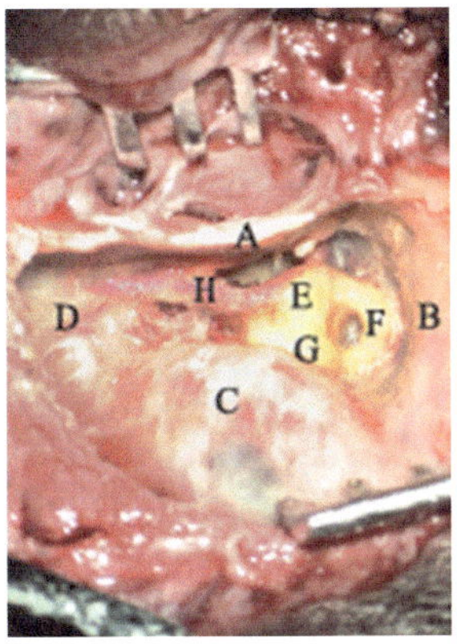

A. Posterior wall of the EAC
B. Tegmen mastoideum
C. Sigmoid sinus
D. Digastric ridge
E. Lateral semicircular canal
F. Superior semicircular canal
G. Posterior semicircular canal
H. Mastoid segment of the facial nerve

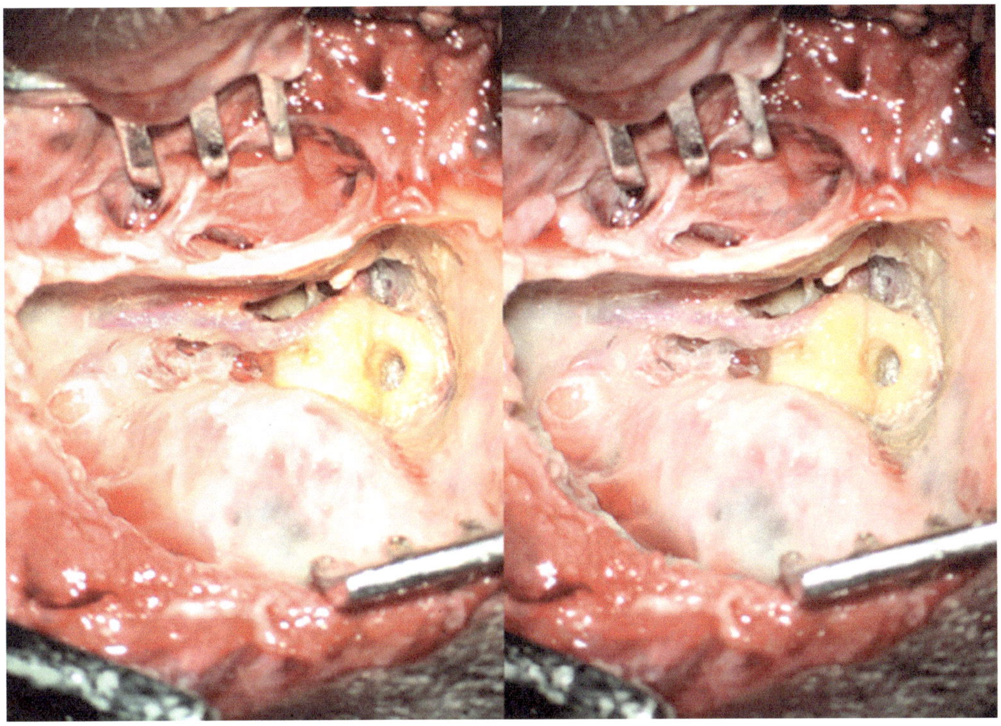

Fig. 4.42 Skeletonization of the mastoid; exposure of the sigmoid sinus (left)
Drill away the mastoid air cells, skeletonize the mastoid, and the dense bone covering the sigmoid sinus can be seen. Gradually thin down the bone until it is semitransparent, and then further skeletonize the three semicircular canals, the mastoid segment of the facial nerve and the digastric ridge. The spatial relationships and relative sizes of these anatomical landmarks can be observed, and this three-dimensional information should be fully considered throughout the dissection
Instruments: large-sized cutting burs, medium-sized diamond burs

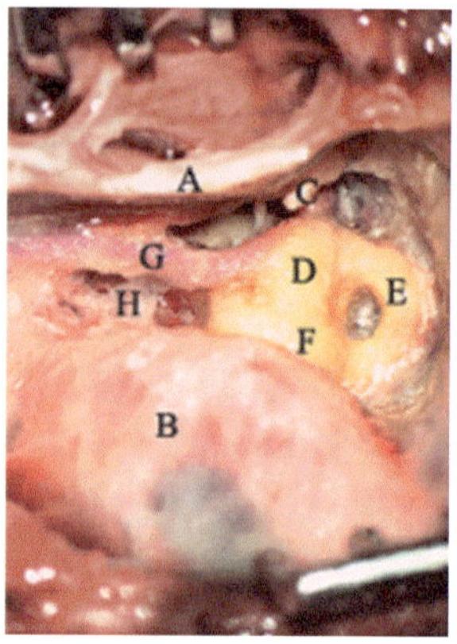

A. Posterior wall of the EAC
B. Sigmoid sinus
C. Short process of the incus
D. Lateral semicircular canal
E. Superior semicircular canal
F. Posterior semicircular canal
G. Mastoid segment of the facial nerve
H. Bony wall of the jugular bulb

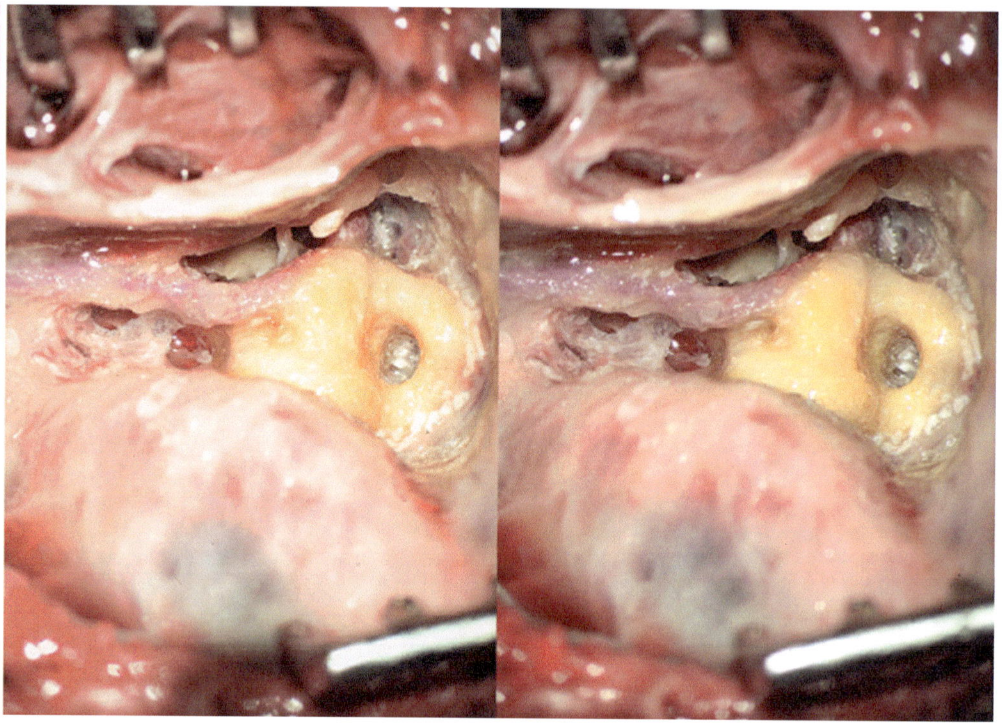

Fig. 4.43 Dissection of air cells inferior to the bony labyrinth and retro-facial air cells (left)
The jugular bulb is located medial to the mastoid segment of the facial nerve and digastric ridge, inferior to the posterior semicircular canal ampullary end and the hypotympanum. The sizes and positions of jugular bulbs are variable. First, exploration of the jugular bulb is performed gradually following the sigmoid sinus; next, to explore the position of the jugular bulb, the mastoid segment of the facial nerve and posterior semicircular canal are used as anatomical landmarks. The bone is gradually thinned down progressing inward
Instruments: medium-sized diamond burs

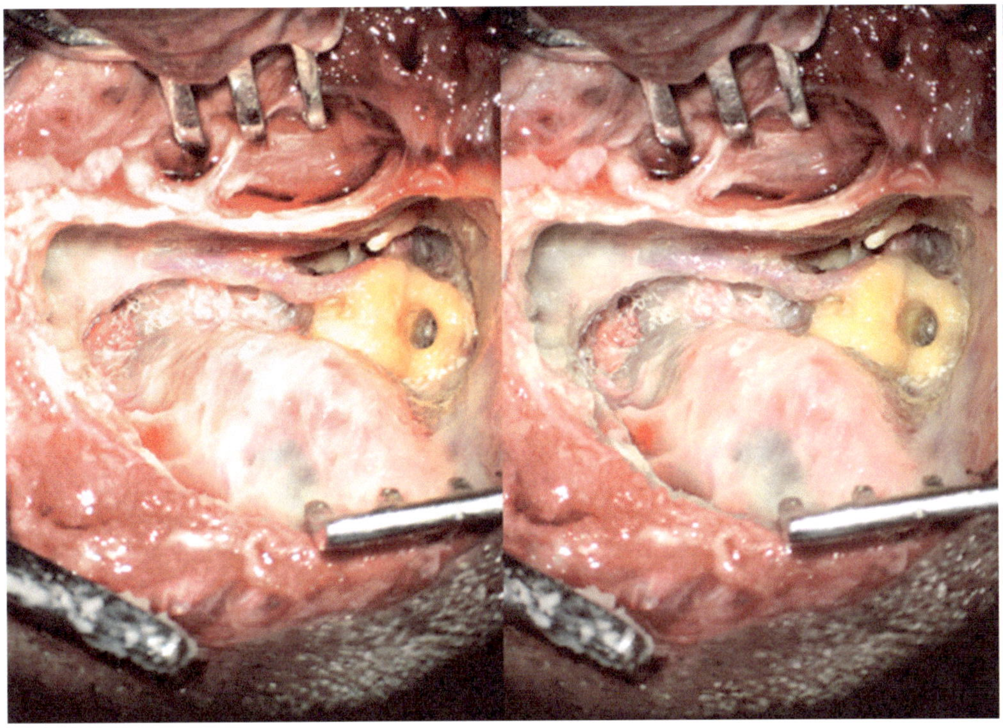

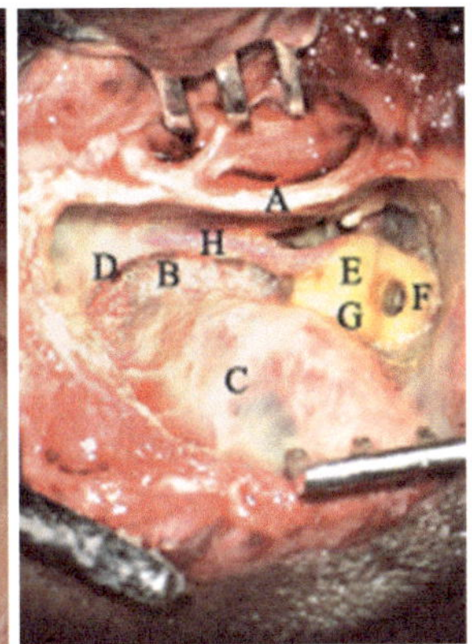

A. Posterior wall of the EAC
B. Retro-facial air cells
C. Sigmoid sinus
D. Digastric ridge
E. Lateral semicircular canal
F. Superior semicircular canal
G. Posterior semicircular canal
H. Mastoid segment of the facial nerve

Fig. 4.44 Exposure of the bone lateral to the jugular bulb (left)
The lower posterior bone over the jugular bulb is thinned down following the sigmoid sinus; the lateral bone over the jugular bulb is thinned down following the mastoid segment of the facial nerve and digastric ridge; the superior and lateral bone over the jugular bulb is then thinned down, taking the posterior semicircular canal ampullary end as the upper boundary. The position of the jugular bulb can then be identified. If the sigmoid sinus is located anteriorly, the sigmoid sinus should be skeletonized first and then the bone over it should be dissected completely until it can be retracted to widen the operative field. The vascular wall of the jugular bulb is very thin; the bone over it should be gently dissected and not drilled, in order to avoid injury to the jugular bulb
Instruments: medium-sized diamond burs

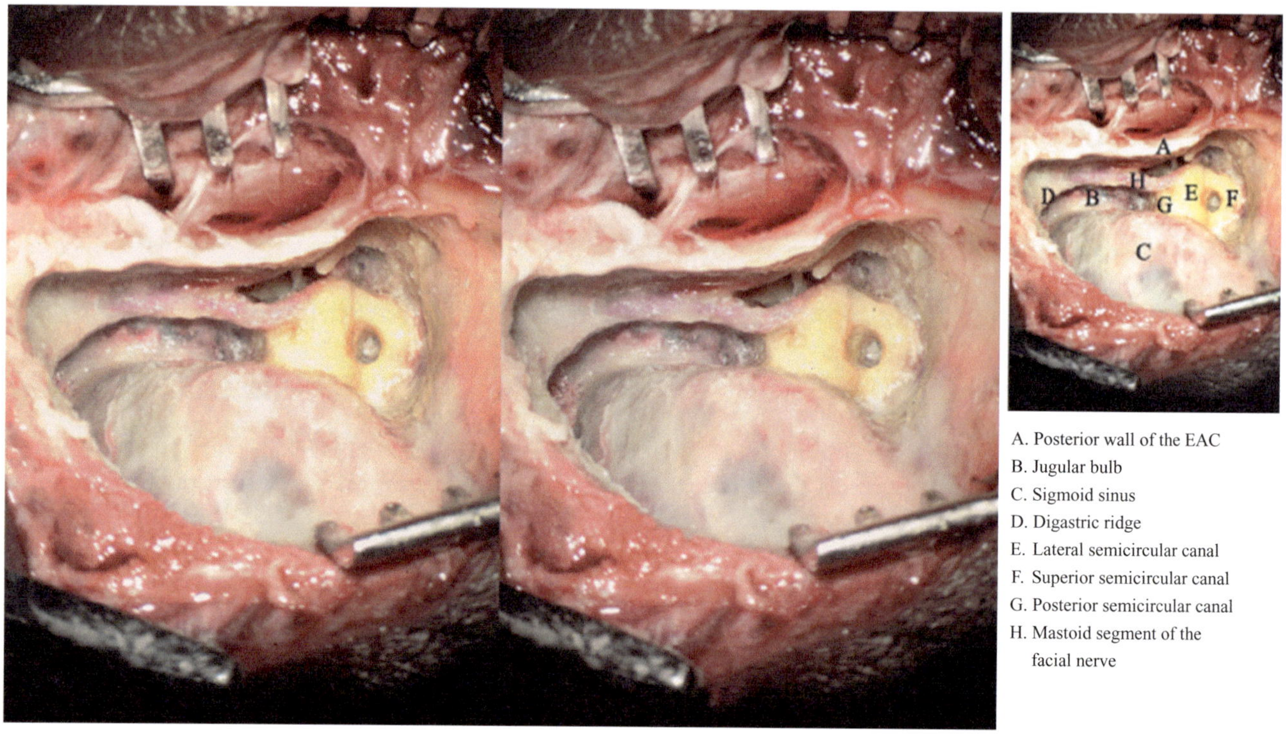

A. Posterior wall of the EAC
B. Jugular bulb
C. Sigmoid sinus
D. Digastric ridge
E. Lateral semicircular canal
F. Superior semicircular canal
G. Posterior semicircular canal
H. Mastoid segment of the facial nerve

Fig. 4.45 Exposure of the jugular bulb (left)
The lateral air cells over the jugular bulb are removed completely and the bone over it is thinned down to expose the bulb. The full length of the sigmoid sinus can be seen. The bottom end of the sigmoid sinus turns forward and upward, then expands and arches upward to form the jugular bulb. The intimate relationship between the jugular bulb and the mastoid segment of the facial nerve, hypotympanum, posterior semicircular canal, sigmoid sinus, posterior fossa dura, and digastric ridge can be observed
Instruments: medium-sized diamond burs

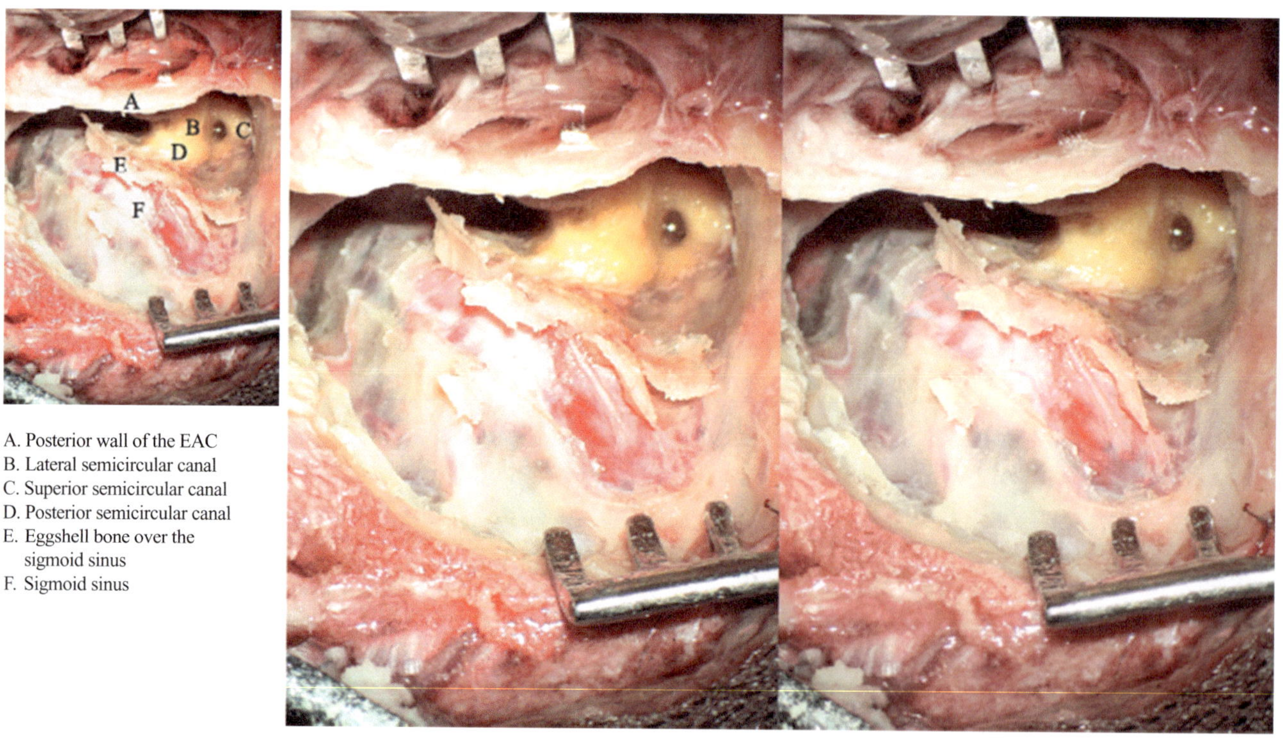

A. Posterior wall of the EAC
B. Lateral semicircular canal
C. Superior semicircular canal
D. Posterior semicircular canal
E. Eggshell bone over the sigmoid sinus
F. Sigmoid sinus

Fig. 4.46 Expose the sigmoid sinus
To train one's abilities in accurate operative technique and use of the bur, the bone over the sigmoid sinus should be thinned down gradually using a large diamond bur until it is very thin and compressible. The eggshell bone plate is dissected off the sigmoid sinus using a middle-ear elevator, to expose the vessel wall completely
Instruments: large-sized diamond burs, middle ear elevator

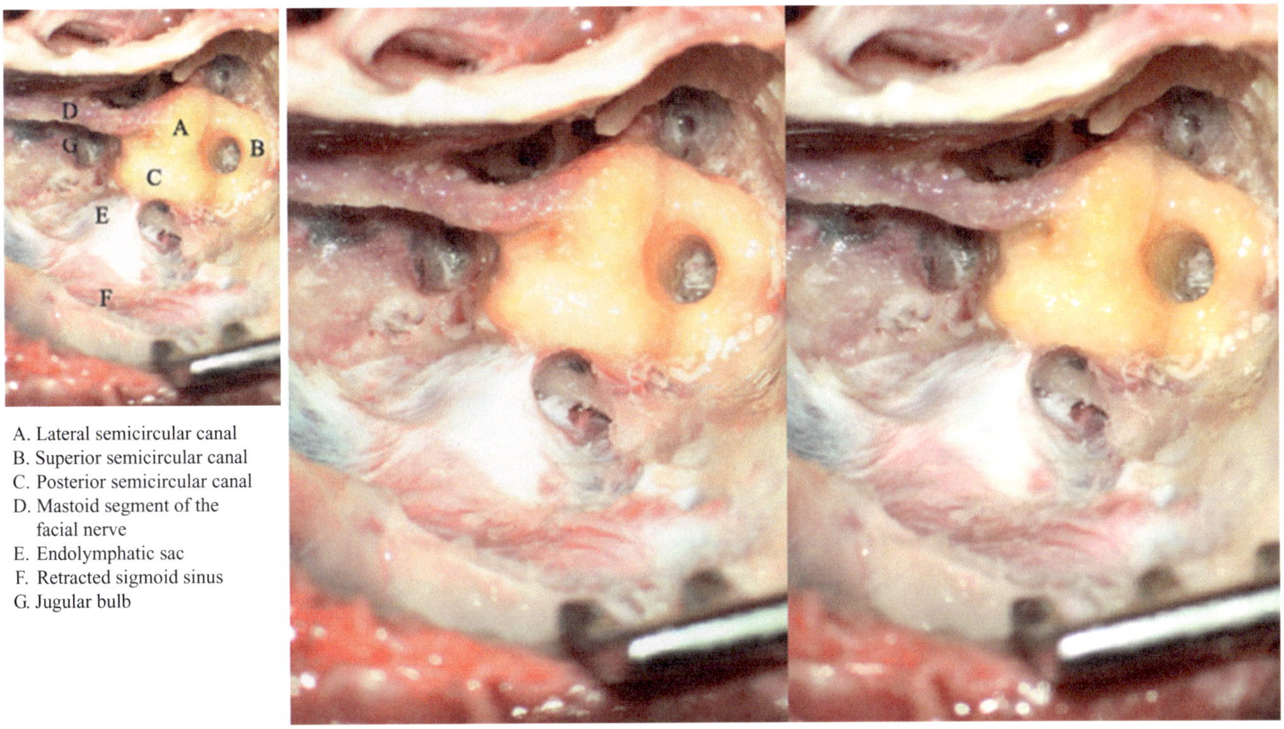

A. Lateral semicircular canal
B. Superior semicircular canal
C. Posterior semicircular canal
D. Mastoid segment of the facial nerve
E. Endolymphatic sac
F. Retracted sigmoid sinus
G. Jugular bulb

Fig. 4.47 Dissection of sigmoid sinus, jugular bulb, and the posterior fossa plate (left)
The bone over the sigmoid sinus, jugular bulb, and posterior fossa plate is thinned down further, the last eggshell bone over the sigmoid sinus is removed and the sigmoid sinus then retracts. Retraction of the sigmoid sinus exposes the white endolymphatic sac, with the pink facial nerve and yellow bony labyrinth lying deep in the mastoid cavity
Instruments: large- or medium-sized diamond burs, middle ear elevator

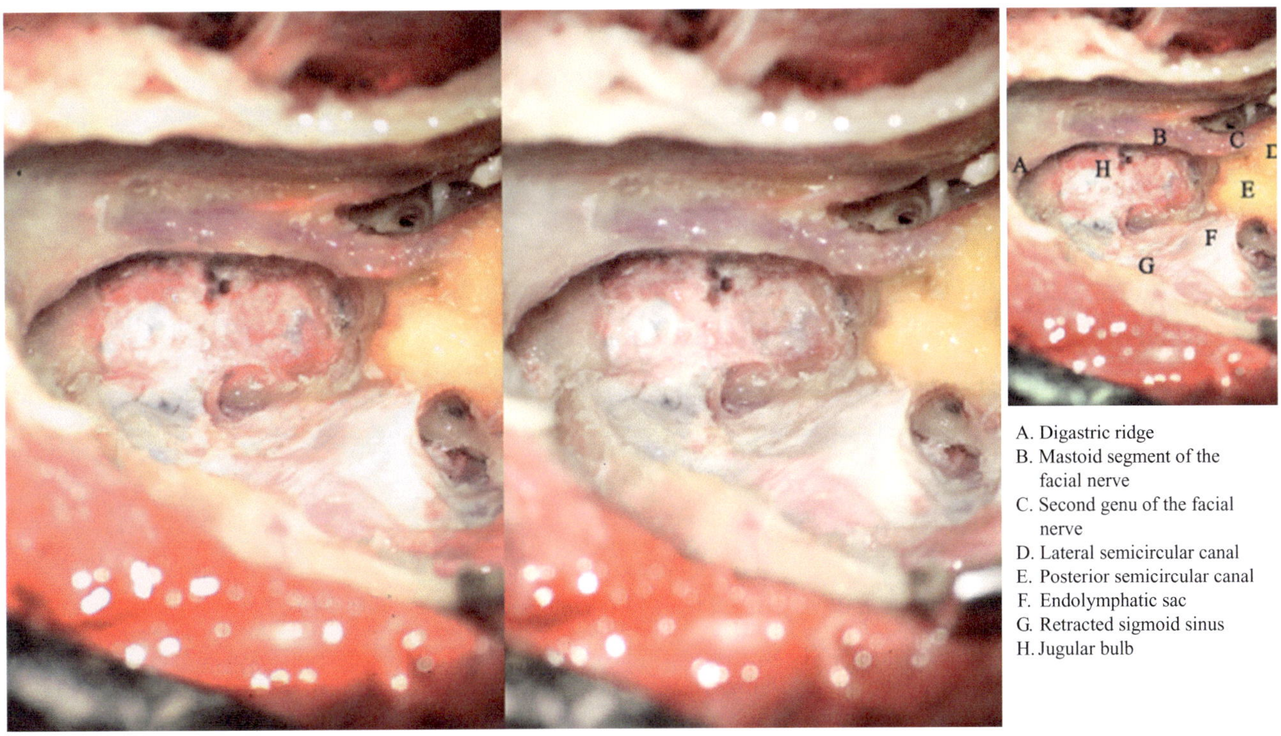

A. Digastric ridge
B. Mastoid segment of the facial nerve
C. Second genu of the facial nerve
D. Lateral semicircular canal
E. Posterior semicircular canal
F. Endolymphatic sac
G. Retracted sigmoid sinus
H. Jugular bulb

Fig. 4.48 Exposure of the whole jugular bulb (left)
The bone over the jugular bulb has been removed completely. The relationships between the jugular bulb and its landmarks are identified: EAC medial end, hypotympanum floor, promontory (the oval window and open scala tympani can be seen through the facial recess), posterior semicircular canal ampullary end, IAC external end superiorly, mastoid segment of the facial nerve anteriorly, digastric ridge inferolaterally, sigmoid sinus, endolymphatic sac and posterior fossa dura posteriorly
Instruments: medium-sized diamond burs, middle ear elevator

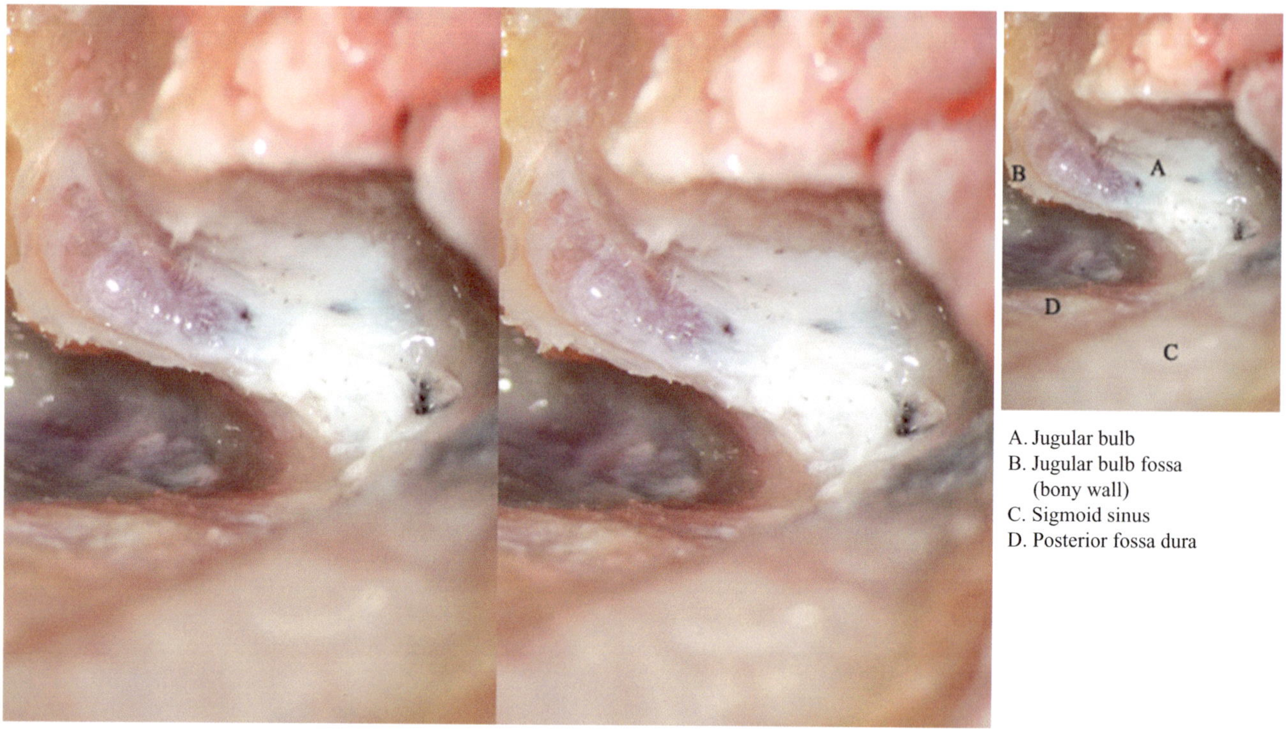

A. Jugular bulb
B. Jugular bulb fossa (bony wall)
C. Sigmoid sinus
D. Posterior fossa dura

Fig. 4.49 Jugular bulb (right)
In this picture, the full length of the right sigmoid sinus and jugular bulb can be seen. The jugular bulb sits in the jugular fossa; the walls are thin and semitransparent, and surgery should be performed carefully to avoid injury to the thin bulb wall

Anatomy of the Tympanic Cavity

Bao-chun Sun and Song Gao

Six Walls of the Tympanic Cavity

1. Outer wall, also called the membranous wall: consists of two parts, the pars tensa, lateral to the mesotympanum, and the pars flaccida, lateral to the epitympanum (attic).
2. Inner wall, also called the labyrinthine wall or the outer wall of the inner ear. The prominence in the middle of the inner wall is called the promontory, in which lies the basal turn of the cochlea. The small hollow posterosuperior to the promontory is called the oval window niche. Its anteroposterior diameter is 3.3 mm and its height is 1.8 mm. At the bottom of the oval window niche is the oval window, which has an area of about 3.2 mm^2 and is closed by the stapedial footplate and annular ligament. There is a fovea in the posterior aspect of the promontory called the round window niche, at the depth of which is the round window, closed by the round window membrane, with an area of 2 mm^2. It lies in a coronal plane perpendicular to that of the stapedial footplate and seals off the tympanic end of the cochlear canal. The cochleariform process is located slightly above the front of the oval window. It contains the tympanic end of the semicanal for the tensor tympani muscle as it turns laterally through a right angle to exit the process, then attaches to the inner side of the junction of the manubrium and neck of the malleus.
3. Anterior wall, also called the carotid wall: the lower part of the anterior wall is separated from the carotid artery by a very thin bony lamella, which may be deficient. The upper part of the anterior wall has two openings, of which the upper one is the opening of the semicanal for the tensor tympani muscle and the lower one is the tympanic opening of the Eustachian (auditory) tube.
4. Posterior wall, also called the mastoid wall: wider above than below, the vertical part of the facial nerve passes through its medial side. The upper part of the posterior wall has the aditus and the superior tympanum, which are connected with the mastoid antrum via the aditus ad antrum. The prominence of the anterior end of the lateral semicircular canal sits on the floor of the aditus and just above this is the incudal fossa, which accommodates the short process of the incus. There is a vertical ridge in the wall that separates the two parts of the posterior tympanum: the facial recess laterally from the sinus tympani medially. Lying on the facial nerve canal, at the level of the oval window, is the pyramidal process, from which the stapedius tendon emerges to attach to the neck of the stapes; the chorda tympani enters the middle ear via a canaliculus, positioned between the pyramidal eminence and the tympanic sulcus.
5. Superior wall, also called the tegmen tympani: separates the tympanum from the middle cranial fossa and extends backward as the tympanic antrum plate.
6. Inferior wall, also called the jugular wall: a narrow thin bone lamella separates the tympanum from the jugular bulb; its anterior part is the posterior wall of the carotid canal. It contains a foramen through which the tympanic branch of the glossopharyngeal nerve (Jacobson's nerve) passes.

Tympanum Contents

1. Auditory ossicles: a chain of three ossicles that are the smallest bones in the human body; the malleus, incus, and stapes.
2. Ossicular ligaments: superior, anterior, and lateral ligaments of the malleus, superior and posterior ligaments of the incus, and the annular ligament of the stapes. The ligaments jointly secure and suspend the ossicles in the tympanum.
3. Tympanic muscles: (1) the tensor tympani muscle arises from the cartilaginous part of the auditory tube, the greater wing of the sphenoid bone and the wall of the canal for the tensor tympani muscle, and its tendon passes at a right angle through the cochleariform process to insert at the junction of the handle and neck of the malleus. Its movement is controlled by a branch from the mandibular division of the trigeminal nerve. When the tensor tympani muscle contracts, it pulls the manubrium inward and increases the tympanic membrane tension to prevent excessive vibration of the tympanic membrane and subsequent damage to the inner ear. (2) the stapedius muscle arises within the pyramidal eminence in the posterior wall of the tympanum; its tendon protrudes out of the pyramidal eminence, passing forward to insert into the posterior part of the neck of the stapes. Its movement is controlled by a small branch of the facial nerve; when the stapedius muscle contracts, it pulls the superstructure backward, which tilts and fixes the stapedial footplate to reduce excessive vibration in the inner ear.

Recesses of the Tympanic Cavity and Tympanic Diaphragm

Recesses of the tympanic cavity: the mucosa of the tympanic cavity covers the ossicles and ligaments and forms many small mucosal recesses, which communicate with the tympanic cavity. (1) Anterior and posterior recesses of the malleus are located between the head of the malleus, the anterior wall of the tympanic cavity and the anterior and superior ligaments of the malleus, or behind the superior ligament of the malleus; (2) Superior and inferior recesses of the incus are located above and below the short process of the incus;

(3) Superior recess of the tympanic membrane, also called Prussak's space, is located between the flaccid part of the tympanic membrane and the neck of the malleus; the upper boundary is the lateral ligament of the malleus and the lower boundary is the lateral process of the malleus; (4) Anterior and posterior recesses of the tympanic membrane are separately located between the tympanic membrane and the anterior and posterior folds of the malleus.

Tympanic diaphragm: the mesotympanum and epitympanum are not freely connected, but are separated by the tympanic diaphragm consisting of the head and neck of the malleus, the body and short process of the incus, anterior and lateral ligaments of the malleus, posterior ligament of the incus, the inner and outer incudal folds, the fold of the tensor tympani muscle and the malleal folds. The tympanic diaphragm contains the anterior and posterior isthmuses to connect the mesotympanum and epitympanum. Due to the existence of various recesses and mucosal folds in the tympanum, the channel between the middle and upper tympanum is narrow, and can easily be blocked when the mucous membrane is swollen, which results in various pathological changes. However, the recesses and mucosal folds of the tympanum can also limit the spread of pathological changes, including infection and cholesteatoma.

Mucous Membrane of the Tympanum

The walls, ossicles, muscle tendons, ligaments, and nerves of the tympanum are covered with mucous membrane. The mucous membrane connects that of the Eustachian tube anteriorly and the mastoid, antrum, and air cells posteriorly. The mucous membrane of the middle ear is cuboidal or low columnar ciliated posteriorly, and columnar ciliated or pseudo-stratified columnar ciliated anteriorly.

Blood Vessels and Nerves of the Tympanum

Blood vessels of the tympanum: arterial blood of the tympanum is mainly supplied by the external carotid artery. The anterior tympanic branch of the maxillary artery mainly supplies the front part of the tympanum, and the stylomastoid branch of the posterior auricular artery mainly supplies the rear part of the tympanum and the mastoid process. The superior tympanic and superficial petrosal branches of the middle meningeal artery supply the roof and medial wall of the tympanum. The inferior branch of the ascending pharyngeal artery supplies the lower part of the tympanum and the tensor tympani muscle. The tympanic branch of the internal carotid artery supplies the front wall of the tympanum. The outer layer of the tympanic membrane is supplied by the deep tympanic branch of the maxillary artery, and the inner layer of the tympanum is supplied by the anterior tympanic and stylomastoid arteries.

The nerves of the tympanum mainly include: (1) the tympanic plexus, which consists of the tympanic branch of the glossopharyngeal nerve (Jacobson's nerve) and the upper and lower carotico-tympanic nerves from the carotid sympathetic nerve. It is located on the promontory surface, and serves the sensation of the tympanum, Eustachian tube and mucous membrane of the mastoid air cell system; (2) nerve to the tensor tympani muscle; (3) the facial nerve passes from front to back in the medial wall, then vertically down in the posterior wall of the tympanum. The chorda tympani branches off the facial nerve from the lower half of the vertical segment and passes upwards and forward through a canaliculus, then between the malleus handle laterally and the long process of the incus medially, exits the middle ear via the petrotympanic fissure, and finally connects with the lingual nerve to supply the sense of taste to the anterior two-third of the tongue.

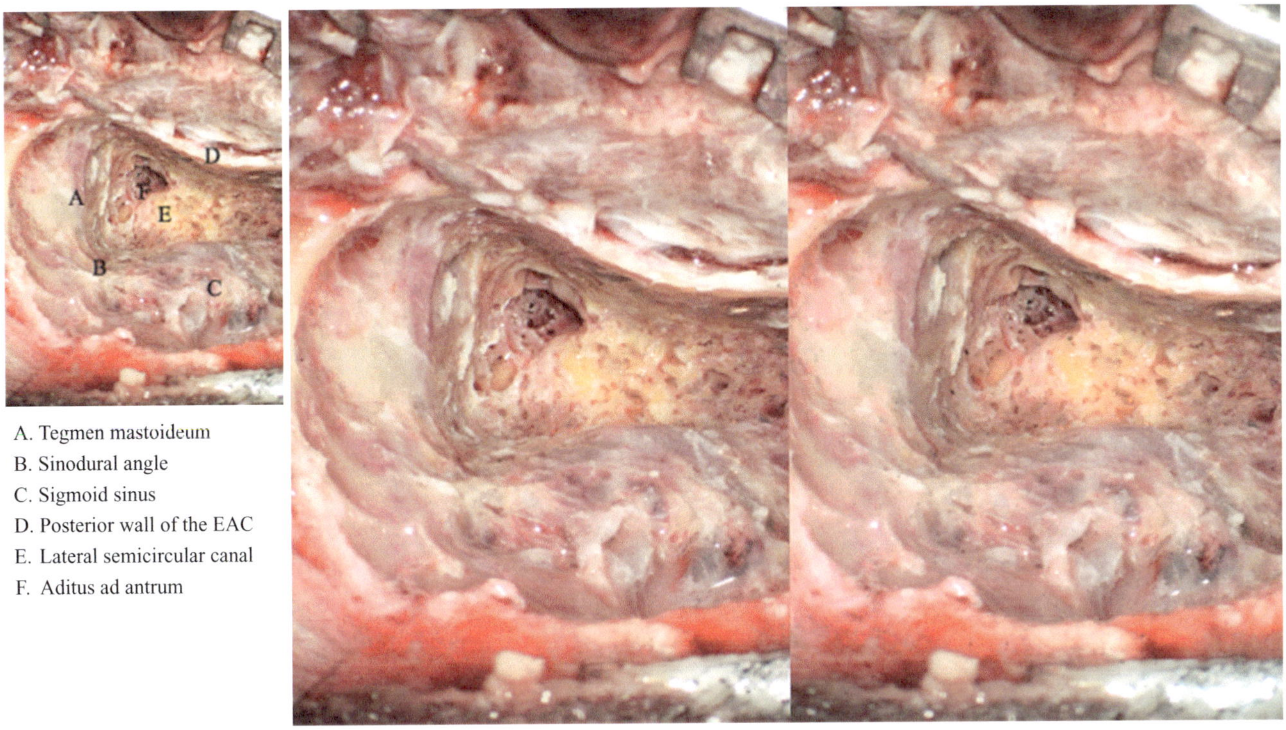

A. Tegmen mastoideum
B. Sinodural angle
C. Sigmoid sinus
D. Posterior wall of the EAC
E. Lateral semicircular canal
F. Aditus ad antrum

Fig. 4.50 Open the mastoid cavity; widen the aditus ad antrum (right) Open the mastoid cavity widely, including the aditus ad antrum, expose the short process of the incus, and open the epitympanum. Before epitympanotomy, deepen the sinodural angle and open the mastoid cavity as required to expose the target structures. *Hints: (1) Maintain the integrity of the bony walls of the mastoid cavity. (2) The progression of drilling should proceed from outside to inside to avoid damage to the deep tissues. (3) Use continuous irrigation during drilling to keep the field clear*
Instruments: large-sized cutting burs, medium-sized diamond burs

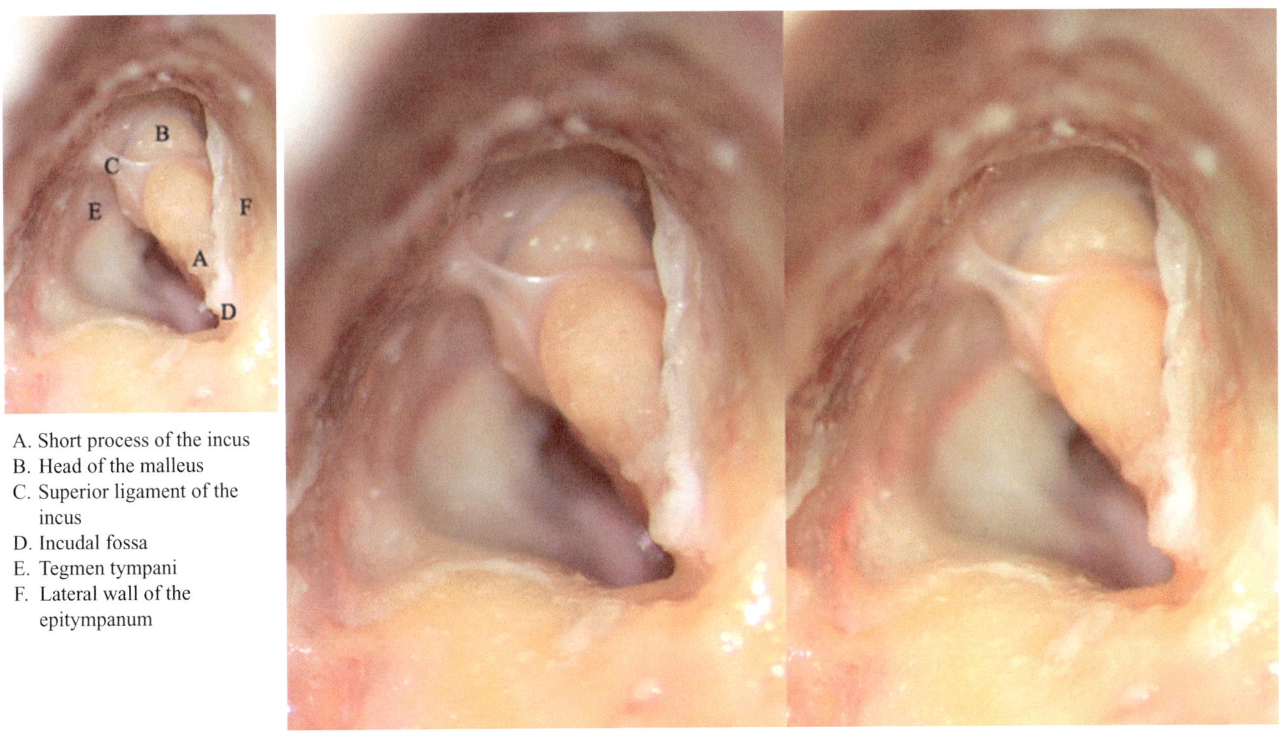

A. Short process of the incus
B. Head of the malleus
C. Superior ligament of the incus
D. Incudal fossa
E. Tegmen tympani
F. Lateral wall of the epitympanum

Fig. 4.51 Posterior part of the epitympanum (right)
Overview of the epitympanum: the tegmen tympani of the middle fossa is superior, the incudal fossa and lateral semicircular canal are inferior, and the wall of the external ear canal is lateral. Identify the incudomalleal joint, incus body, short process of the incus, superior and posterior ligaments of the incus, and the superior fold of the malleus. The key to enlarging the aditus ad antrum is to select the appropriate drills. It is recommended to use a drill with a diameter of 1/2 to 2/3 the width of the aditus, which is efficient and safe
Instruments: medium-sized diamond burs

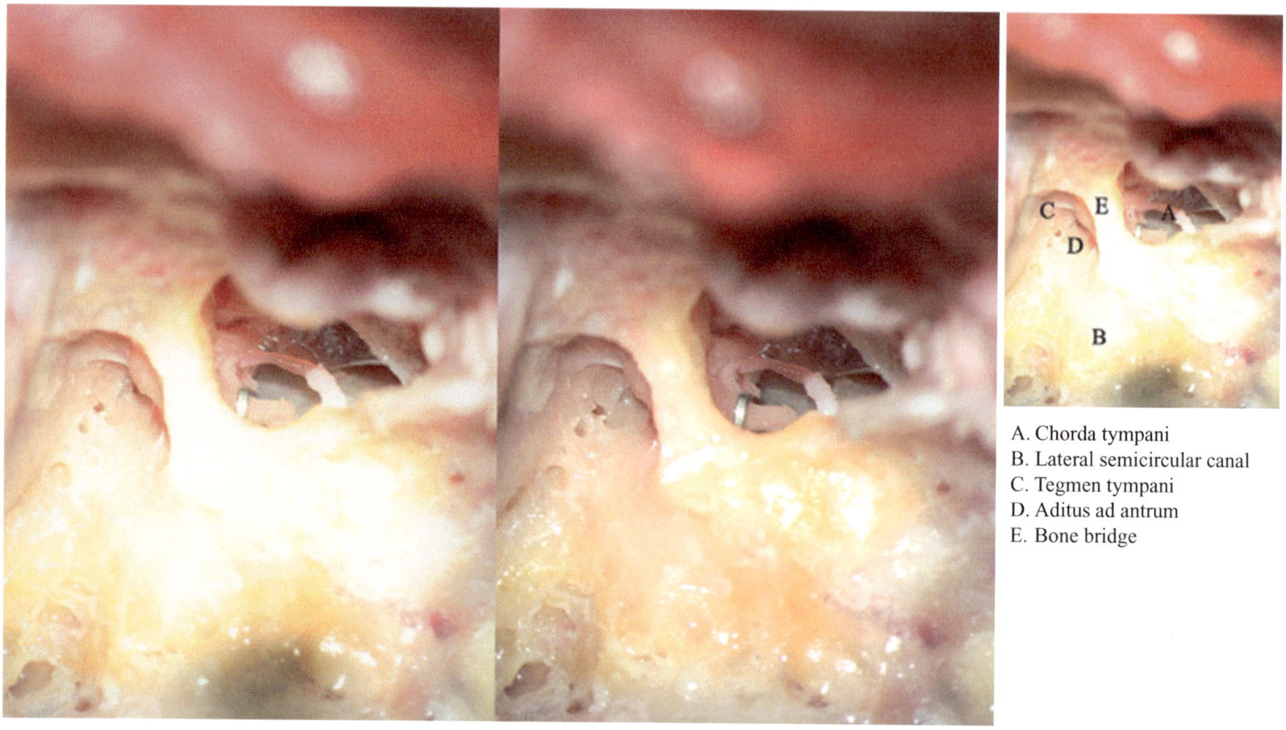

A. Chorda tympani
B. Lateral semicircular canal
C. Tegmen tympani
D. Aditus ad antrum
E. Bone bridge

Fig. 4.52 Exposure of bone bridge (right)
Remove the posterior and superior walls of the EAC from outside to inside; part of the lateral wall of the epitympanum is retained, which is the bone bridge. The ossicular chain is located deep to the bone bridge, which is formed by the anterior and posterior buttresses together
Instruments: medium-sized cutting and diamond burs

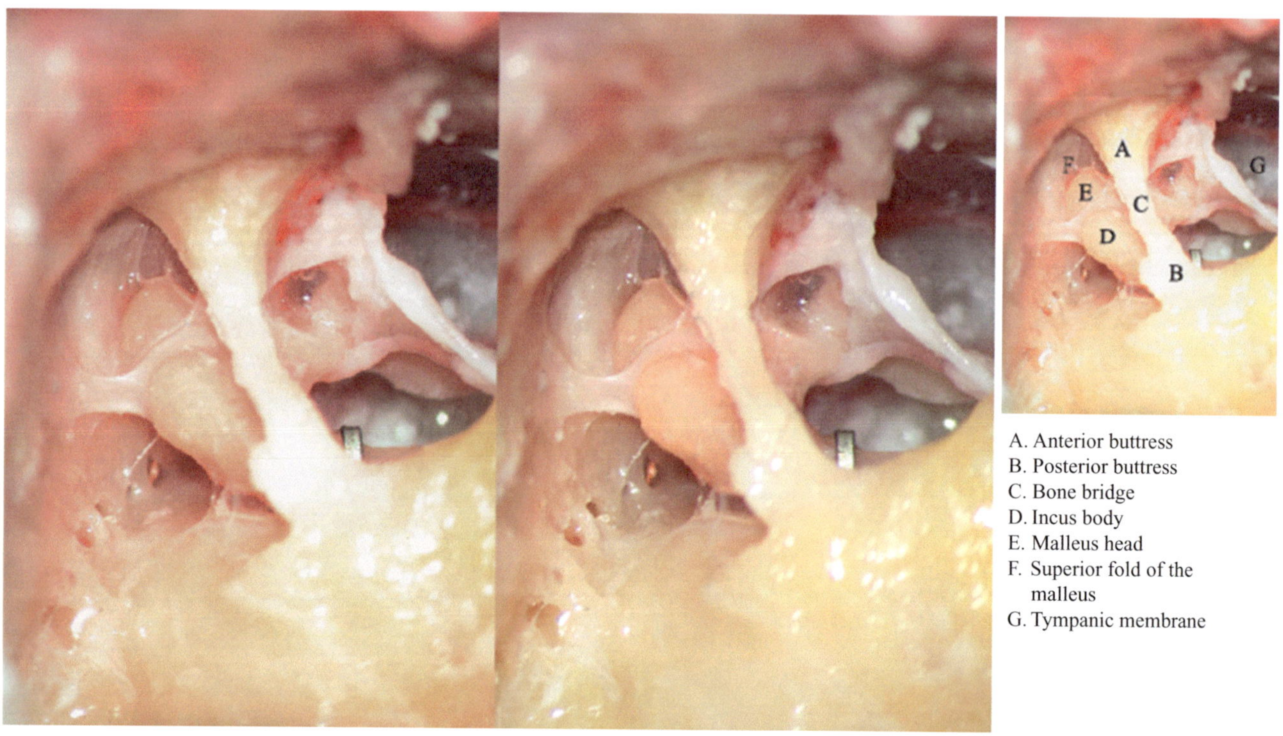

A. Anterior buttress
B. Posterior buttress
C. Bone bridge
D. Incus body
E. Malleus head
F. Superior fold of the malleus
G. Tympanic membrane

Fig. 4.53 Bone bridge and tympanum (right)
The bone bridge is located lateral to the ossicular chain, and its anterior end is part of the tympanic scutum. Drill carefully around the bone bridge using a medium-sized diamond bur until it is thin enough to curette away with a hook. The bone bridge should not be removed using a drill as it might damage the ossicular chain and inner ear
Instruments: medium-sized diamond burs

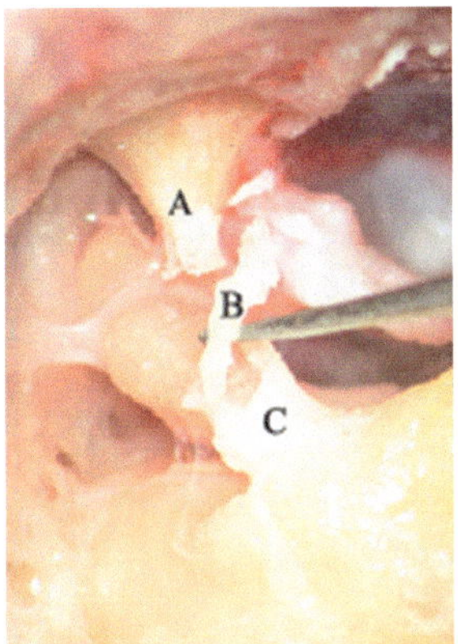

A. Anterior buttress
B. Separated bone bridge
C. Posterior buttress

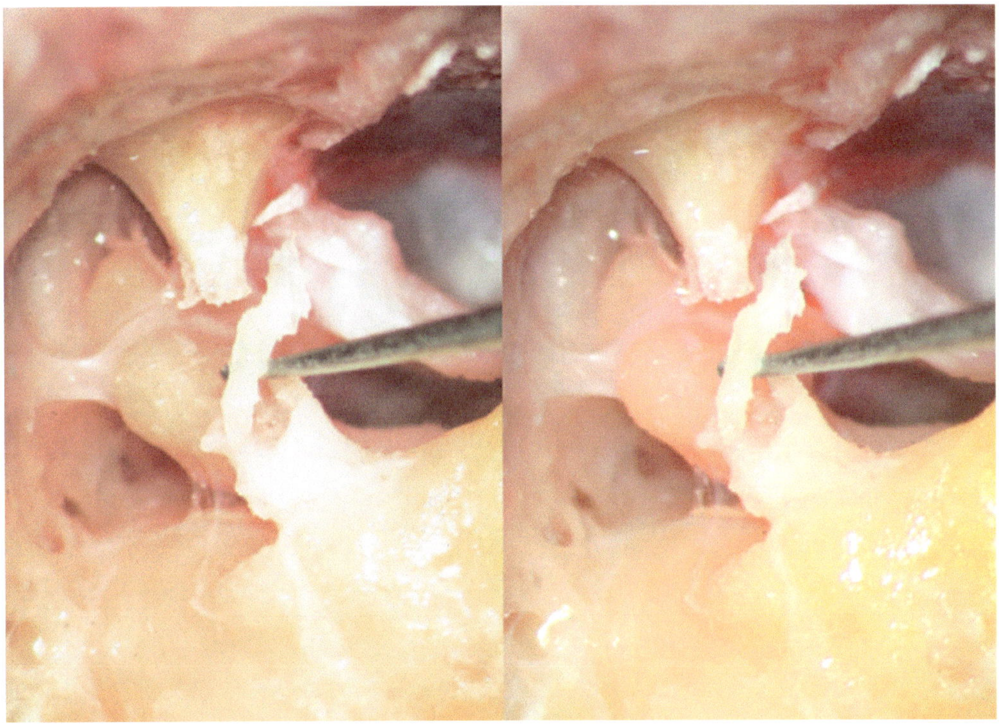

Fig. 4.54 Removal of the bone bridge (right)
Remove the bone bridge, exposing the tympanum and its contents. Using a hook provides better control than using a drill for this step

Instruments: hook

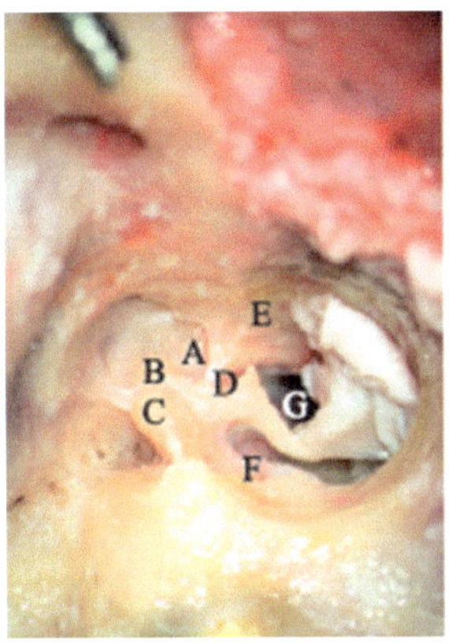

A. Anterior epitympanic recess
B. Malleus head
C. Incus body
D. Superior recess of tympanic membrane
E. Anterior wall of the EAC
F. Chorda tympani
G. Tympanic opening of the Eustachian tube

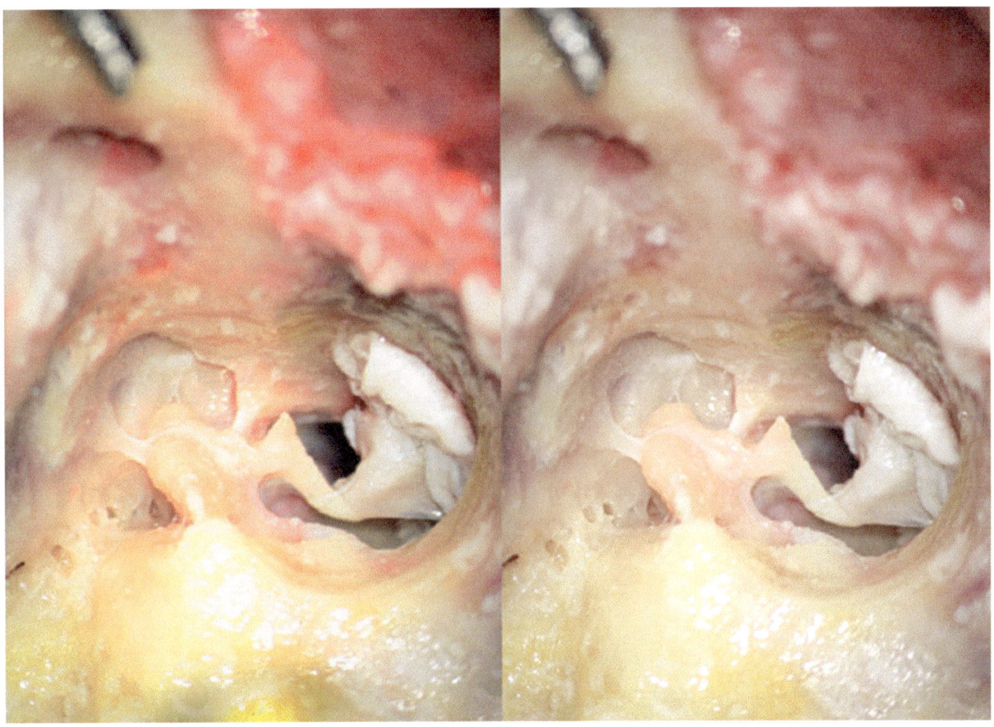

Fig. 4.55 Tympanic cavity (right)
Remove the bone bridge, then drill down the remnants of the posterior buttress, releasing the drum. Expose: (1) the ossicular chain and the chorda tympani, between the handle of the malleus and long process of the incus. (2) ossicular ligaments that stabilize the ossicles, lateral ligament of the malleus, superior and posterior ligaments of the incus, (3) recesses of the tympanic cavity, anterior epitympanic recess, superior recess of tympanic membrane (Prussak's space). *Hints: Drilling the anterior buttress should not proceed beyond the anterior wall of the EAC to avoid damage to the mandibular fossa*
Instruments: medium-sized diamond burs

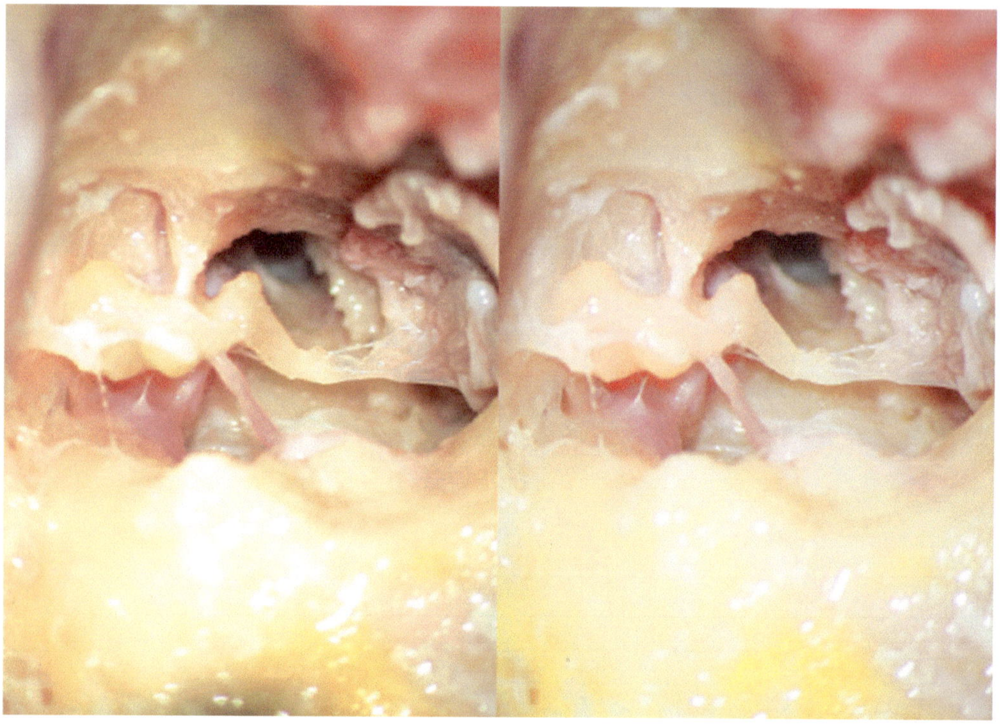

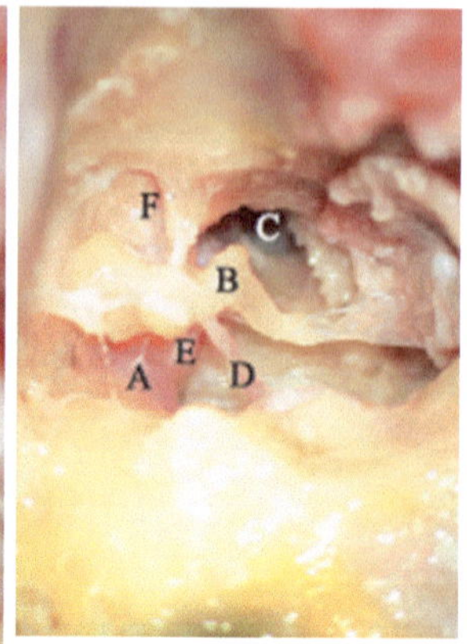

A. Facial nerve canal
B. Malleus
C. Tympanic opening of the Eustachian tube
D. Chorda tympani
E. Cochleariform process
F. Anterior epitympanic recess

Fig. 4.56 Removal of incus (right)
Separate the incudomalleal joint and incudostapedial joint with a right-angle hook and remove the incus. Expose the ligaments and folds around the malleus: the superior ligament of the malleus, superior fold of the malleus, lateral ligament of the malleus, and tensor tympani tendon. The facial nerve canal lies medial to the head of the malleus and above the cochleariform process
Instruments: right-angle hook, Hartmann ear forceps

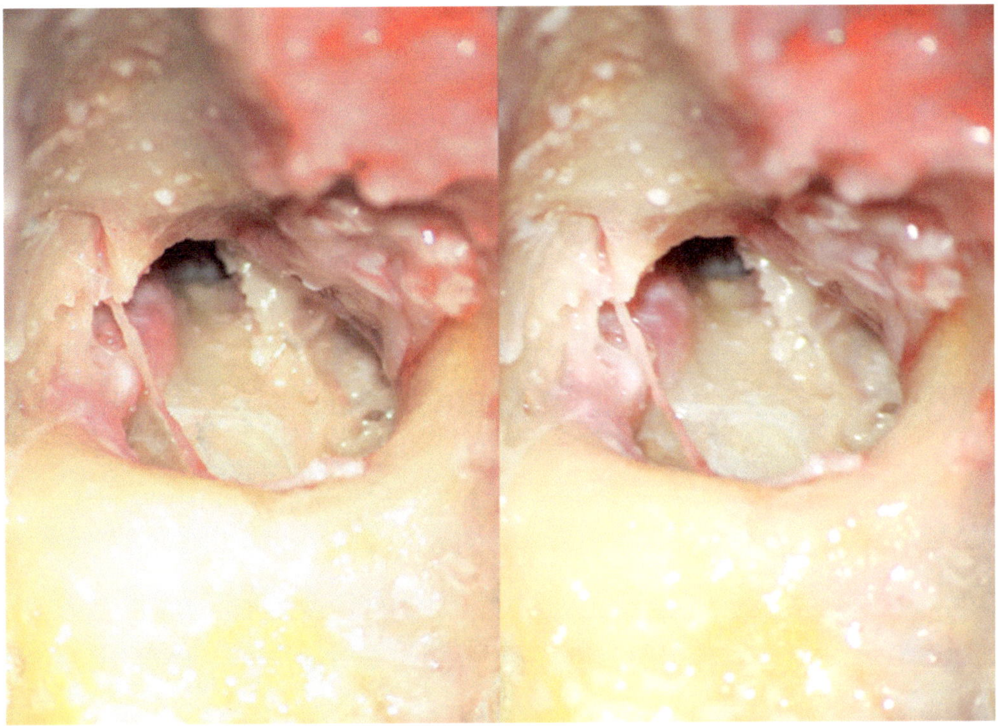

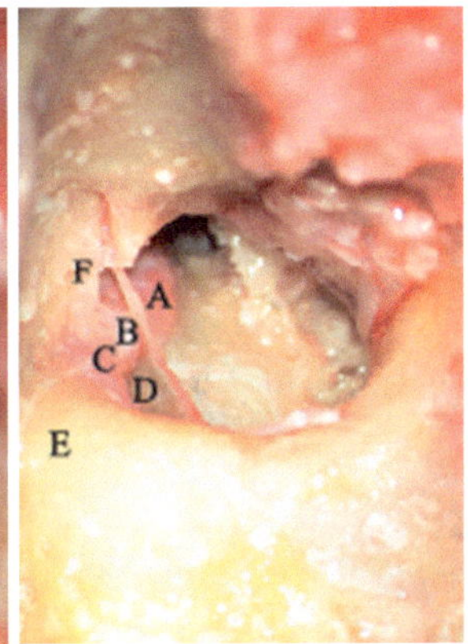

A. Semicanal for the tensor tympani muscle
B. Cochleariform process
C. Facial nerve canal
D. Oval window niche
E. Lateral semicircular canal
F. Cog

Fig. 4.57 Removal of malleus (right)
Cut the tensor tympani tendon and separate the tympanic membrane from the handle to remove the malleus. The semicanal for the tensor tympani muscle lies in the superior part of the tympanic cavity. The cochleariform process and the horizontal segment of the facial nerve are posterior to the semicanal. Sometimes the horizontal segment of the facial nerve and the semicanal for the tensor tympani muscle appear to be connected directly. In fact, the horizontal segment of the facial nerve runs medial to the tensor tympani muscle. Sometimes there is a vertical bony spur pointing down from the tegmen tympani to the epitympanum, at the level of the processus, known as the "cog." The epitympanum is divided into two parts by the cog; the front part is called the anterior epitympanum. It is a cholesteatoma-prone site
Instruments: Hartmann ear forceps, middle ear elevator

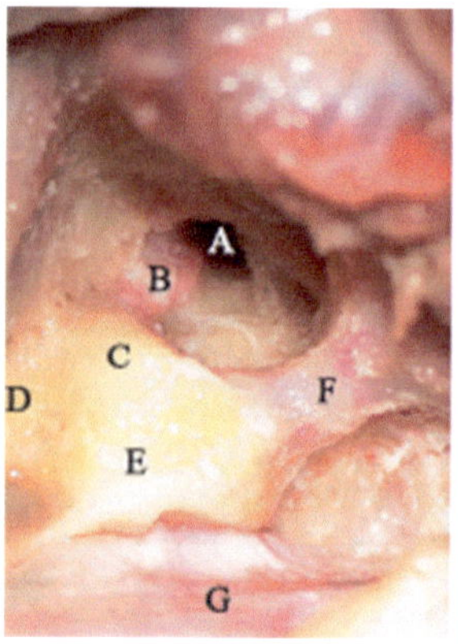

A. Tympanic opening of Eustachian tube
B. Cochleariform process
C. Lateral semicircular canal
D. Superior semicircular canal
E. Posterior semicircular canal
F. Vertical segment of the facial nerve
G. Posterior fossa dura

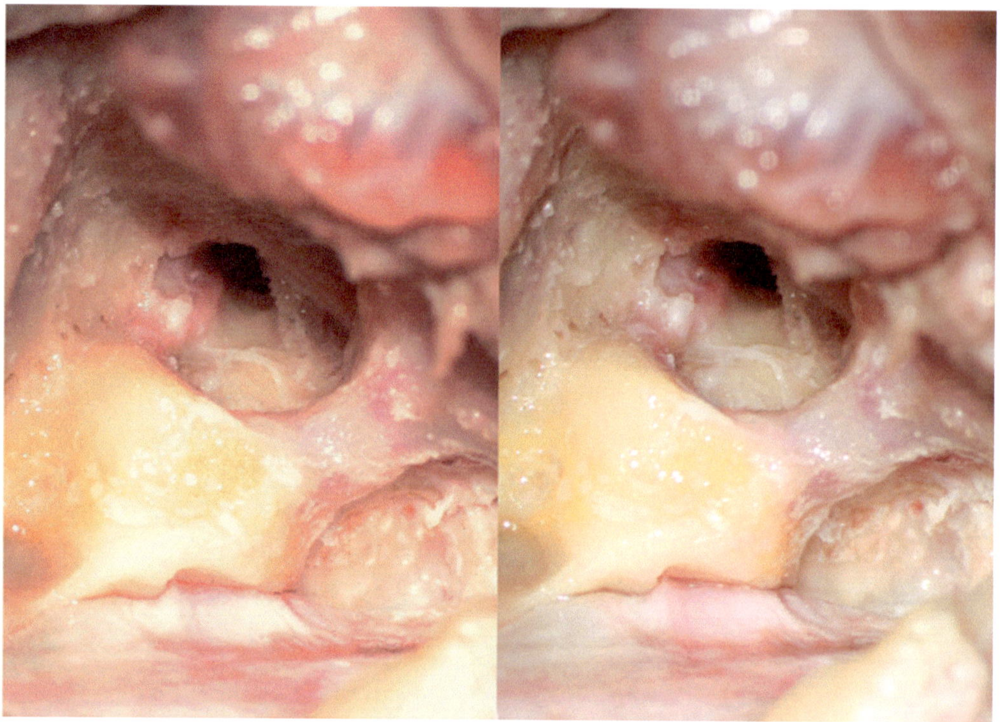

Fig. 4.58 Removal of chorda tympani (right)
The chorda tympani arises from the posterior wall of the EAC and runs forward between the handle of the malleus and the long process of the incus, then passes into the infratemporal fossa through the petrotympanic fissure. Cut the chorda tympani and remove the tympanic component
Instruments: ophthalmic scissors

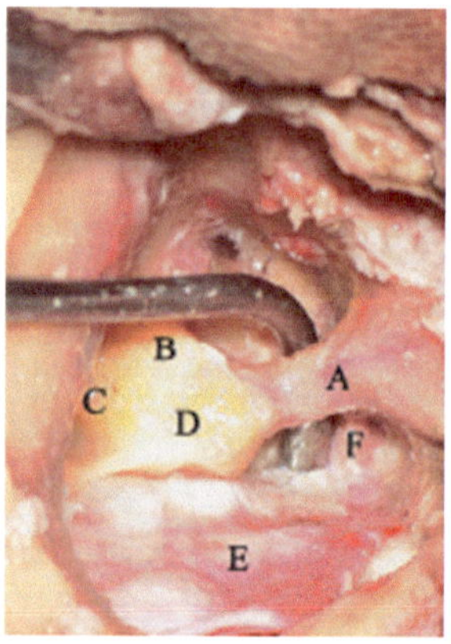

A. Vertical segment of the facial nerve
B. Lateral semicircular canal
C. Superior semicircular canal
D. Posterior semicircular canal
E. Posterior fossa dura
F. Jugular bulb

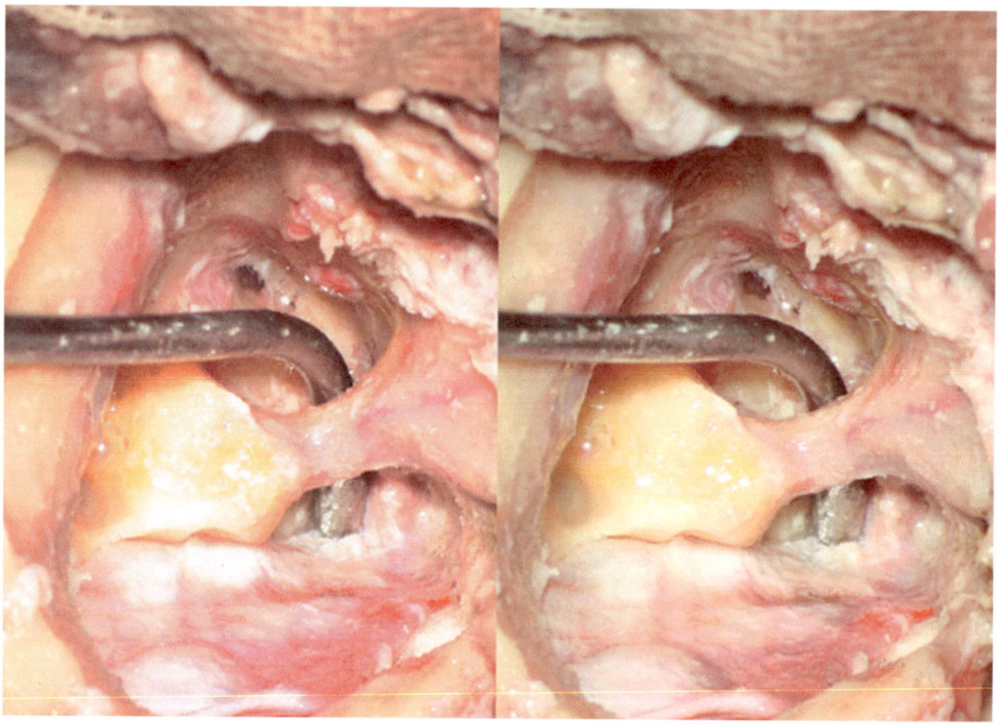

Fig. 4.59 Removal of air cells medial to the facial nerve (right)
The jugular bulb is the only important structure medial to the vertical segment of the facial nerve. Removal of a glomus tympanicum tumor may require removal of bone medial to the facial nerve to avoid injury to the nerve
Instruments: medium-sized diamond burs

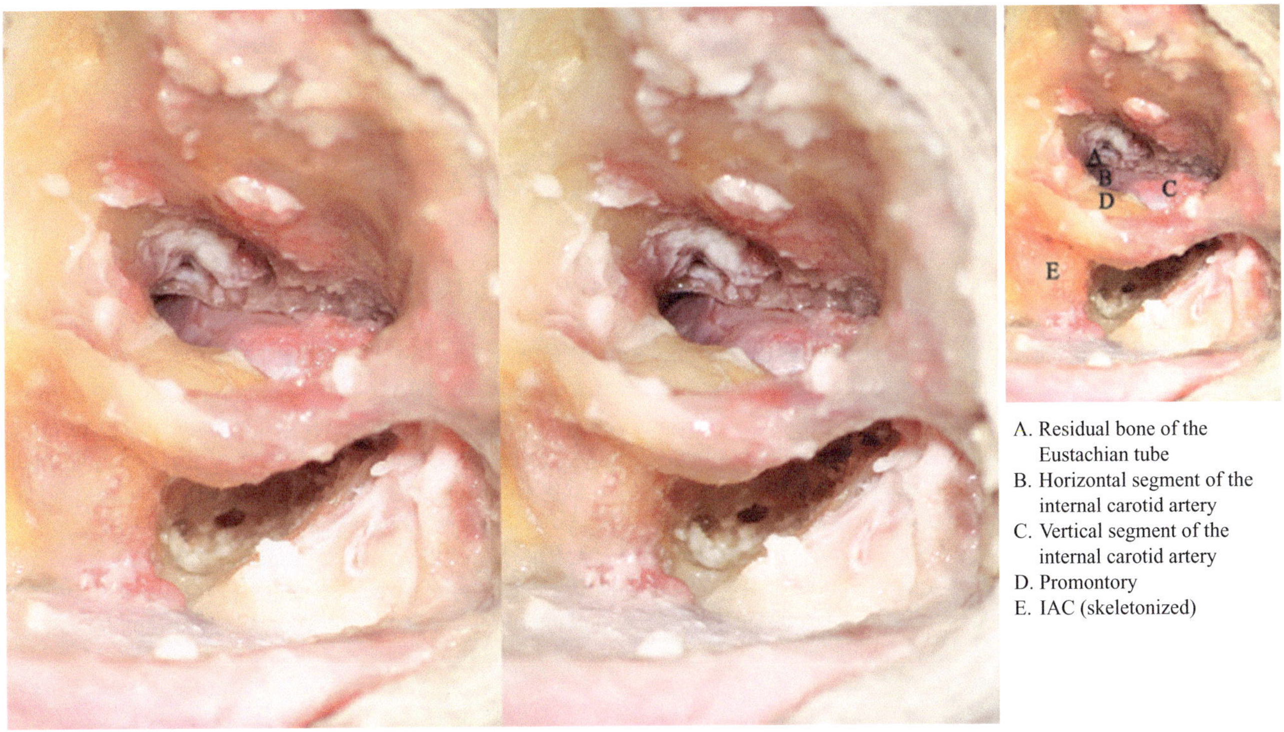

A. Residual bone of the Eustachian tube
B. Horizontal segment of the internal carotid artery
C. Vertical segment of the internal carotid artery
D. Promontory
E. IAC (skeletonized)

Fig. 4.60 Exposure of the IAC and internal carotid artery (right)
The internal carotid artery enters the temporal bone through the carotid canal in the inferior surface of the petrous portion and runs upwards anteromedial to the cochlea. It then turns forward into the horizontal segment of the internal carotid artery. The bone plate between the internal carotid artery and the Eustachian tube is very thin or may be deficient. Drill away the bone anterior to the promontory and inferior to the tympanic opening of the Eustachian tube, exposing the vertical and horizontal segments of the internal carotid artery
Instruments: medium-sized diamond burs

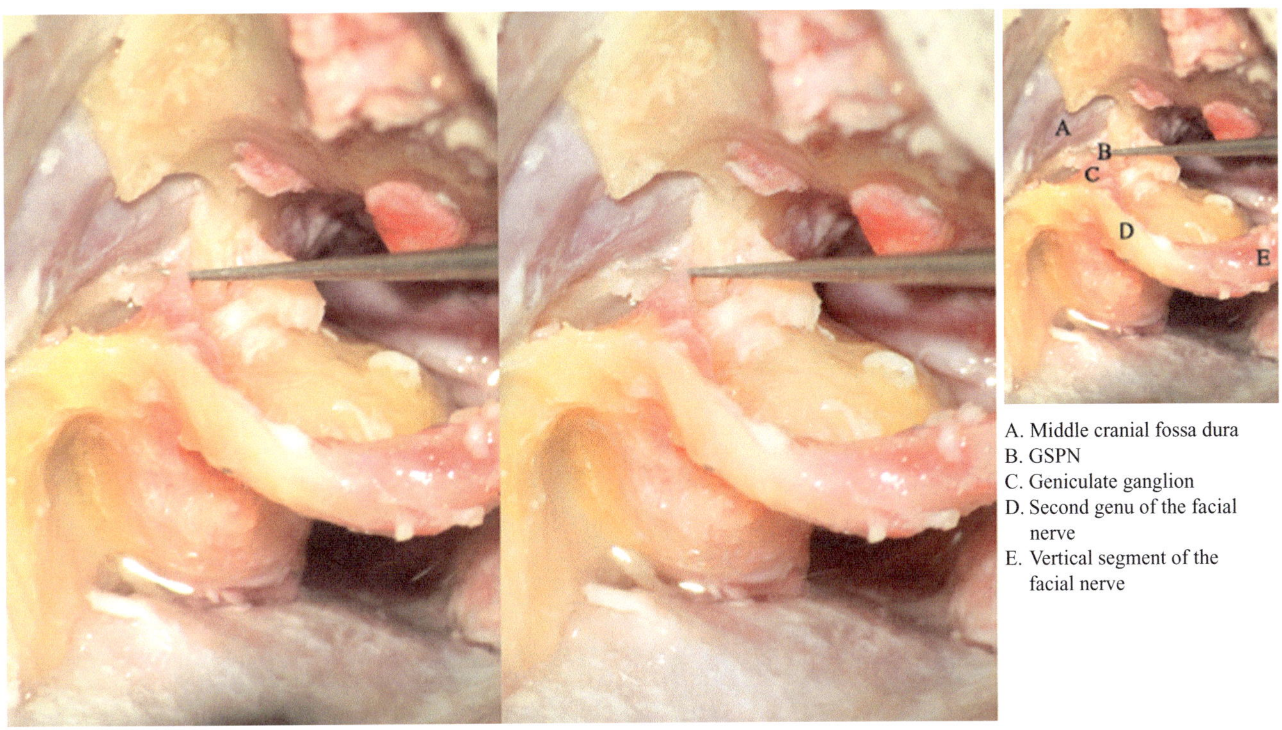

A. Middle cranial fossa dura
B. GSPN
C. Geniculate ganglion
D. Second genu of the facial nerve
E. Vertical segment of the facial nerve

Fig. 4.61 Greater superficial petrosal nerve (GSPN, right)
Remove the tegmen tympani, and trace along the horizontal segment of the facial nerve to expose the geniculate ganglion. Remove bone anterolateral to the geniculate ganglion to further expose the GSPN, which enters into the pterygopalatine ganglion. Postganglionic fibers are distributed in the lacrimal gland, nasal mucous gland, and nasal vascular wall
Instruments: right-angle hook, medium- and small-sized diamond burs

Anatomy of the Ossicular Chain

Chang Guo

The three auditory ossicles are the malleus, incus, and stapes, the last of which is the smallest bone in the human body. They form the ossicular chain that connects the tympanic membrane with the oval window and incorporates two joints. The ossicular chain mediates sound transmission from the tympanic membrane to the fluid of the inner ear. The chain forms a lever mechanism: the axis of motion is around a line joining the anterior malleal ligament to the short process of the incus; the long arm of leverage is the malleus handle and the short arm is the long process of the incus. The ossicular chain mass is almost equal on each side of the axis of motion; vibration of the tympanic membrane is transferred to the tip of the malleus handle and moves it inward, which in turn rotates the head of the malleus and the body of the incus around the axis. The long process of the incus and the handle of the malleus are both located below the axis and move in the same direction.

The acoustic impedance matching system of the middle ear is formed by the tympanic membrane, ossicular chain, and oval window and is an effective transducer of sound for hearing in humans. The acoustic impedance of inner ear lymph is 3800 times more than that of air, so 99.9% of sound energy will be lost when conducted from air to fluid. The loss is equivalent to 32.5 dB of sound energy. The middle ear compensates for the loss of sound energy through the following mechanisms: first, by the difference between the effective vibration area of the tympanic membrane and stapes footplate, the gain of sound pressure can be improved by as much as 25 dB; second, the leverage effect of the ossicular chain can improve sound pressure about 1.3 times, providing a gain of 2.3 dB; and third, the curved membrane provides a gain of 6 dB. Therefore, the acoustic impedance matching mechanism of the middle ear can compensate for almost all of the sound energy lost during sound conduction from air to fluid.

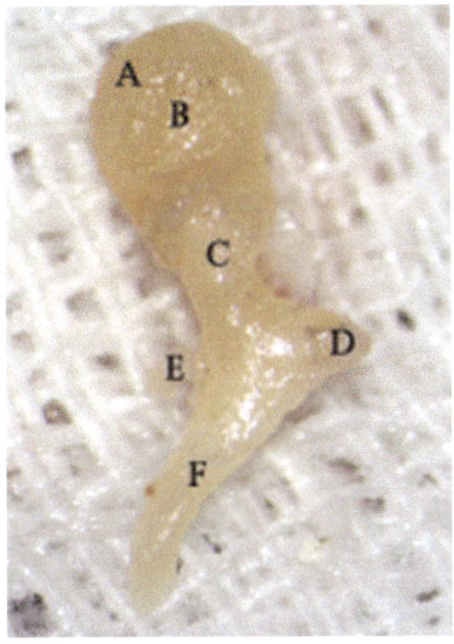

A. Head of the malleus
B. Articular surface
C. Neck of the malleus
D. Lateral process of the malleus
E. Anterior process of the malleus
F. Handle of the malleus

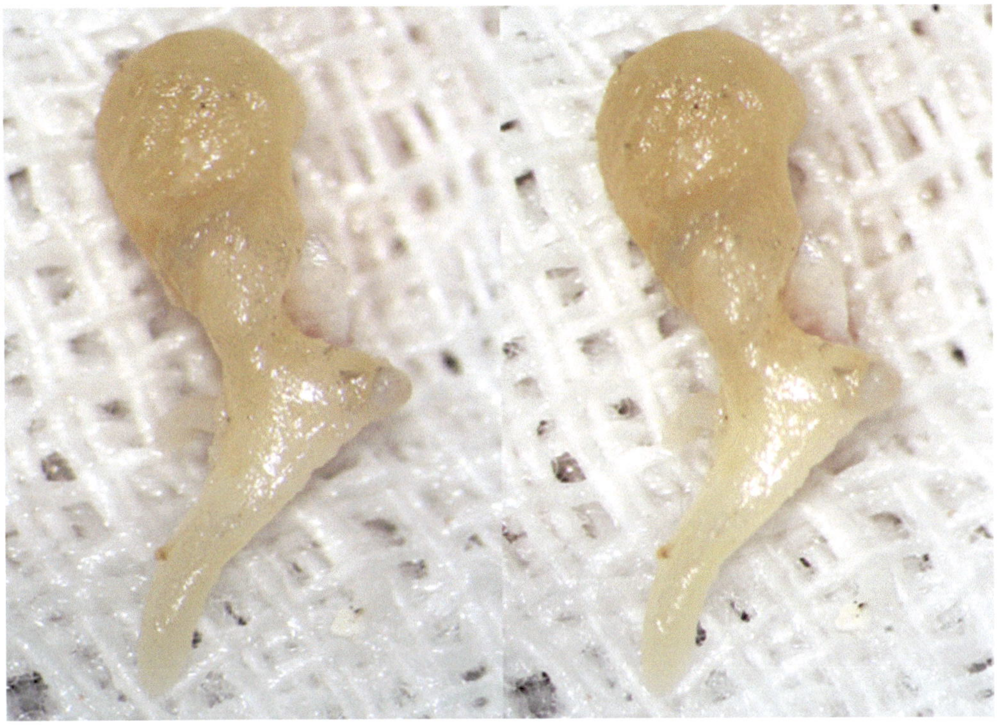

Fig. 4.62 Malleus (right)
The malleus has head, neck, anterior and lateral processes, and a handle (manubrium). The head is about 3.5 mm in height; the handle is about 4.6 mm long, and the angle between the handle and neck is about 130°. The head of the malleus, located in the epitympanum, articulates with the incus through a U-shaped articular surface. The neck is a narrow section below the head and joins it to the handle. The handle's lateral surface is attached to the tympanic membrane and its tip corresponds to the umbo of the tympanic membrane. The anterior process protrudes forward from the neck to connect with the anterior malleal ligament. The lateral process sits on the outer surface of the upper end of the handle and attaches to the anterior and posterior malleal folds

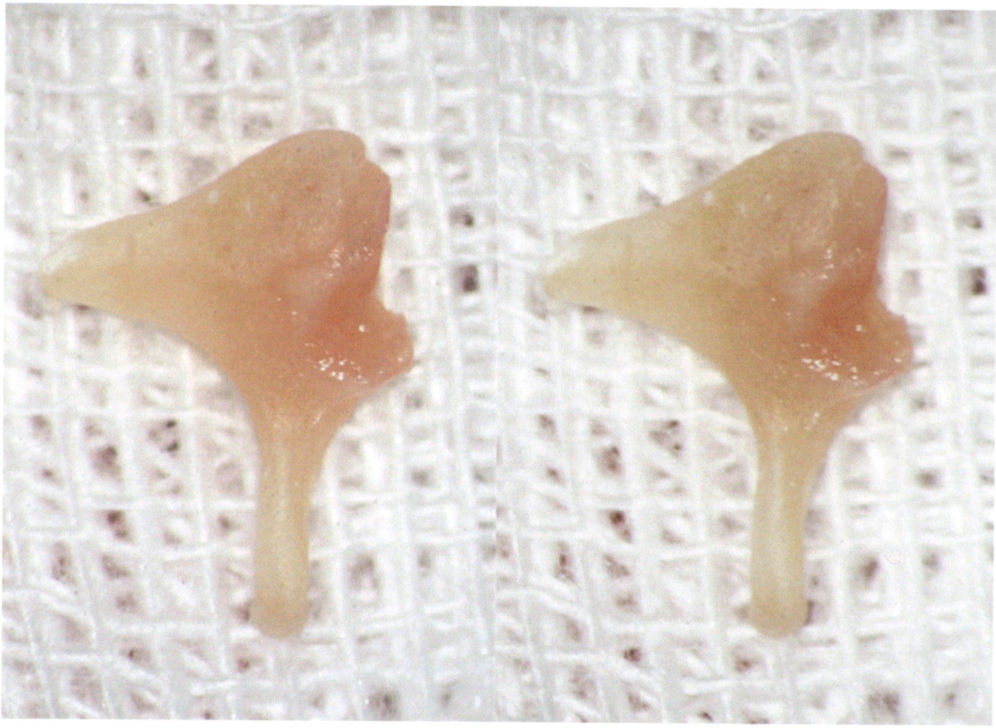

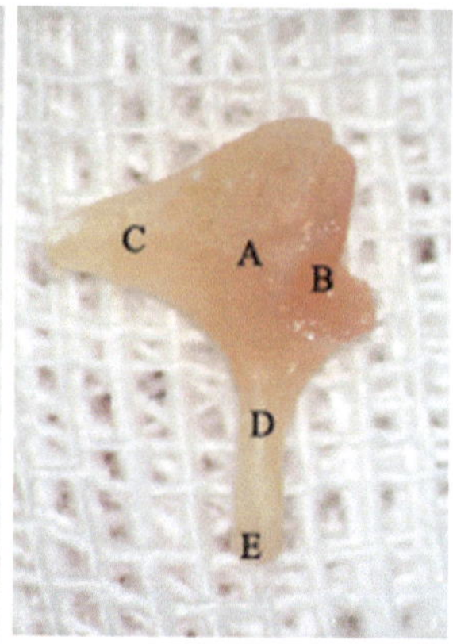

A. Body of the incus
B. Articular surface
C. Short process of the incus
D. Long process of the incus
E. Tip of long process with lenticular process on medial surface

Fig. 4.63 Incus (right)
The incus has a body, short and long processes, and connects the malleus and stapes. The body is about 2 mm wide; the long process is about 7 mm long and the short one is about 5 mm long. The angle between the long and short processes is about 100°. The body, located in the epitympanum, articulates with the malleus via its anterior saddle-shaped articular surface. The short process sits in the fossa incudis, located at the bottom of the aditus ad antrum. The long process sits posteromedial to the malleus handle. Its terminal end curves inward, then forms the lenticular process, which articulates with the stapes head

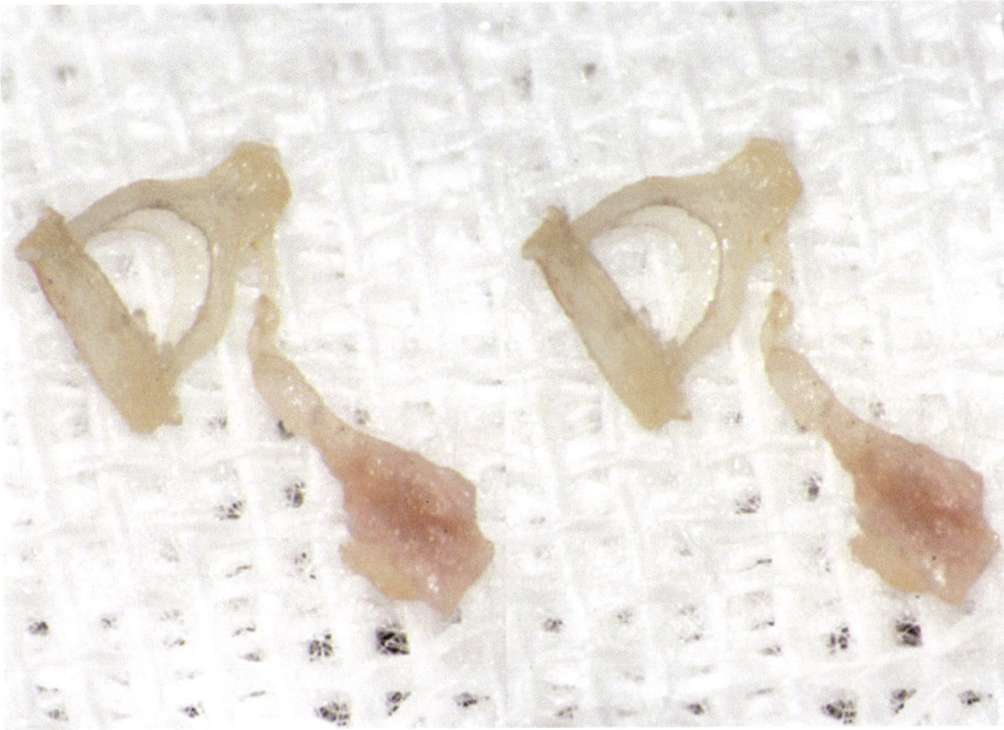

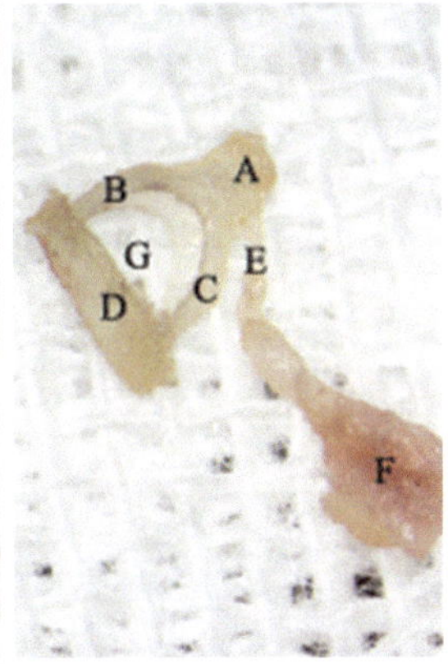

A. Head of the stapes
B. Anterior crus
C. Posterior crus
D. Footplate of the stapes
E. Stapedius tendon
F. Stapedius muscle
G. Obturator foramen

Fig. 4.64 Stapes
The stapes, shaped like a stirrup, is the smallest ossicle. It has a head, neck, anterior and posterior crura, and footplate. The stapes is about 3.2 mm in height, and its footplate is about 2.9 mm long and 1.3 mm wide. The head sits laterally and articulates with the lenticular process of the incus. The tendon of the stapedius muscle attaches to the posterior surface of the neck The anterior crus is straight and slightly shorter than the posterior crus, which is slightly curved. The footplate is a thin oval plate that seals the oval window via its annular ligament. The stapedius muscle is located in the bone deep to the vertical segment of the facial nerve; its tendon passes through the pyramidal process to reach the neck of the stapes. The obturator foramen is the opening surrounded by the anterior and posterior crura and the footplate

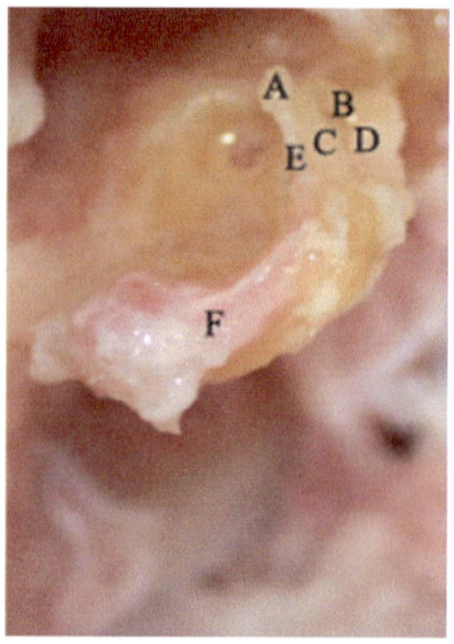

A. Head of the stapes
B. Anterior crus
C. Posterior crus
D. Footplate of the stapes
E. Stapedius tendon
F. Stapedius muscle

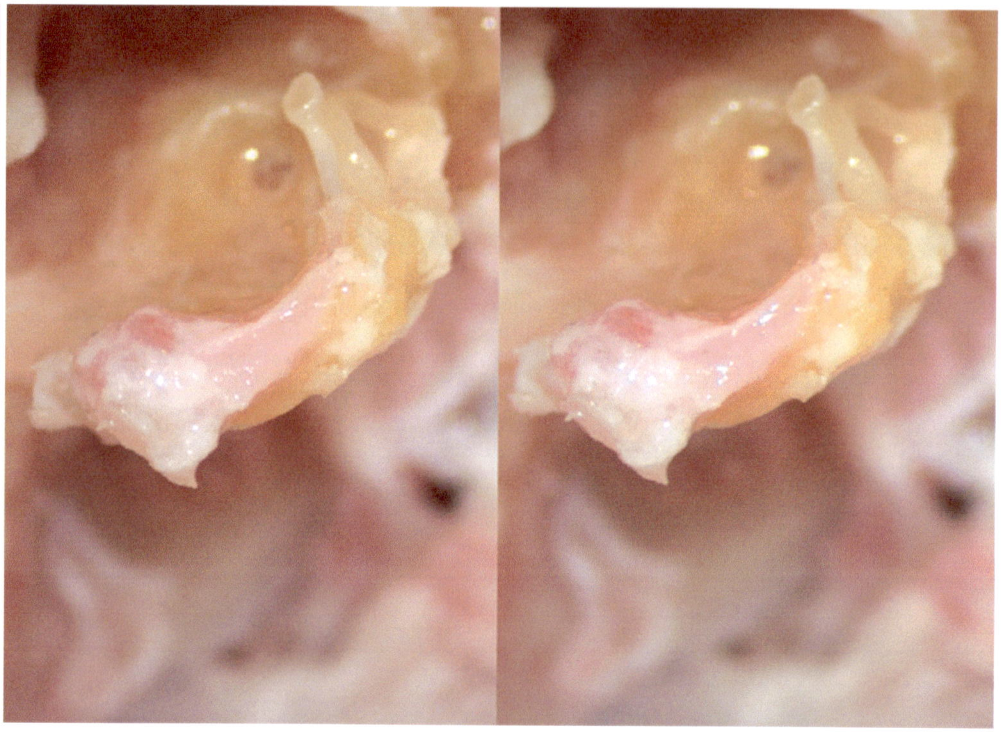

Fig. 4.65 Stapes and stapedius muscle (left)
Through a retroauricular approach, the stapedius muscle can be exposed by moving the vertical segment of the facial nerve forward and drilling the bone medial to the nerve. The stapedius muscle is located deep to the bony vertical facial nerve canal and posterior to the pyramidal process. The stapedius tendon passes through the tip of the process and attaches to the posterior surface of the stapes neck. The stapedius muscle acts as an antagonist to the tensor tympani muscle. It pulls back on the head of the stapes, tilting the footplate on its posterior edge and moving its anterior part laterally. The facial nerve supplies the stapedius muscle via its stapedial branch, providing the efferent arc of the stapedial reflex

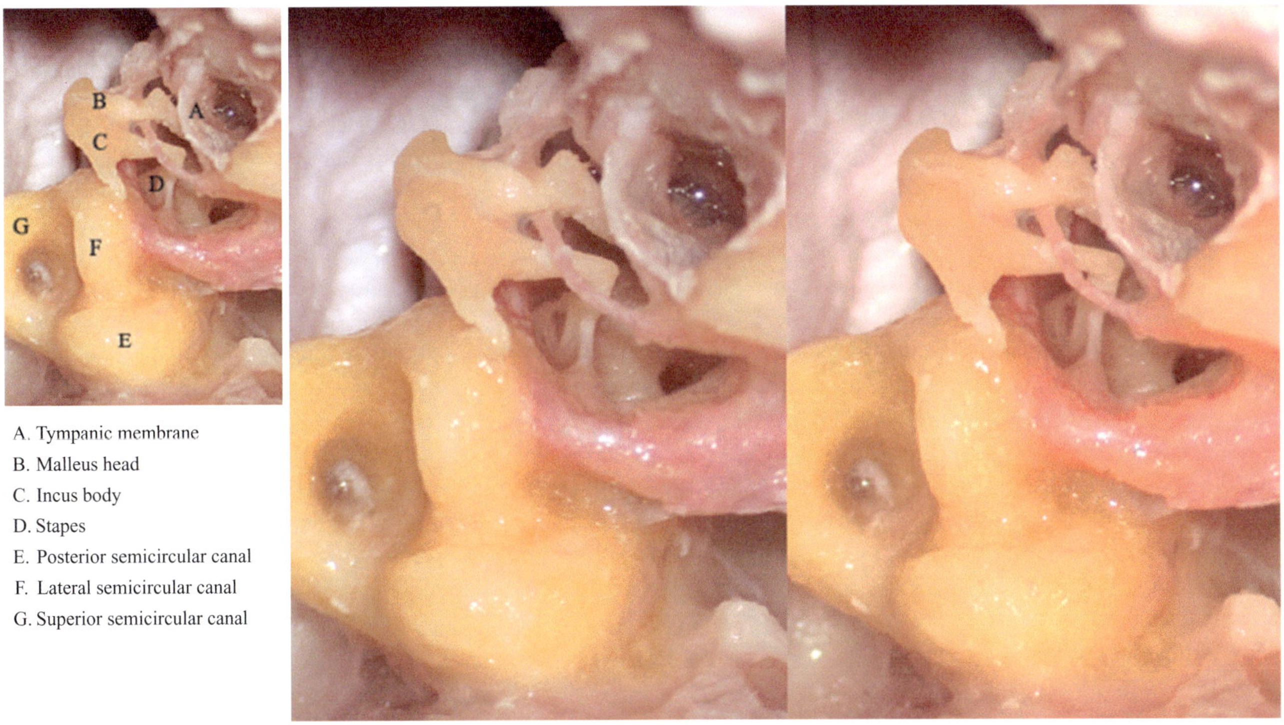

A. Tympanic membrane
B. Malleus head
C. Incus body
D. Stapes
E. Posterior semicircular canal
F. Lateral semicircular canal
G. Superior semicircular canal

Fig. 4.66 Ossicular chain
The three auditory ossicles form the ossicular chain that is supported by joints and ligaments. The malleus handle is directly attached to the tympanic membrane. The head of the malleus articulates with the body of the incus. The short process of the incus is located in the fossa incudis, which is anterolateral to the lateral semicircular canal. The lenticular process of the incus articulates with the head of the stapes. The stapes footplate covers the oval window. The stapedius tendon passes through the pyramidal process, then attaches to the stapes neck

Anatomy of the Round Window Niche and Cochlear Aqueduct

Kun Ma and Vincent C Cousins

Located postero-inferiorly in the medial wall of the tympanic cavity is the round window niche, which has an ovoid shape with an average width of 1.66 mm and a depth of 1.34 mm. The plane of the opening of the round window niche is almost perpendicular to that of the round window. The round window membrane is usually obscured by the edge of the niche. To expose the round window, the anterior and superior bony edges of the niche must be partly drilled off. The round window membrane is very thin, and consists of three layers: the lateral mucosa, which is continuous with the middle ear mucosa, the middle connective tissue layer, and the thin interior intima. The round window membrane is normally around 2 mm^2 in an average area, 70 μm thick, with a 1.14 mm transverse diameter and 1.65 mm vertical diameter. The mean distance from the inferior margin of the round window membrane to the proximal posterior ampullary nerve is around 1.19 mm and from the umbo to the round window is 3.44 mm. The round window membrane is essential to maintain the proper physiological functions of the middle and inner ear. If ruptured, it may cause a range of conditions including sudden deafness, permanent sensorineural deafness, and perilymph fistula. Healing after rupture may lead to an increase in thickness, decrease in flexibility, malposition, and changes in permeability or compliance.

The cochlear aqueduct sits below the inferior border of the IAC, between it and the jugular bulb and has a length of 10 mm. It lies in the triangular fossa between the anteromedial jugular fossa, the inferior petrous bone, and the carotid foramen, and is situated next to the petrosal ganglion of the pharyngeal nerve. It has a tight external aperture and a funnel-shaped internal opening at the lower edge of the round window, separated from the basal turn of the cochlea by a limiting membrane that prevents cerebrospinal fluid from communicating directly with perilymph.

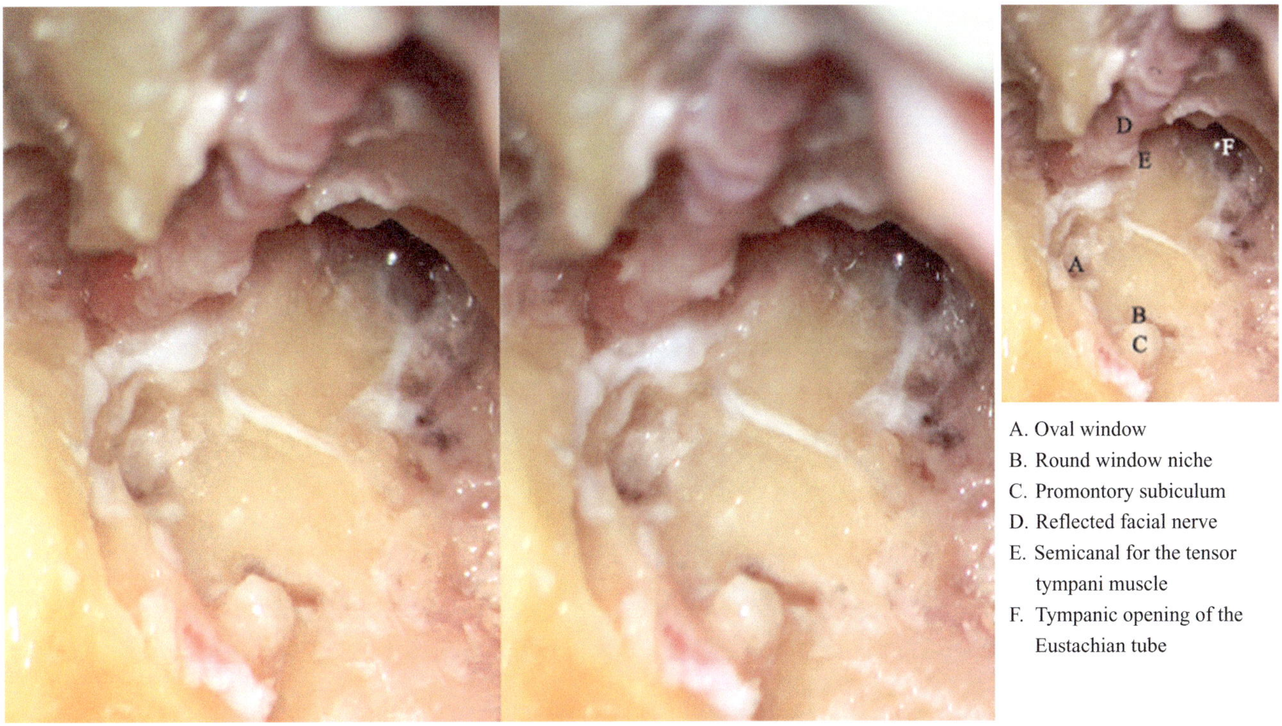

A. Oval window
B. Round window niche
C. Promontory subiculum
D. Reflected facial nerve
E. Semicanal for the tensor tympani muscle
F. Tympanic opening of the Eustachian tube

Fig. 4.67 Exposure of the round window niche after anterior displacement of the facial nerve (right)
After removal of the middle ear structures and re-routing of the facial nerve anteriorly, the oval window, promontory, round window in the medial wall of the tympanum and the tympanic ostium of the Eustachian tube in the anterior wall of the tympanum can be identified. During round window surgery, the anterosuperior bony edge of the niche usually needs to be drilled away to obtain adequate exposure of the round window. Removal of too much bone from the edge of the niche should be avoided so as not to damage the round window membrane or accidentally open the scala tympani. The mean depth of the niche is 1.34 mm
Instruments: small-sized diamond burs

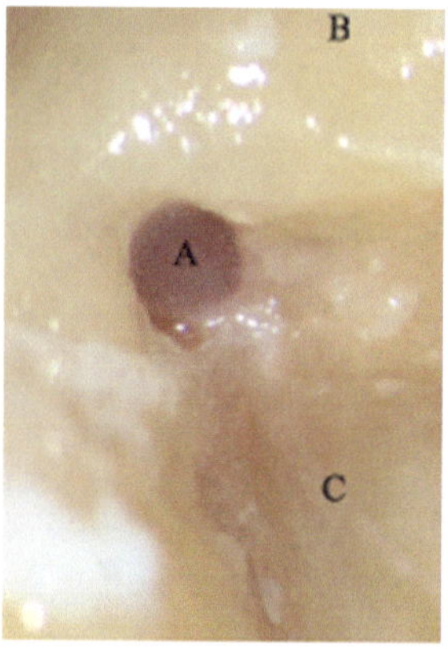

A. Round window membrane
B. Promontory
C. Cochlear aqueduct

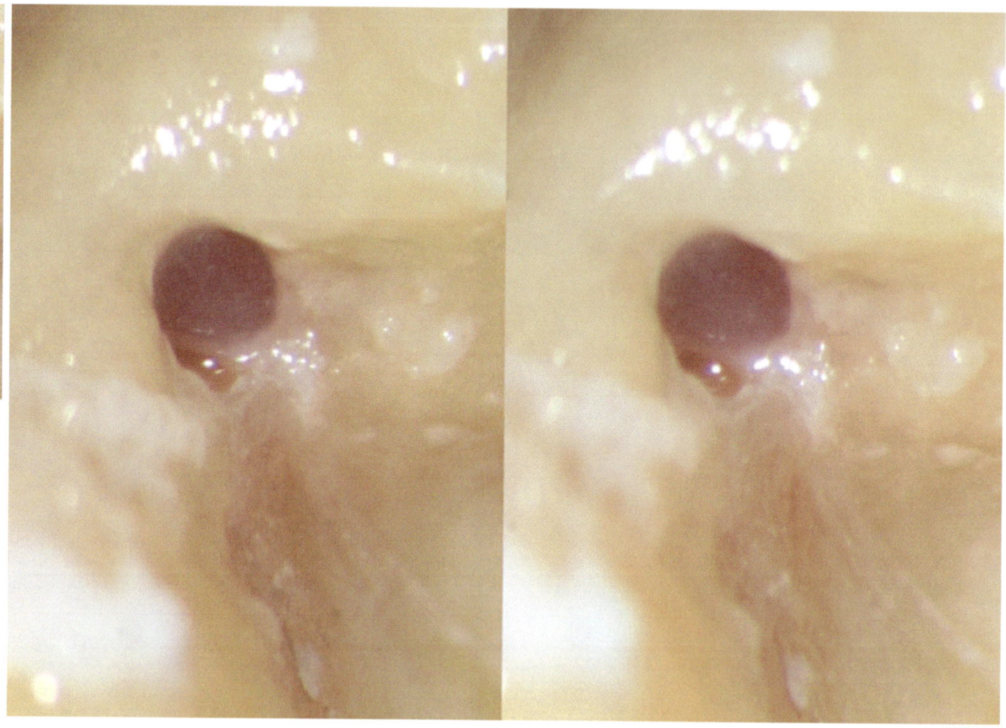

Fig. 4.68 The round window and internal opening of the cochlear aqueduct (right)
The round window is deep within the niche and covered by a membrane that seals off the blunt end of the scala tympani of the cochlea. When tympanic mucosal folds covering the niche have been removed and the anterosuperior bony edge of the round window niche has been partly drilled way, the very thin, tensile, translucid membrane will be exposed. With further drilling of the inferior and medial bony edges of the round window niche, the very small and fine cochlear aqueduct is seen

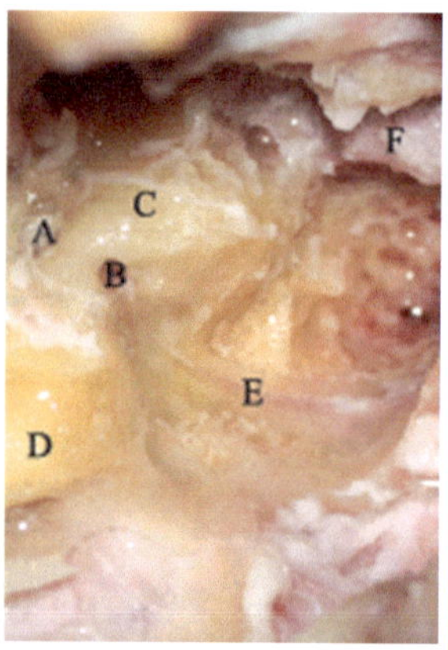

A. Oval window
B. Round window membrane
C. Promontory
D. Posterior semicircular canal
E. Cochlear aqueduct
F. Internal carotid artery

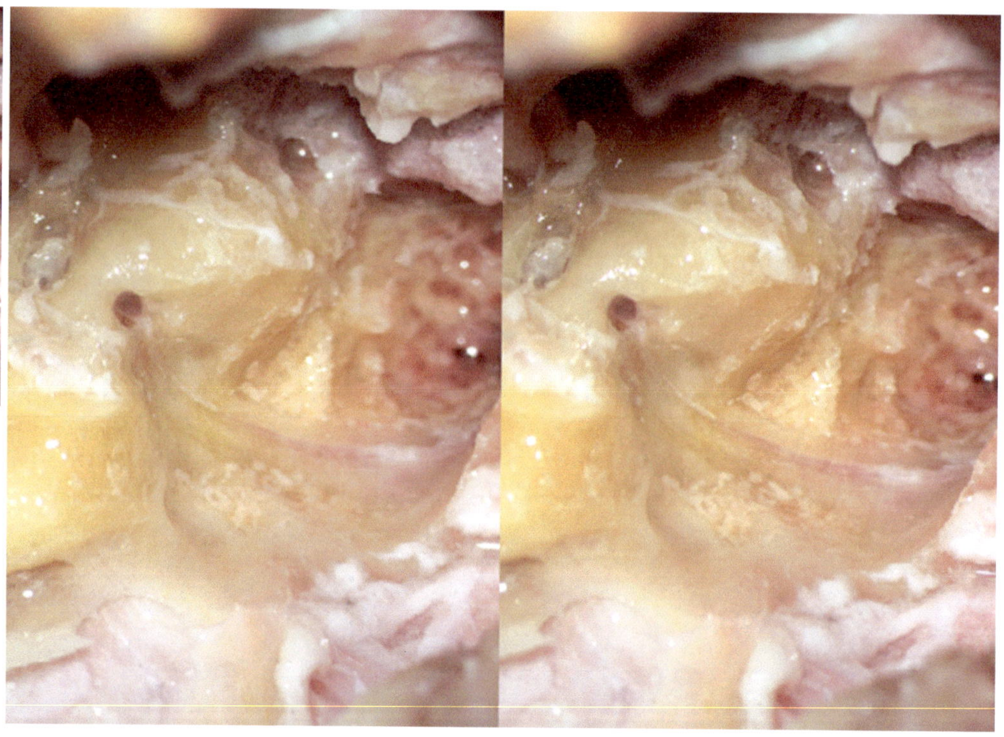

Fig. 4.69 Whole course of cochlear aqueduct (right)
The round window membrane serves as an anatomical landmark to identify the upper end of the cochlear aqueduct. Drilling inferior and medially from that point allows exposure of the full length of the aqueduct. The cochlear aqueduct is divided into the petrous segment and otocyst segment by the pars isthmus with a full length of around 12.9 mm. Its inner opening lies next to the round window, while the external aperture is located in the triangular bone fossa between the medial walls of the jugular fossa and carotid foramen
Instruments: small-sized diamond burs

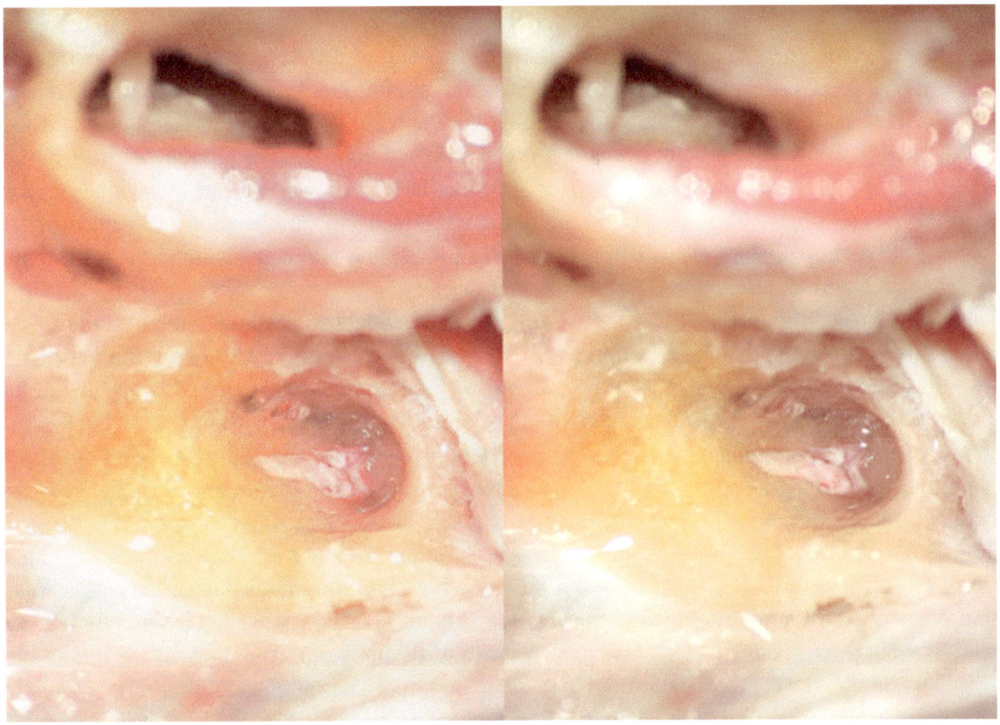

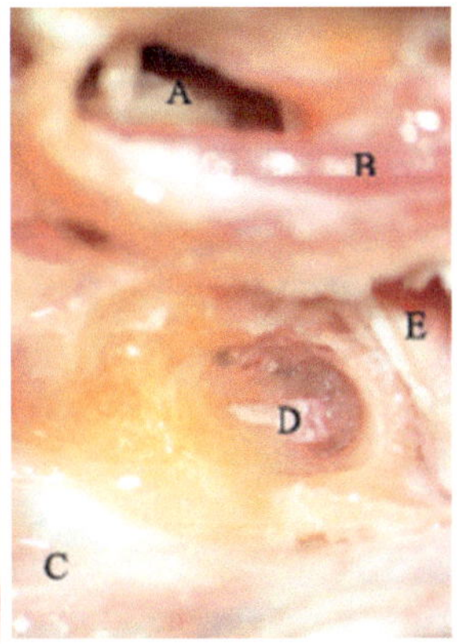

A. Promontory
B. Vertical segment of the facial nerve
C. Dura mater of the posterior cranial fossa
D. External aperture of the cochlear aqueduct
E. Opened jugular bulb

Fig. 4.70 External aperture of cochlear aqueduct (right)
The jugular bulb can serve as a landmark. When the bone superior and medial to the jugular bulb has been drilled away, the external aperture of the cochlear aqueduct will be exposed, with a funnel-like shape and an average width of 2.64 mm. The 9th, 10th, and 11th cranial nerves lie inferior and medial to the cochlear aqueduct, particularly the ninth nerve which lies only 0.70–1.56 mm from the external aperture. Once the cochlear aqueduct has been identified, special care must be taken not to damage the ninth nerve below
Instruments: small-sized diamond burs

Anatomy of the Cochlea

Zhan-guo Jin

The cochlea resembles a nautilus shell. It consists of a bony duct or tube that spirals around a central axis anterior to the vestibule and contains the auditory sense organ. It makes 2.5–2.75 turns around its axis, has a height of 5 mm at its apex, a width of 9 mm at its base, and a length of 30–33 mm. The left and right cochleae spiral in opposite directions.

The anatomical relationships of the cochlea are complex. Anteriorly are the internal carotid artery and the tympanic opening of the Eustachian tube. Superiorly are the tensor tympani muscle, the prominence of the horizontal canal of the facial nerve, and the labyrinthine segment of the facial nerve. Behind are the vestibule and fundus of the IAC. The basal turn of the cochlea protrudes into the middle ear as the promontory.

The cochlear axis (the modiolus) is a hollow bony tube that contains the auditory nerve. The bony spiral lamina protrudes from the bony axis along the length of the cochlea and gives attachment to the basement membrane as it passes across to the lateral wall of the cochlea. The bony spiral lamina and the basement membrane together divide the cochlea into upper and lower cavities. The upper cavity is further divided into two parts by the vestibular membrane (or Reissner's membrane), so the cross-section of the cochlea is divided into three cavities: scala vestibuli (superiorly), scala media, and scala tympani (inferiorly). The scala media is also called the membranous duct of the cochlea; it contains endolymph and both of its ends are closed. The cochlear cupula is the blind end of the cochlear duct at the apex of the cochlea. The basal or vestibular end of the duct is joined to the saccule via the ductus reuniens. The basal end of the scala vestibuli is closed by the stapes footplate in the oval window; the apical end of the scala vestibuli communicates with the scala tympani via the helicotrema around the cochlear cupula. The basal end of the scala tympani is closed by the round window membrane. The internal aperture of the cochlear aqueduct is in the lower wall of the scala tympani near the round window; its external aperture is located in the triangular fossa in the bone between the jugular fossa and the internal carotid artery.

The helicotrema is bounded by the hamulus of the spiral lamina; it forms the junction of the scala vestibuli and scala tympani. The cochlear diameter becomes smaller toward its apex, the bony spiral lamina gradually narrows as the basilar membrane gradually widens. The vibration amplitude and natural frequency of the basilar membrane also change from base to apex, as do the acoustic waves of different frequencies along the length of the cochlea. High-frequency sounds are sensed at the base and low-frequency sounds are sensed at the apex. Rosenthal's canal is located at the junction of the cochlear axis and the bony spiral lamina and contains the cochlear spiral ganglion. The spiral ganglion is the first-order neuron of the cochlear nerve. It is comprised of two types of neurons: Type I accounts for 90–95% of the total cochlear spiral ganglion cells and are bipolar neurons; Type II accounts for the remaining 5–10% and are pseudounipolar neurons. The outer layer of the cochlear nerve is composed of nerve fibers from the organ of Corti in the basilar and middle turns of the cochlea, which transmit the nerve impulses generated by the stimulation of medium- and high-frequency sounds. The nerve fibers of the apical turn of the cochlea run in the central axis of the cochlear nerve and transmit impulses caused by low-frequency sounds. In addition, the terminal cochlear nerve fibers have only 1.5 turns while the cochlea has 2.5–2.75 turns.

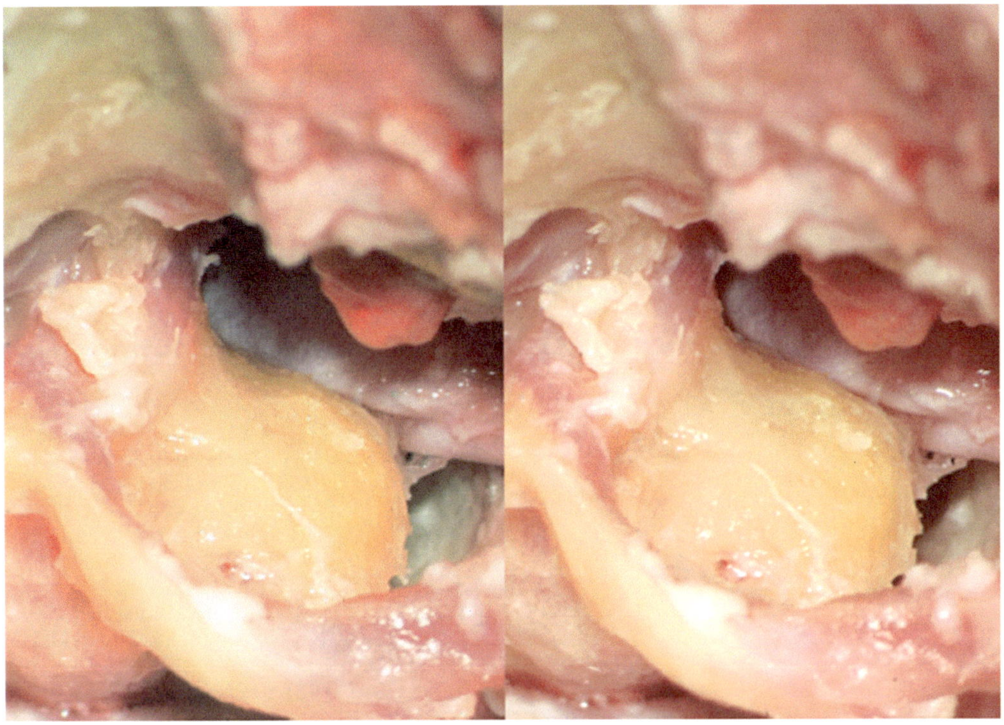

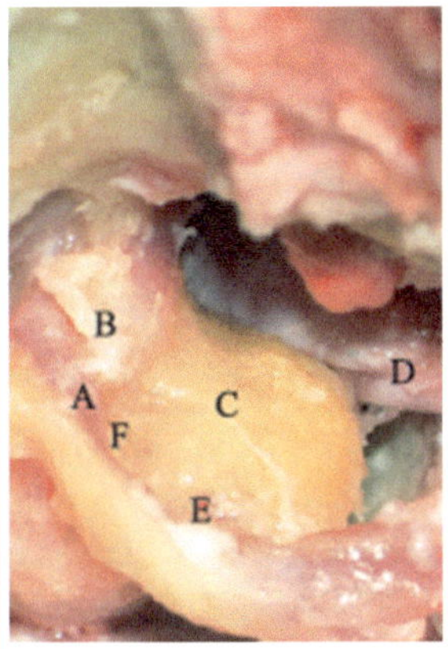

A. Horizontal segment of the facial nerve
B. Cochleariform process
C. Promontory
D. Internal carotid artery
E. Round window niche (part only)
F. Oval window (part only)

Fig. 4.71 Resection of the tympanic structures (right)
After resection of the posterior wall of the EAC and the outer wall of the tympanic cavity, the cavity including its anterior component is exposed. One can see the promontory of the medial wall of the tympanic cavity. The round window niche is located directly behind the promontory and the oval window is above it and behind the upper part of the promontory. The horizontal segment of the facial nerve, cochleariform process, and semicanal for the tensor tympani muscle are superior to the promontory. The internal carotid artery has been exposed in front of the promontory. The thin bone plate that separates the internal carotid artery and Eustachian tube is seen. Dissection in the region of the tympanic opening of the Eustachian tube must be gentle, to avoid damage to the internal carotid artery
Instruments: tapering diamond burs, middle ear scissors, middle ear elevator

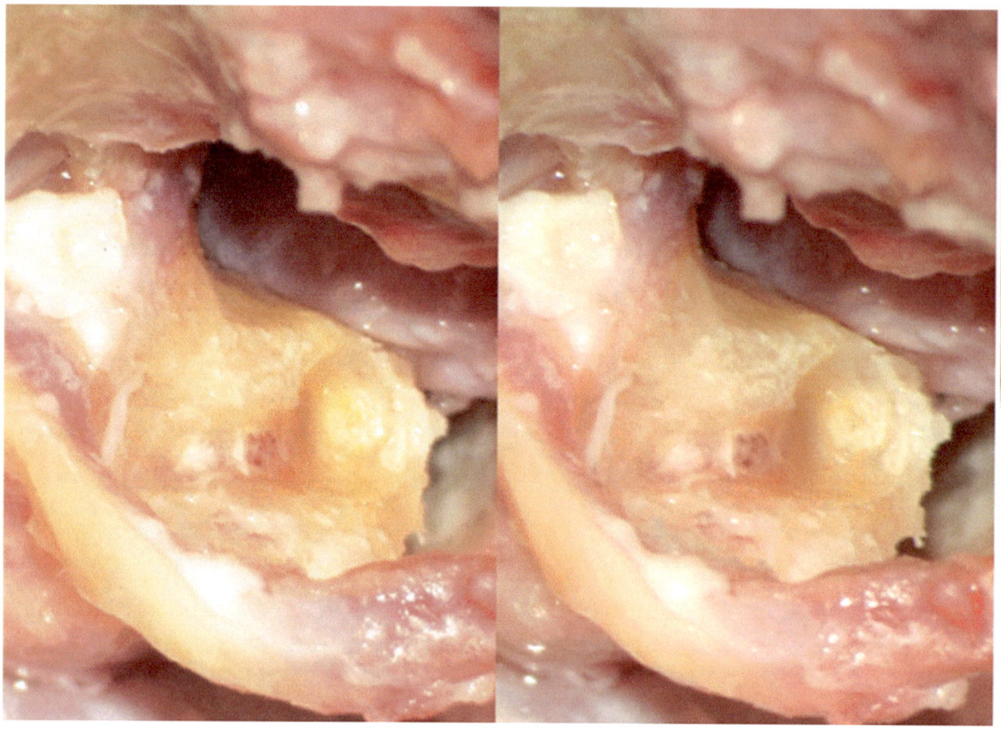

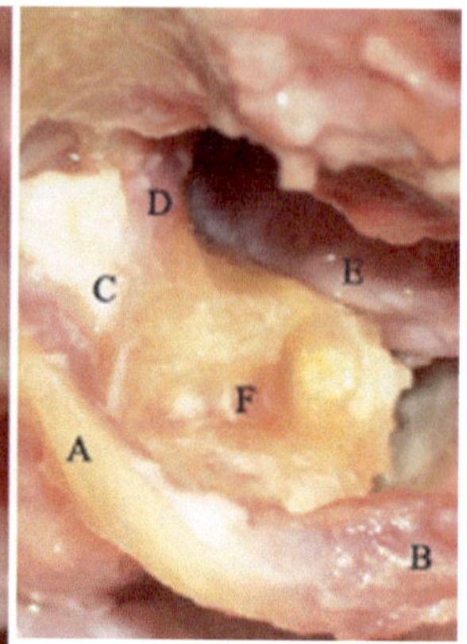

A. Remnant of the horizontal semicircular canal
B. Vertical segment of the facial nerve
C. Cochleariform process
D. Semicanal for the tensor tympani muscle
E. Internal carotid artery
F. Basilar turn of the cochlea

Fig. 4.72 Resection of the promontory, part of the basilar turn of the exposed cochlea (right)
The round window membrane forms the closed end of the scala tympani of the cochlea. Drilling away bone from the lower part of the promontory reveals the basal turn of the cochlea. *Hint: drill parallel to the line of the basal turn, layer by layer, to expose the translucent cochlear bony wall*
Instruments: medium- and small-sized diamond burs

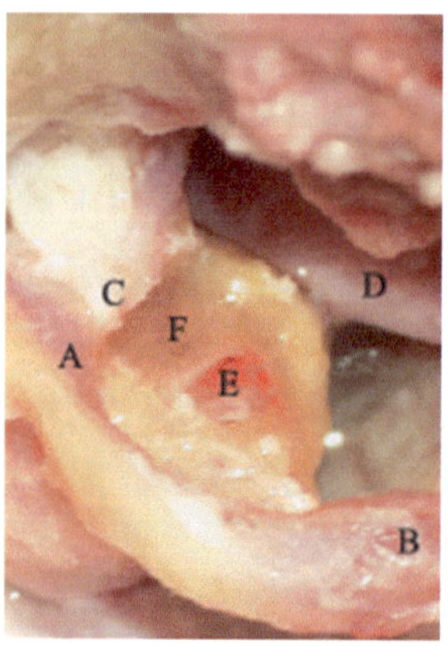

A. Horizontal segment of the facial nerve
B. Vertical segment of the facial nerve
C. Cochleariform process
D. Internal carotid artery
E. Basilar turn of the cochlea
F. Bone wall of the middle turn of cochlea

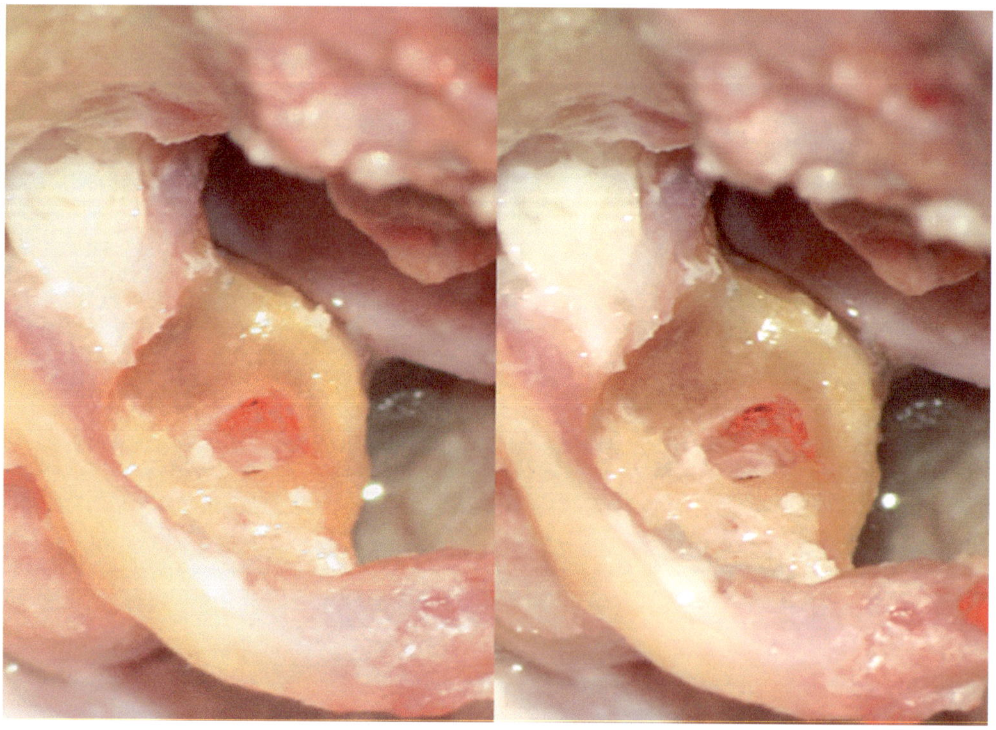

Fig. 4.73 Expose the basal turn of the cochlea (right)
Using the round window niche as an anatomical landmark, drill parallel to the spiral direction of the cochlea, layer by layer, to remove promontory bone and reveal the basal turn of the cochlea. Starting at the basal turn, drill away the bone layer by layer from the lateral and superior surfaces along the line of the lumen to expose it all the way to the apex
Instruments: medium- and small-sized diamond burs

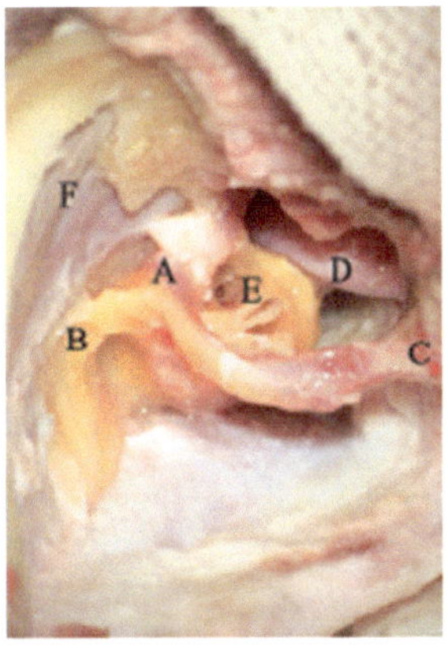

A. Geniculate ganglion
B. Remnants of the superior semicircular canal
C. Stylomastoid foramen
D. Internal carotid artery
E. Cochlea
F. Dura of the middle cranial fossa

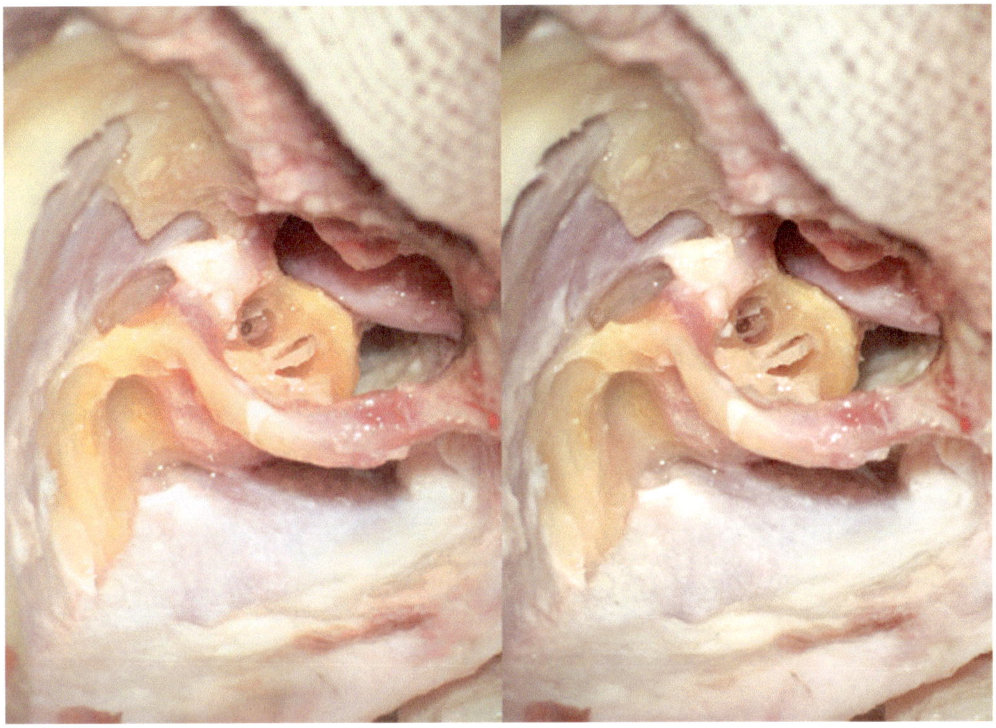

Fig. 4.74 Completely open the cochlea and its surrounding structures (right)
At the front of the cochlea is the internal carotid artery; above it from front to back are the tympanic opening of the Eustachian tube and the semicanal for the tensor tympani muscle, cochleariform process, and the horizontal segment of the facial nerve. The fundus of the IAC is behind and medial to the cochlea. The remnants of the superior semicircular canal can be seen in the Figure. The geniculate ganglion is separated from the middle cranial fossa by a thin plate of bone, and the GSPN passes forward from this below the dura. The internal carotid artery may be dehiscent at the lower edge of the promontory as a developmental anomaly or maybe exposed from trauma or form a pseudoaneurysm and be exposed to the middle ear cavity
Instruments: medium and tapering diamond burs

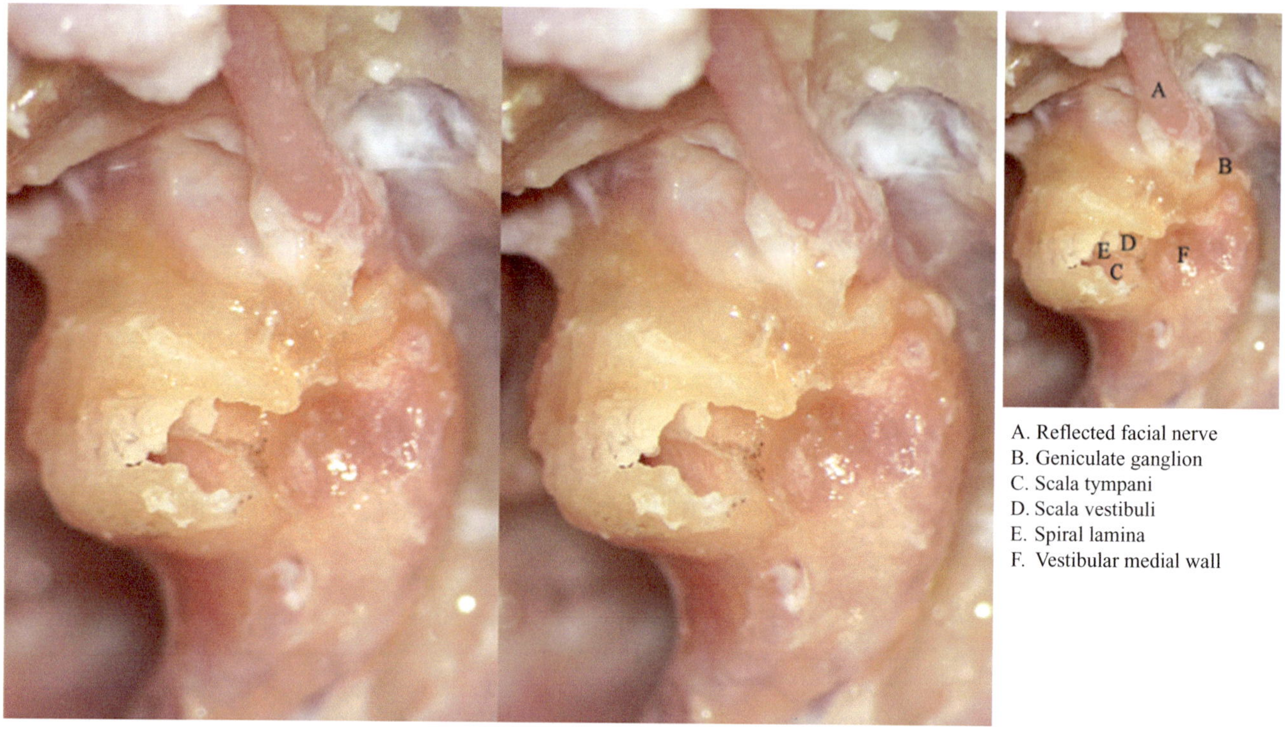

A. Reflected facial nerve
B. Geniculate ganglion
C. Scala tympani
D. Scala vestibuli
E. Spiral lamina
F. Vestibular medial wall

Fig. 4.75 Expose the basilar turn of the cochlea (left)
Reflect the facial nerve forward, remove the semicircular canals and vestibule, drill off the bone below the labyrinth, and skeletonize the IAC. One sees the outline of the IAC medially and the outline of the cochlea externally. The picture shows the left cochlea. The scala vestibuli, scala tympani, spiral lamina, basilar membrane, and the cochlear axis are seen at the center of the cochlea
Instruments: hook, tapering diamond burs

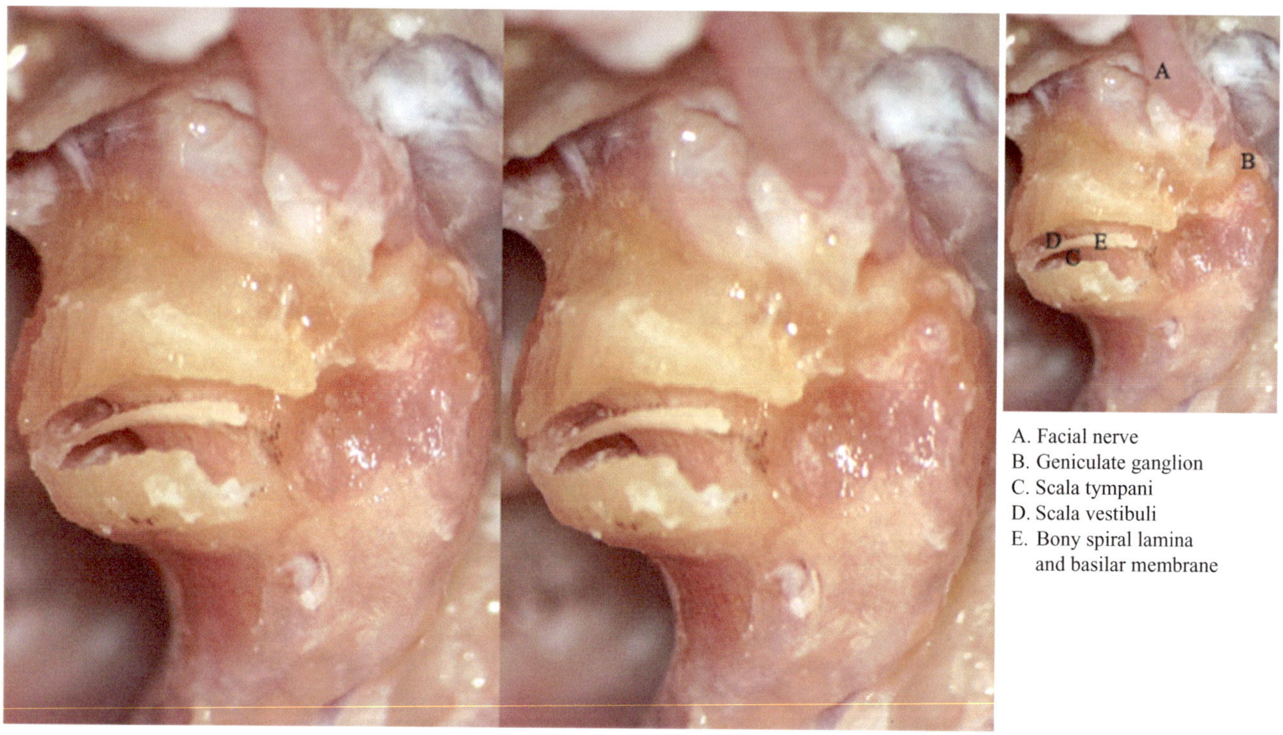

A. Facial nerve
B. Geniculate ganglion
C. Scala tympani
D. Scala vestibuli
E. Bony spiral lamina
and basilar membrane

Fig. 4.76 Open the basal turn of the cochlea (left)
Carefully remove the outer wall of the cochlea to reveal its internal structure, showing the bony spiral lamina and the basilar membrane, which divide the cochlea into the upper chamber (the scala vestibuli and scala media) and the lower chamber (the scala tympani)
Instruments: hook, tapering diamond burs

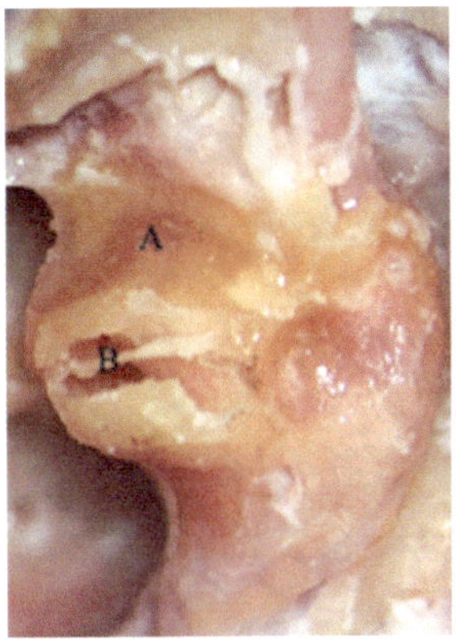

A. Bony wall of the middle and apical turns of the cochlea
B. Basal turn of the cochlea

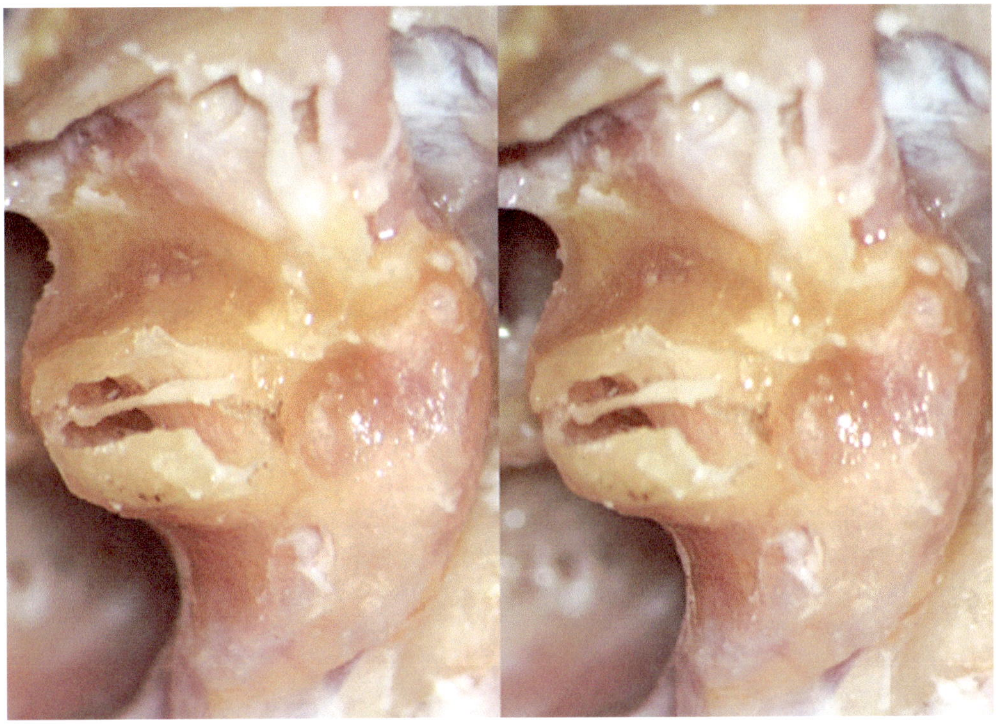

Fig. 4.77 Remove the bone wall of the middle and apical turns of the cochlea (left)
With the opened basal turn of the cochlea as an anatomical landmark, drill as described above, following the spiral direction of the cochlea, to expose the bony wall of the middle and apical turns of the cochlea

Instruments: tapering diamond burs

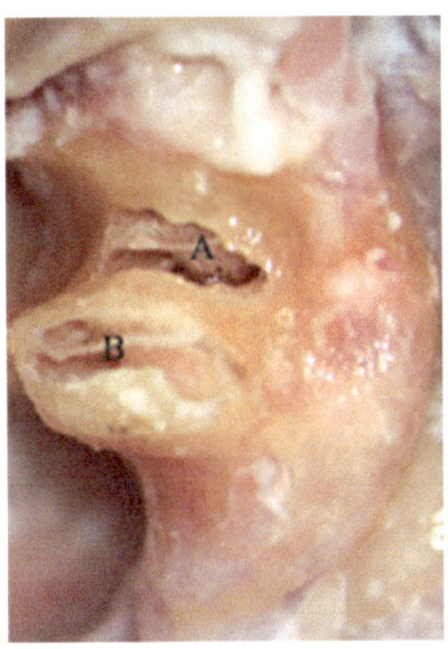

A. Middle turn of the cochlea
B. Basal turn of the cochlea

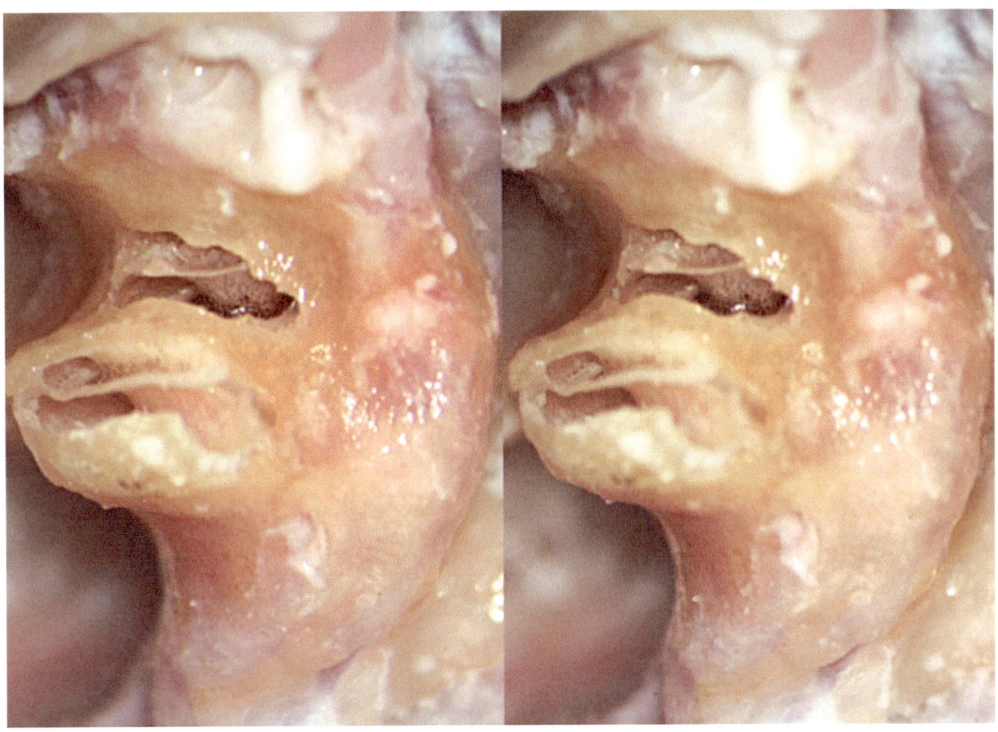

Fig. 4.78 Open the middle turn of the cochlea (left)
Using a tapered diamond bur, remove the bony wall of the middle turn of the cochlea layer by layer, revealing its internal structure as well as the cochlear axis (modiolus)

Instruments: tapering diamond burs

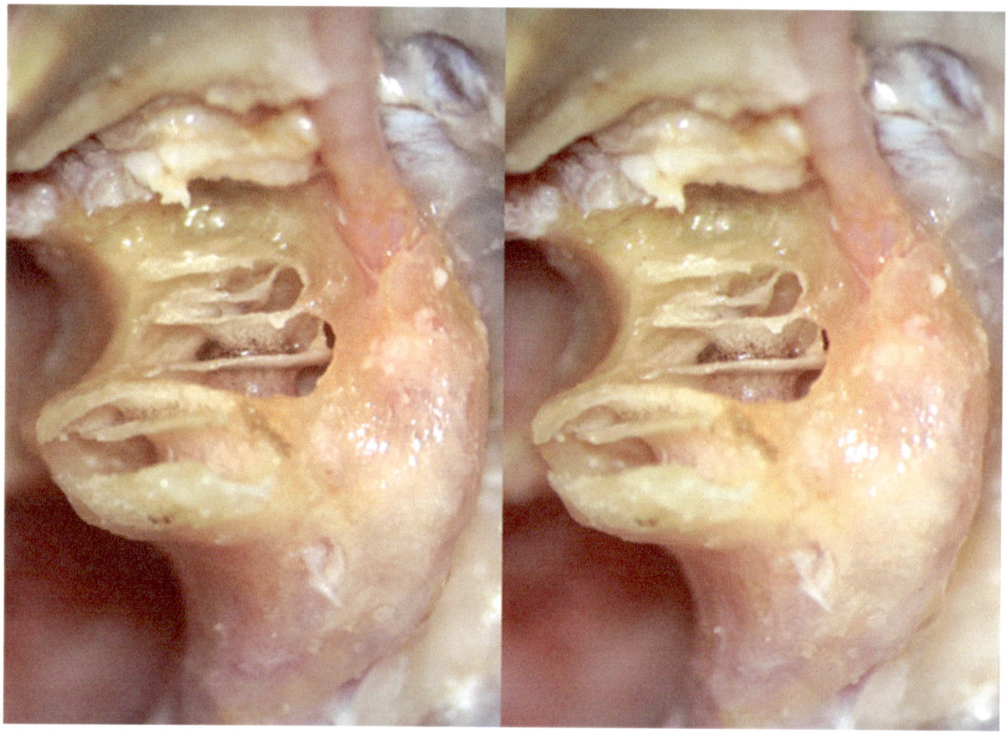

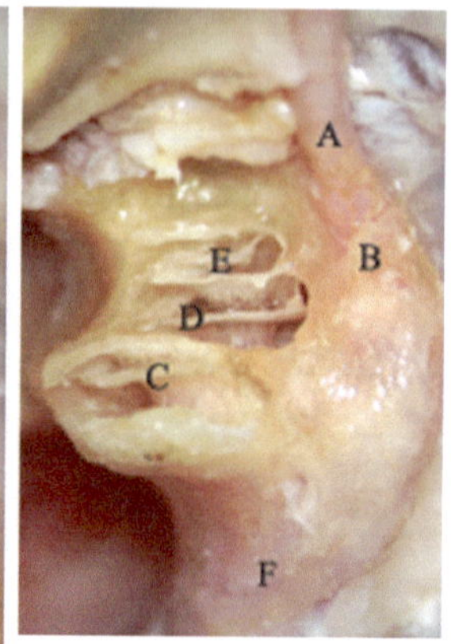

A. Reflected horizontal segment of the facial nerve
B. Geniculate ganglion
C. Basal turn of the cochlea
D. Middle turn of the cochlea
E. Apical turn of the cochlea
F. Outline of the IAC

Fig. 4.79 Expose the internal structure of the cochlea (left)
The lateral wall of the cochlea has been completely resected and the internal structure of the cochlea revealed. The cochlear axis (modiolus) with a rotation of 2.5–2.75 turns is located at the center of the cochlea

Instruments: tapering diamond burs

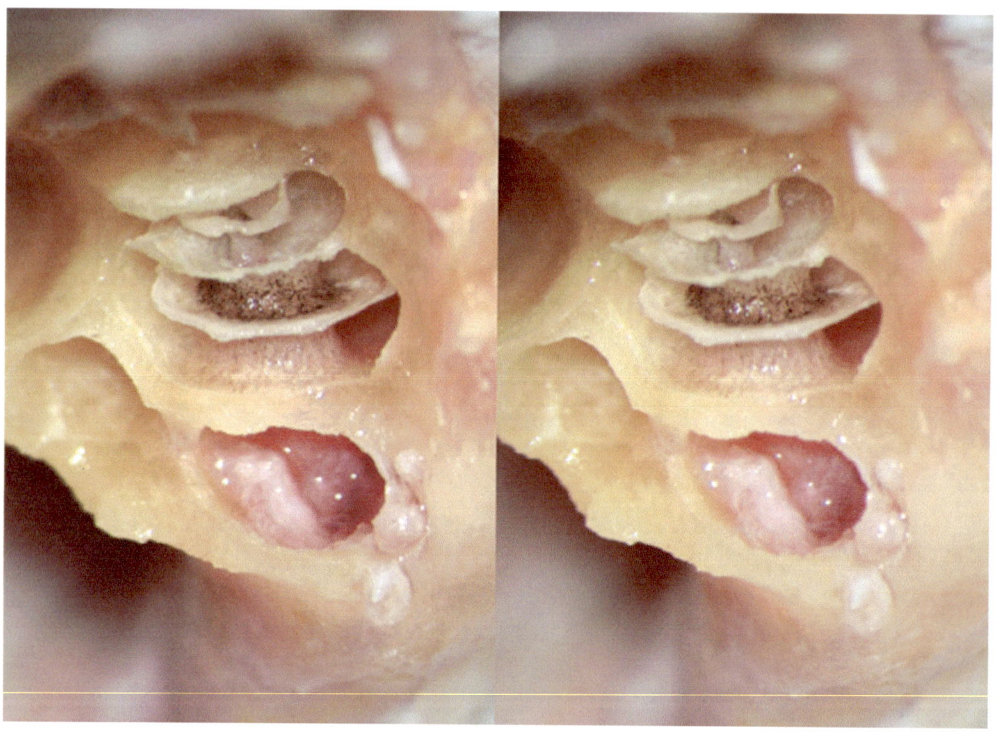

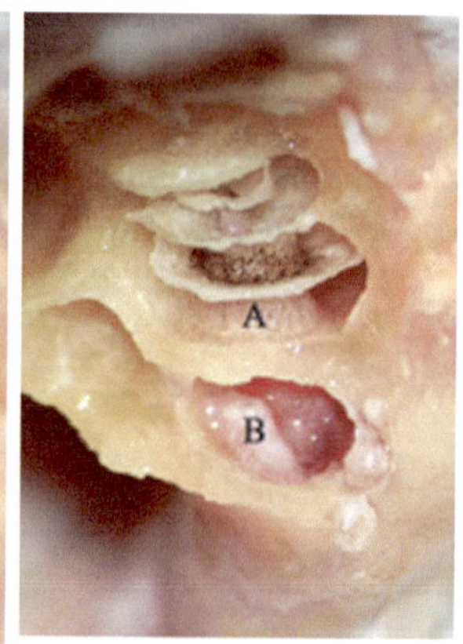

A. Modiolus
B. Acoustic nerve

Fig. 4.80 Drill off the bony wall of the modiolus (left)
Use a tapered diamond bur to remove the lateral bony wall of the modiolus. Note that the modiolus is a hollow bone tube that contains the cochlear fibers

Instruments: hook, tapering diamond burs

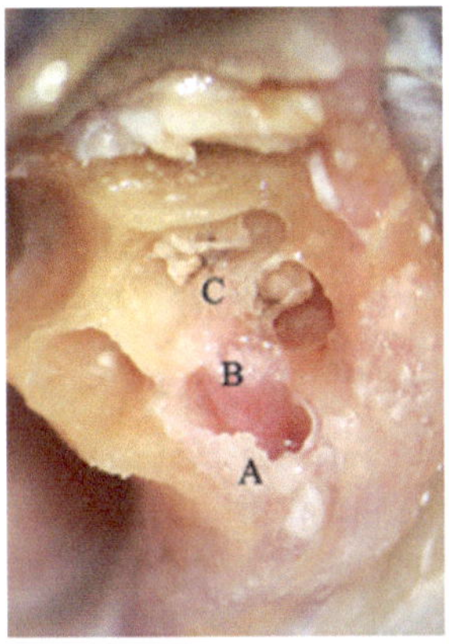

A. Cochlear nerve fibers distributed in the basal turn of cochlea
B. Cochlear nerve fibers distributed in the middle turn of cochlea
C. Area of the helicotrema

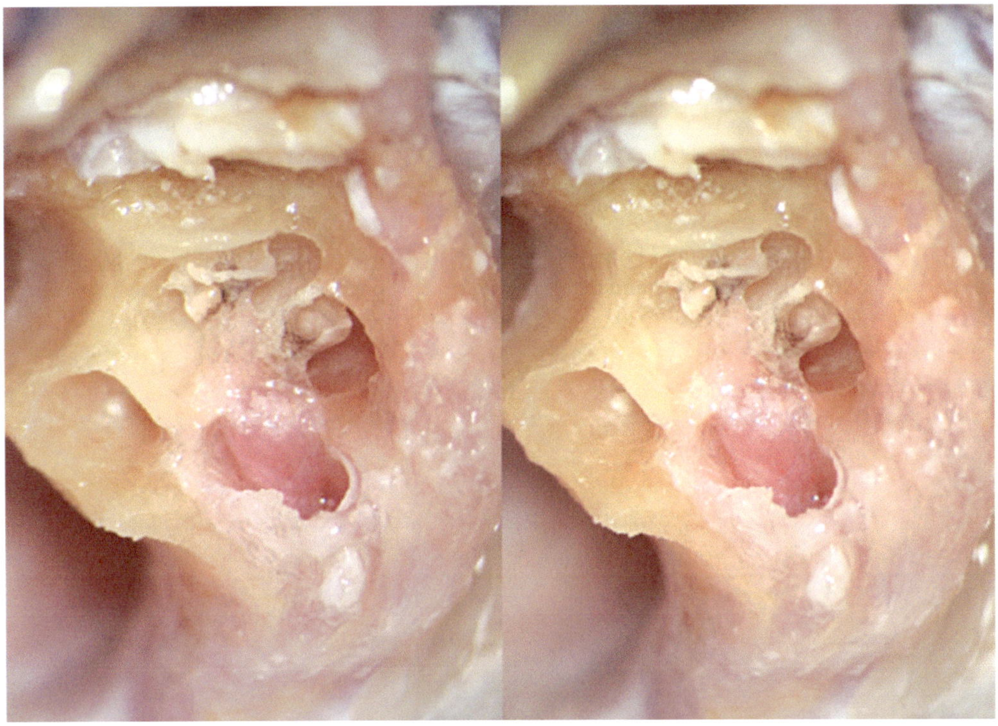

Fig. 4.81 Expose cochlear nerve fibers (left)
Completely remove the lateral wall of the modiolus, revealing the cochlear nerve (fibers). The cochlear spiral ganglion is located in Rosenthal's canal. The peripheral process of the cochlear spiral ganglion cells passes through small canals in the osseous spiral lamina to the organ of Corti. The central processes converge in the modiolus to form the cochlear nerve, which then passes into the fundus of the IAC. The central fibers in the nerve carry impulses produced by low-frequency sounds and the peripheral fibers carry those produced by high-frequency sounds
Instruments: tapering diamond burs

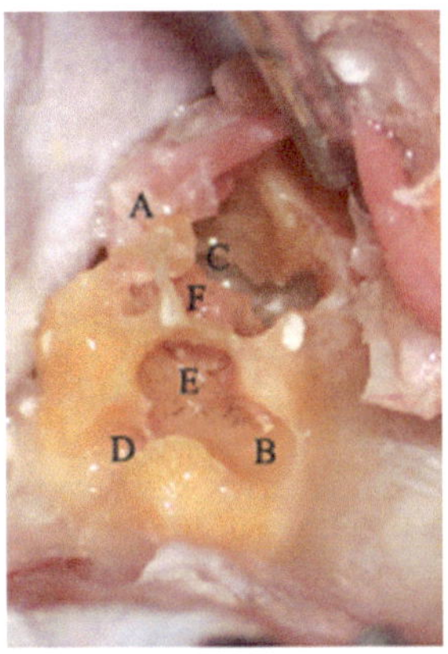

A. Geniculate ganglion
B. Ampullary part of the posterior semicircular canal
C. Cochlea
D. Common crus
E. Utricular recess
F. Saccular recess

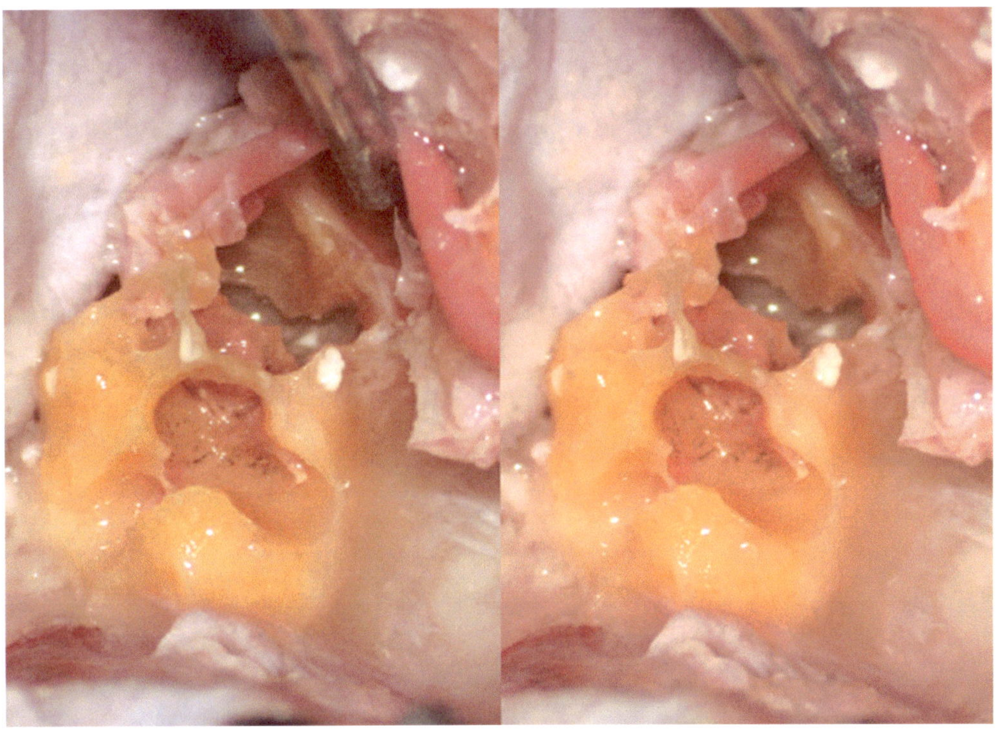

Fig. 4.82 Cochlea and vestibule (right)
Reflect the facial nerve forward, and drill away the bony walls of the semicircular canals, vestibule, and cochlea. The inner wall of the vestibule presents the vestibular crest, which separates the utricular and saccular recesses containing the utricle and saccule, respectively. The vestibular cavity communicates with the scala vestibuli inferiorly and contains perilymph
Instruments: medium tapering diamond burs

Cochlear Implantation

Chao-chan Cai and Feng Xin

Under normal conditions, action potentials generated by vibration of the basilar membrane in human hair cells induce hearing on arrival at the auditory center of the brain via the auditory nerve. Sensory hearing loss is caused by functional impairment or loss of hair cells in the inner ear, as the action potentials that stimulate the auditory center are not generated. Neural or central hearing loss is caused by disabilities of the auditory nerves, auditory pathways, or auditory center. Cochlear implants are designed to treat sensory hearing loss. Auditory brainstem implantation may work in some cases of deafness resulting from damaged auditory nerves but with intact upper auditory pathways from the brain stem and above.

Currently, the most widely used cochlear implants are produced by Cochlear Ltd. of Australia, MED-EL Ltd. of Austria, and Advanced Bionics Ltd. of America (AB). These manufacturers offer various models of implants. Domestic Chinese cochlear implants produced by Nurotron of Hangzhou, and Listent of Shanghai are also widely used in clinical practice.

Although the configuration of the various brands and models of cochlear implants differs, the implant systems always consist of external (microphone, sound processor, transmitter coil) and internal (receiver–stimulator, cochlear electrodes, reference electrode) components. Cochlear implantation is the process of inserting the internal components into the human body. Its basic steps include resection of the mastoid, exposure of the facial recess, fashioning of an implantation region for the receiver–stimulator (R/S), cochlear fenestration, insertion of electrodes, and closure of the operative site.

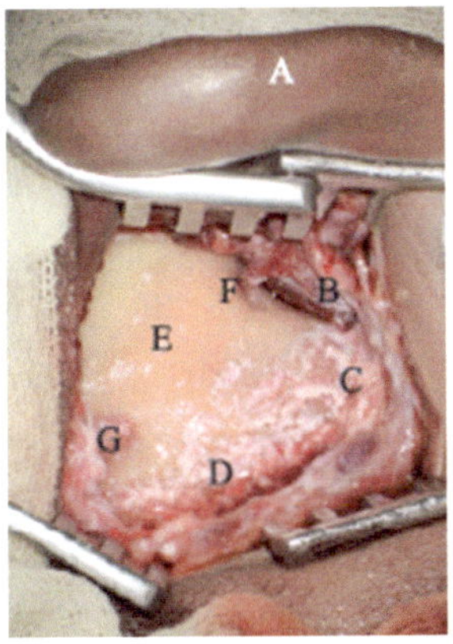

A. Auricle
B. Flap of the EAC
C. Mastoid tip
D. Posterior border of the mastoid
E. Temporal line
F. Cribriform area
G. Parietal incisura

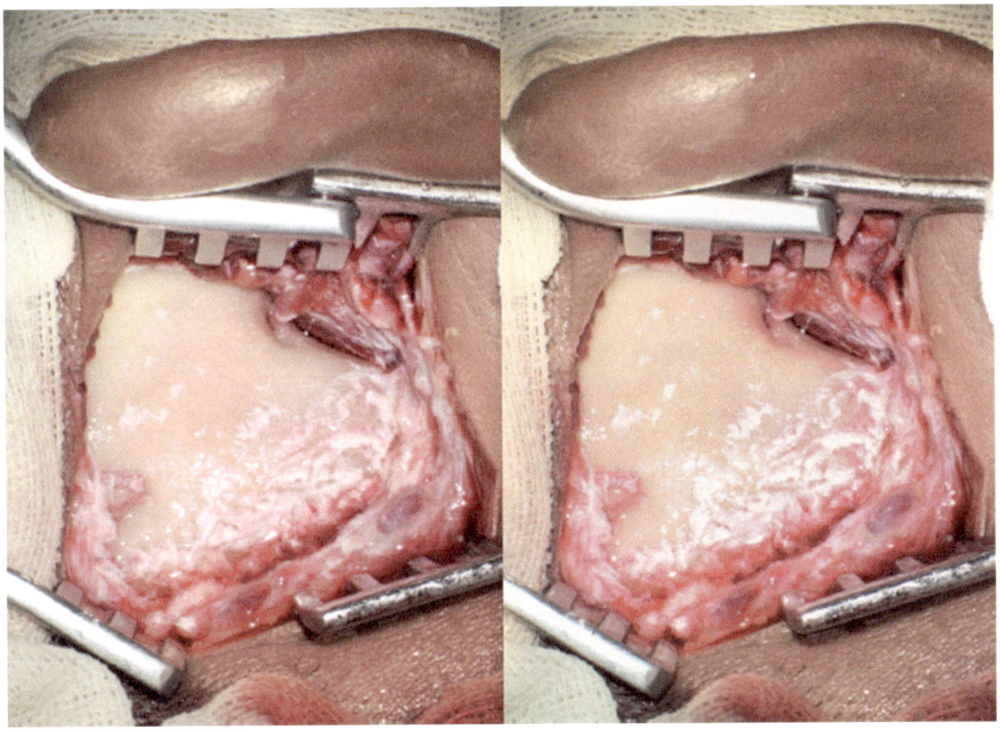

Fig. 4.83 The postauricular incision (right)
Make an arc incision posterior to the auricle, extending from just superior to the apex of the mastoid tip to a point inferior to the upper edge of the attachment of the auricle. The distances between the incision and the postauricular sulcus are: top 0.5 cm, middle 1.5–2.0 cm, and behind the lobule 1.2 cm. Incise the skin and subcutaneous tissues down to the mastoid bone, separating the flap with a periosteal elevator, and expose the mastoid area with the aid of a self-retaining mastoid retractor. *Important anatomical marks: posterior wall of the EAC, suprameatal spine, cribriform area, temporal line, mastoid tip, parietal incisura etc. Instruments: scalpel, periosteal elevator, mastoid retractor*

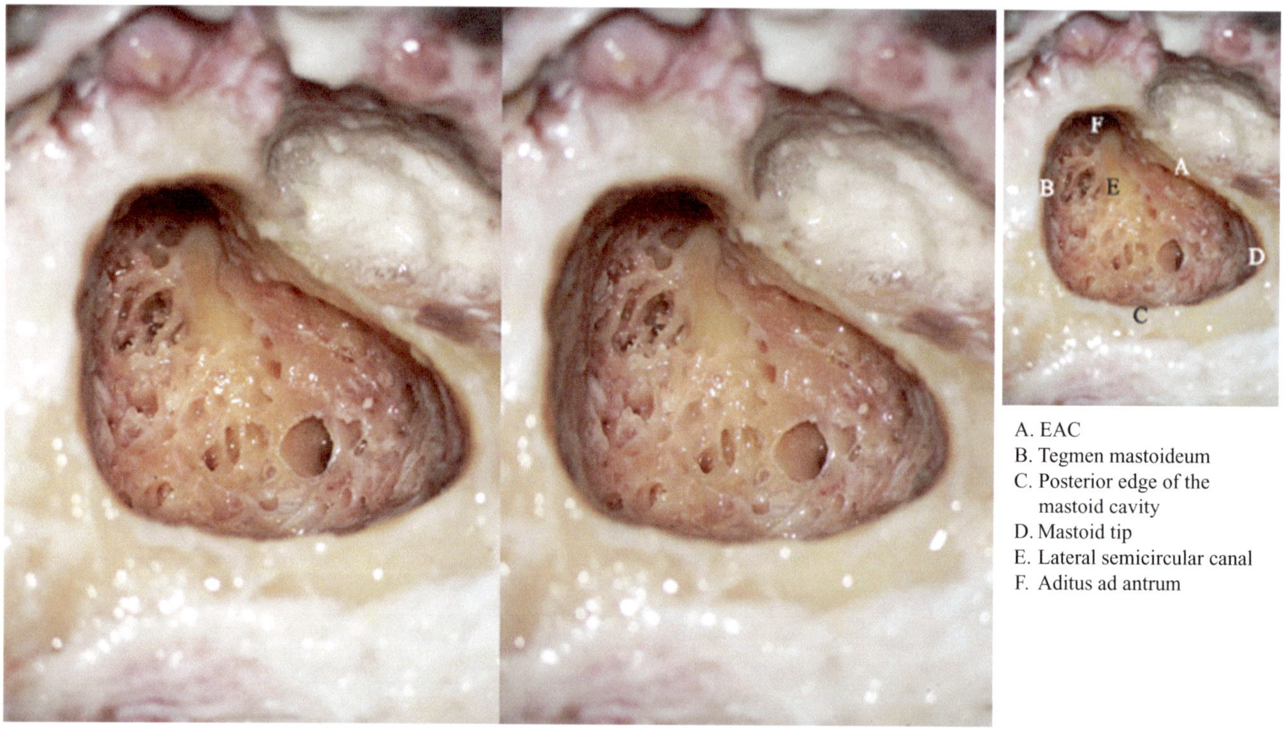

A. EAC
B. Tegmen mastoideum
C. Posterior edge of the mastoid cavity
D. Mastoid tip
E. Lateral semicircular canal
F. Aditus ad antrum

Fig. 4.84 Mastoidectomy (right)
Most patients undergoing cochlear implantation have normal mastoids, enabling straightforward exposure of the important structures in the operative field. Detailed procedures: drill away the air cells of the mastoid, revealing the aditus ad antrum and the tympanic antrum, identify the lateral semicircular canal and the short process of the incus, thin the posterior wall of the EAC, and expose the posterior and inferior parts of the mastoid cavity, but only as required. The cortical bone in the edges of the mastoid cavity must be retained with some overhang, to assist stabilization of the electrode cables
Instruments: large-sized cutting burs, medium-sized diamond burs

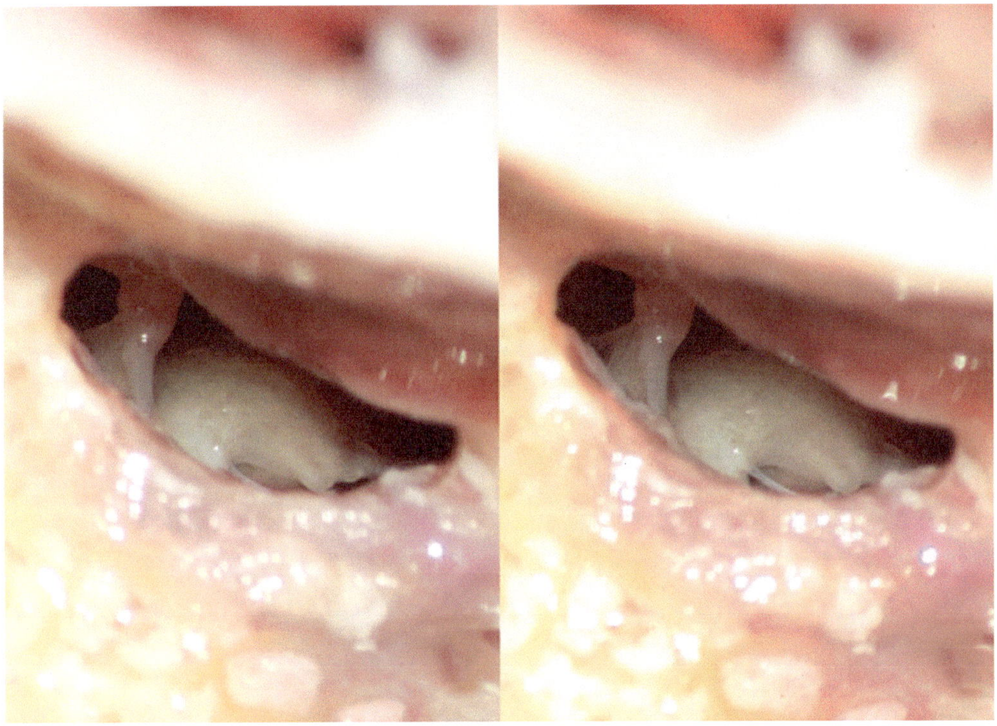
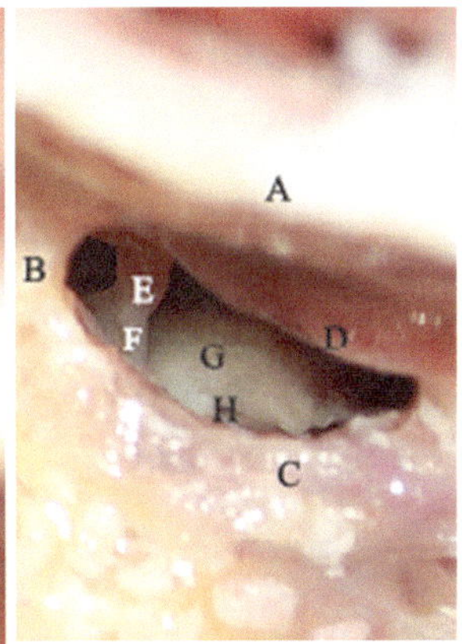

A. Posterior wall of the EAC
B. Incus buttress
C. Vertical portion of the fallopian canal
D. Chorda tympani canal
E. Incudostapedial joint
F. Stapedius tendon
G. Promontory
H. Round window niche

Fig. 4.85 Open the facial recess (right)
Minimally invasive cochlear implantation employs minimal but adequate instrumentation to preserve cochlear function. It is necessary to open the facial recess sufficiently to expose the round window niche in all directions. Drill away the overhanging lip of the round window niche to expose the round window membrane
Instruments: medium- and small-sized diamond burs, right-angle hook

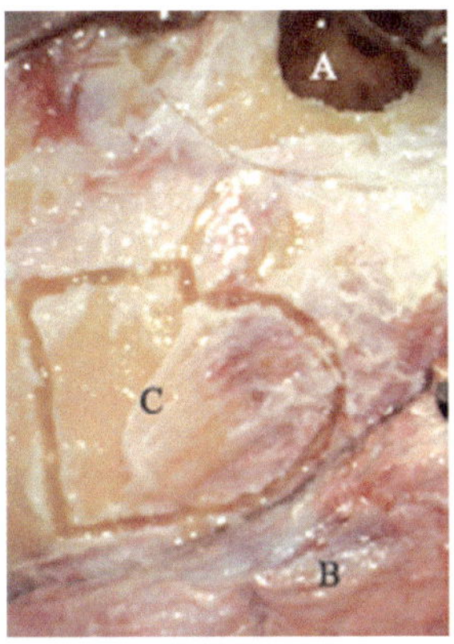

A. Mastoid cavity
B. Sub-occipital muscle
C. R/S bed marked out

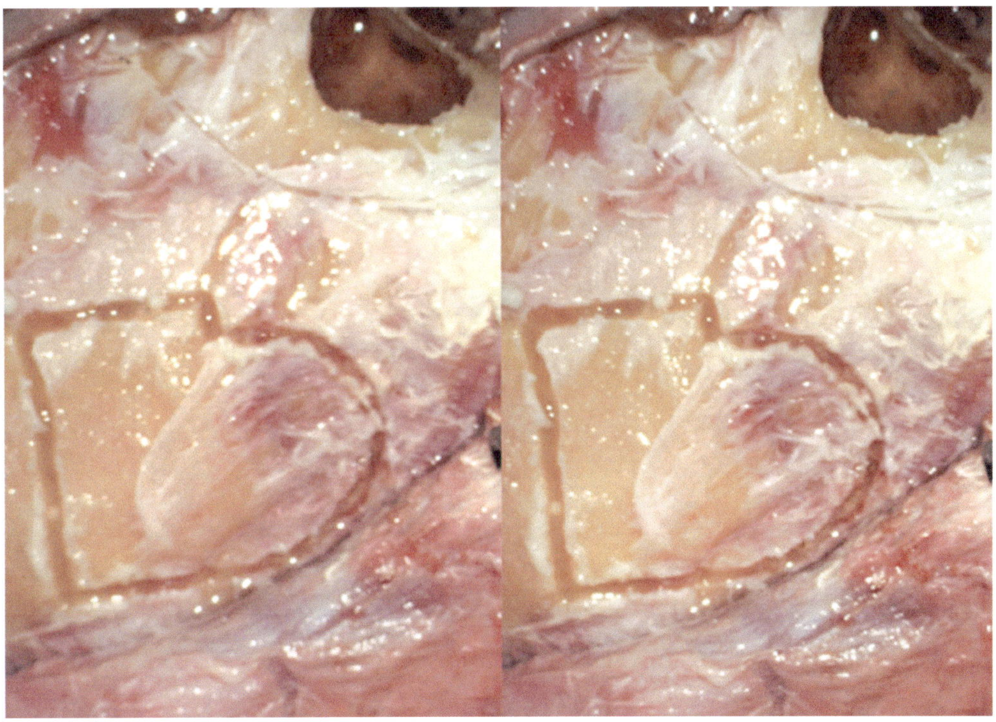

Fig. 4.86 Preparation of the bony bed for receiver/stimulator (right, MED-EL)
The center of the implant bed is located posterosuperior to the opened mastoid. The distance between the receiver/stimulator (R/S) and mastoid cavity should be more than 1.5 cm. The implanted bed shown here is suitable for implanting the body of MED-EL C40+ and the Pulsar series
Instruments: small-sized cutting burs, implant template

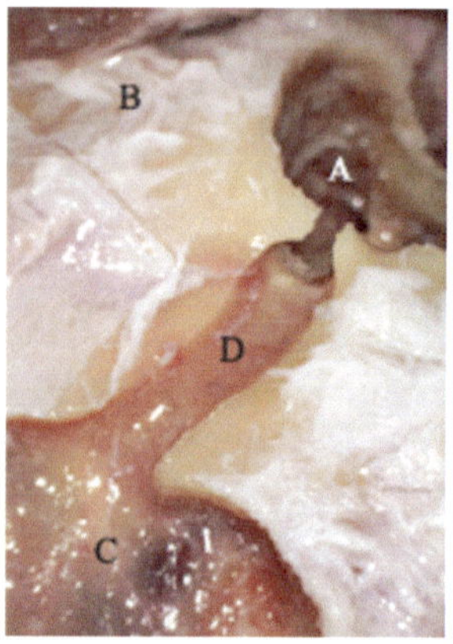

A. Mastoid cavity
B. Squamous portion of the temporal bone
C. Implant bed
D. Trough for electrode cable

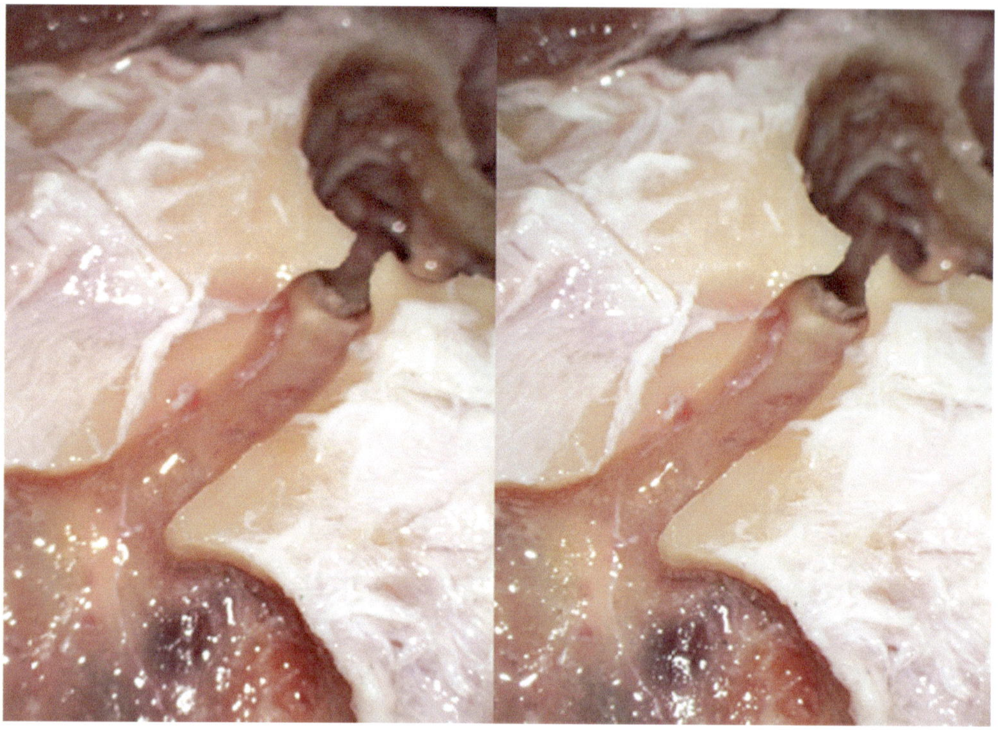

Fig. 4.87 Drill out the implant bed and electrode trough (right)
Drill out the implant bed carefully with a diamond bur until the template can be well seated into it, then drill the trough for the electrode cable connecting the implant bed and the mastoid cavity using a medium cutting bur. As a child's skull is thinner, the inner table of the skull may need to be removed down to expose the dura. Adult patients have thicker skulls and the inner table can be retained after adequate bone removal to allow proper seating of the R/S and electrode cable
Instruments: medium-sized diamond burs, elevator, implant body template

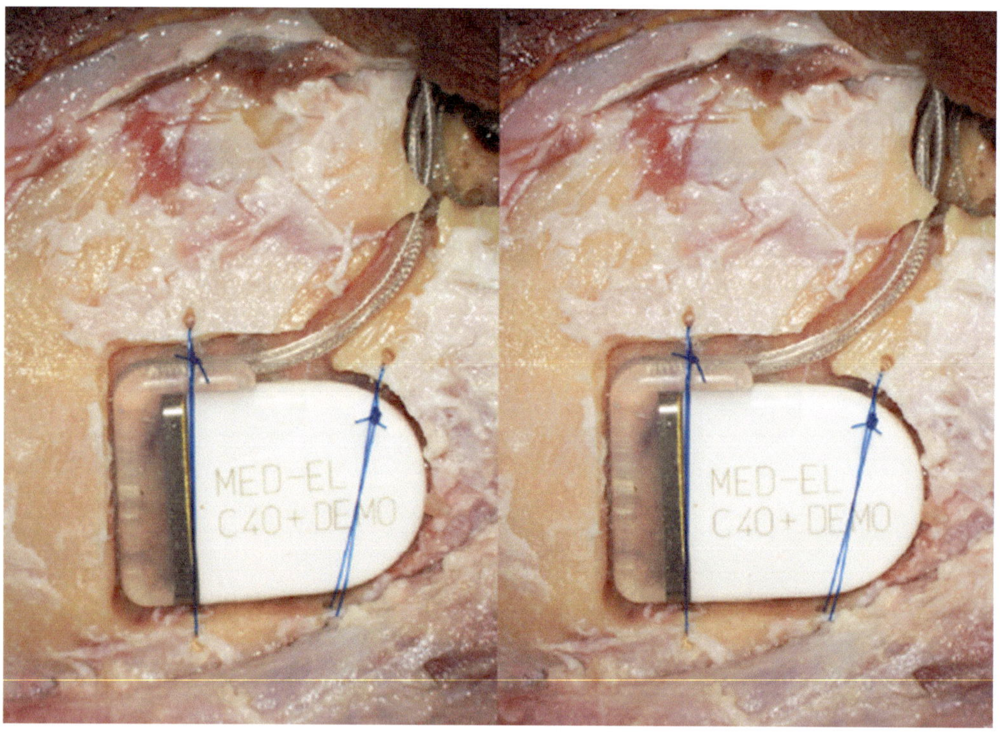

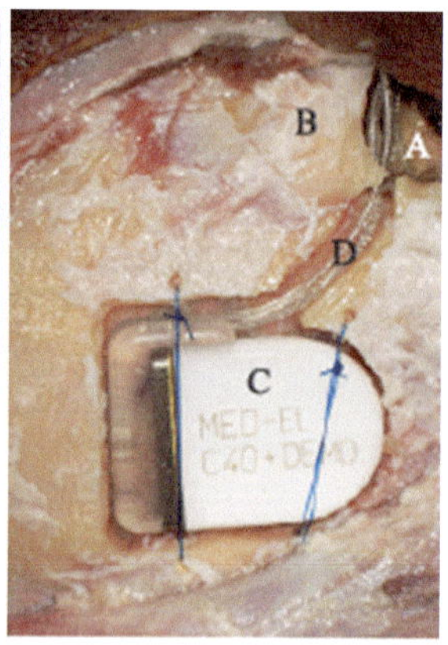

A. Mastoid cavity
B. Squamous portion of the temporal bone
C. MED-EL C40+ R/S imbedded and fixed
D. Electrode cable in the trough

Fig. 4.88 Embedded MED-EL (Austria) R/S (model, right)
Embed the MED-EL implant (model) and electrode cable. The MED-EL series of implants (Pulsar, C40+) usually require fixation with sutures

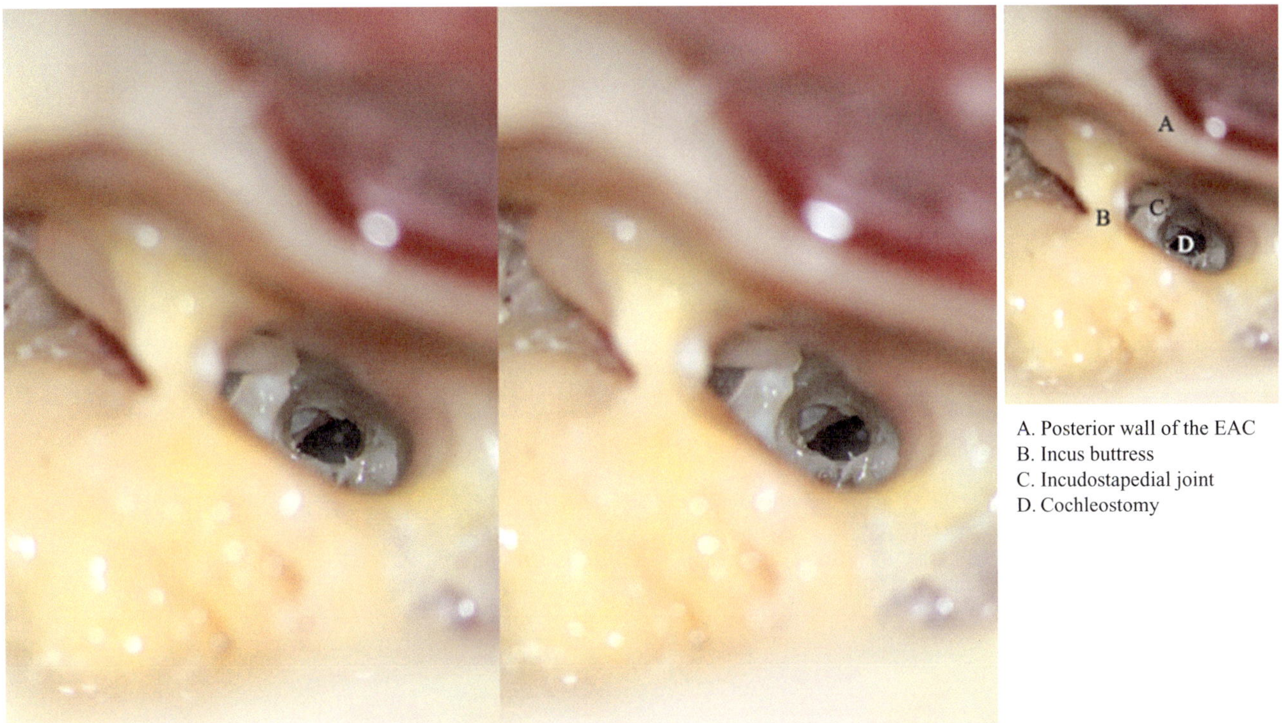

A. Posterior wall of the EAC
B. Incus buttress
C. Incudostapedial joint
D. Cochleostomy

Fig. 4.89 Cochleostomy (right)
The facial recess is opened to provide a good view of the promontory and allow the cochleostomy into the basal turn of the cochlea. It is important to note that the cochlea should be opened after the R/S has been implanted and fixed in place (if necessary) and closed immediately after the electrode array has been inserted. This is to minimize the exposure time and the level of interference with the inner ear, to assist in retaining as much residual hearing as possible
Instruments: small-sized diamond burs

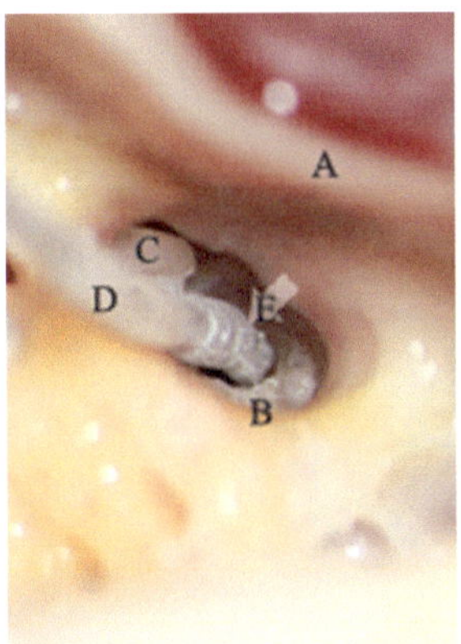

A. Posterior wall of the EAC
B. Inner edge of the facial recess
C. Long process of the incus
D. Electrode array of the implant
E. Insertion limit point of electrode array

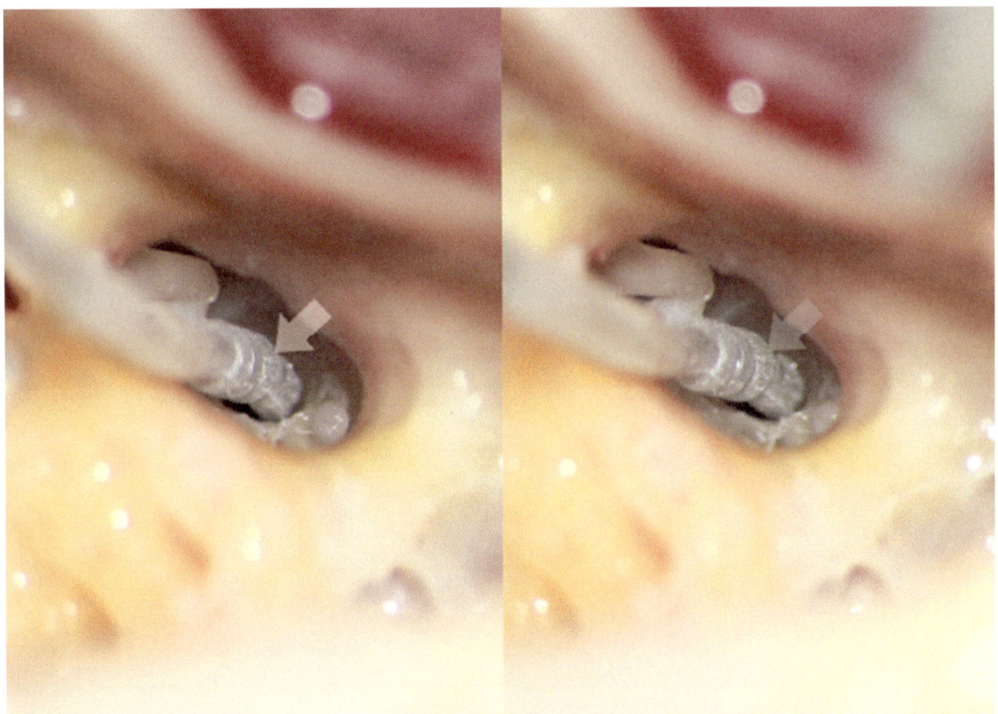

Fig. 4.90 Insertion of the electrode array (right)
Insert the electrode array using the electrode fork and electrode tweezers. This is the Australian Cochlear straight electrode array; the insert portion has three circular ribs. Insertion is stopped when the first rib sits at the rim of the cochleostomy; then the opening is sealed with small pieces of temporalis muscle
Instruments: electrode fork, electrode tweezers

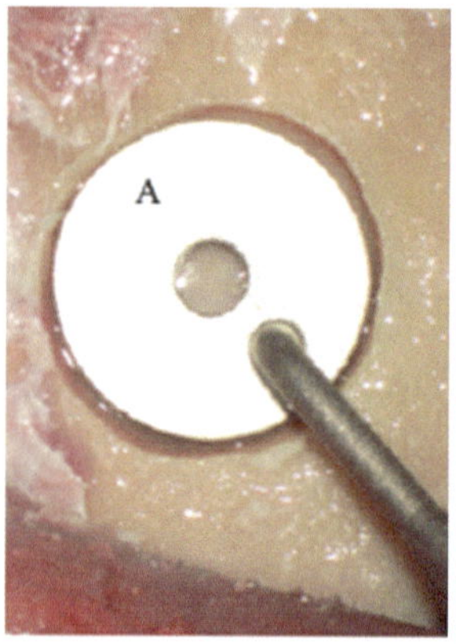

A. Round implant template

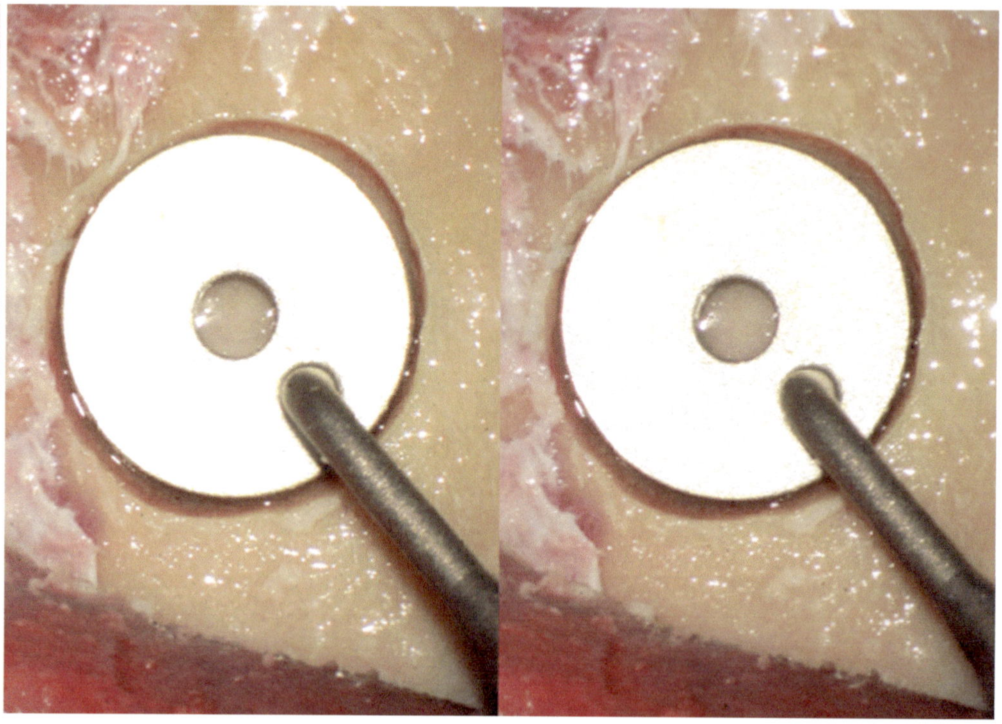

Fig. 4.91 Round bony bed for Implants (left)
The implant templates of the Australian Cochlear freedom model and American AB 90K model are round. The techniques for making the implant beds are as described previously

Instruments: medium-sized diamond burs

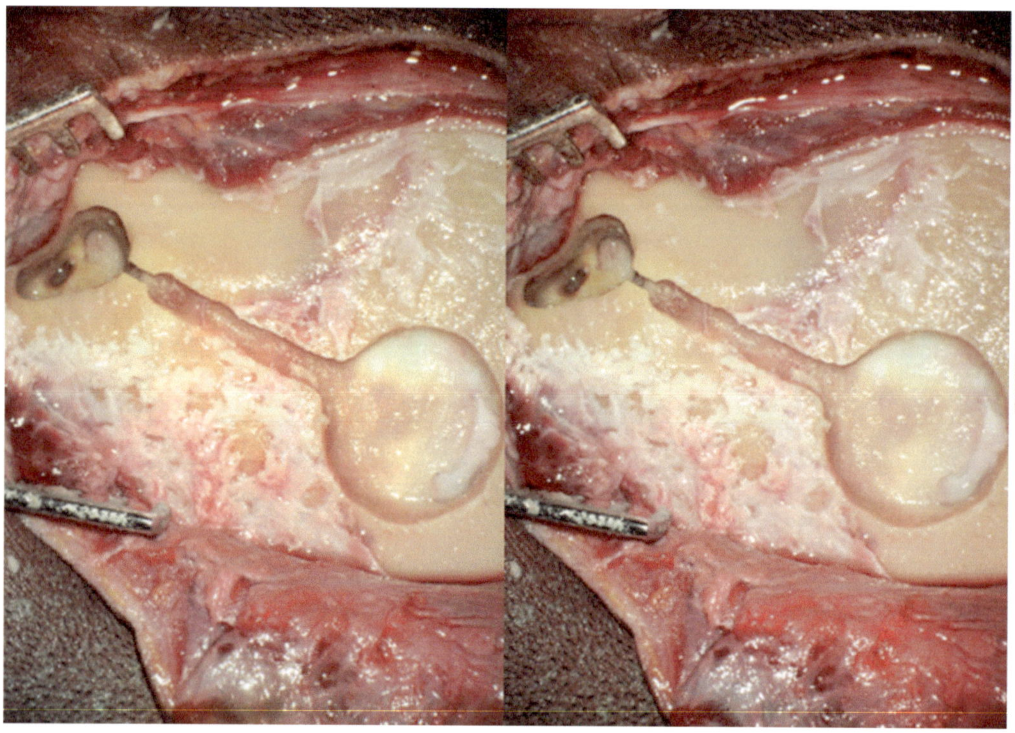

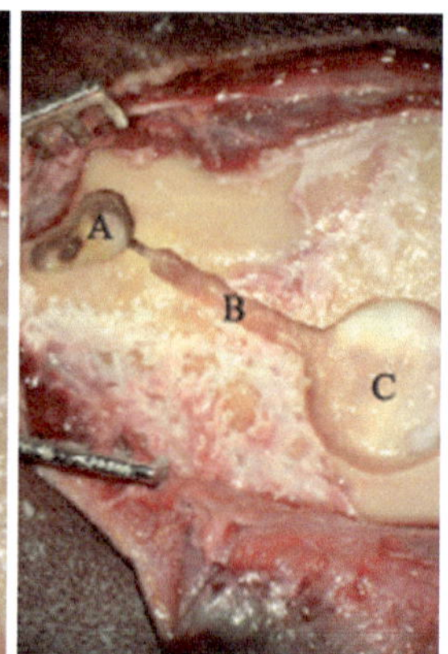

A. Mastoid cavity
B. Trough for electrode array
C. Bony bed for R/S

Fig. 4.92 Drilling trough for electrode array (left)
Drill a trough for the electrode array, which connects the implant bed with the mastoid cavity

Instruments: medium-sized cutting burs

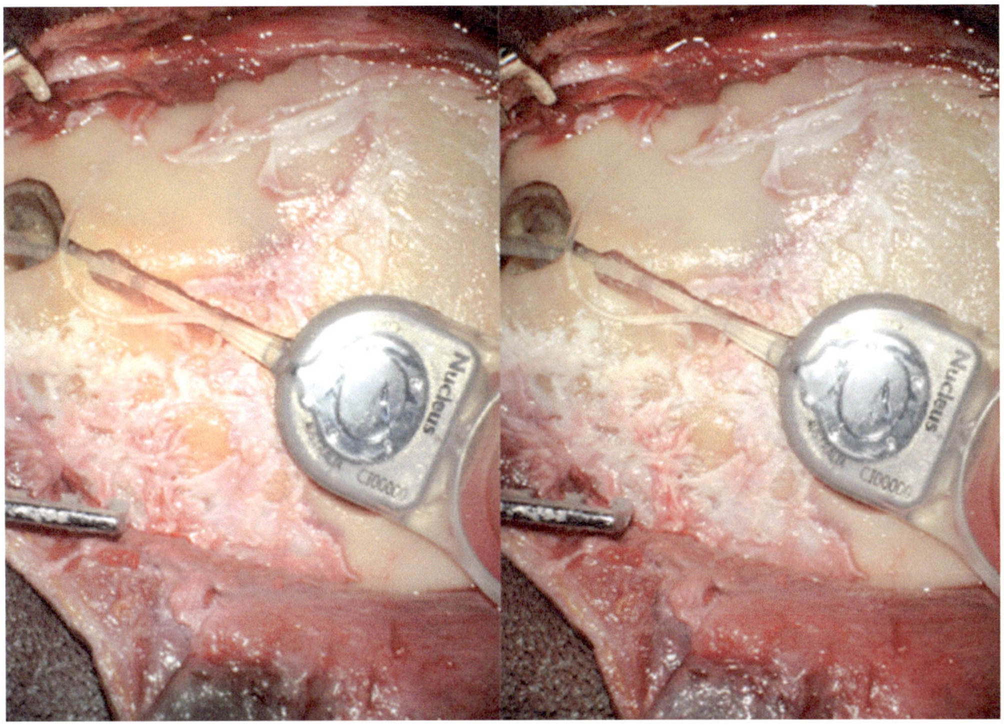

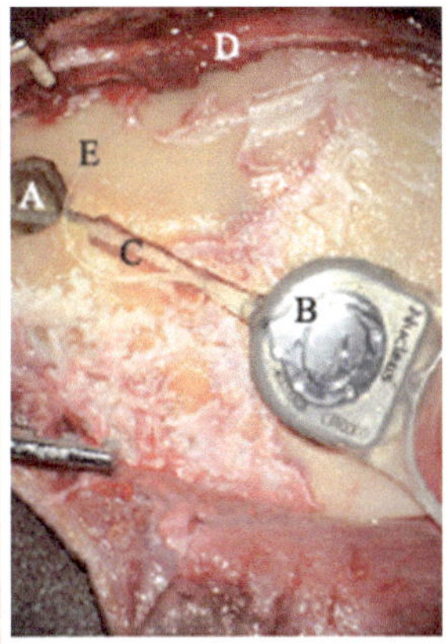

A. Mastoid cavity
B. R/S
C. Electrode array in trough
D. Temporalis muscle
E. Reference electrode

Fig. 4.93 Cochlear Nucleus implant (left)
Cochlear implant and electrode in situ after implantation has been completed. The reference electrode is placed under the temporalis muscle above the level of the upper edge of the auricle

Instruments: elevator, tissue forceps

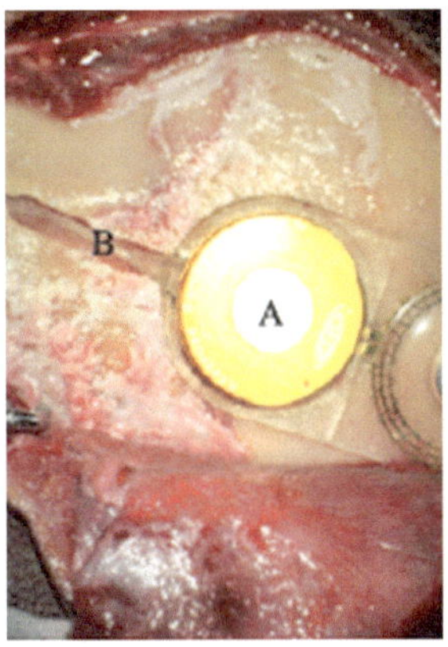

A. AB R/S
B. Trough containing the electrode array

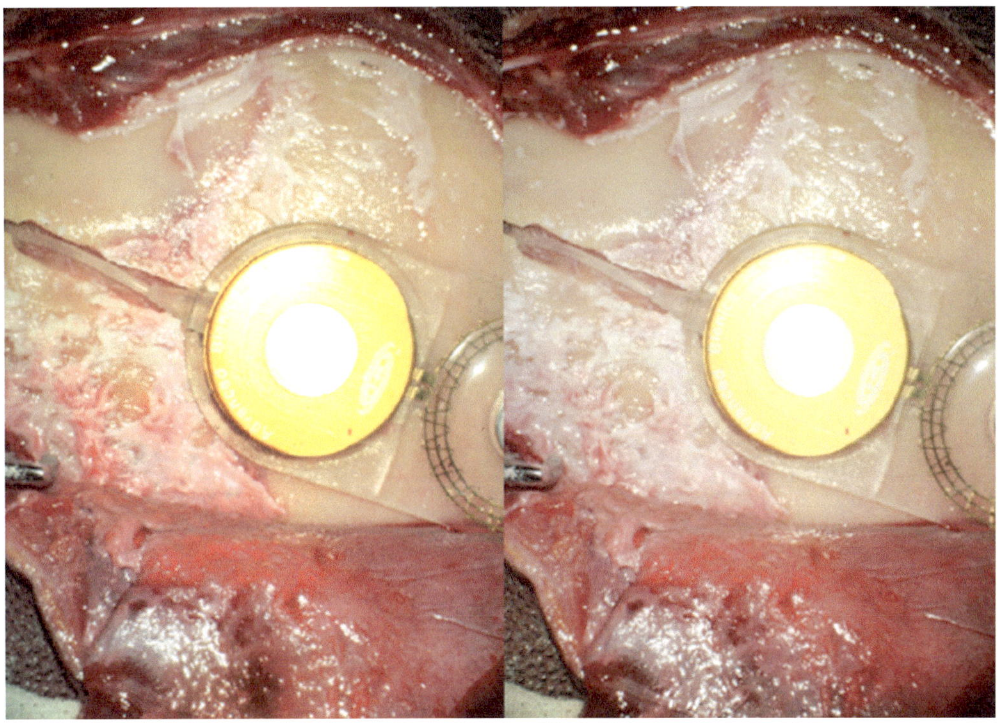

Fig. 4.94 Advanced Bionics (AB) implant (left)
Implant AB R/S and electrode

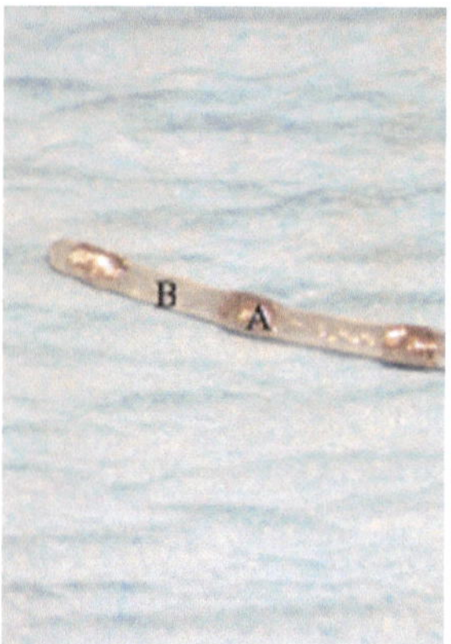

A. Electrode contact point
B. Contact separation zone

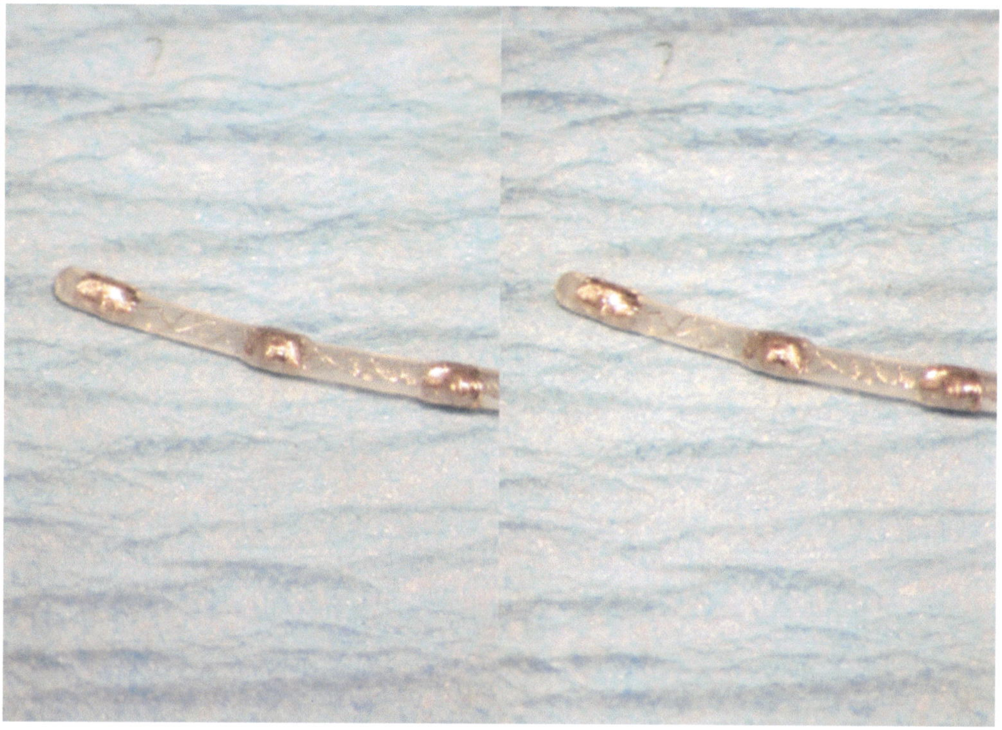

Fig. 4.95 The tip of the electrode and the electrode contact point
The electrode is a flexible cord made up of 12–24 electrode contact points (multichannel cochlear implant). The electrode contains a number of guide wires, each of which is connected to an electrode point. The guide wires are arranged in a "Z" or wavy format, which avoids fractures of the electrode

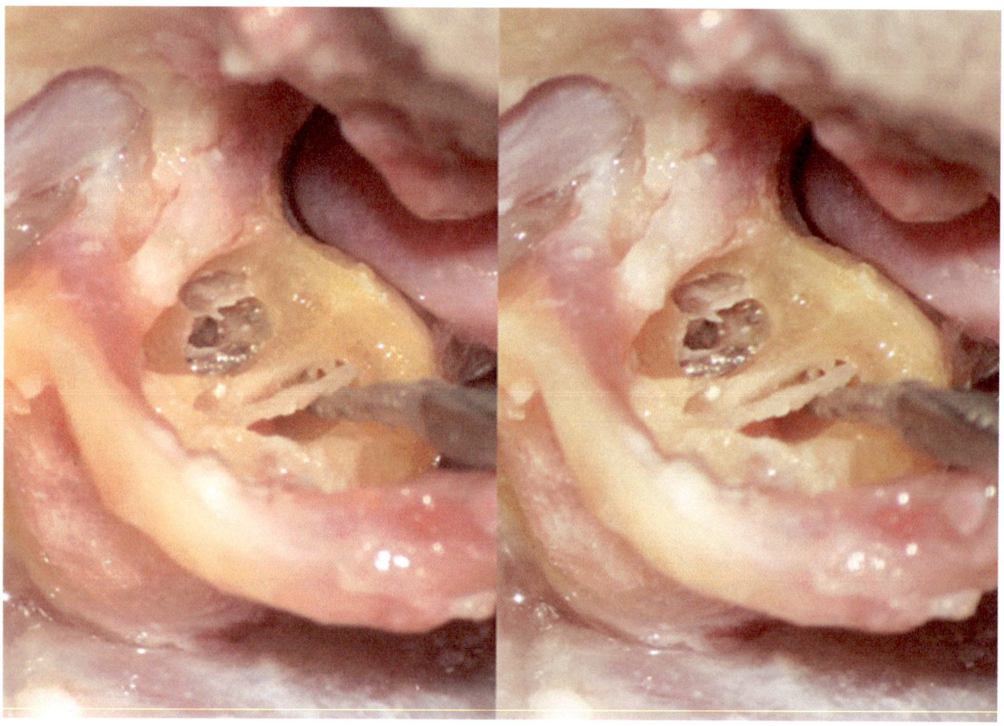

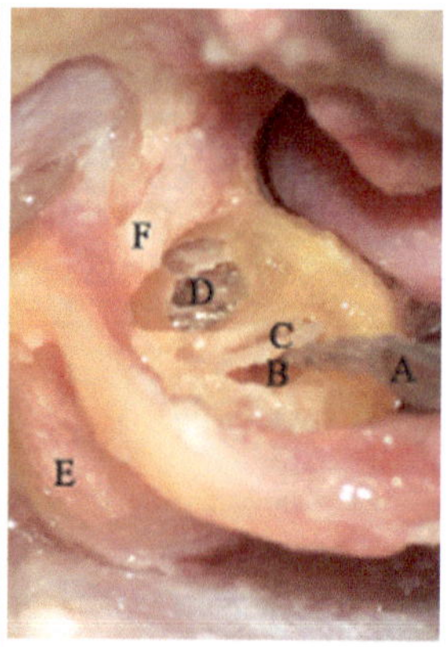

A. Electrode of a cochlear implant
B. Scala tympani
C. Scala vestibuli
D. Middle turn and cupula of the cochlea
E. IAC
F. Cochleariform process

Fig. 4.96 Location of electrode in cochlea (right)
Remove the structures of the middle ear and skeletonize the IAC. Open the lateral wall of the cochlea, and insert the electrode into the scala tympani of the basal turn of the cochlea. The electrode is rotated into the cochlea along the lumen of the scala tympani

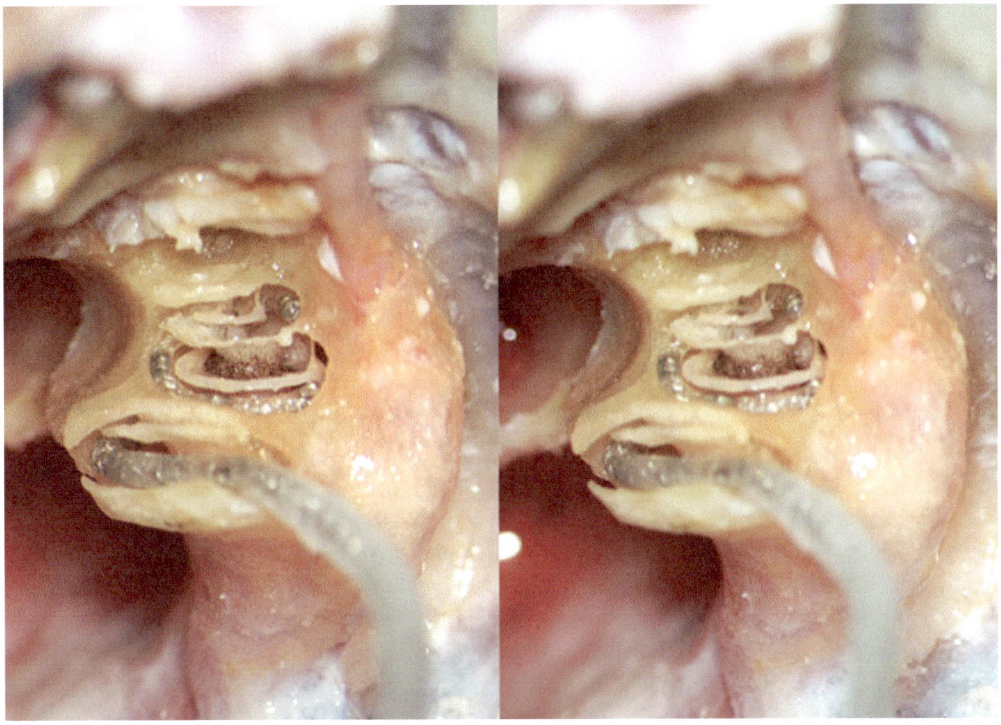

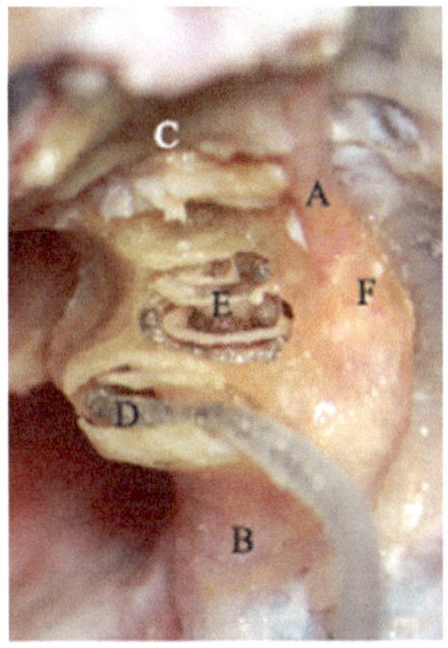

A. Re-routed facial nerve
B. IAC
C. Posterior wall of the mandibular fossa
D. Electrode
E. Middle and apical turn of the cochlea
F. Geniculate ganglion

Fig. 4.97 Location of electrode in cochlea (left)
(As with the Type A approach to the infratemporal fossa, the facial nerve has been re-routed forward.) Open the outer wall of the cochlea, and insert the electrode into the scala tympani of the basal turn of the cochlea. The electrode is rotated into the middle and apical turns of the cochlea along the lumen of the scala tympani

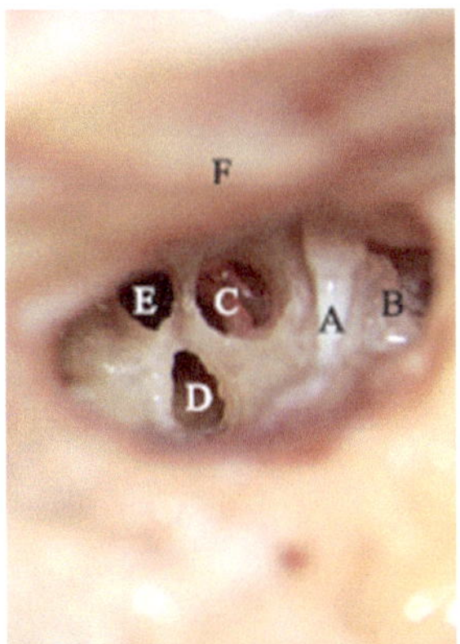

A. Stapedius tendon
B. Anterior crus of the stapes
C. Cochleostomy anterior to the round window niche
D. Round window
E. Cochleostomy antero-inferior to the round window
F. Posterior wall of the EAC

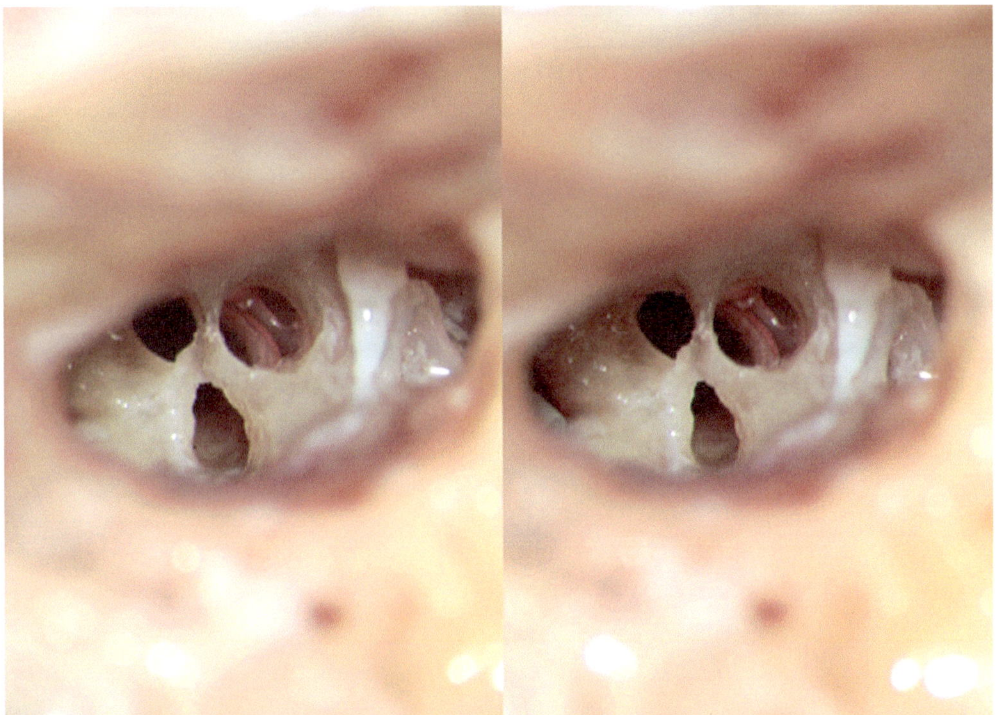

Fig. 4.98 Cochleostomy (left)
The traditional cochleostomy site is anterior to the round window niche. There is a good view of the scala tympani in most situations, but sometimes this approach may disrupt the basilar membrane and scala vestibuli, causing loss of residual hearing. Insertion via the round window allows placement of the electrode array into the scala tympani. A cochleostomy anterior and inferior to the round window will also ensure that the electrode is kept inside the scala tympani

Vibrant Soundbridge Implantation

Xu-kun Yan and Xue Gao

Hearing loss can affect the threshold of hearing and also reduce the audible dynamic range. The function of a conventional hearing aid is to capture and amplify the sound, and transmit the amplified signal through the earmold or directly through the hearing aid to the acoustic structure of the middle ear. This will have a better effect for patients with an increased auditory threshold, but a limited effect on a narrowed audible dynamic range. A variety of new hearing-aid devices are designed to compensate for the shortcomings of traditional hearing aids, one of which is the Vibrant Soundbridge (VSB).

The VSB is an implantable middle ear auditory prosthesis in two parts, the external auditory processor (AP) and the vibrant ossicular reconstructive prosthesis (VORP), which is implanted. The AP includes a microphone, digital signal processor, regulator, and a battery. The VORP includes electromagnetic induction receiving coils, modems, wires, and a floating mass transducer (FMT). The VSB collects acoustic signals through the AP and converts them into electrical signals, which are sent by electromagnetic induction to the receiving coils and decoded by the modem, thus driving FMT vibration. By driving the ossicular chain or direct vibration of the round window membrane, the FMT causes a mechanical vibration signal to be conducted into the inner ear, stimulating hair cells to produce hearing. The VSB can provide stimulus signals from 250 to 8000 Hz. Each 1-micron displacement of the FMT can provide 120 dB of sound pressure level (SPL) gain. Both hearing threshold and audible dynamic range are improved by the VSB in patients with moderate to severe hearing loss.

The VSB implantation method is similar to that of a cochlear implant. The basic steps include: mastoidectomy, preparation of the implant bed posterosuperior to the mastoid, and opening of the facial recess. The differences are: (1) VSB requires the scalp thickness covering the implant to be less than 7 mm. If the scalp is too thick it will interfere with signal transduction from the AP to the VORP; (2) The facial recess opening needs to be larger in VSB than for cochlear implantation.

The diameter of the FMT is 1.8 mm and its height is 2.3 mm. It also has a titanium clip for fixation. The facial recess needs to be opened sufficiently to allow FMT insertion into the tympanic cavity. The VSB was originally designed to improve the hearing of patients with moderate to severe sensorineural deafness. After the success of FMT implantation to the round window, its application was extended to patients with conductive and mixed deafness. Specific VSB indications are: age older than 18 years (the implant age can be lower in patients with external and middle ear deformities); the benefit from traditional hearing aids is limited, or there are contraindications to the use of traditional hearing aids; external and middle ear deformities; bilateral moderate to severe sensorineural, conductive or mixed deafness that has been stable for more than 2 years; sequelae of chronic otitis media, open mastoid cavity, absence of ossicular chain and otosclerosis not amenable to traditional stapes surgery.

Contraindications include retrocochlear deafness, central deafness, active middle ear infection, chronic hydrops of the inner ear, tympanic membrane perforation with recurrent infection of the middle ear, progressive hearing loss of more than 15 dB over 2 years, and patients with inappropriate expectations of hearing recovery.

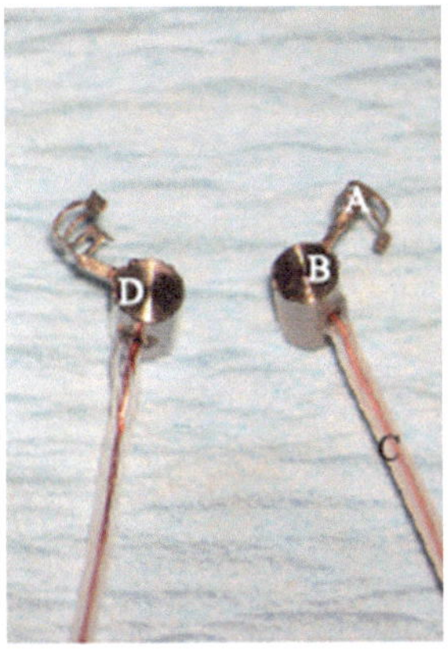

A. Titanium clip
B. Floating mass transducer prosthesis (for left ear)
C. Conducting wire
D. Floating mass transducer prosthesis (for right ear)

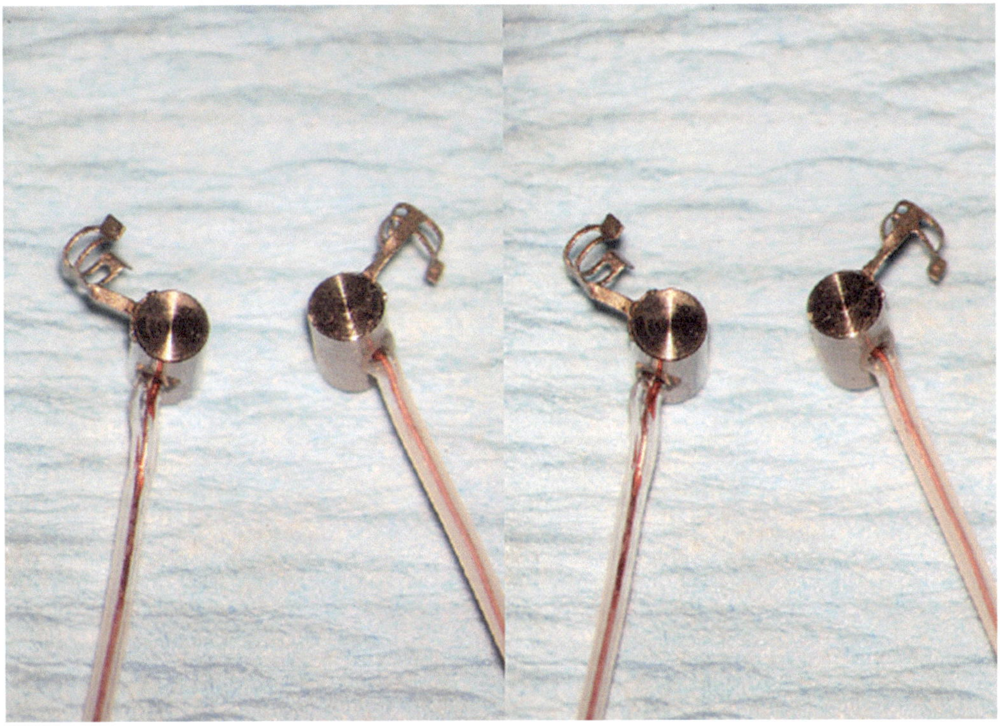

Fig. 4.99 Floating mass transducer (FMT)
The FMT is an electromagnetic induction device with a cylindrical titanium shell that is bound tightly to the conductive coil. There is a permanent rare earth metal magnet in the shell. When the coil outside the shell is electrified, it generates a variable magnetic field, and thence mechanical vibration. The FMT vibration stimulates the ossicular chain and round window membrane to vibrate together, thus stimulating the inner ear

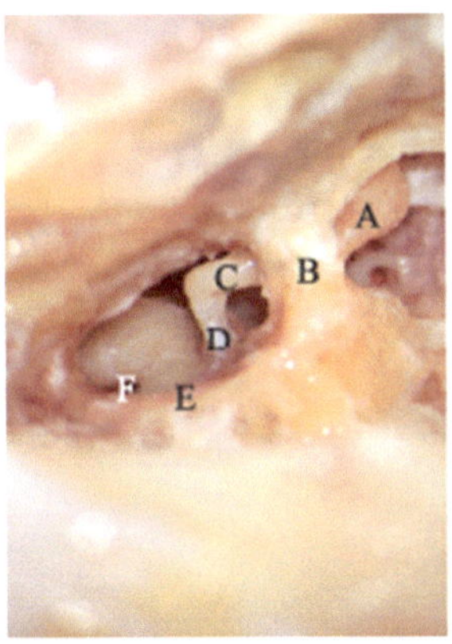

A. Short process of the incus
B. Incus buttress
C. Long process of the incus
D. Stapedius tendon
E. Vertical segment of the facial nerve canal
F. Round window niche

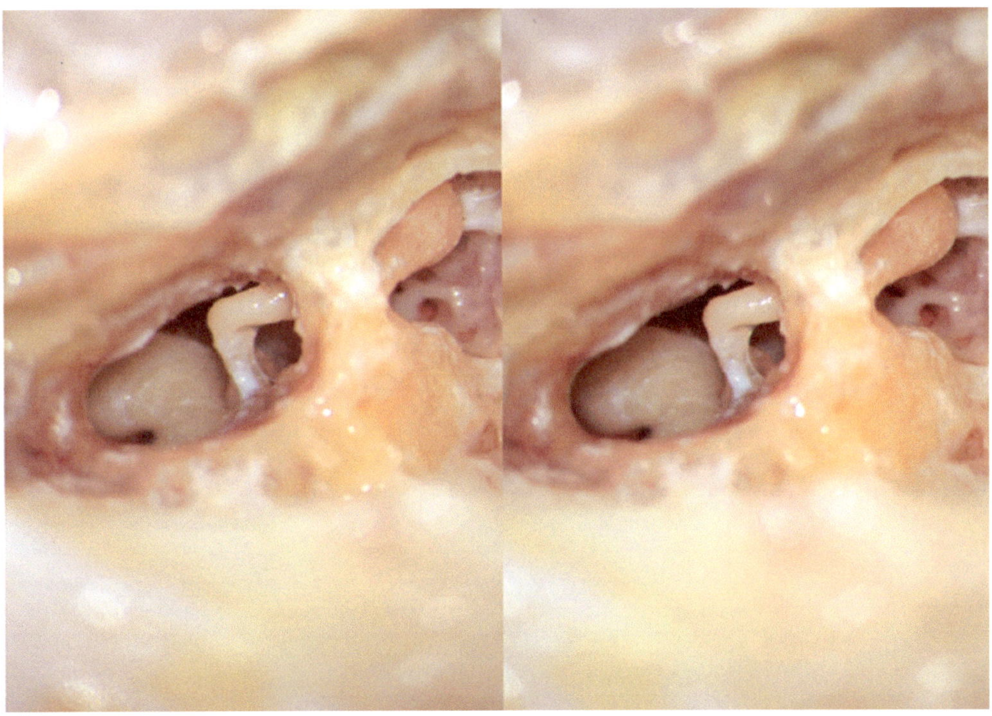

Fig. 4.100 Open facial recess (left)
After mastoidectomy, open the facial recess until the incudostapedial joint is fully exposed

Instruments: large-sized cutting burs, medium-sized diamond burs, right-angle hook

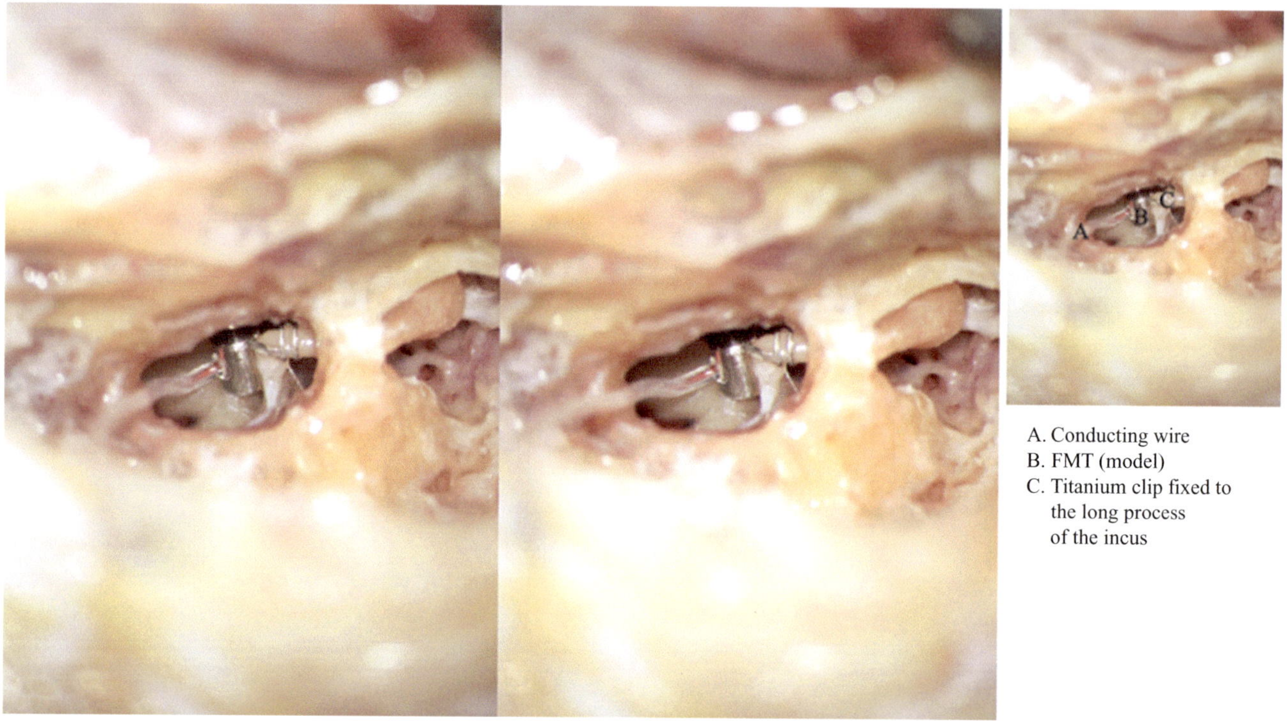

A. Conducting wire
B. FMT (model)
C. Titanium clip fixed to the long process of the incus

Fig. 4.101 Stapes vibration plasty (left)
Place the FMT into the tympanic cavity through the facial recess. Note the angle and position of the FMT with the incus and stapes. Observe whether the FMT is appropriate for the incus and stapes. Make sure that the long axis of the FMT is parallel to the long axis of the stapes
Instruments: right-angle hook, small-sized diamond burs

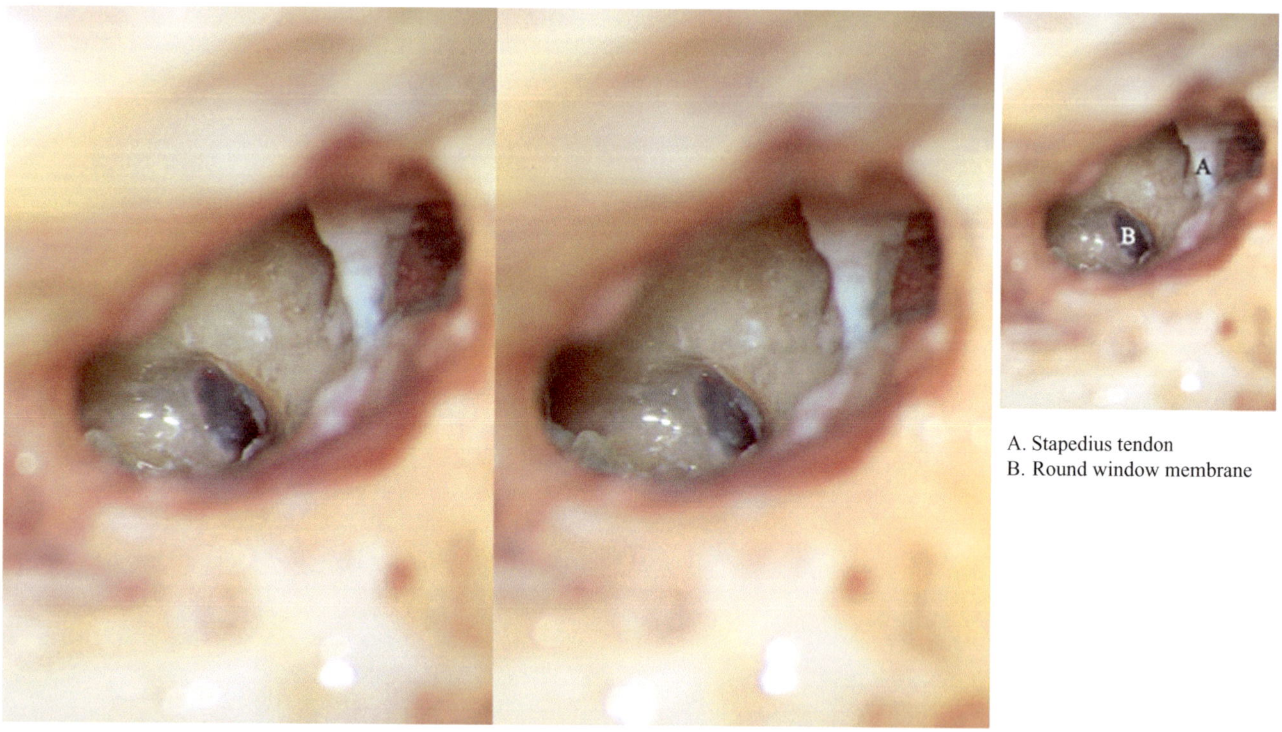

A. Stapedius tendon
B. Round window membrane

Fig. 4.102 Round window vibration plasty (left)
As well as connecting to the ossicular chain, the FMT can also be affixed to the round window niche by a round window vibration plasty, to vibrate the round window membrane directly. Enlarge the facial recess inferiorly until the round window niche is fully revealed. Remove the anterosuperior bony margin of the niche to reveal the round window membrane. Note that the bony margin cannot be completely removed. Leave a small circle of bony margin to accommodate and fix the FMT
Instruments: small-sized diamond burs

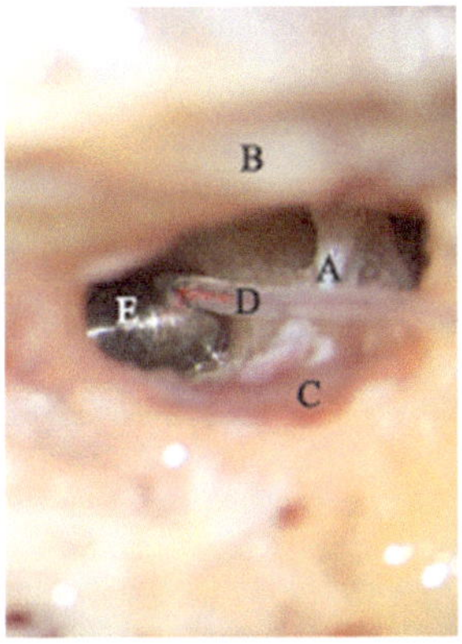

A. Stapedius tendon
B. Posterior EAC wall
C. Vertical facial nerve canal
D. Conducting wire
E. FMT (model)

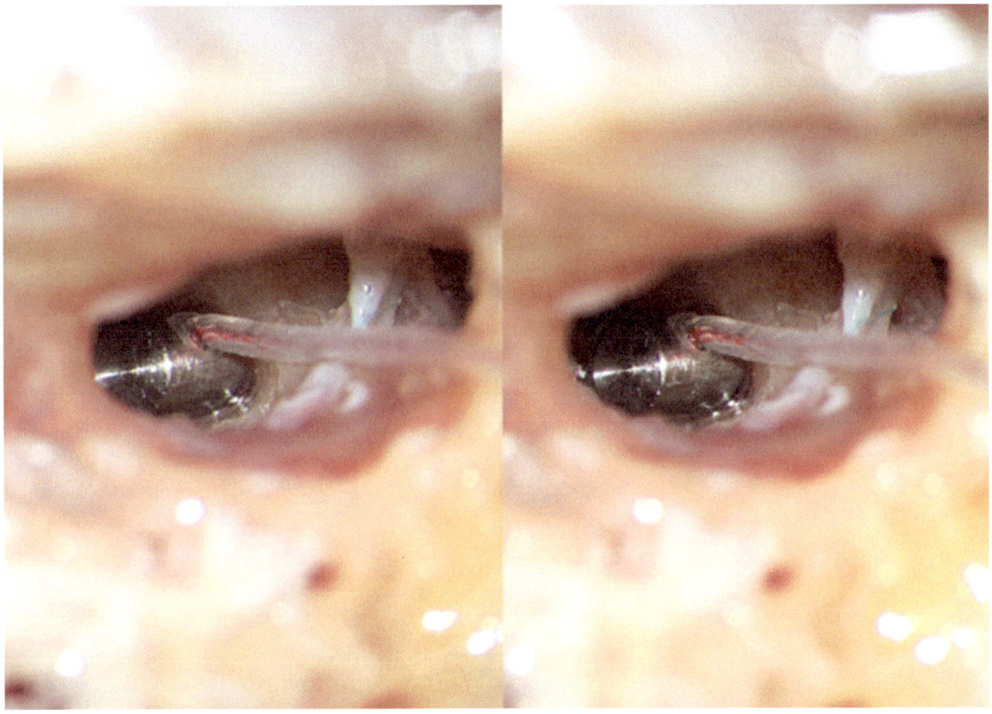

Fig. 4.103 Cochlear window vibration plasty (left)
Cut off the titanium clip of the FMT. Place the end without the titanium clip on the round window membrane after its full exposure. Adjust the FMT so that it sits perpendicular to the round window membrane; some bone from the hypotympanum may need to be removed to ensure correct positioning. During surgery, a disc of fascia 2 mm in diameter and 0.1–0.2 mm thick should be placed over the round window membrane to protect it and improve the coupling of the FMT with the membrane
Instruments: small-sized diamond burs, right-angle hook

Suggested Reading

Bai S-l. Systematic anatomy. Beijing: People's Medical Publishing House; 2001.

Brackmann D-E, Shelton C, Arriaga M-A. Otologic surgery. 4th ed. Philadelphia: Elsevier Medicine; 2015.

Dai P, Han D-y, Cousins VC, et al. Stereo operative atlas of micro ear surgery. Singapore: Springer; 2017.

Gulya A-J. Gulya and Schuknecht's anatomy of the temporal bone with surgical implications. New York: Informa Healthcare USA; 2007.

Huang X-z, Wang J-b. Practice of otorhinolaryngology. Beijing: People's Medical Publishing House; 1999.

Huang X-z, Wang J-b, Kong W-j. Practical otolaryngology-head and neck surgery. 2nd ed. Beijing: People's Medical Publishing House; 2008.

Jiang S-c. Ear anatomy and temporal bone histopathology. Beijing: People's Military Medical Press; 1999.

Jiang S-c, Gu R. Otology. Shanghai: Shanghai Science and Technology Publishing House; 2002.

Jiang S-c, Yang W-y, Gu R. Otorhinolaryngology—head and neck surgery. 2nd ed. Beijing: People's Medical Publishing House; 2007.

Mansour S, Magnan J, Ahmad H-h, Nicolas K, Louryan S. Comprehensive and clinical anatomy of the middle ear. 2nd ed. Switzerland: Springer; 2019.

Sanna M, Khrais T, Falcioni M, et al. The temporal bone: a manual for dissection and surgical approaches. New York: Thieme; 2005.

Wang Z-m. Ear microsurgery. Shanghai: Shanghai Science and Education Publishing House; 2004.

Yang W-y, Zhai S-q. Head and neck anatomy and temporal bone surgery. Beijing: People's Military Medical Publishing House; 2002.

5 Translabyrinthine Approach

Hong-lei Zhang, Qi Li, Yu-bin Ji, and Pu Dai

Surgical Procedures Using the Translabyrinthine Approach

The translabyrinthine approach is the most direct microsurgical route to expose the internal auditory canal (IAC) and cerebellopontine angle (CPA) from the side of the skull. This route is not affected by the anatomical limitations associated with the middle cranial fossa approach and provides access to the sigmoid sinus and jugular bulb. It also avoids retraction of the cerebellar hemisphere, thus minimizing adverse effects on the brain.

The operations that can be carried out through the translabyrinthine approach are as follows:

1. Labyrinthectomy
2. Vestibular neurotomy
3. Acoustic neuroma resection
4. Facial nerve decompression
5. Resection of intratemporal facial nerve tumor
6. Resection of other lesions of the IAC and CPA when preservation of hearing is not possible, such as in the case of neurofibromatosis type II, meningioma, glomus jugulare tumor, and petrosal adenoma
7. Resection of petroclival meningioma
8. Resection of petrosal cholesteatoma, cholesterol granuloma, etc. without hearing preservation

H.-l. Zhang (✉)
Department of Otolaryngology Head and Neck Surgery, Air Force Medical Center, PLA, Beijing, China

Q. Li
Department of Otolaryngology Head and Neck Surgery, Children's Hospital of Nanjing Medical University, Nanjing, China

Y.-b. Ji
Department of Otolaryngology Head and Neck Surgery, Beijing Tsinghua Changgung Hospital, Beijing, China

P. Dai
College of Otolaryngology Head and Neck Surgery, Chinese PLA General Hospital, Beijing, China

Related Anatomical Structures

1. The vestibule is a slightly oval-shaped space located between the cochlea anteriorly and the semicircular canals posteriorly and contains the utricle and saccule.
2. Osseous semicircular canals: three canals in the petrous bone, which each comprise two-thirds of a circle, are perpendicular to each other and located posterior and superior to the vestibule with which they communicate. These canals are named the superior, lateral, and posterior semicircular canals, according to their position in relation to the vestibule.
3. Single crus: the posterior and non-ampullated end of the lateral semicircular canal, which joins the vestibule separately.
4. Common crus: the posterior end of the superior semicircular canal and the superior end of the posterior semicircular canal, which are both non-ampullated, join to form the common crus, which opens into the vestibule through a single bony opening.
5. Endolymphatic sac: a cystic structure located in the subdural space of the posterior cranial fossa, which communicates with the distal end of the endolymphatic duct.
6. Endolymphatic duct: it is an inverted j-shaped tube contained within the bony vestibular aqueduct, which communicates anteriorly with the utricle, which is part of the membranous labyrinth in the vestibule, and posteriorly with the endolymphatic sac. These structures contain endolymph.
7. IAC: a bony neurovascular channel in the petrous bone, containing the facial nerve, cochlear nerve, vestibular nerves, nervus intermedius, and labyrinthine arteries and veins. The outer end of the IAC is called the fundus and abuts the medial vestibular wall. The inner opening of the IAC is called the porus.
8. Horizontal crest: the horizontal crest is a crest of bone in the wall of the fundus, which separates the facial and superior vestibular nerves above from the cochlear and inferior vestibular nerves below.

P. Dai et al. (eds.), *Stereoscopic Anatomical Atlas of Ear Surgery*, https://doi.org/10.1007/978-981-16-0927-5_5

9. Vertical crest: also known as Bill's bar. A vertical bony crest in the wall of the fundus that separates the facial nerve and the superior vestibular nerve.
10. Lower cranial nerves: the common name for cranial nerves IX to XII. These four nerves are the lowest of the cranial nerves, and their nerve roots arise close to each other. Cranial nerves IX, X, and XI pass out of the skull through the jugular foramen, while cranial nerve XII exits through its own foramen. Paralysis of nerves IX–XI leads to dysphagia, dysphonia, aspiration, and inability to raise the shoulder.

Anatomy Overview

1. Skin-osteoperiosteal flap. The skin incision is made 2–4 cm behind the retroauricular sulcus. Usually, with larger tumors the incision is made more posteriorly, to assist with opening of the dura mater of the posterior cranial fossa and better expose the CPA.
2. Enlarged mastoidectomy. A standard canal-wall-up mastoidectomy is performed, with extra bone removed 2 cm posterior to the sigmoid sinus and 2 cm above the middle cranial fossa floor. Skeletonize the sigmoid sinus and remove bone from its surface or retain a plate of bone over its mid-portion (so-called Bill's island). The bone covering the posterior cranial fossa between the sigmoid sinus and the bony labyrinth is completely drilled away. Bone is removed from the surface of the sigmoid sinus, and from the adjacent middle cranial fossa dura, to create the sinodural angle. The short process of the incus, the mastoid roof (tegmen mastoideum), the sigmoid sinus, and the vertical segment of the facial nerve are identified, and an extended mastoidectomy is performed. *Hints: (1) A "Bill's island" of bone protects the sigmoid sinus when the labyrinth is removed. When the sigmoid sinus is positioned anteriorly, a sufficient amount of the bone plate on the surface of the sigmoid sinus should be removed to enlarge the field of vision. (2) Extensive removal of bone covering the middle cranial fossa (above the tegmen) and the posterior cranial fossa (posterior to the sigmoid sinus) is the key to fully reveal the IAC and CPA.*
3. Skeletonize the jugular bulb and facial nerve. The lower boundary of the labyrinthine resection is the roof of the jugular bulb, which must be identified and skeletonized. The lateral semicircular canal and ampulla of the posterior semicircular canal are closely related to the horizontal segment, the second genu, and the vertical segment of the facial nerve, so the facial nerve needs to be accurately identified and skeletonized before removing the labyrinth.
4. Removal of the semicircular canals and vestibule. The vestibule and three semicircular canals are adjacent to the middle cranial fossa floor, posterior cranial fossa dura mater, facial nerve, cochlea, and other important structures. Therefore, it is necessary to first define the spatial relationships between the anatomical structures, and then to define the peripheral boundaries of the planned resection; finally, the vestibule and semicircular canals should be removed using a safe technique and appropriate instruments. Overview of the operation: (1) Contour the three semicircular canals and expose their "blue line". (2) Skeletonize the vertical segment of the facial nerve. (3) Remove the lateral semicircular canal from anterior to posterior (preserve the anterior inferior segment of the ampulla to protect the horizontal segment and second genu of the facial nerve). (4) Remove the posterior semicircular canal from inferior to superior (Care should be taken to protect the vertical segment of facial nerve when removing the ampullary end of the posterior semicircular canal). (5) Remove the superior semicircular canal from anterior to posterior, parallel to the middle fossa dura (preserve the anteromedial segment of the ampullary end to protect the labyrinthine segment of the facial nerve).
5. Open the vestibule and protect its medial wall so as not to damage the lateral end of the IAC. *Hints: (1) The medial wall of the vestibule forms the lateral end of the IAC, and careful removal of bone is required to avoid entering the canal directly. (2) The superior semicircular canal is the upper boundary of the IAC and a landmark for the superior vestibular nerve; the preserved medial wall of the ampulla of the superior semicircular canal can also protect the labyrinthine segment of the facial nerve.*
6. Skeletonize the IAC. After resection of the labyrinth, the upper and lower boundaries of the IAC are confirmed at the level of the ampullae of the superior and posterior semicircular canals, respectively. Remove bone from the back of the IAC and gradually skeletonize it, leaving only a thin layer of bone on the surface of the dural lining. To adequately expose the IAC and the CPA, the bone should be removed from 270 degrees of its circumference. *Hints: (1) The lower limit of bone removal under the IAC is the cochlear aqueduct and jugular bulb. The cochlear aqueduct can be identified after the removal of air cells. The deep surface of the cochlear aqueduct points to the neural part of the jugular foramen below, and the glossopharyngeal nerve is medial to the aqueduct. (2) Be careful when removing bone from the upper lip of the IAC to avoid damaging the facial nerve, which runs along the upper anterior part of the canal.*
7. Identify the IAC segment of the facial nerve. Remove the thin bone pieces of the medial vestibular wall (i.e., the lateral end of the IAC) and open the dura mater of the canal; the facial nerve is in front of the vertical crest and above the horizontal crest at the lateral end of the

IAC. The bone is further removed, and the labyrinthine segment of the facial nerve is exposed.

8. Open the dura mater of the posterior cranial fossa. The dura mater of the posterior cranial fossa is incised to reveal the IAC segment of the facial nerve extending to the CPA. The extent of incision of the dura mater of the posterior cranial fossa depends on the extent of exposure required, and the incision may begin near the sigmoid sinus if a larger surgical area is required. Close attention should be paid when cutting the dura mater, to preserve the petrosal vein.
9. Tumor resection. In acoustic neuroma resection, the tumor can be removed from lateral to medial along the IAC once the course of the facial nerve is confirmed at the lateral end of the canal. For larger tumors, intracapsular resection can be used to reduce the size of the tumor and then removal of the residue from surrounding structures, such as the facial nerve and brainstem is undertaken, until the tumor has been completely removed.
10. Closure of the surgical cavity. At the completion of acoustic neuroma resection, dura mater defects, the IAC, and the mastoid cavity are usually obliterated with strips of abdominal fat, and the aditus entrance is filled with temporal muscle to close the operative cavity.

Purpose and Requirements of Anatomical Dissection

1. Master the use of drill bits of different types and sizes
2. Identify the outline of the mastoid cavity wall, the facial nerve canal, and the sigmoid sinus
3. Understand the spatial relationship between the lateral end of the IAC and the inner ear
4. Understand the anatomy of the facial nerve in terms of its vertical, horizontal, labyrinthine, IAC, and CPA segments

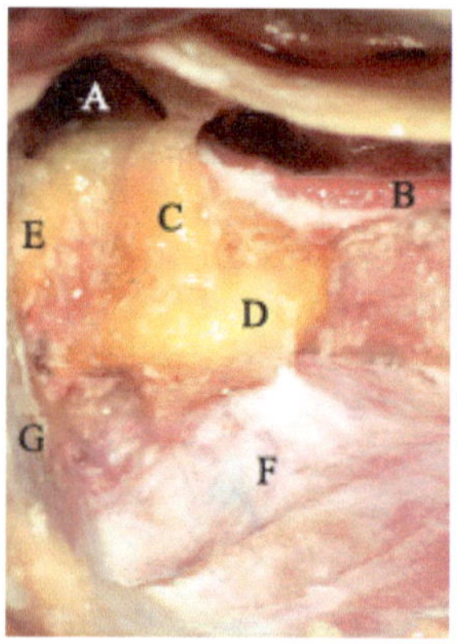

A. Aditus ad antrum
B. Mastoid segment of the facial nerve
C. Lateral semicircular canal
D. Posterior semicircular canal
E. Superior semicircular canal
F. Dura mater of the posterior fossa
G. Dura mater of the middle fossa

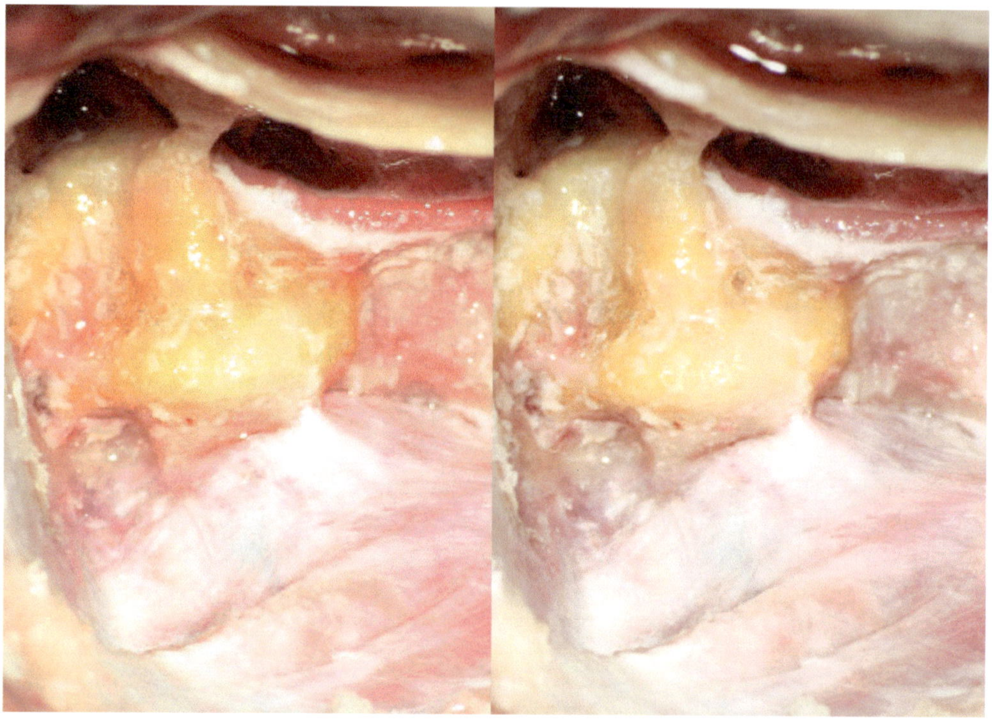

Fig. 5.1 Skeletonization of the mastoid cavity and the semicircular canals (right)
The mastoid cavity is enlarged and contoured. The bony plates over the middle and posterior fossa dura are resected to reveal the bony labyrinth, and the three semicircular canals are skeletonized. If a far-advanced sigmoid sinus and a high jugular bulb are encountered, it is necessary to resect the bone over these structures to enlarge the surgical field. *Hints: Careful technique is required to avoid damaging the thin and weak vascular walls of the sigmoid sinus and jugular blub*
Instruments: large- or medium-sized cutting burs and diamond burs, small-sized diamond burs, elevator, bone rongeur

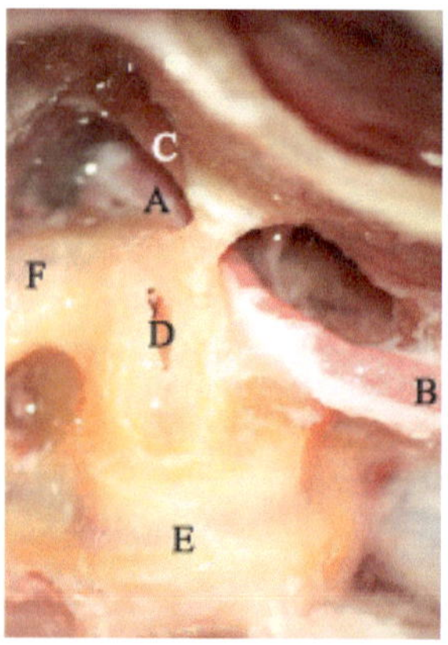

A. Tympanic segment of the facial nerve
B. Mastoid segment of the facial nerve
C. Short process of the incus
D. Lumen of the lateral semicircular canal and membranous labyrinth
E. Posterior semicircular canal
F. Superior semicircular canal

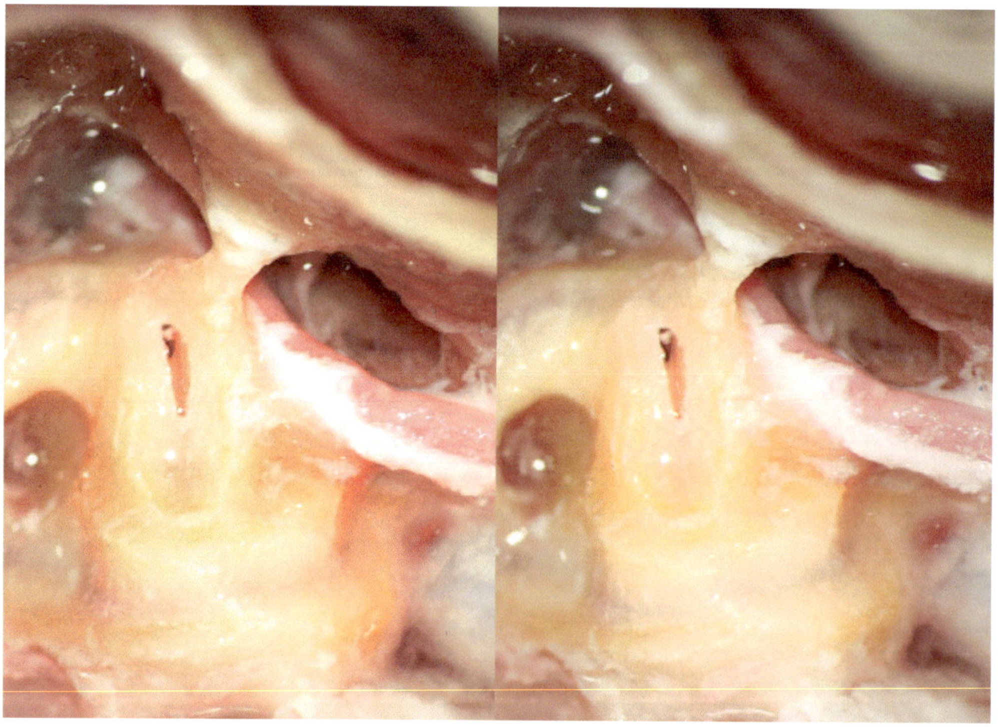

Fig. 5.2 Appearance of the "blue lines" of the superior and posterior semicircular canal. Opening the lateral semicircular canal (right)
Based on their skeletonization, the three semicircular canals are polished along the canal direction using a diamond bur to expose the "blue lines." Carefully observe the spatial relationships of the three semicircular canals. The lumens of the three semicircular canals are exposed by polishing and opening the "blue lines," and the morphological features of the membranous labyrinth within the canals are observed. *Hints: When the lumen of the lateral semicircular canal is opened, the anterior and medial walls of the canal ampulla must be preserved to protect the geniculate ganglion, tympanic segment, and pyramidal segment of the facial nerve*
Instruments: medium- and small-sized diamond burs

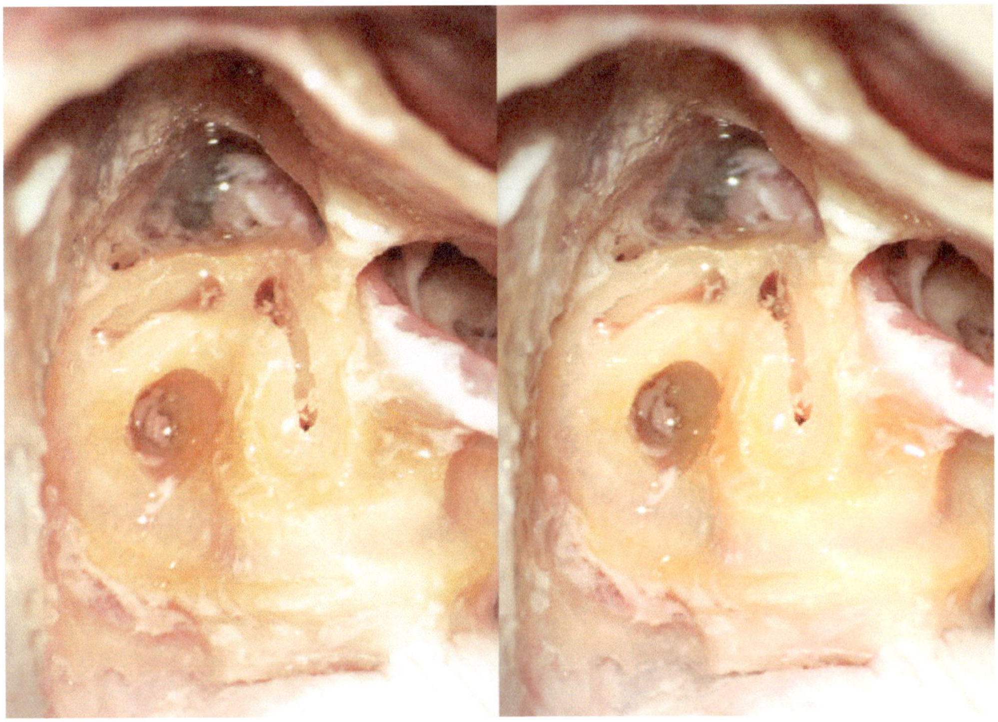
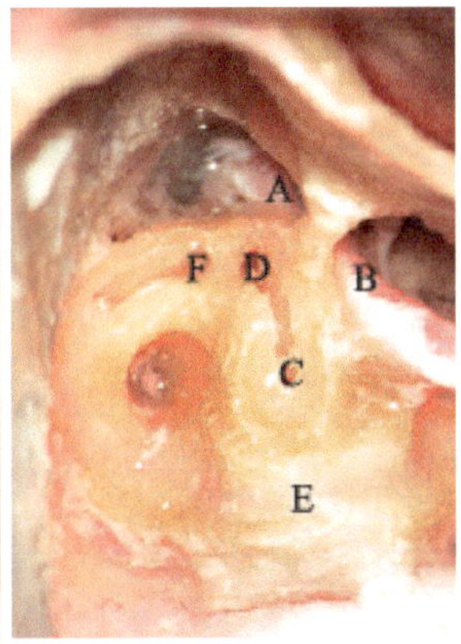

A. Tympanic segment of the facial nerve
B. Pyramidal segment of the facial nerve
C. Posterior single crus of the lateral semicircular canal
D. Lateral semicircular canal ampulla
E. Posterior semicircular canal
F. Superior semicircular canal ampulla

Fig. 5.3 Opening the superior semicircular canal (right)
After opening the lateral semicircular canal to expose its lumen, ampulla, and posterior single crus, the lateral bony wall of the superior semicircular canal is removed layer by layer along its curve using a medium-sized diamond bur until the lumen, ampulla, and common crus are exposed. *Hints: Care should be taken to avoid damaging the dura mater of the middle fossa above the superior semicircular canal. The medial wall of the superior semicircular canal ampulla should be preserved, as it will aid identification of the upper limit of the IAC*
Instruments: medium-sized diamond burs, micro-hook

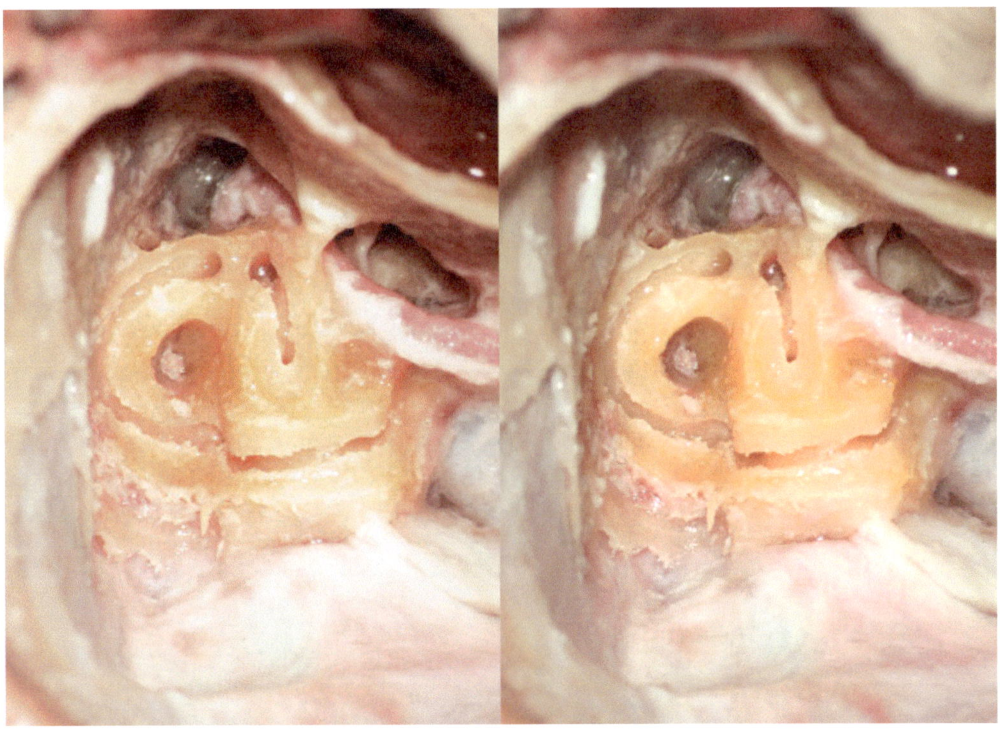
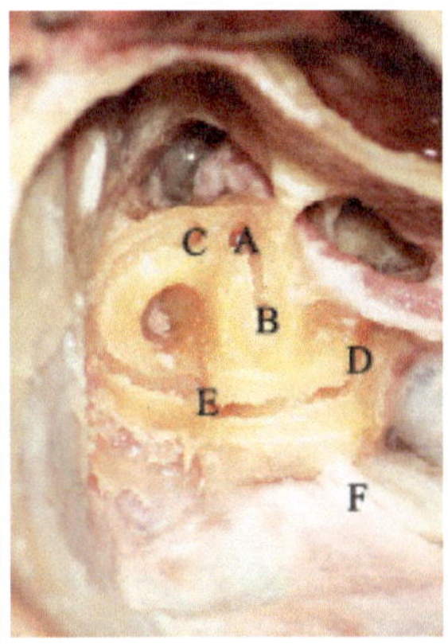

A. Lateral semicircular canal ampulla
B. Posterior single crus of the lateral semicircular canal
C. Superior semicircular canal ampulla
D. Posterior semicircular canal ampulla
E. Common crus
F. Endolymphatic sac

Fig. 5.4 Opening the posterior semicircular canal (right)
The bone of the posterior semicircular canal is removed layer by layer along the curve of the canal to expose the membranous labyrinth and ampulla. After the bone is removed, it can be seen that the superior and posterior semicircular canals join together to form the common crus. The endolymphatic sac is located between the two layers of posterior fossa dura mater located at the rear of the posterior semicircular canal, and below the backward extension of a line passing through the lateral semicircular canal. The endolymphatic sac is whiter than the dura mater
Instruments: medium-sized diamond burs, micro-hook

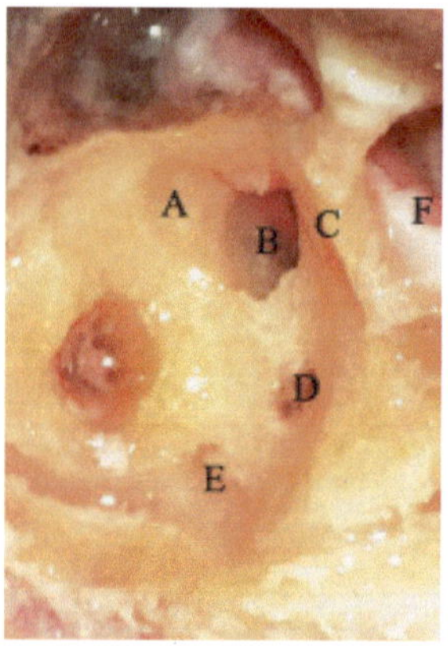

A. Medial wall of the superior semicircular canal ampulla
B. Vestibule
C. Inferior wall remnant of the lateral semicircular canal
D. Posterior single crus of the lateral semicircular canal
E. Common crus
F. Pyramidal segment of the facial nerve

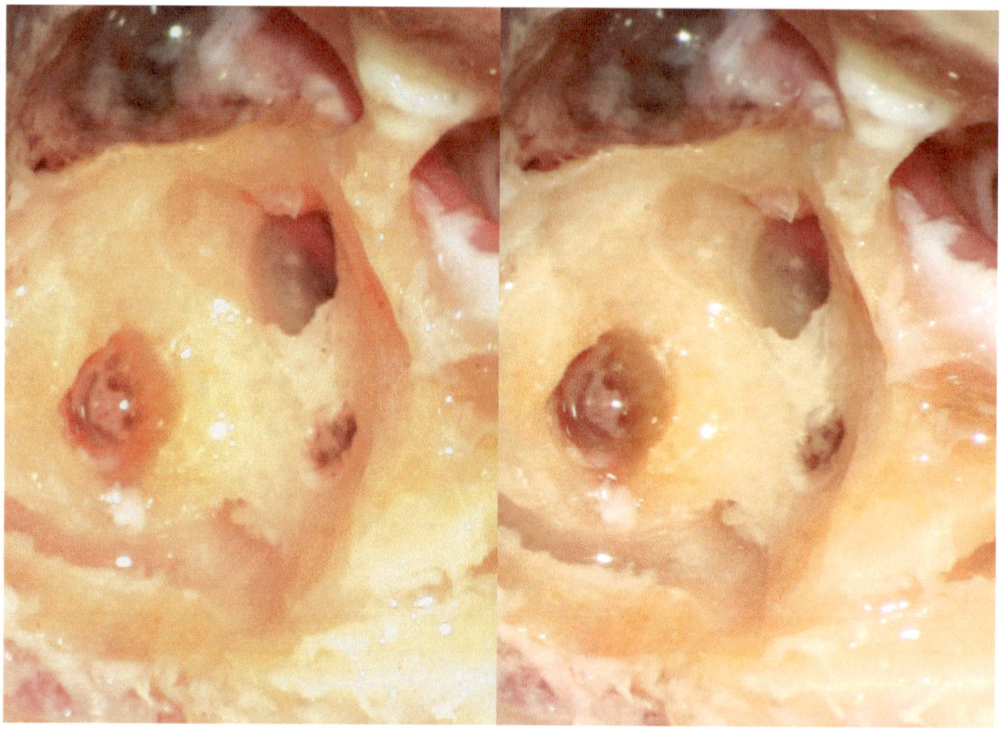

Fig. 5.5 Opening the vestibule (right)
The bone of the three semicircular canals is further removed to expose the three ampullae, common crus, and posterior single crus; then, the vestibule is located and opened. *Hints: The bone should be removed layer by layer, from front to back, without penetrating deeply with the drill so as not to damage the vestibular medial wall or the nerves in the IAC*
Instruments: medium-sized diamond burs

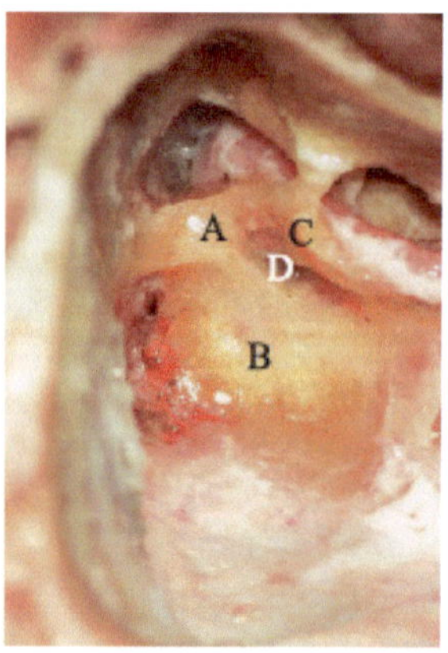

A. Medial wall of the superior semicircular canal ampulla
B. Lateral wall of the IAC (the fundus)
C. Inferior wall remnants of the lateral semicircular canal
D. Medial wall of the vestibule

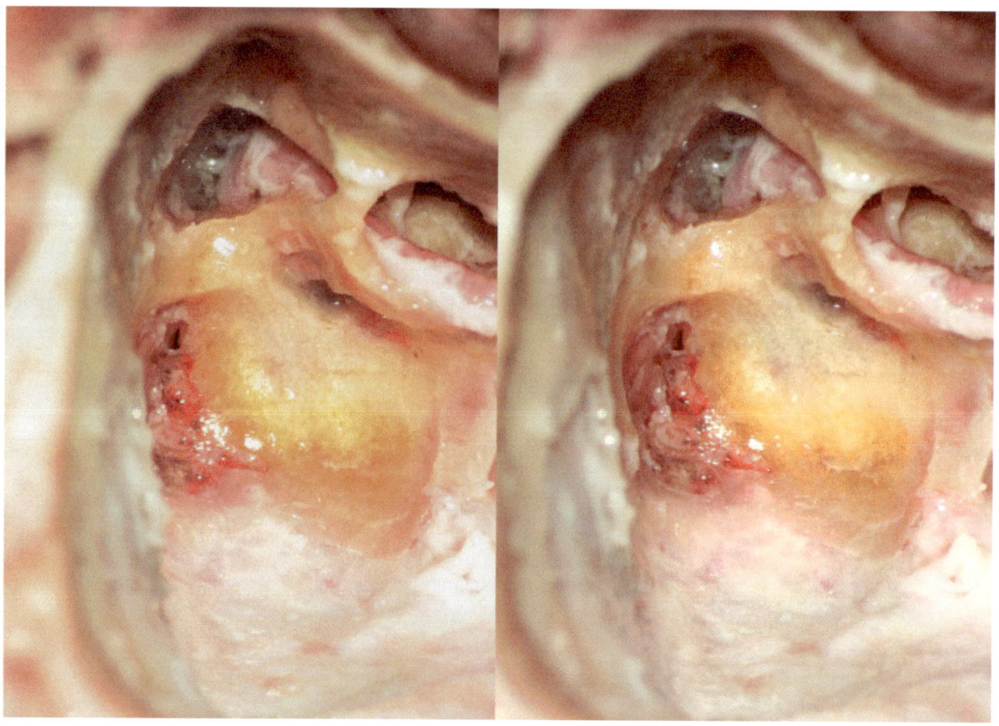

Fig. 5.6 Resection of the vestibule (right)
Using a medium-sized cutting bur, the labyrinthine bone and remnants of the posterior fossa bony plate between the superior and inferior boundaries of the IAC are removed, to expose the vestibular medial wall. The superior boundary of the IAC is at the level of a line connecting the tympanic segment of the facial nerve and the sinodural angle. The inferior boundary is parallel to the superior boundary at the level of a line running from the intersection of the pyramidal and vertical segments of the facial nerve to the posterior fossa. *Hints: Carefully observe the three semicircular canals, the macula sacculi, and the macula utriculi during the procedure. The facial nerve must be protected during the removal of the lateral bone of the IAC fundus*
Instruments: medium-sized cutting burs and diamond burs, elevator, hemostatic forceps

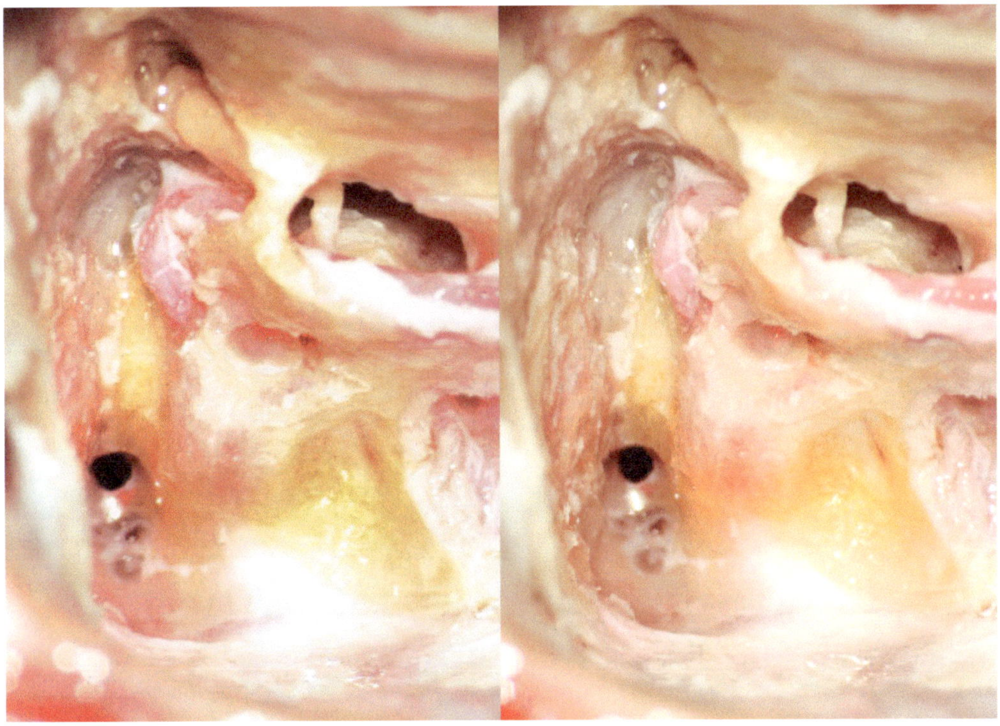

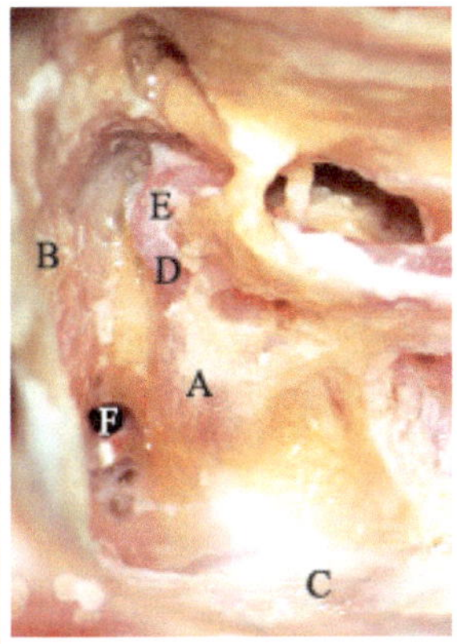

A. IAC
B. Bony plate of the middle fossa
C. Dura mater of the posterior fossa
D. Labyrinthine segment of the facial nerve
E. Geniculate ganglion
F. Supra-labyrinthine air cells

Fig. 5.7 Skeletonization of the IAC (right)
After the superior and inferior boundaries of the IAC have been confirmed, the bone surrounding the IAC is removed layer by layer from the IAC porus to its fundus. When dissecting these important structures, including the dura mater, facial nerve, jugular bulb, and IAC contents, a diamond bur must be used to help protect them. *Hints: Carefully identify the cochlear aqueduct when the bone of the IAC is removed along its inferior boundary, and protect the jugular bulb below and glossopharyngeal nerve medially Instruments: medium- and small-sized cutting burs, medium- and small-sized diamond burs*

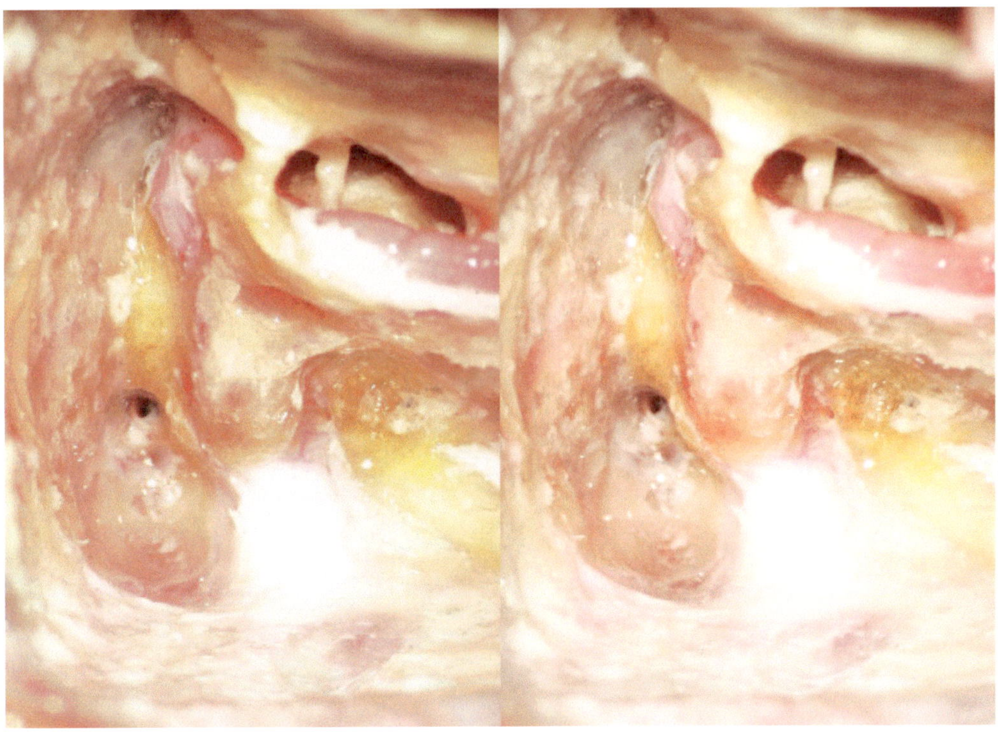

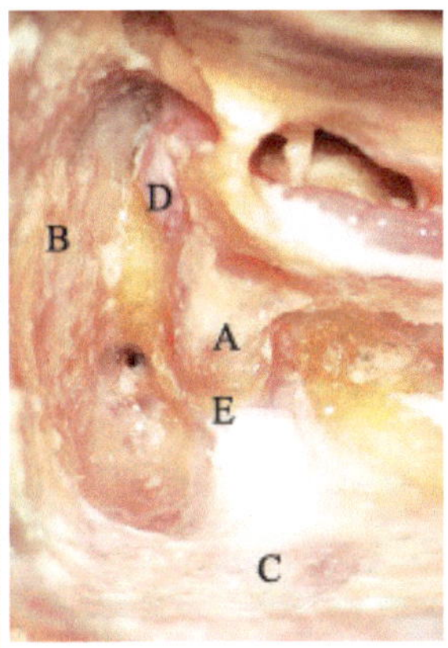

A. IAC
B. Bony plate of the middle fossa
C. Dura mater of the posterior fossa
D. Labyrinthine segment of the facial nerve
E. IAC porus

Fig. 5.8 Skeletonization of the IAC and porus (right)
The bone between the dura mater of the posterior fossa and IAC is further removed using medium- and small-sized diamond burs, to expose the IAC porus. The bone of the wall of the IAC is removed from the upper to the lower boundary for at least 180 degrees, but the range may be extended 270 and even 360 degrees depending on the purpose of the operation. *Hints: The drill should always be parallel to the long axis of the IAC, and bone removal must be carried out layer by layer. Satisfactory exposure will usually allow leaving an eggshell layer of bone over the jugular bulb below, middle fossa dura and superior petrosal sinus above, and the sigmoid sinus behind*
Instruments: medium-sized diamond burs

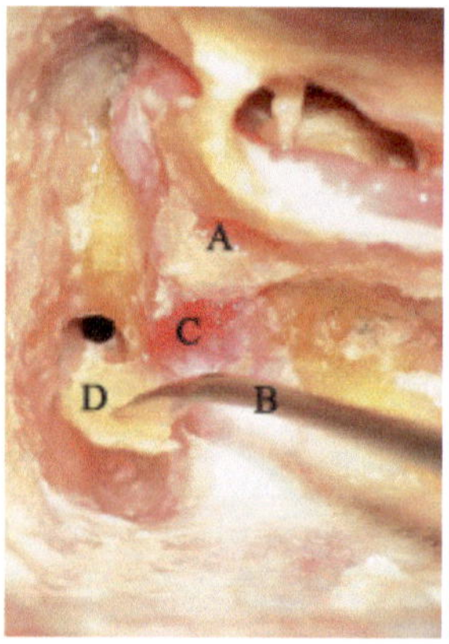

A. Medial wall of the vestibule
B. Middle ear elevator
C. Dura mater of the IAC
D. Thin bony plate elevated from the IAC

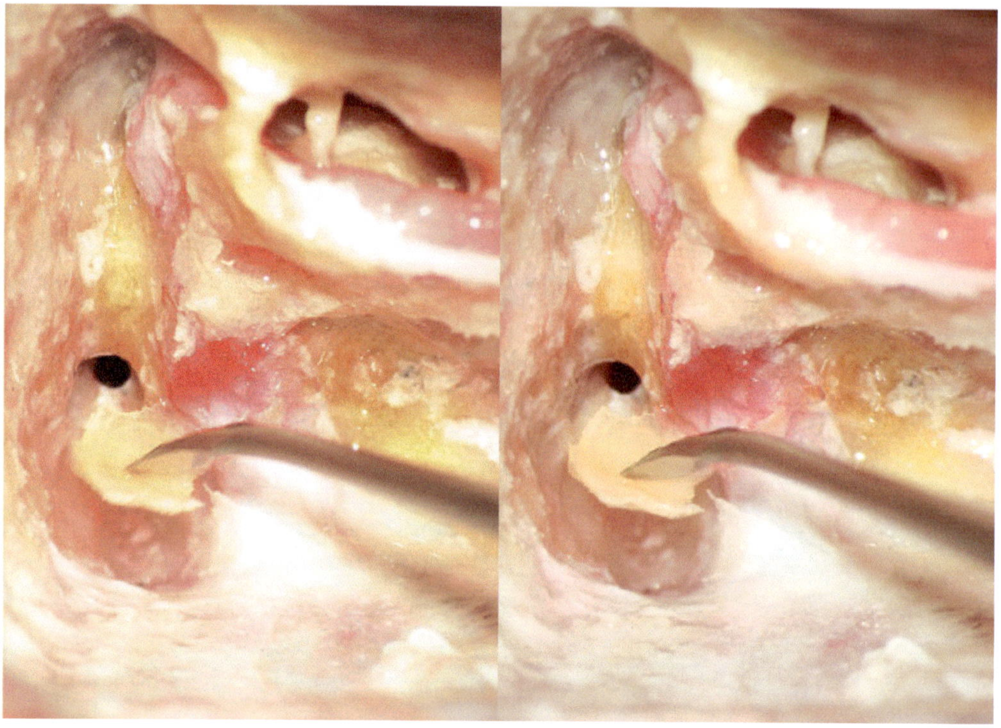

Fig. 5.9 Removing the thin bony plate from the IAC (right)
The thin bony plate is removed from the surface of the IAC to expose the dura mater thereof. During the procedure, a sucker may be placed between the elevator and dura mater to avoid causing damage. Minimal if any suction pressure should be applied to avoid damage to the IAC contents, however
Instrument: middle ear elevator

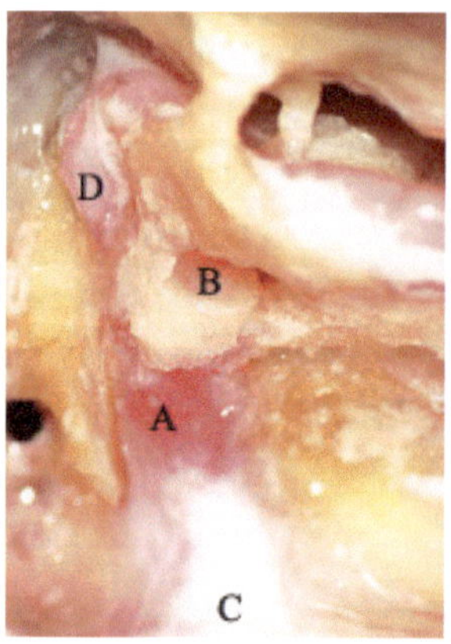

A. Dura mater of the IAC
B. Medial wall of the vestibule
C. Dura mater of the posterior fossa
D. Labyrinthine segment of the facial nerve

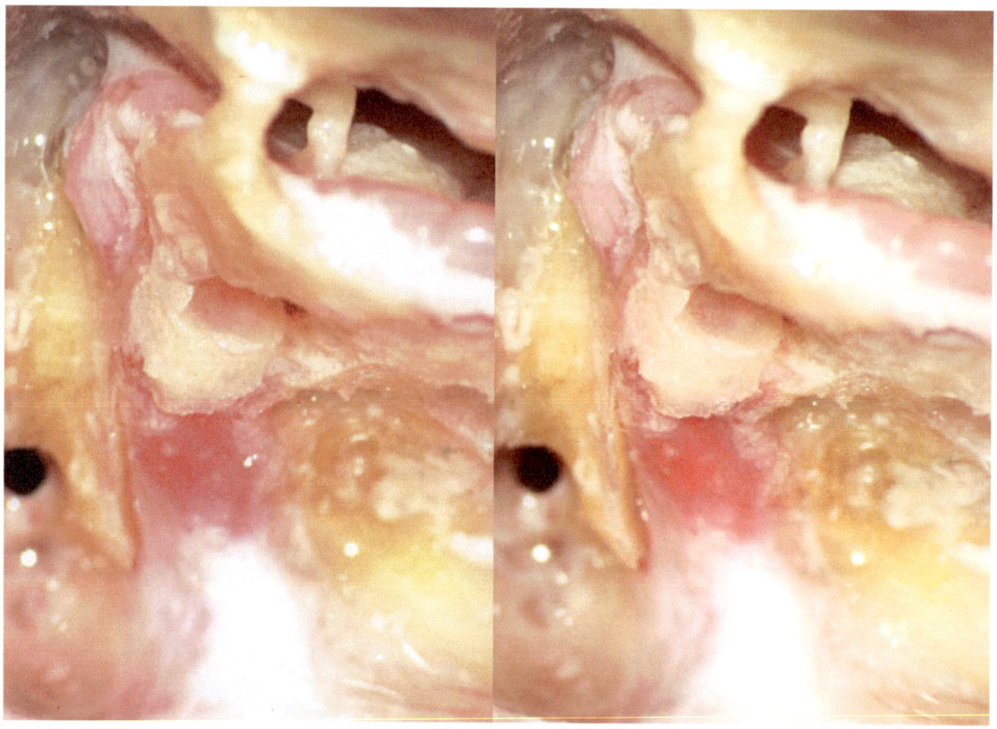

Fig. 5.10 Vestibule, IAC, and facial nerve (right)
The thin bony plate surrounding the IAC is further removed using the elevator and a small diamond bur, to fully expose the dura mater of the canal. The exposed dura mater extends from the porus of the IAC and the posterior fossa posteriorly, forward to the IAC fundus. *Hints: The labyrinthine segment of the facial nerve and the dura mater should be fully protected during the operation*
Instruments: middle ear elevator, small-sized diamond burs

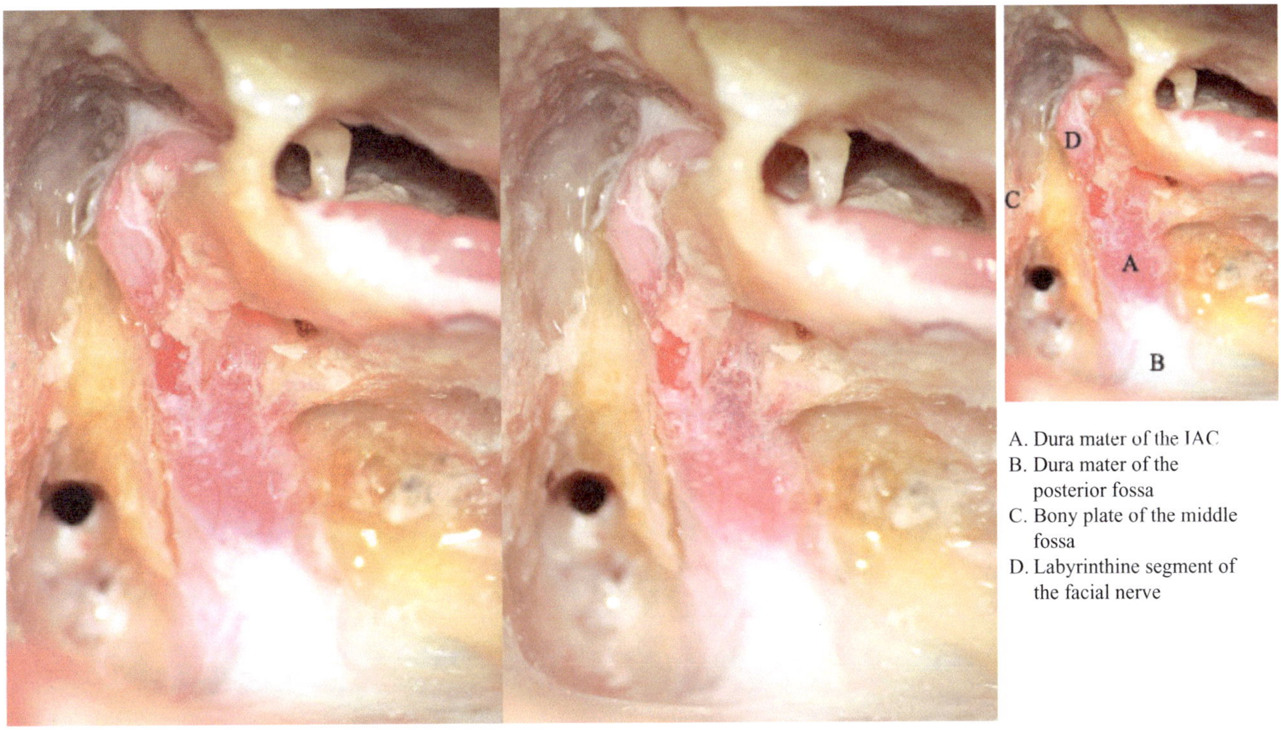

A. Dura mater of the IAC
B. Dura mater of the posterior fossa
C. Bony plate of the middle fossa
D. Labyrinthine segment of the facial nerve

Fig. 5.11 Exposure of the full length of the IAC (right)
The remnant bone located behind the IAC fundus is further removed using a small-sized diamond bur and the dura mater of the IAC is fully exposed. The opening range of the canal seen here extends for 180 degrees
Instruments: small-sized diamond burs

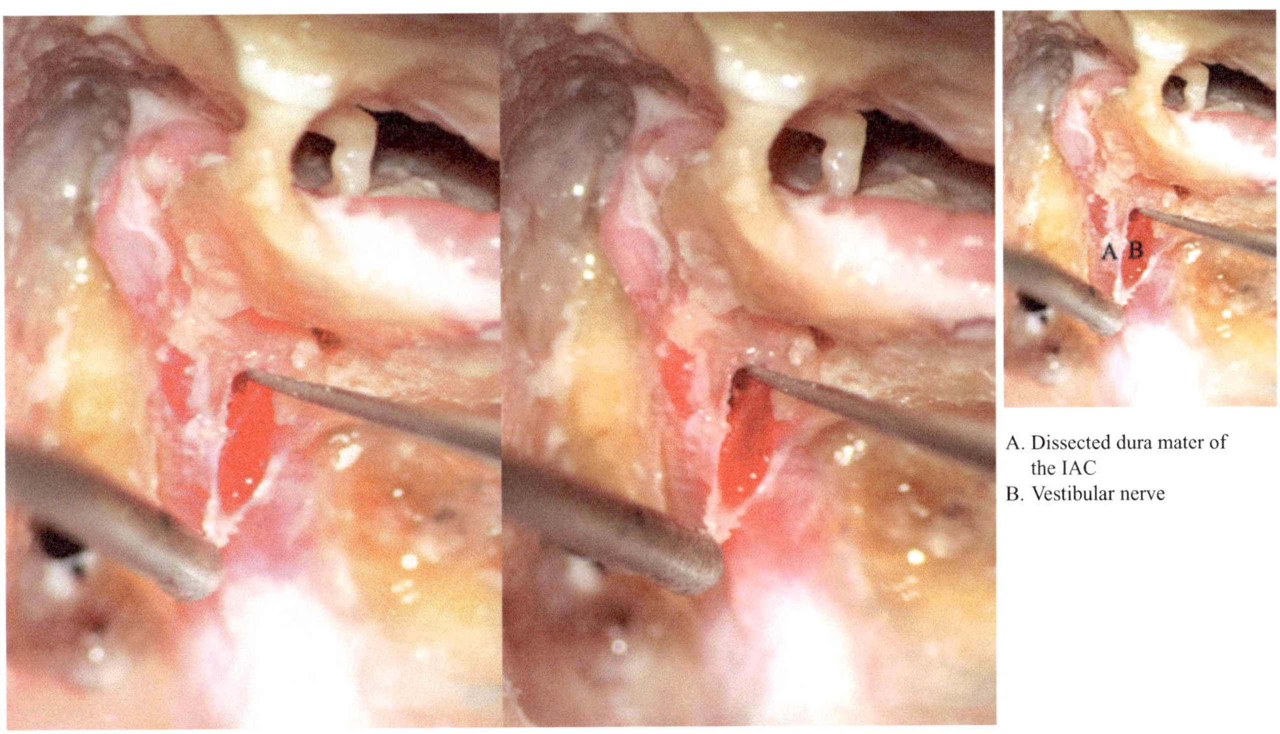

A. Dissected dura mater of the IAC
B. Vestibular nerve

Fig. 5.12 Incision of the dura mater of the IAC (right)
The dura mater of the IAC is opened along its longitudinal axis using a straight needle or sharp knife. The vestibular nerve is the first structure seen after the incision of the dura mater. During the operation, because of the uncertainty regarding the location of the facial nerve, which may be compressed by an acoustic neuroma, the dura mater is always incised along the lower edge of the IAC to avoid damaging the facial nerve
Instruments: straight needle or sharp knife

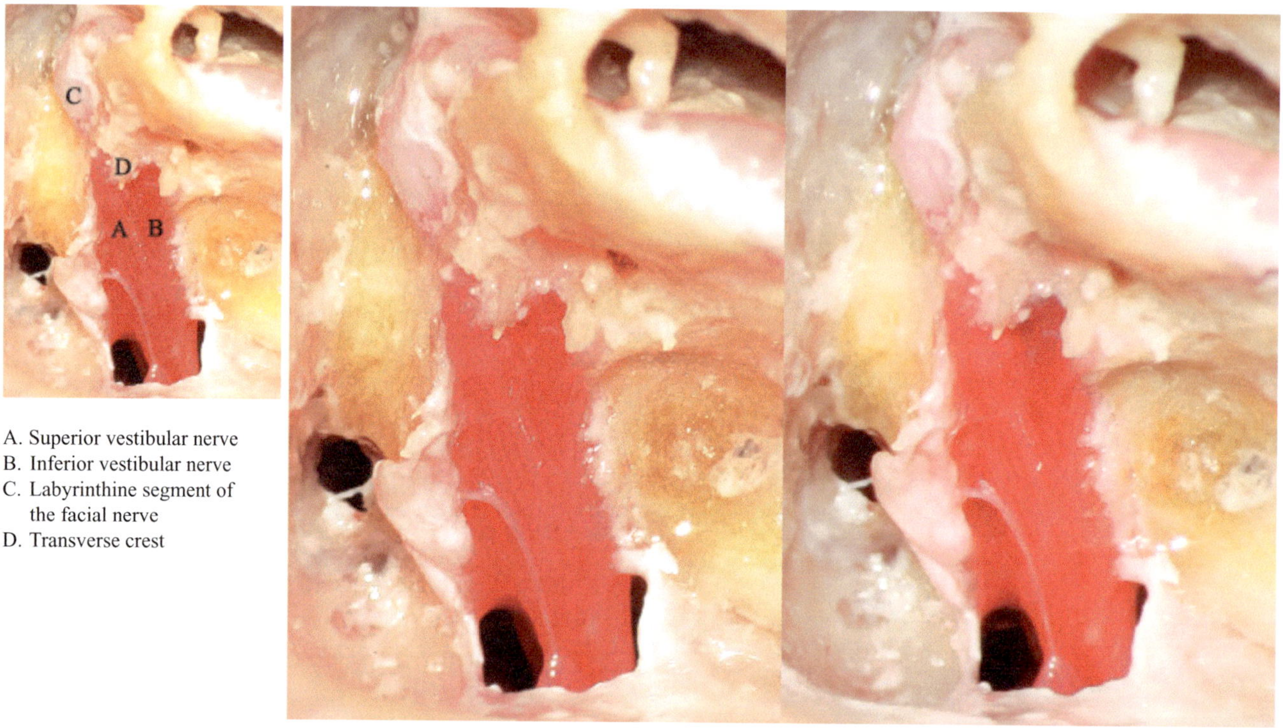

A. Superior vestibular nerve
B. Inferior vestibular nerve
C. Labyrinthine segment of the facial nerve
D. Transverse crest

Fig. 5.13 Exposure of the vestibular nerve inside the IAC (right)
The posterior dura mater of the IAC is resected to fully open the canal. The vestibular nerve, with its superior and inferior branches, is the most posterior structure in the IAC. The superior vestibular nerve, which supplies the ampullae of the lateral and superior semicircular canals and the utricle, is thicker than the inferior vestibular nerve, which supplies the posterior semicircular canal ampulla and the saccule. The superior vestibular and inferior vestibular nerves are separated by the transverse crest laterally in the IAC
Instruments: hook, middle ear elevator, ophthalmic scissors

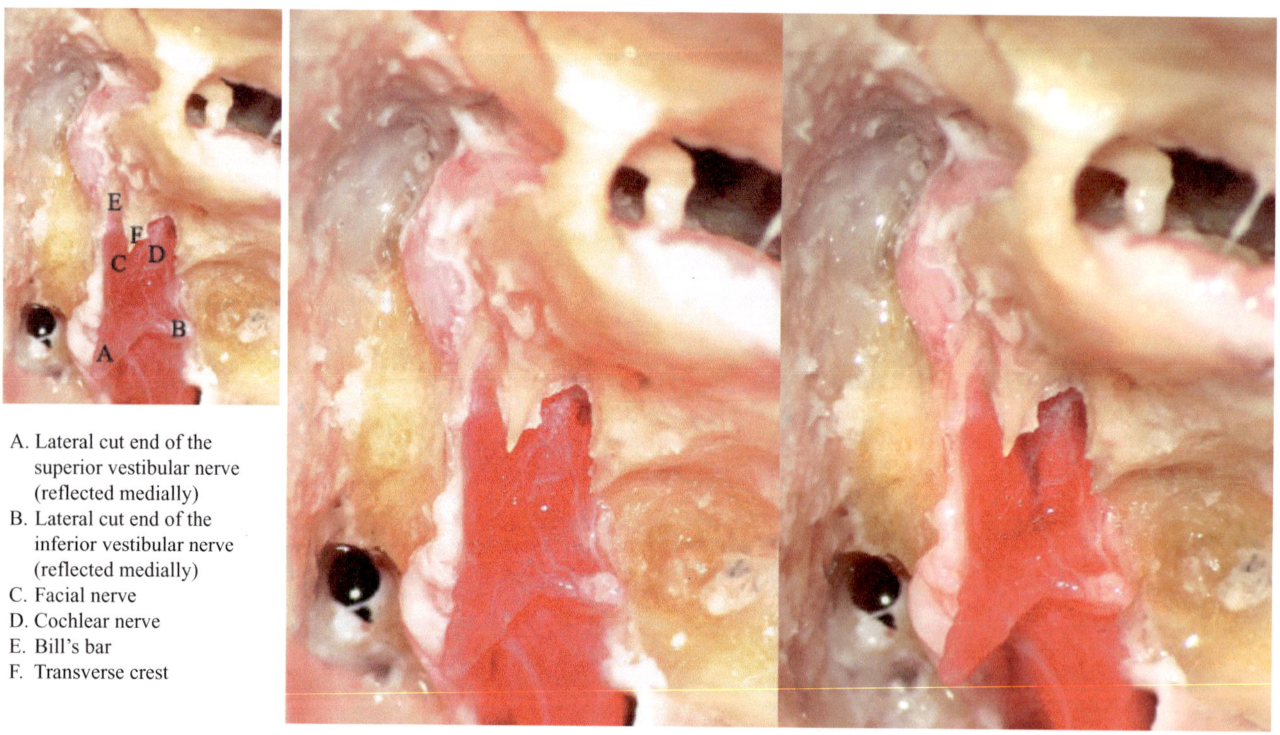

A. Lateral cut end of the superior vestibular nerve (reflected medially)
B. Lateral cut end of the inferior vestibular nerve (reflected medially)
C. Facial nerve
D. Cochlear nerve
E. Bill's bar
F. Transverse crest

Fig. 5.14 Isolating and sectioning the vestibular nerve (right)
The superior and inferior vestibular nerves are isolated from the IAC fundus; the facial nerve is located anterior and superior, and the cochlear nerve anterior and inferior, in the canal. The IAC fundus is divided into superior and inferior parts by the transverse crest. Bill's bar is located between the facial nerve and superior vestibular nerve
Instruments: hook, middle ear elevator

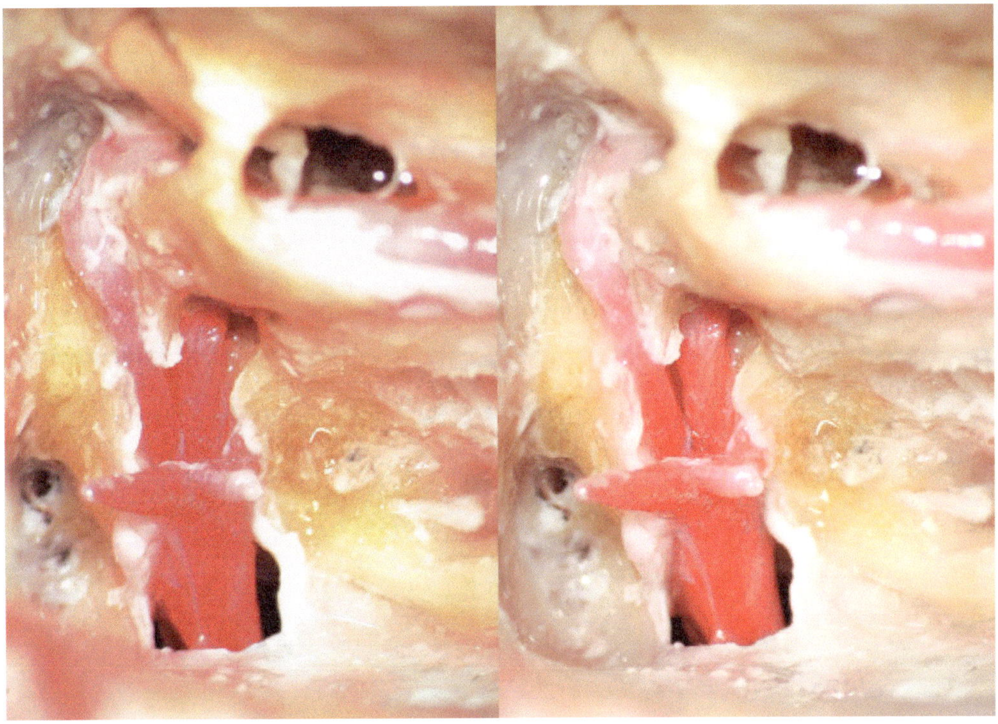

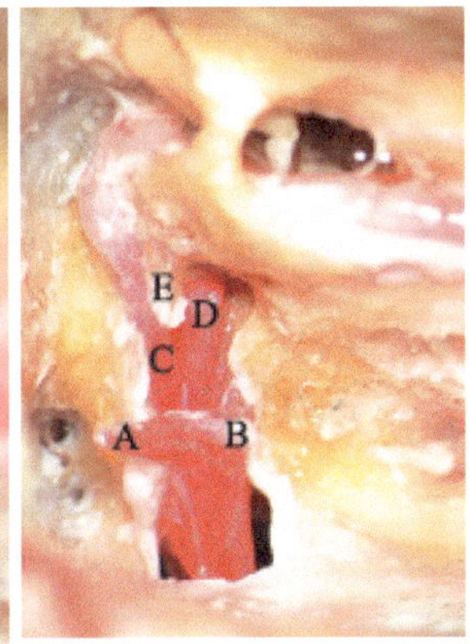

A. Lateral cut end of the superior vestibular nerve (reflected medially)
B. Lateral cut end of the inferior vestibular nerve (reflected medially)
C. Facial nerve
D. Cochlear nerve
E. Transverse crest

Fig. 5.15 Structures in the IAC (right)
Bill's bar is removed using a small-sized diamond bur and the labyrinthine segment of the facial nerve is exposed. The facial nerve is exposed from the geniculate ganglion to the meatal segment, and the nerves in the IAC can then be observed clearly
Instruments: small-sized diamond burs, right-angle hook

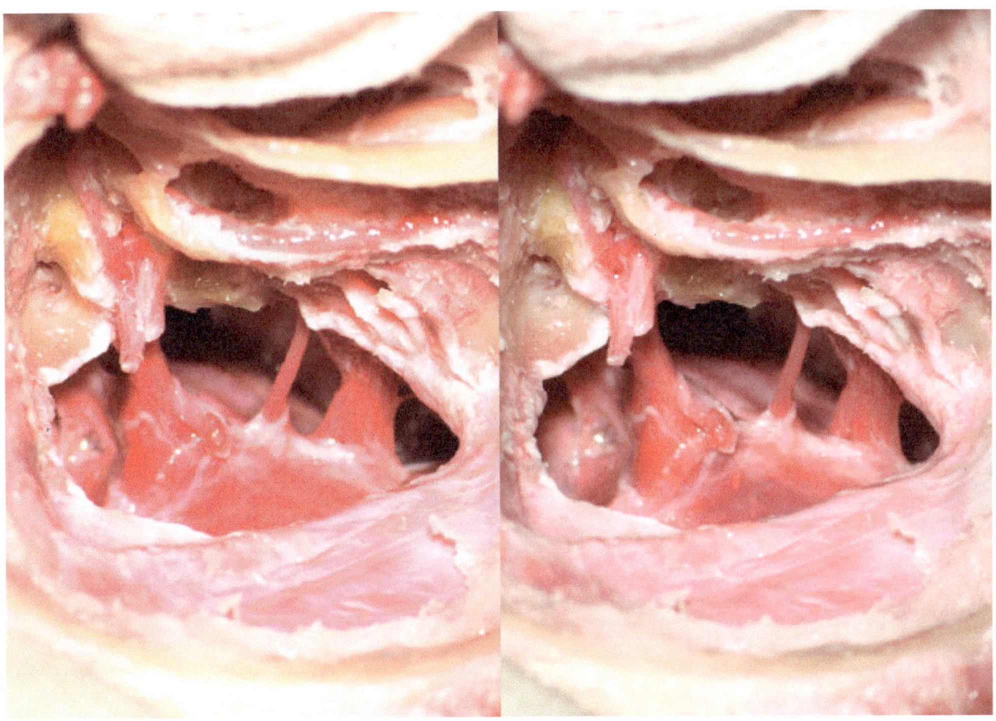

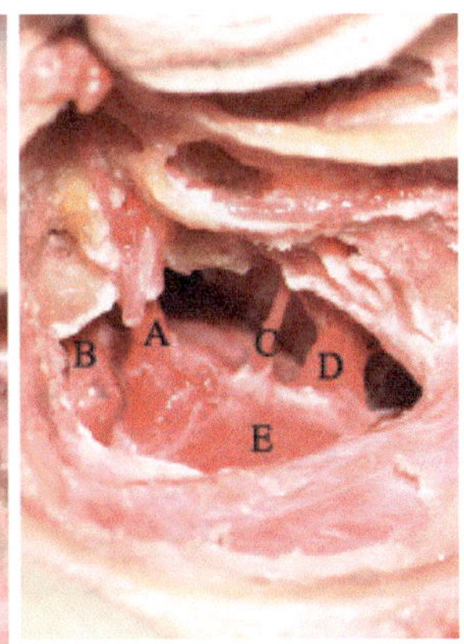

A. Facial-acoustic nerve tract
B. Trigeminal nerve
C. Glossopharyngeal nerve
D. Vagus and accessory nerves
E. Cerebellum

Fig. 5.16 Opening the CPA (right)
The dura mater of the posterior fossa is fully exposed and resected using ophthalmic scissors, to expose the CPA and the structures therein. From above to below, the pontine exit of the trigeminal nerve, pontobulbar sulcus exit of the facial nerve tract, and medulla oblongata exit of the glossopharyngeal, vagus, and accessory nerves
Instruments: medium-sized diamond burs, ophthalmic scissors

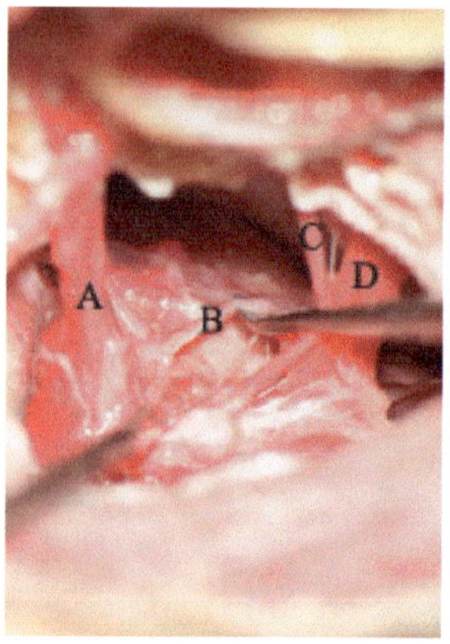

A. Facial-acoustic nerve tract
B. Anterior inferior cerebellar artery
C. Glossopharyngeal nerve
D. Vagus and accessory nerves

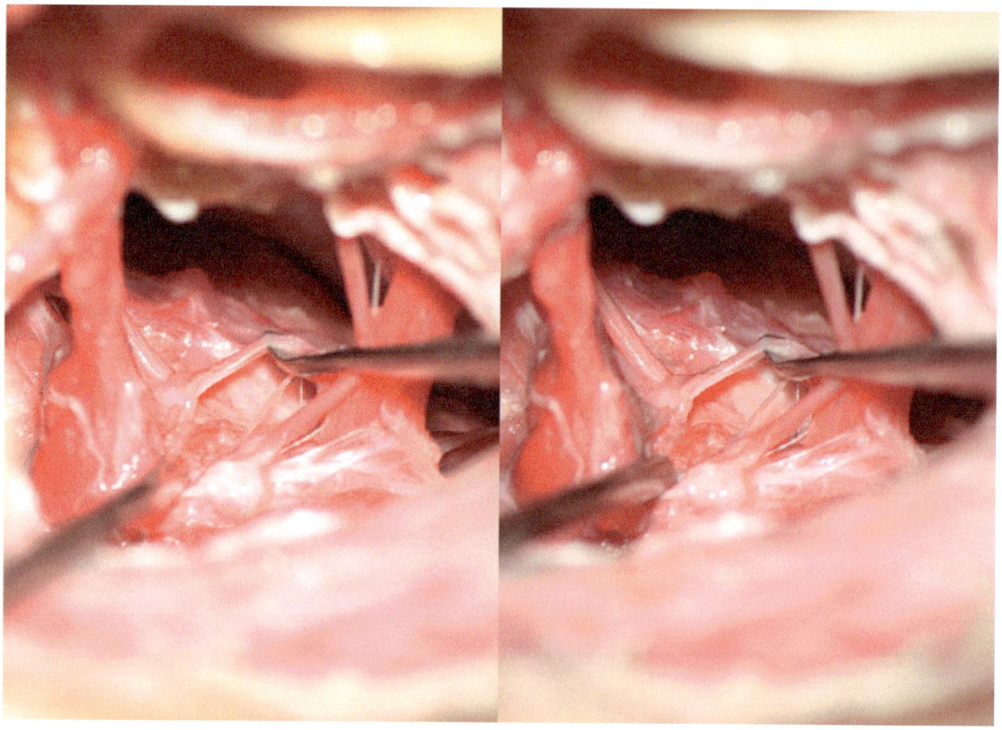

Fig. 5.17 Anterior inferior cerebellar artery (right)
The anterior inferior cerebellar artery, which arises from the basilar artery, almost always passes between the facial and vestibular nerves, but occasionally passes on the ventral or dorsal side of the facial-acoustic nerve tract. It sends off branches to supply the anterior inferior part of the cerebellum and the facial-acoustic nerve root zone. It also gives off a labyrinthine artery that supplies the inner ear. The figure shows that the anterior inferior cerebellar artery is lifted by the elevator as it passes from the medial side of the facial-acoustic nerve tract

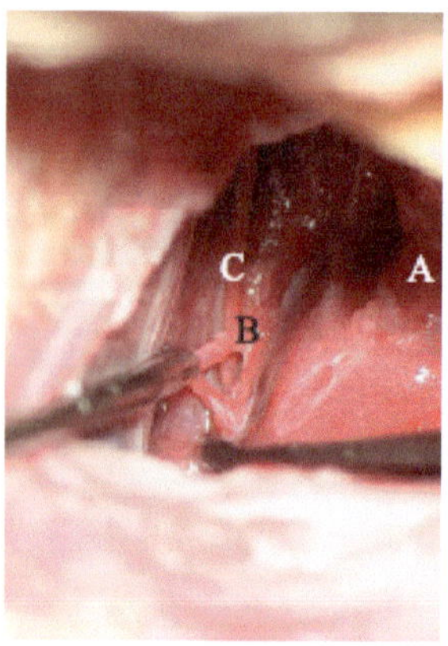

A. Trigeminal nerve root
B. Superior cerebellar artery
C. Trochlear nerve

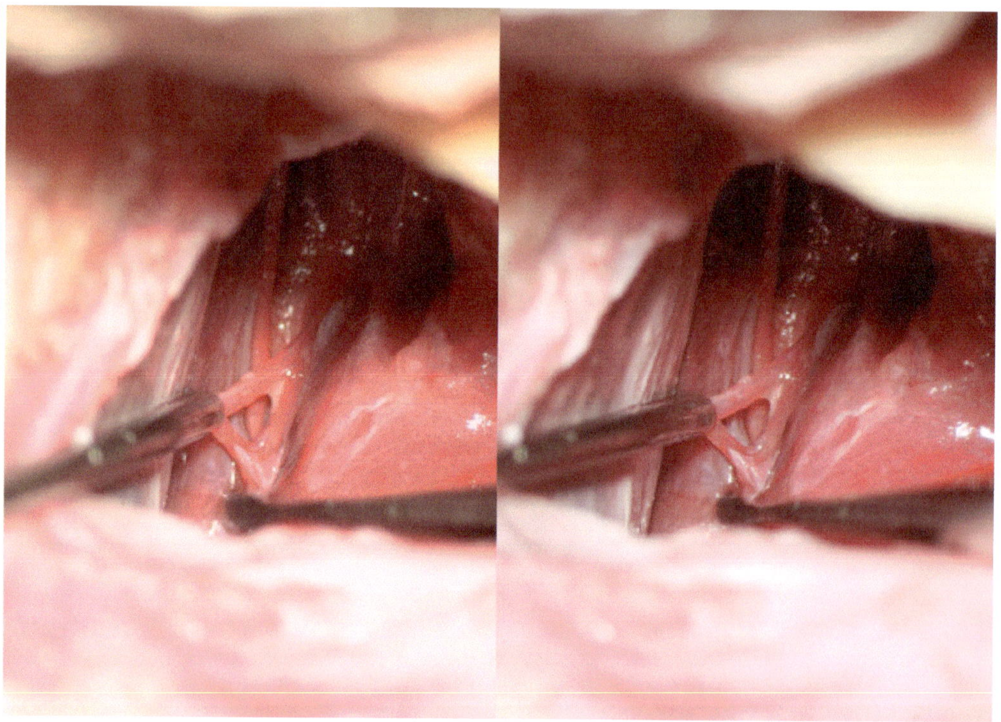

Fig. 5.18 Superior cerebellar artery and trochlear nerve (right)
Below the tentorium of the cerebellum, the superior cerebellar artery and trochlear nerve arise from the basilar artery and dorsal part of the midbrain, respectively. The superior cerebellar artery supplies part of the mesencephalon, the pons, and the superior part of the cerebellum. Brainstem necrosis may result if the superior cerebellar artery or its branches are damaged during surgery. One important cause of trigeminal neuralgia is intimate contact between the superior cerebellar artery and trigeminal nerve

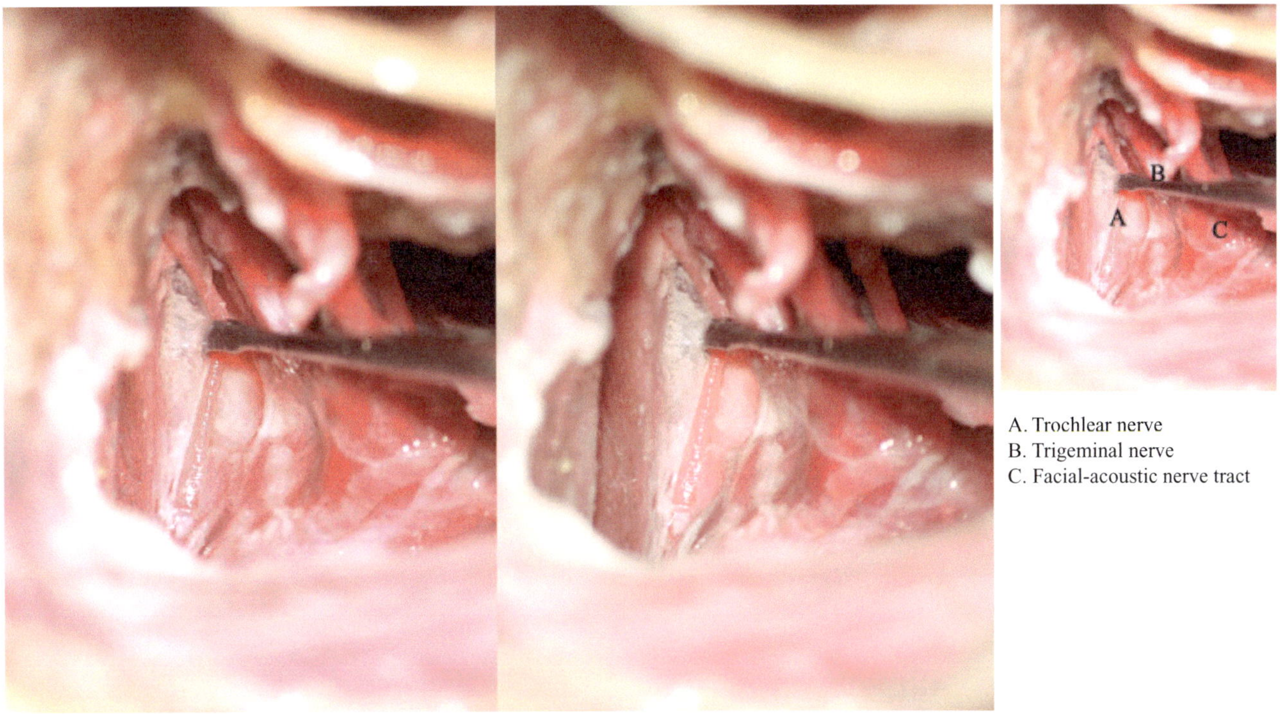

A. Trochlear nerve
B. Trigeminal nerve
C. Facial-acoustic nerve tract

Fig. 5.19 Cranial nerves IV, V, VII, and VIII (right)
The four cranial nerves from top to bottom are IV (trochlear nerve), V (trigeminal nerve), VII (facial nerve), and VIII (vestibulocochlear)

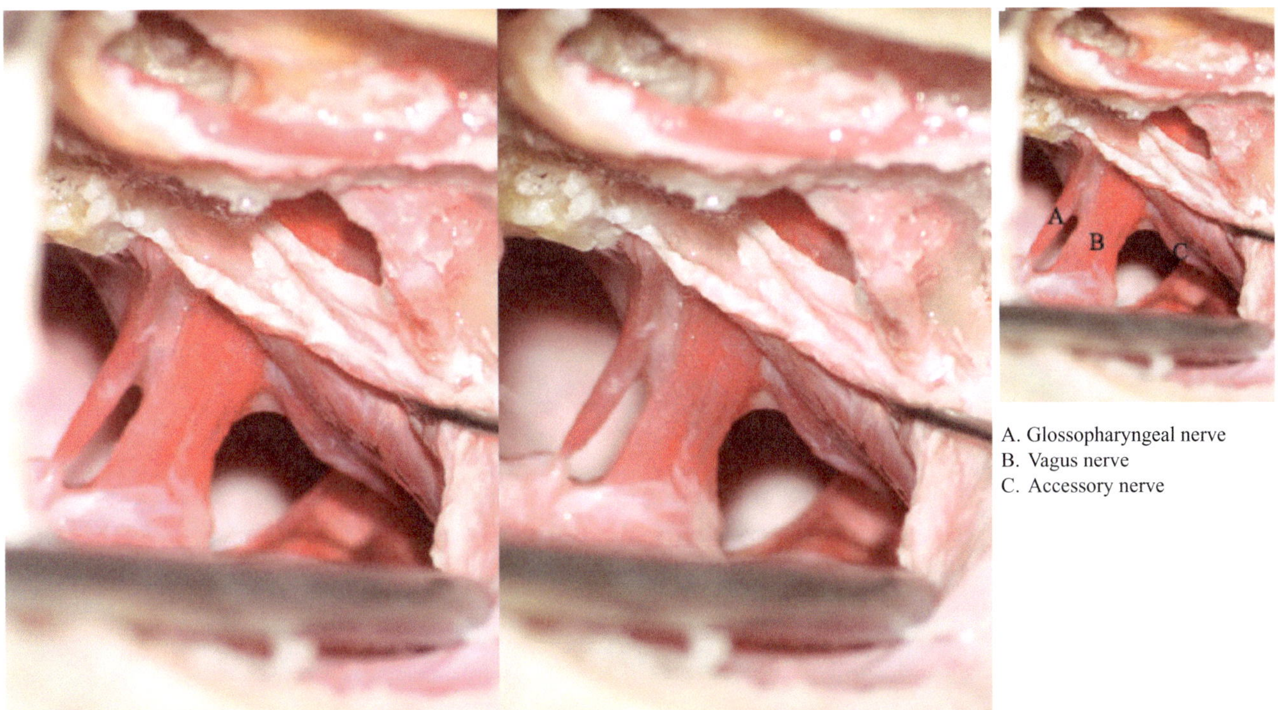

A. Glossopharyngeal nerve
B. Vagus nerve
C. Accessory nerve

Fig. 5.20 Cranial nerves IX, X, and XI (right)
By retracting the dura mater of the posterior fossa, cranial nerves IX (glossopharyngeal nerve), X (vagus nerve), and XI (accessory nerve), which arise from the medulla oblongata, can be well exposed, but the hypoglossal nerve is difficult to see because it is positioned much lower

Suggested Reading

Brackmann D-E, Shelton C, Arriaga M-A. Otologic surgery. 4th ed. Philadelphia: Elsevier Medicine; 2015.

Charabi S, Mantoni M, Tos M, et al. Cystic vestibular schwannomas: neuroimaging and growth rate. J Laryngol Otol. 1994;108(5):375–9.

Glasscock M-E, Hays J-W. The translabyrinthine removal of acoustic and other cerebellopontine angle tumors. Ann Otol Rhinol Laryngol. 1973;82(4):415–27.

Gulya A-J. Gulya and Schuknecht's anatomy of the temporal bone with surgical implications. New York: Informa Healthcare USA; 2007.

House W-F. Surgical exposure of the internal auditory canal and its contents through the middle, cranial fossa. Laryngoscope. 1961;71:1363–85.

Jackler R-K, Brackmann D-E. Neurotology. 2nd ed. Philadelphia: Elsevier Mosby; 2004.

Naguib M-B, Saleh E, Cokkeser Y, et al. The enlarged translabyrinthine approach for removal of large vestibular schwannomas. J Laryngol Otol. 1994;108(7):545–50.

Sanna M, Khrais T, Falcioni M, et al. The temporal bone: a manual for dissection and surgical approaches. New York: Thieme; 2005.

Middle Cranial Fossa Approach

6

Yi Jiang, Guo-jian Wang, and Vincent C Cousins

Surgical Procedures Using the Middle Cranial Fossa Approach

The middle cranial fossa (MCF) approach is used during temporal craniotomy to expose the anterior and posterior regions of the temporal bone and petrous apex. Depending on the degree of exposure required, an extended MCF approach or trans-petrosal approach with progressive removal of the petrous barrier can be used. The MCF approach may be used for the following procedures and conditions:

1. Facial nerve decompression (geniculate ganglion, labyrinthine and internal auditory canal segments) when hearing can be preserved
2. Facial nerve neuroma
3. Acoustic neuroma within the internal auditory canal (IAC)
4. Petrous bone cholesteatoma and cholesterol granuloma
5. Vestibular neurectomy
6. Meningoencephalocele (radical resection and repair of dura and tegmen)
7. Petroclival meningioma resection
8. Upper clival and petrous apex chordoma resection
9. Eustachian tube reconstruction
10. MCF schwannoma resection
11. Cavernous hemangioma resection
12. Excision of trigeminal nerve roots
13. Superior semicircular canal dehiscence (resurfacing and plugging)
14. Cochlear implantation (rarely)

Related Anatomical Structures

1. Tegmen: a flat area of bone in the lateral part of the MCF floor that separates the middle ear cleft from the MCF contents. The tegmen is divided into tympanic and mastoid sections according to the structures that it covers. It can be identified after elevating the temporal lobe.
2. Greater superficial petrosal nerve (GSPN): a branch projecting from the geniculate ganglion that passes through the GSPN sulcus and eventually merges with the pterygopalatine ganglion. The GSPN runs parallel to the long axis of the petrous bone and is medial to the middle meningeal artery. Tracing the GSPN posteriorly to the facial hiatus and geniculate ganglion can help locate the inner ear when using the MCF approach.
3. Foramen spinosum: located lateral to the foramen ovale, the foramen spinosum allows passage of the middle meningeal artery and the meningeal branch of the mandibular nerve.
4. Middle meningeal artery: an artery originating from the maxillary branch of the external carotid artery. Extending from the maxillary artery, it passes through the foramen spinosum intracranially then divides into two branches that supply the basal dura of the cortex and calvarium.
5. Internal auditory canal (IAC): a bony neurovascular channel in the petrous bone containing the facial nerve, cochlear nerve, vestibular nerve, intermediate nerve, labyrinthine artery and vein. When observed using the middle fossa approach, the IAC lies beneath the line that bisects the angle between the long axis of the superior semicircular canal and the GSPN.
6. Facial hiatus: an opening in the temporal bone through which the GSPN passes anteriorly from the geniculate ganglion to the GSPN sulcus.
7. Geniculate ganglion: at the point of termination of its labyrinthine segment, the facial nerve thickens and bends laterally then back toward its horizontal segment. This

Y. Jiang (✉)
Department of Otolaryngology Head and Neck Surgery, Shanghai Ninth People's Hospital, Shanghai Jiao Tong University School of Medicine, Shanghai, China

G.-j. Wang
College of Otolaryngology Head and Neck Surgery, Chinese PLA General Hospital, Beijing, China

V. C. Cousins
Department of Ear Nose and Throat Surgery, Alfred Hospital, Melbourne, Australia

Department of Surgery, Monash University, Melbourne, Australia

P. Dai et al. (eds.), *Stereoscopic Anatomical Atlas of Ear Surgery*, https://doi.org/10.1007/978-981-16-0927-5_6

thicker genu is the geniculate ganglion. Absence of the bone over the geniculate ganglion results in direct contact with the dura of the middle fossa in 5–15% of cases.

8. Arcuate eminence: a smooth bony elevation medial to the tegmen mastoideum. The arcuate eminence serves as a marker of the superior semicircular canal and guides one using the MCF approach to the inner ear.
9. Superior petrosal sinus: a sinus located in the superior petrosal sulcus of the petrous bone attached to the tentorium. It connects medially with the posterior end of the cavernous sinus and laterally with the junction of the transverse and sigmoid sinuses. The petrosal veins join the superior petrosal sinus.

Anatomy Overview

1. Incision: a 7–8 cm curved incision is begun in the preauricular area and extended superiorly with the flap based anteriorly. The skin, subcutaneous tissue, and periosteum are incised. The temporalis muscle is elevated from the temporal fossa and a retractor is placed to expose the temporal squama.
2. Temporal craniotomy: an approximately 4 × 3 cm craniotomy is created with two-thirds anterior and one-third posterior to the middle zygomatic root/anterior EAC wall. The inferior edge of the bone window should be near the zygoma and level with the floor of the MCF. *Hints: A cutting bur is used to begin the temporal craniotomy, and diamond burs should be used when close to the dura. Before elevating the bone flap, the temporal bone and underlying dura should be carefully separated using a blunt raspatory.*
3. Elevation of the dura from the floor of the middle fossa: carefully separate the dura from the underlying temporal bone with a blunt raspatory to avoid laceration. Identify the middle meningeal artery and expose the floor of the middle fossa with a brain spatula. Identifiable landmarks include the foramen spinosum edge behind the middle meningeal artery, the GSPN with the facial nerve hiatus, and the arcuate eminence. If the temporal lobe is difficult to lift, further elevation of the dura over the parietal and occipital lobes may be required. *Hints: In 5–15% of cases, the geniculate ganglion of the facial nerve is exposed. Dural elevation should be performed gently using identified landmarks to prevent damage to the facial nerve. In surgery, stimulation of the GSPN may assist identification of the geniculate ganglion via retrograde current passage to reach the facial nerve.*
4. IAC exposure: adequately expose the landmarks on the floor of the MCF. Identify the orientation of the IAC within the surgical field. Complete bone removal with diamond burs, drill around the medial porus acousticus, as this area contains more surrounding bone that can be safely removed compared to the lateral fundus of the IAC, access to which is more restricted. *Hints: Exercise caution to avoid injury to the superior petrosal sinus, which lies within the superior petrosal sulcus of the petrous ridge, when exposing the IAC. The labyrinthine portion of the facial nerve lies between the basal turn of the cochlea and the superior semicircular canal. Use an appropriately sized bur and drill parallel to the superior semicircular canal. Avoid injury to the ampulla of the superior semicircular canal and the cochlea, which are near the posterior and anterior edges of the facial nerve, respectively. The angle formed by the superior semicircular canal and the IAC is 45–60° and can be used to locate the IAC. It is recommended that the canal is not blue-lined due to the risk of opening the inner ear.*
5. Exposing the nerves in the IAC: identifying the IAC begins with bone removal just lateral to the petrous ridge. Once the porus of the IAC has been exposed, continue removing the bone in that area, progressing laterally toward the fundus until the IAC is sufficiently exposed. The fundus separates the IAC from the vestibule and cochlea, which are in close proximity to each other. Medially, there are no delicate structures near the IAC except the endolymphatic sac. In total, 75% of the IAC circumference can be dissected. Laterally, an eggshell thin bone plate over the top of the canal is elevated to expose the dura. Carefully identify the labyrinthine segment of the facial nerve and the superior vestibular nerve, the cochlear nerve, the inferior vestibular nerve, the intermedius nerve, and the labyrinthine artery in the IAC. Bill's bar is a useful landmark during this procedure. *Hints: The lateral eggshell thin bone plate of the IAC should be retained when dissecting the IAC, to prevent the bur from penetrating the dura and damaging the nerves within. Pneumatized bone may extend over some or all of the IAC and require extensive removal before exposing the canal. This can be assessed with pre-operative CT scans, particularly coronal sections.*

Purposes and Requirements of Anatomical Dissection

1. Skilled use of various bur types
2. Effective drilling technique for the temporal craniotomy
3. Understanding of the correct methodology for elevating the dura
4. Effective use of the brain spatula and adjustable retractor
5. In-depth knowledge of the location and anatomy of the IAC
6. In-depth knowledge of the location and anatomy of the geniculate ganglion, labyrinthine segment, and horizontal segment of the facial nerve

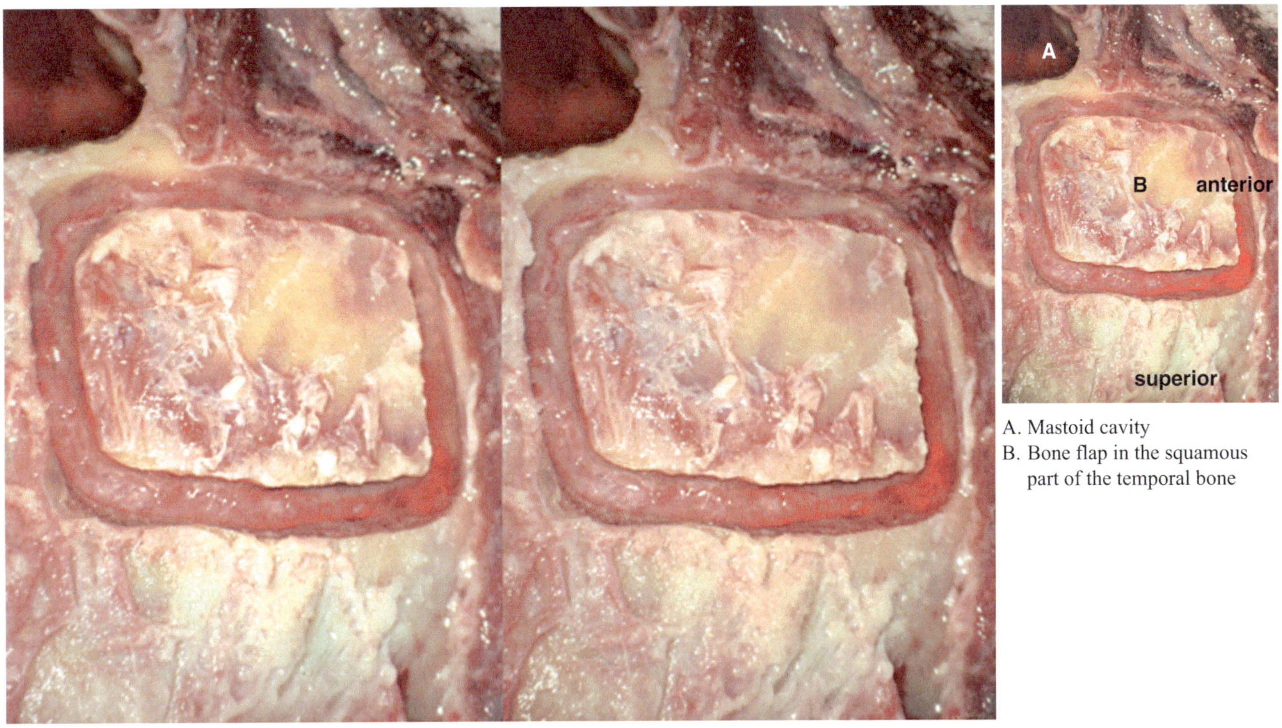

A. Mastoid cavity
B. Bone flap in the squamous part of the temporal bone

Fig. 6.1 Forming a window in the temporal bone (left)
Left temporal bone observed from superior to inferior. An inverted-L shaped incision (7–8 cm × 2 cm) is extended from in front of the tragus. A retractor is used to hold the flap forward and expose the squamous part of the temporal bone. Above the zygomatic arch and temporal line, bone grooves are drilled with a medium-sized cutting bur to form a 3 × 4 cm rectangle. The anterior 2/3 of the rectangle should be in front of the vertical line through the anterior wall of the external auditory canal (EAC)
Instruments: medium-sized cutting burs, small-sized diamond burs, adjustable self-retaining retractor

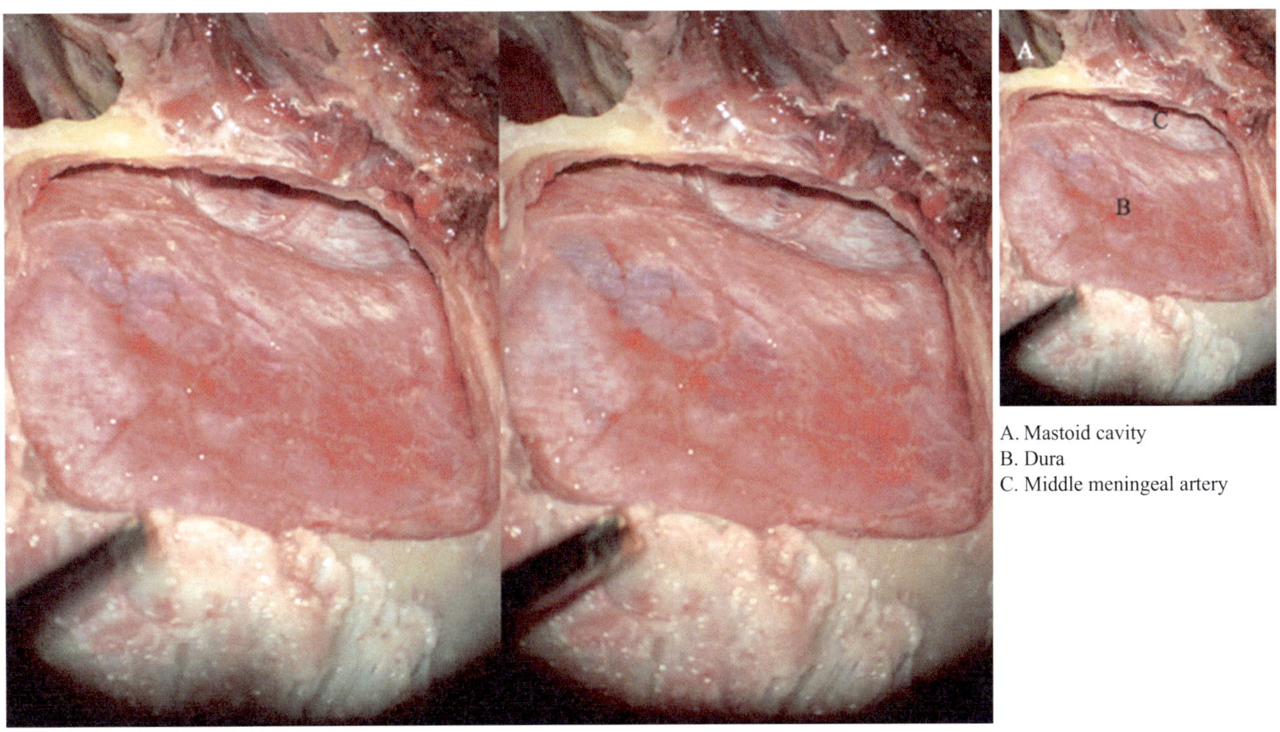

A. Mastoid cavity
B. Dura
C. Middle meningeal artery

Fig. 6.2 Exposing the endocranium of the temporal lobe (left)
The bone flap is removed to form a rectangular window in the temporal bone. Exercise caution to avoid injuring the dura or cerebral tissue during dissection
Instruments: elevator, brain spatula

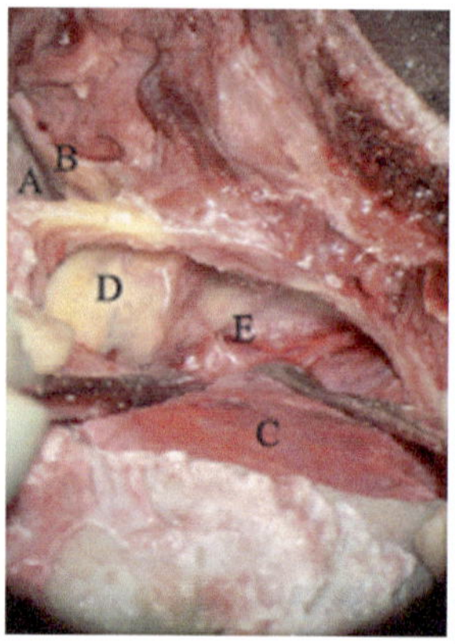

A. Mastoid cavity
B. Posterior wall of the EAC
C. Dura
D. Tegmen mastoideum
E. Sulcus for the middle meningeal artery

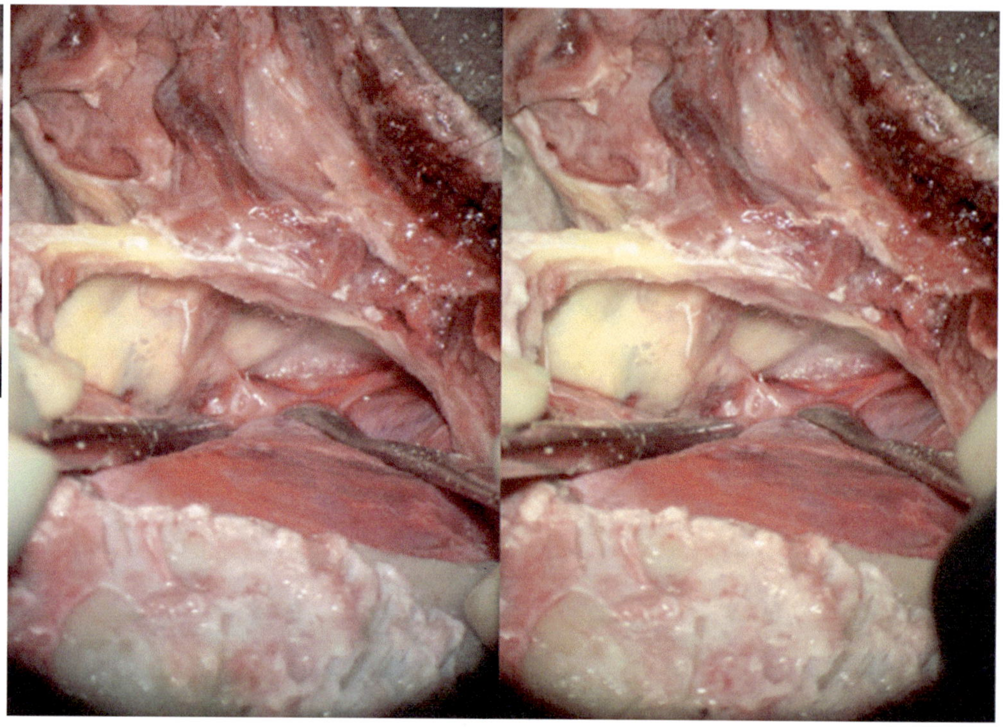

Fig. 6.3 Identifying anatomical landmarks of the middle cranial fossa (left)
An elevator or brain spatula is used to detach the dura of the MCF from the anterior surface of the petrosal bone. Three important anatomical landmarks on the base of the MCF can be identified: the middle meningeal artery (through the foramen spinosum), the GSPN (from the geniculate ganglion), and the arcuate eminence (marking the superior semicircular canal). After dural detachment, the first identifiable landmark is the middle meningeal artery, which can be traced to the foramen spinosum
Instruments: elevator, brain spatula

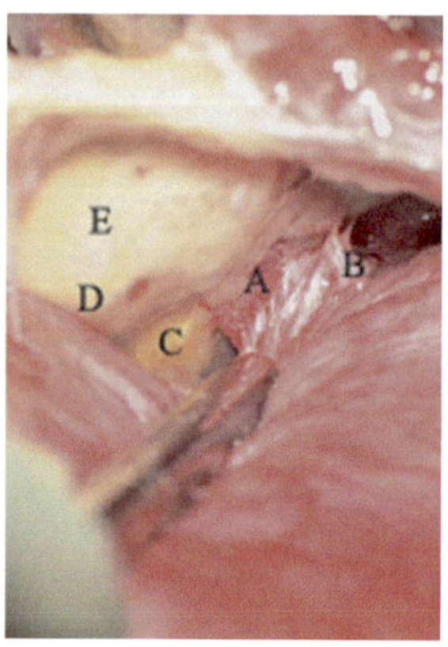

A. Facial hiatus
B. Middle meningeal artery
C. Bone around the cochlea
D. Arcuate eminence
E. Tegmen mastoideum

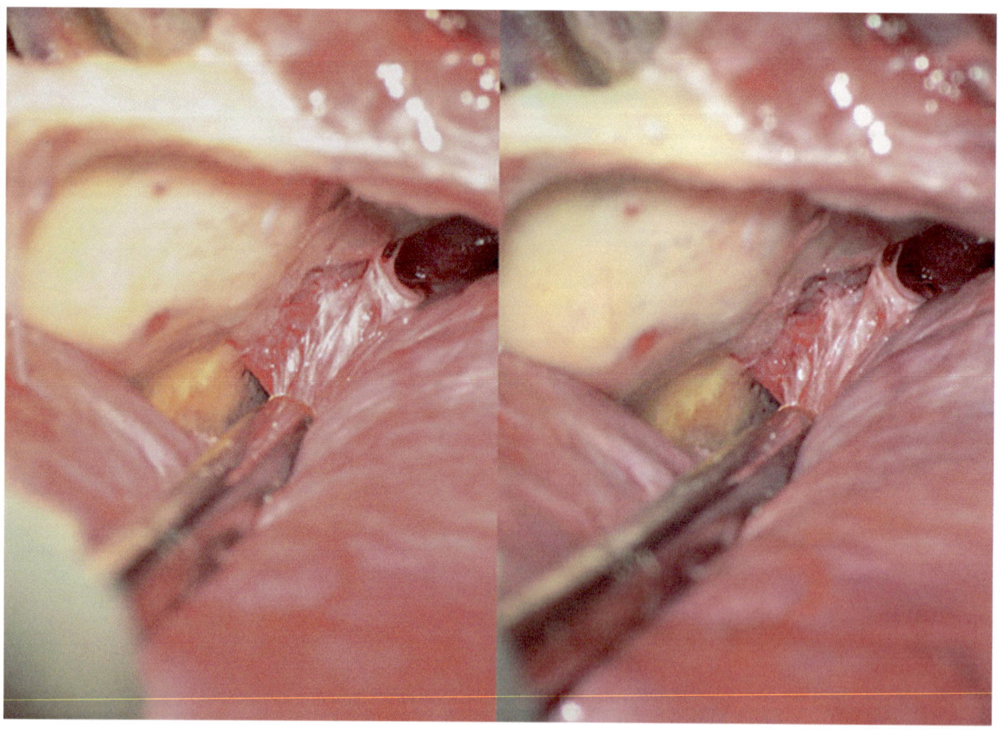

Fig. 6.4 Locating the facial hiatus (left)
The GSPN is the second important anatomical landmark. The nerve is posterior and medial to the middle meningeal artery and emerges from the facial hiatus anteriorly. The dura should be detached from the bone to protect the GSPN. The arcuate eminence, the third important landmark, will be exposed as the dura is detached further posteriorly. The three landmarks are used in combination. Not all patients have an arcuate eminence and not all superior semicircular canals are positioned identically relative to the arcuate eminence. The target structures should be identified and assessed relative to the overall anatomic structure of the cavity
Instruments: elevator, brain spatula

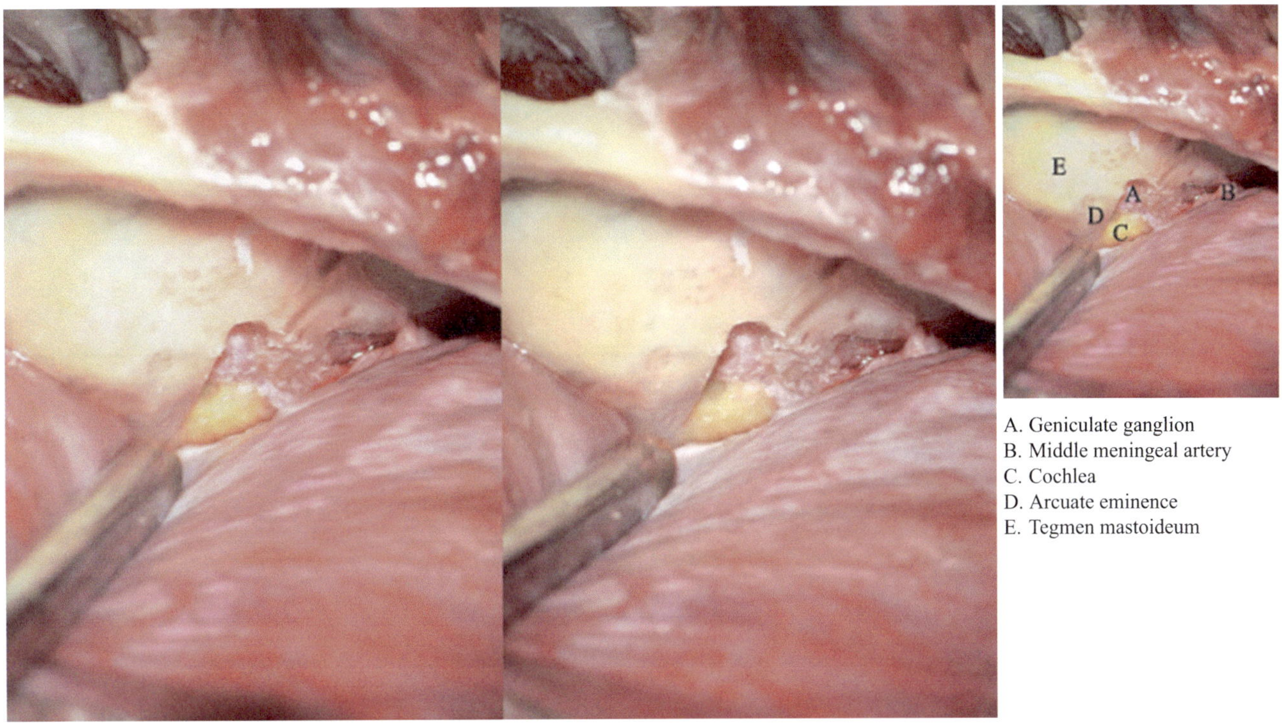

A. Geniculate ganglion
B. Middle meningeal artery
C. Cochlea
D. Arcuate eminence
E. Tegmen mastoideum

Fig. 6.5 Exposing the geniculate ganglion (left)
Once the facial hiatus has been identified, the nearby bone should be drilled carefully to expose the geniculate ganglion. To avoid damaging the geniculate ganglion and GSPN, the bone should be removed at a low drill speed using minimal pressure with continuous irrigation to remove bone dust and cool the bur
Instruments: medium-sized diamond burs

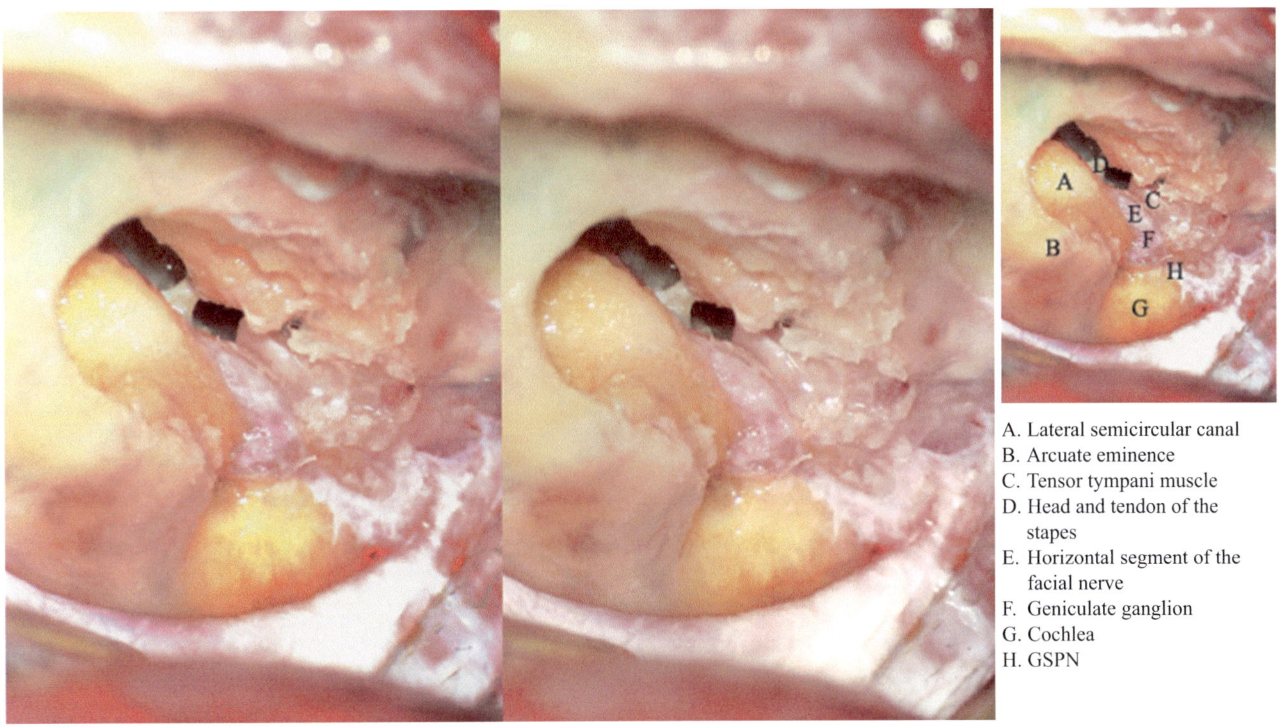

A. Lateral semicircular canal
B. Arcuate eminence
C. Tensor tympani muscle
D. Head and tendon of the stapes
E. Horizontal segment of the facial nerve
F. Geniculate ganglion
G. Cochlea
H. GSPN

Fig. 6.6 Exposing the tympanic cavity and mastoid (left)
Part of the tympanic and tegmen mastoideum is removed to expose the lateral semicircular canal, part of the ossicles, and the horizontal segment of the facial nerve
Instruments: small- and medium-sized diamond burs

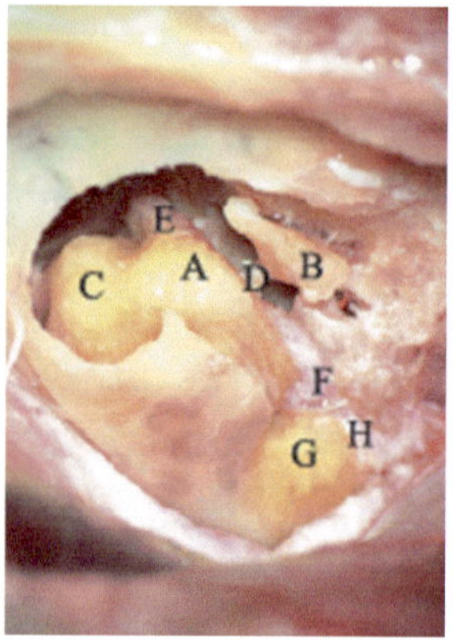

A. Lateral semicircular canal
B. Incudomalleal joint
C. Posterior semicircular canal
D. Head and tendon of the stapes
E. Pyramid segment of the facial nerve
F. Geniculate ganglion
G. Cochlea
H. GSPN

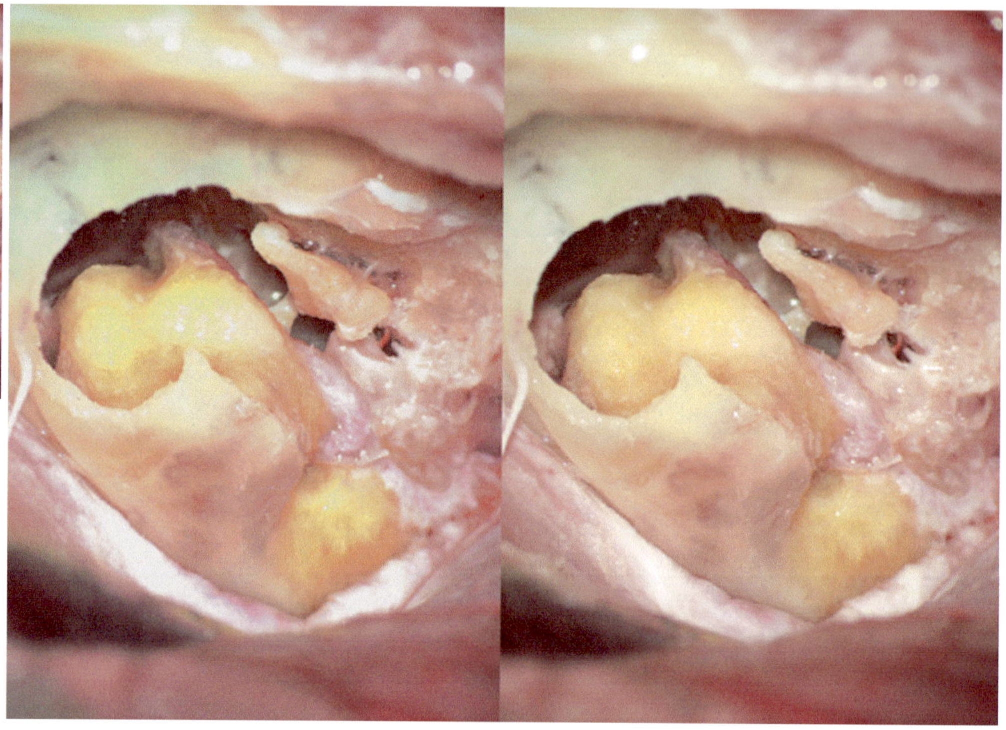

Fig. 6.7 Removing the majority of the tympanic and tegmen mastoideum (left)
The majority of the tympanic and tegmen mastoideum is removed to expose the lateral semicircular canal, posterior semicircular canal, and vertical segment of the facial nerve. The mastoid approach is used to further expose the contents of the epitympanum, including the ossicles
Instruments: medium-sized diamond burs

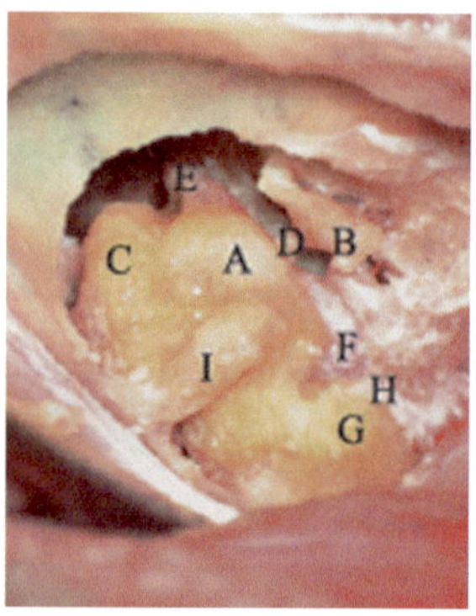

A. Lateral semicircular canal
B. Incudomalleal joint
C. Posterior semicircular canal
D. Head and tendon of the stapes
E. Pyramid segment of the facial nerve
F. Geniculate ganglion
G. Cochlea
H. GSPN
I. Superior semicircular canal

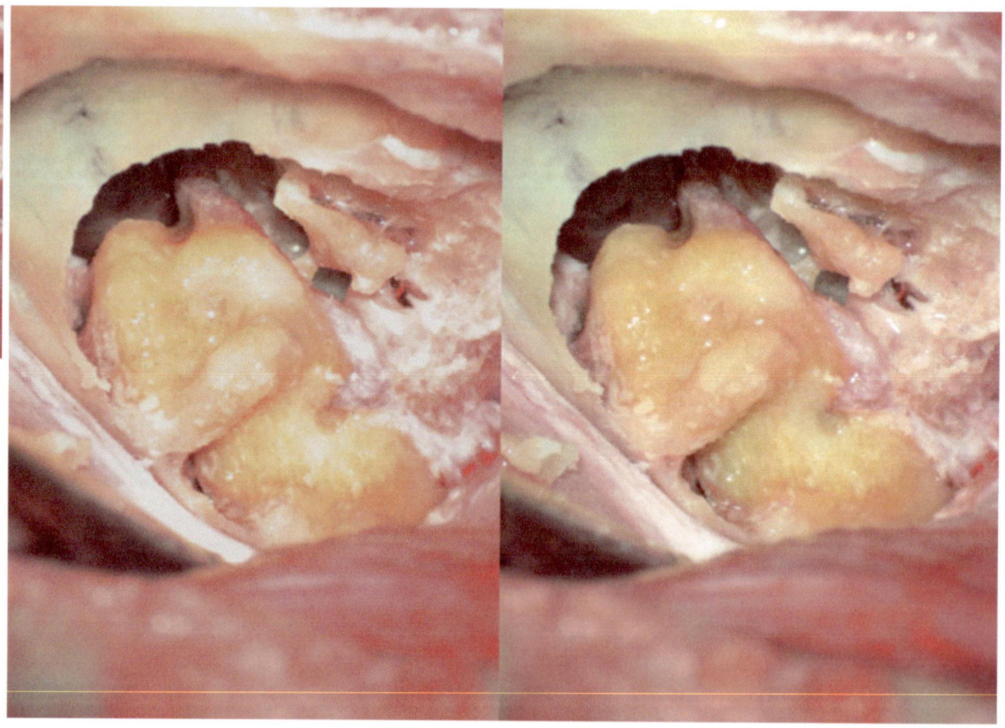

Fig. 6.8 Outlining the superior semicircular canal (left)
The location of the superior semicircular canal is identified based on the position of the posterior and lateral semicircular canals. Outline the superior semicircular canal with a medium-sized diamond bur
Instruments: medium-sized diamond burs

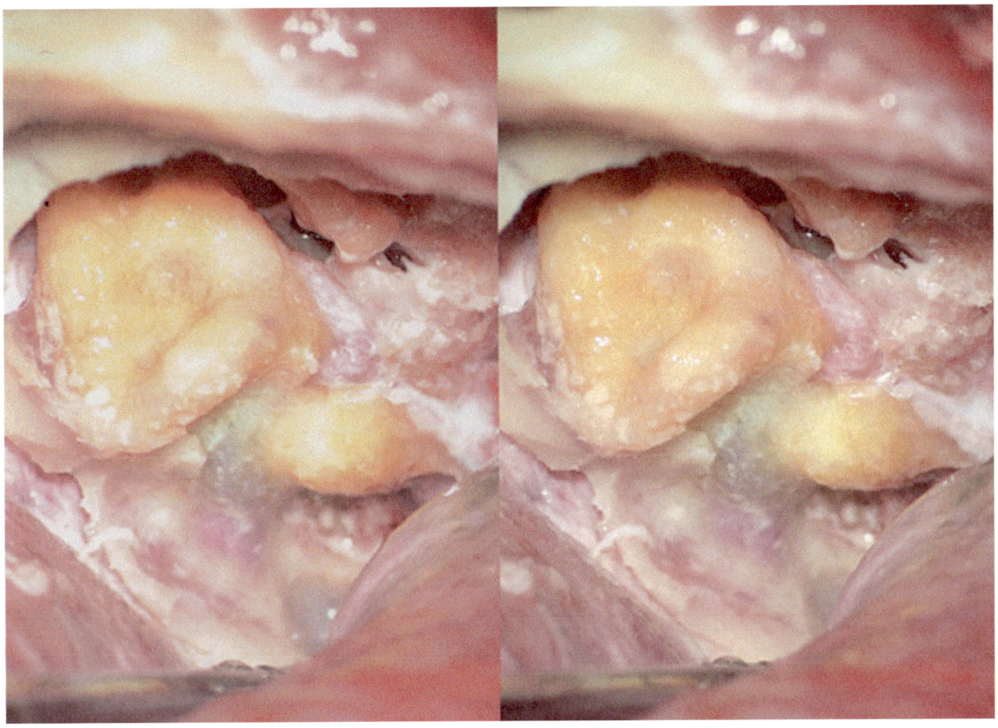

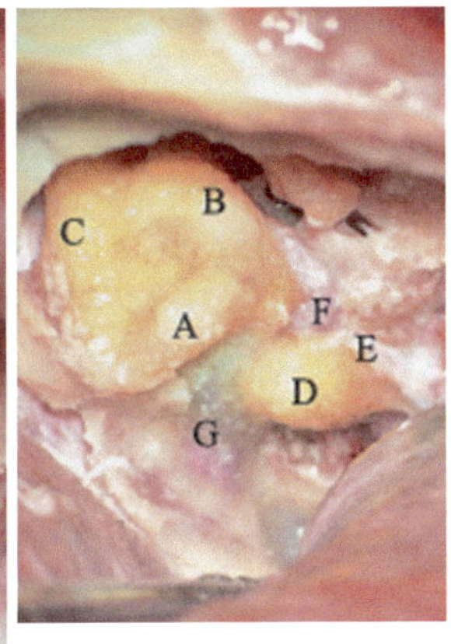

A. Superior semicircular canal
B. Lateral semicircular canal
C. Posterior semicircular canal
D. Cochlea
E. GSPN
F. Geniculate ganglion
G. IAC

Fig. 6.9 Locating the IAC (left)
The IAC is located between the cochlea, superior semicircular canal, and dura of the posterior cranial fossa. The IAC can be exposed using the MCF approach. The superior semicircular canal is posterior, superior and lateral to the IAC. The plane of the superior semicircular canal forms an approximately 60° angle with the IAC. The cochlea is anterior, inferior, and medial to the geniculate ganglion. The air cells of the petrous apex are anterior and medial to the IAC and in close proximity to the cochlea and internal carotid artery
Instruments: small-sized diamond burs

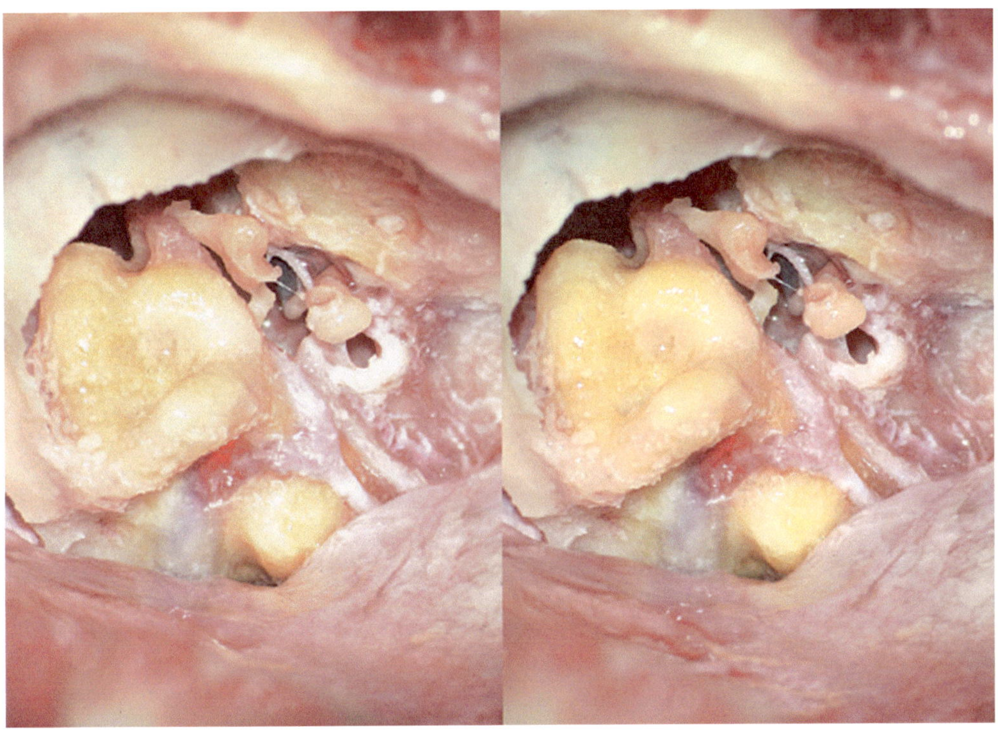

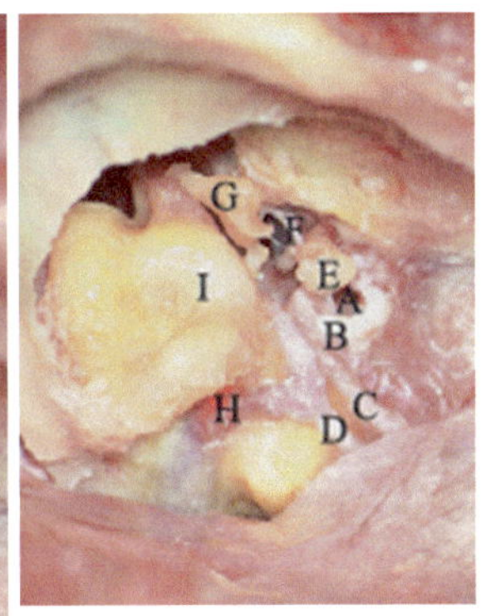

A. Tympanic opening of the Eustachian tube
B. Tensor tympani muscle
C. LSPN
D. GSPN
E. Head of the malleus
F. Chorda tympani
G. Dislocated incus
H. Labyrinthine segment of the facial nerve
I. Lateral semicircular canal

Fig. 6.10 Exposing the labyrinthine segment of the facial nerve (left)
The labyrinthine and IAC segments of the facial nerve are exposed by removing the bone between the geniculate ganglion, cochlea, and superior semicircular canal. The lesser superficial petrosal nerve (LSPN) is exposed by removing the bone lateral to the GSPN. The LSPN and GSPN run parallel. The LSPN is derived from the tympanic branch of the glossopharyngeal nerve, which enters the skull base through the tympanic canaliculus and joins the otic ganglion through foramina in the greater wing of the sphenoid bone. The incudomalleal joint is separated and the incus is disarticulated to expose the horizontal segment of the facial nerve. The bone lateral to the tensor tympani muscle is removed to expose the tympanic opening of the Eustachian tube
Instruments: crochet hook, small-sized diamond burs

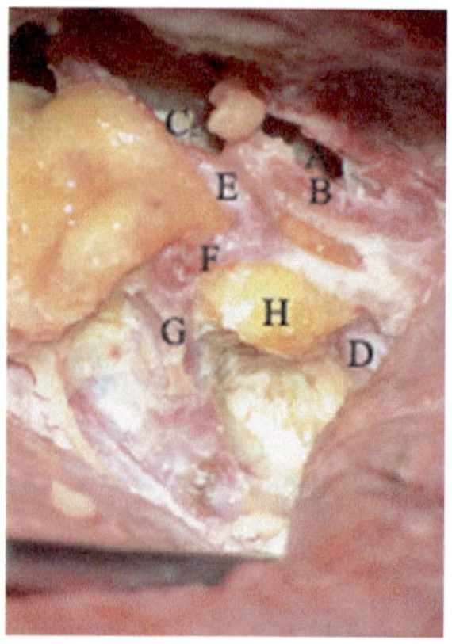

A. Eustachian tube
B. Tensor tympani muscle
C. Head of the stapes
D. Internal carotid artery
E. Horizontal segment of the facial nerve
F. Labyrinthine segment of the facial nerve
G. IAC
H. Cochlea

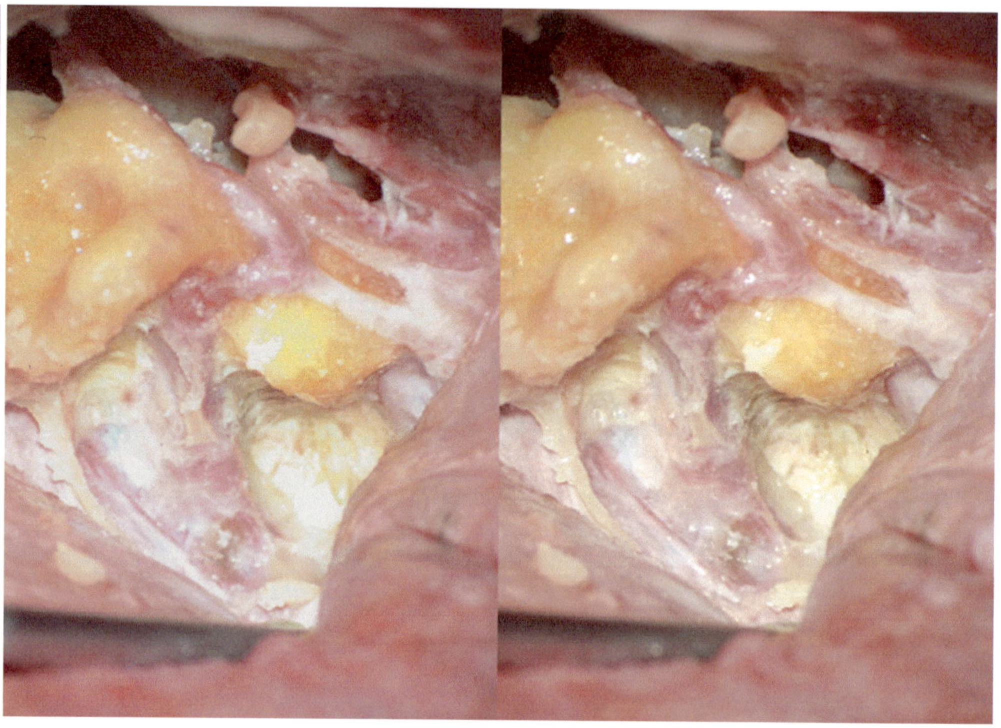

Fig. 6.11 Exposing the horizontal segment of the facial nerve and IAC (left)
The dislocated incus is removed to expose the horizontal segment of the facial nerve. The bone near the IAC and the bone anterior and medial to the basal turn of the cochlea are removed to expose anterior and superior portions of the internal carotid artery
Instruments: crochet hook, medium-sized diamond burs

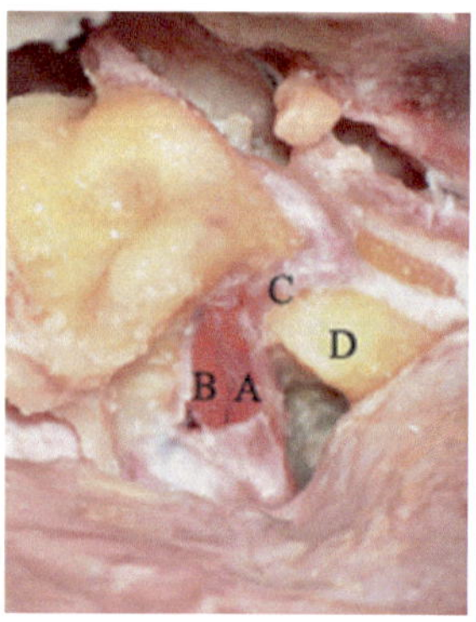

A. IAC segment of the facial nerve
B. Superior vestibular nerve
C. Labyrinthine segment of the facial nerve
D. Cochlea

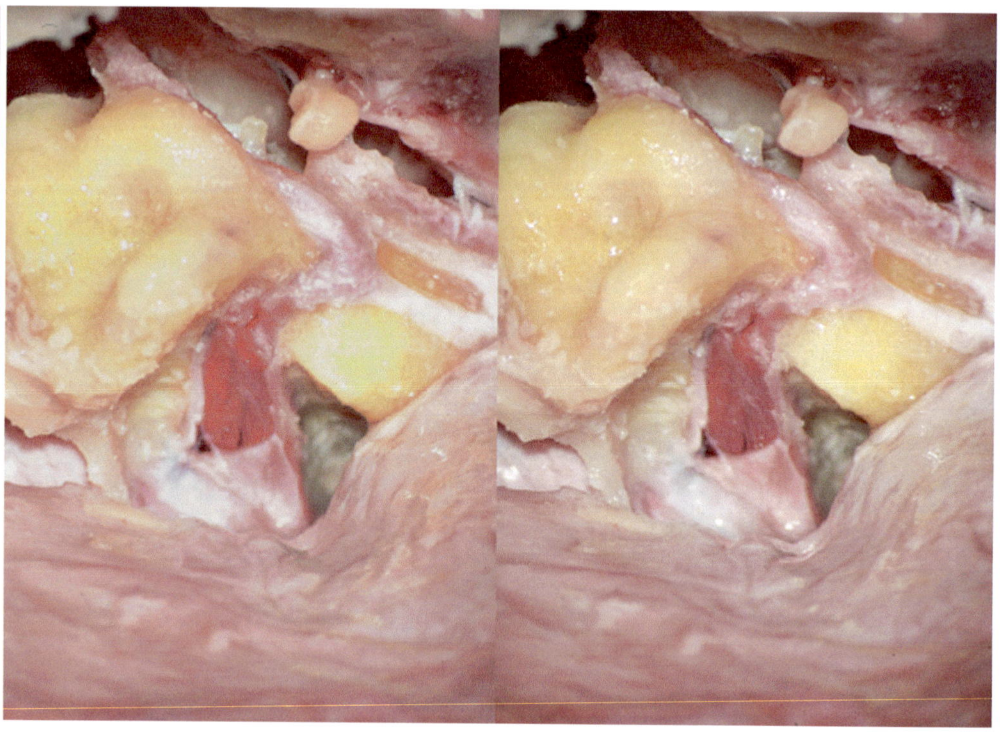

Fig. 6.12 Opening the IAC (left)
The thin bone along the upper wall of the IAC is removed and the dura of the IAC is cut from the lateral end using ophthalmic scissors. Using the MCF approach, the following landmarks can be identified: the facial nerve is located anterior superior and the superior vestibular nerve is located posterior superior. The cochlear nerve is inferior to the facial nerve and the inferior vestibular nerve is inferior to the superior vestibular nerve. Bill's bar is located between the facial nerve and superior vestibular nerve. The horizontal crest is located between the superior and inferior nerves
Instruments: right-angle hook, ophthalmic scissors

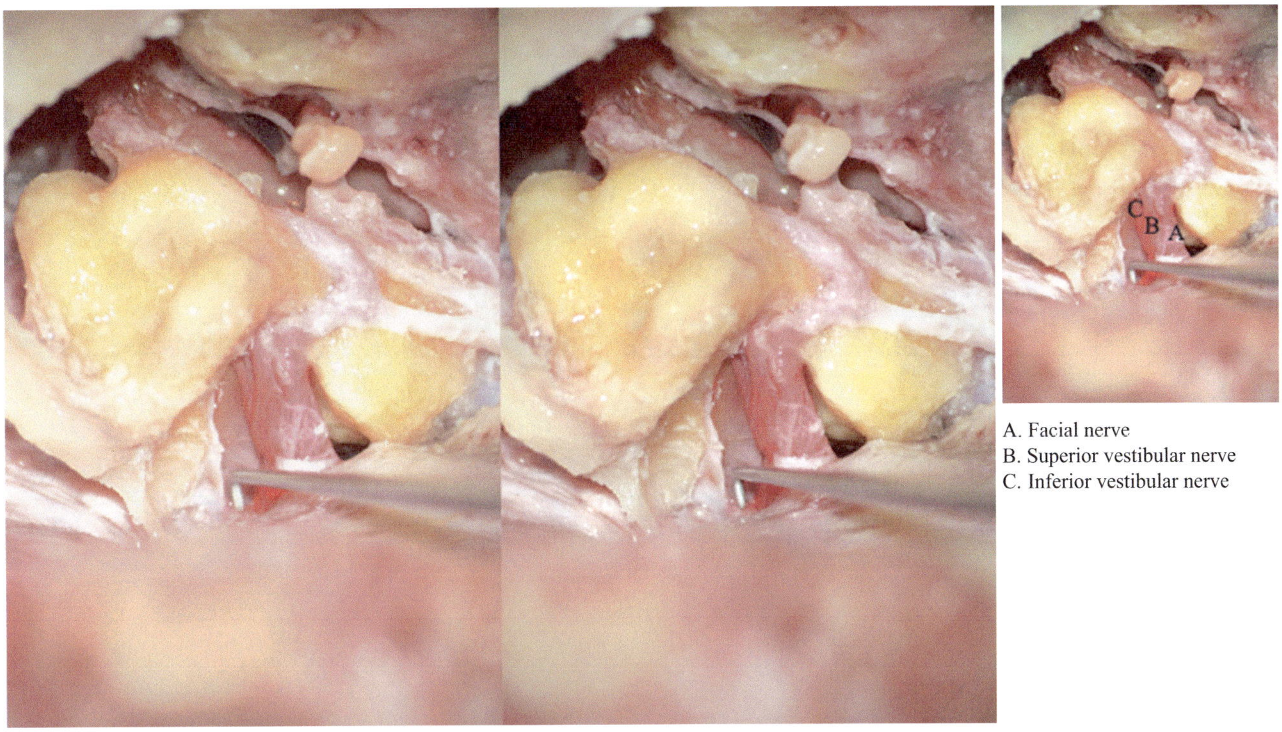

A. Facial nerve
B. Superior vestibular nerve
C. Inferior vestibular nerve

Fig. 6.13 Exposing the inferior vestibular nerve (left)
The facial nerve and superior vestibular nerve are held forward gently with a hook to expose the inferior vestibular nerve beneath the superior vestibular nerve

Instruments: right-angle hook

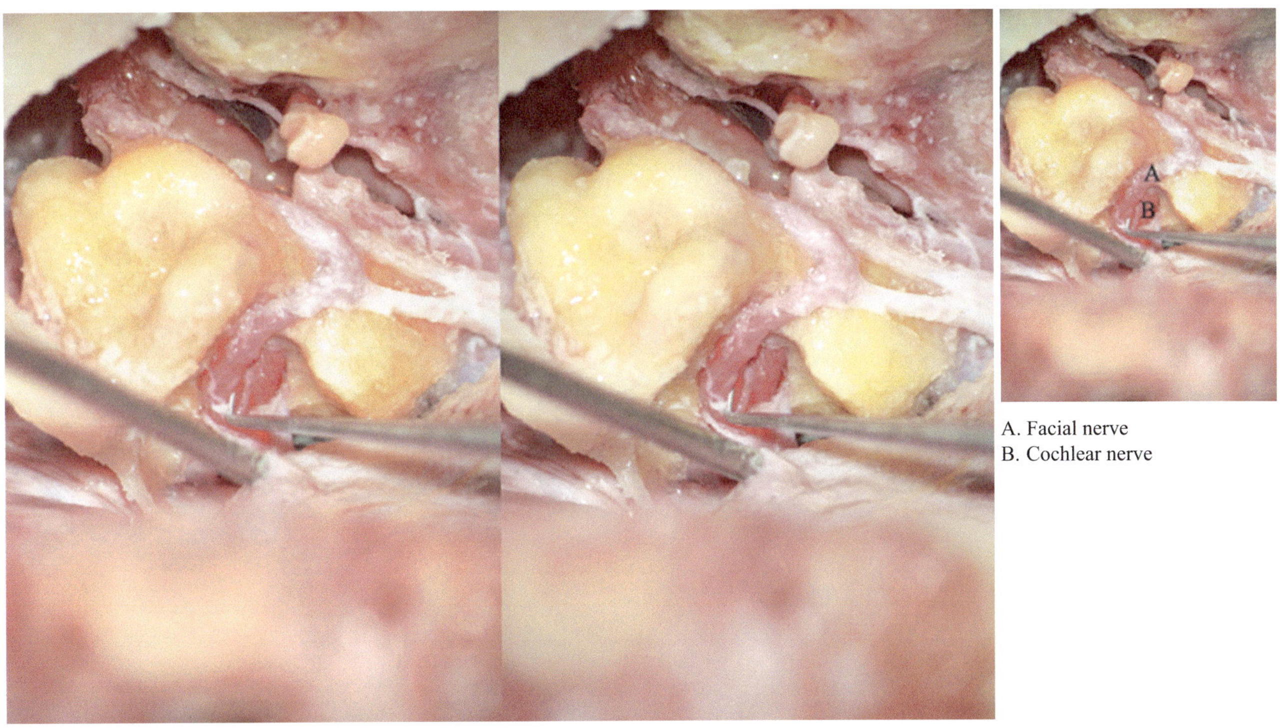

A. Facial nerve
B. Cochlear nerve

Fig. 6.14 Exposing the cochlear nerve (left)
The facial nerve and superior vestibular nerve are held backward gently with a hook to expose the cochlear nerve beneath the facial nerve

Instruments: right-angle hook

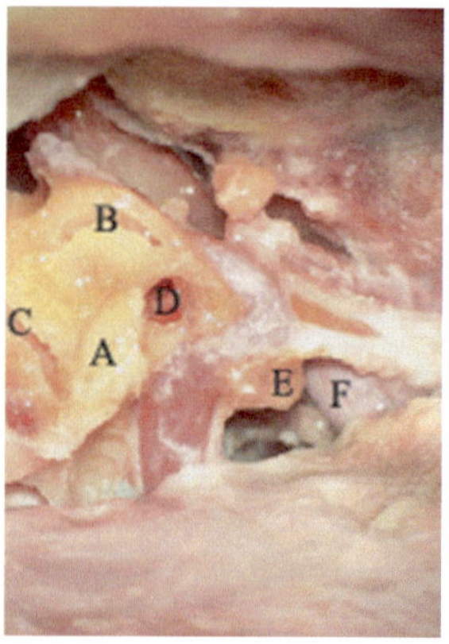

A. Superior semicircular canal (remnant)
B. Lateral semicircular canal (remnant)
C. Posterior semicircular canal (remnant)
D. Vestibule
E. Basal turn of the cochlea
F. Horizontal segment of the internal carotid artery

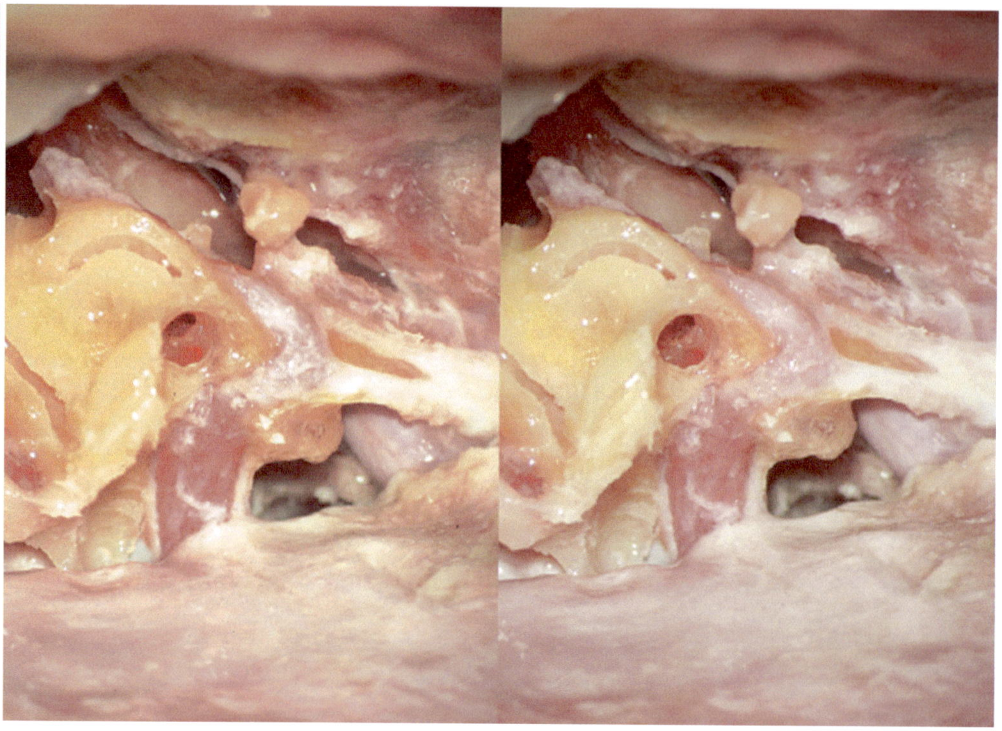

Fig. 6.15 Opening the semicircular canal and vestibule (left)
The three semicircular canals are opened using a medium-sized diamond bur. The canals are arranged in three perpendicular planes. The ampulla and anterior bone of the superior semicircular canal are removed to expose the vestibule
Instruments: small- and medium-sized diamond burs

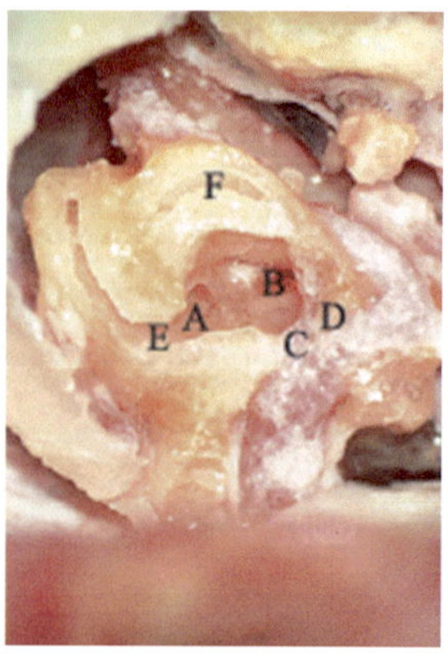

A. Ampulla of the posterior semicircular canal
B. Saccular recess
C. Superior vestibular nerve
D. Bill's bar
E. Common crus
F. Lateral semicircular canal

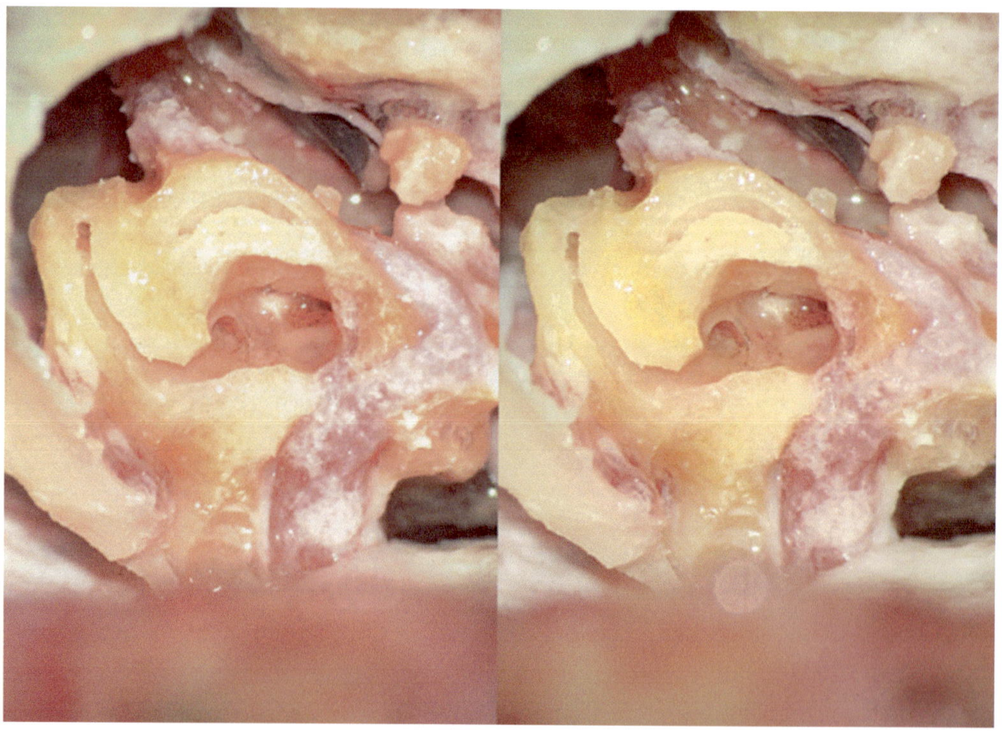

Fig. 6.16 Removing the superior semicircular canal and opening the vestibule (left)
The superior semicircular canal and the posterior medial wall of the vestibule are removed to further expose the vestibule. The anteroinferior region of the vestibular cavity connects to the scala vestibuli of the cochlea, with the oval window sealed by the stapes footplate and its annular ligament. The ampulla of the posterior semicircular canal can be observed in the posterior inferior region of the vestibule. The medial wall of the vestibule also forms the lateral wall of the fundus of the IAC
Instruments: small- and medium-sized diamond burs

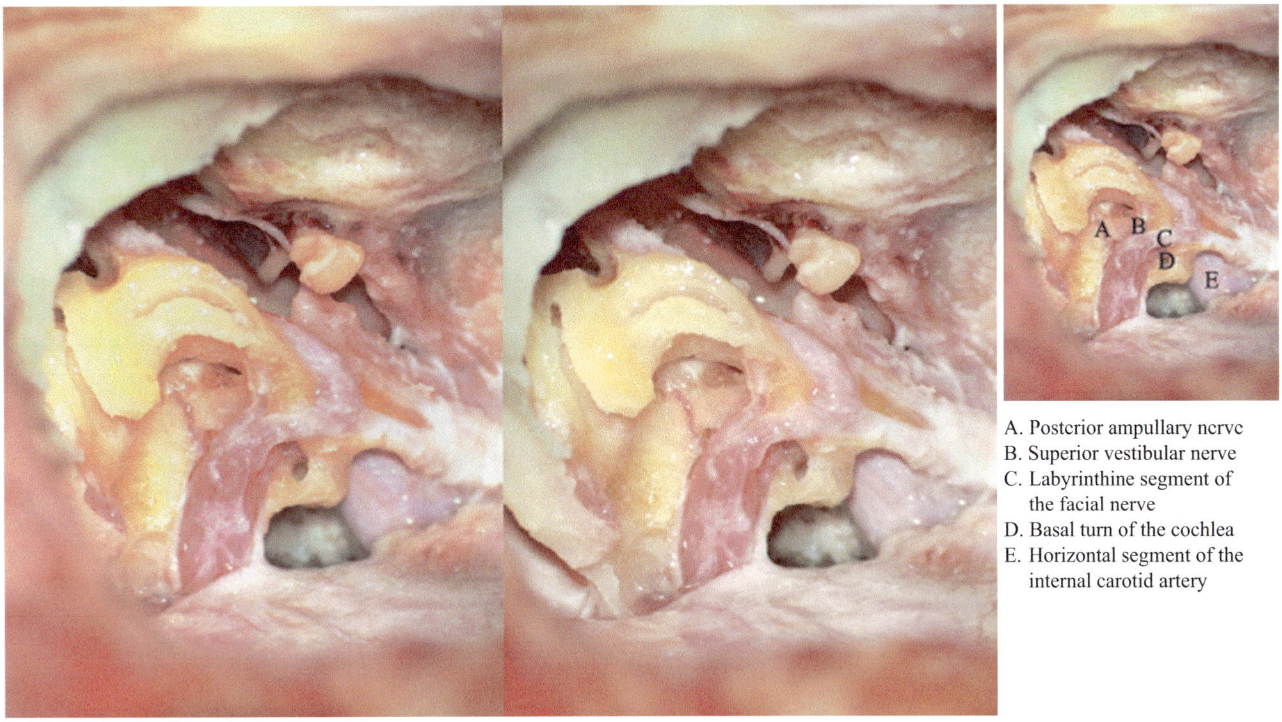

A. Posterior ampullary nerve
B. Superior vestibular nerve
C. Labyrinthine segment of the facial nerve
D. Basal turn of the cochlea
E. Horizontal segment of the internal carotid artery

Fig. 6.17 Exposing the posterior ampullary nerve and opening the basal turn of the cochlea (left)
The posterior ampullary nerve innervates the ampulla of the posterior semicircular canal. The middle part of the posterior wall of the vestibule is removed to expose the posterior ampullary nerve. Part of the cochlear bone is removed to open the basal turn of the cochlea
Instruments: small-sized diamond burs

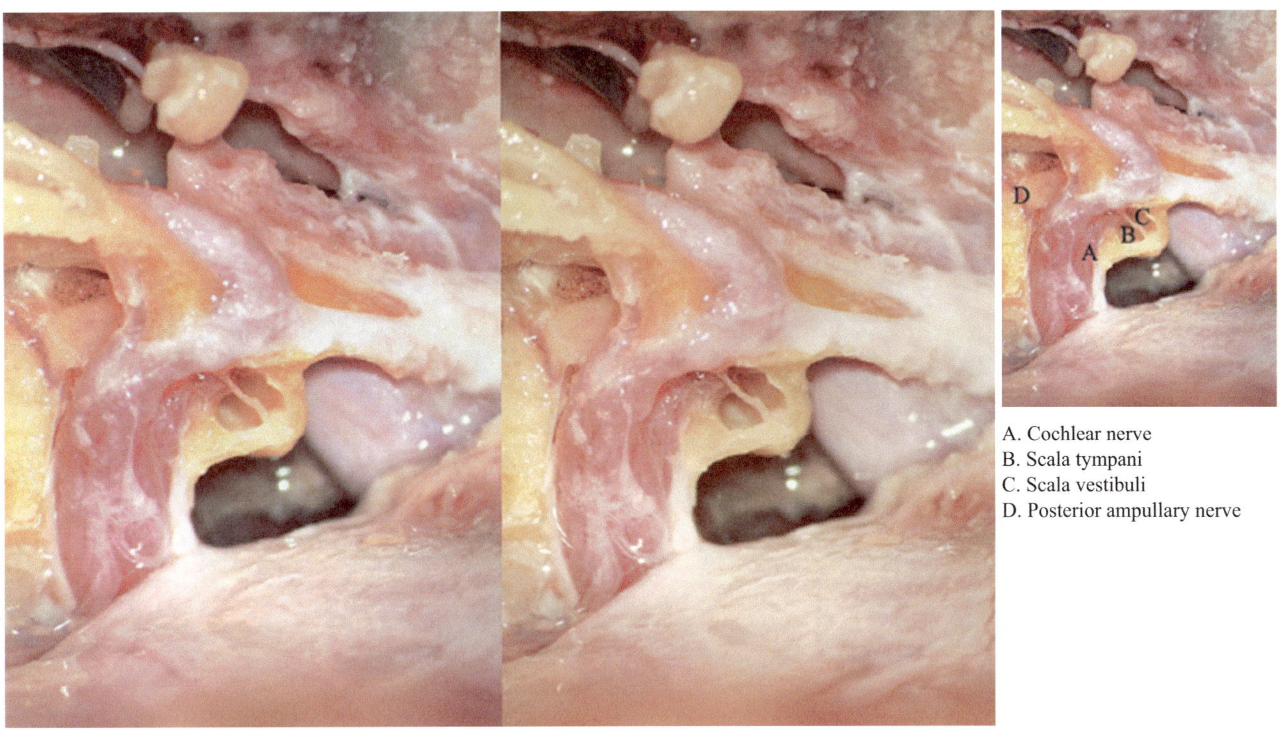

A. Cochlear nerve
B. Scala tympani
C. Scala vestibuli
D. Posterior ampullary nerve

Fig. 6.18 Opening the basal turn of the cochlea (left)
The bony wall is removed to further expose the basal turn of the cochlea. The cochlear duct is separated by the osseous spiral lamina and the basilar membrane into two parts: the scala tympani and the scala vestibuli. The vestibular membrane is very delicate; thus, the scala media is difficult to expose because it lies between the vestibular membrane and the basilar membrane
Instruments: small-sized diamond burs

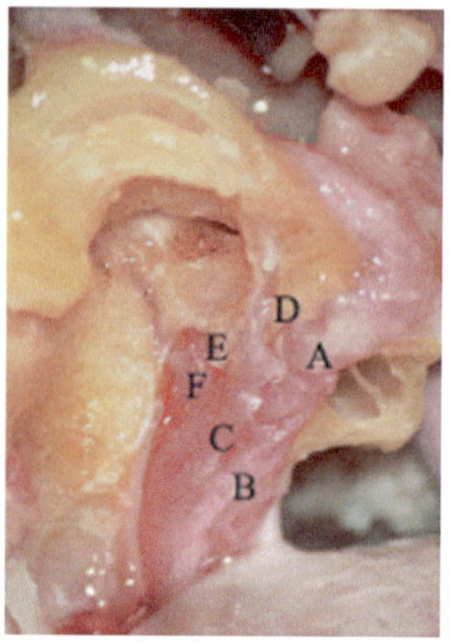

A. Labyrinthine segment of the facial nerve
B. IAC segment of the facial nerve
C. Superior vestibular nerve
D. Bill's bar
E. Transverse crest
F. Inferior vestibular nerve

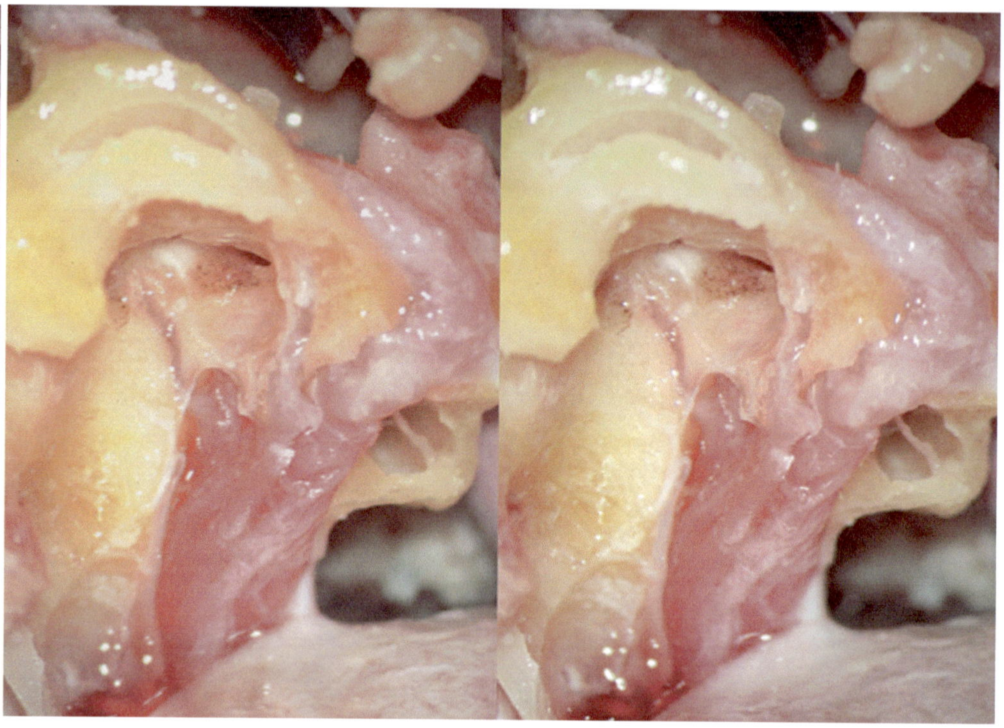

Fig. 6.19 Fundus of the IAC (left)
The fundus of the IAC is separated into superior and inferior segments by the transverse crest. In the superior segment, Bill's bar separates the anterior zone of the facial nerve from the superior vestibular nerve. The labyrinthine segment of the facial nerve travels anterolaterally from the IAC until it reaches the geniculate ganglion. The posterior zone in the upper vestibular area contains the superior vestibular nerve. In the inferior segment, the cochlear nerve sits in the anterior zone, and the saccular nerve of the inferior vestibular nerve sits in the posterior zone. There is a small foramen located posterior-inferiorly toward the inferior vestibular zone, through which the terminal branch of the inferior vestibular nerve, the posterior ampullary nerve, passes
Instruments: small-sized diamond burs

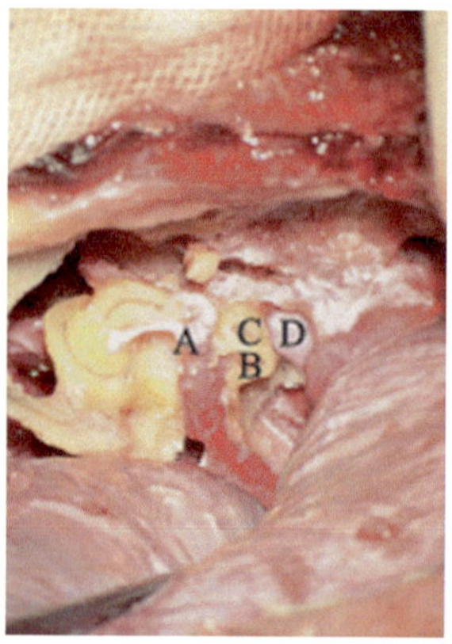

A. GSPN and the geniculate ganglion reflected back towards the vestibule
B. Basal turn of the cochlea
C. Middle turn of the cochlea
D. Horizontal segment of the internal carotid artery

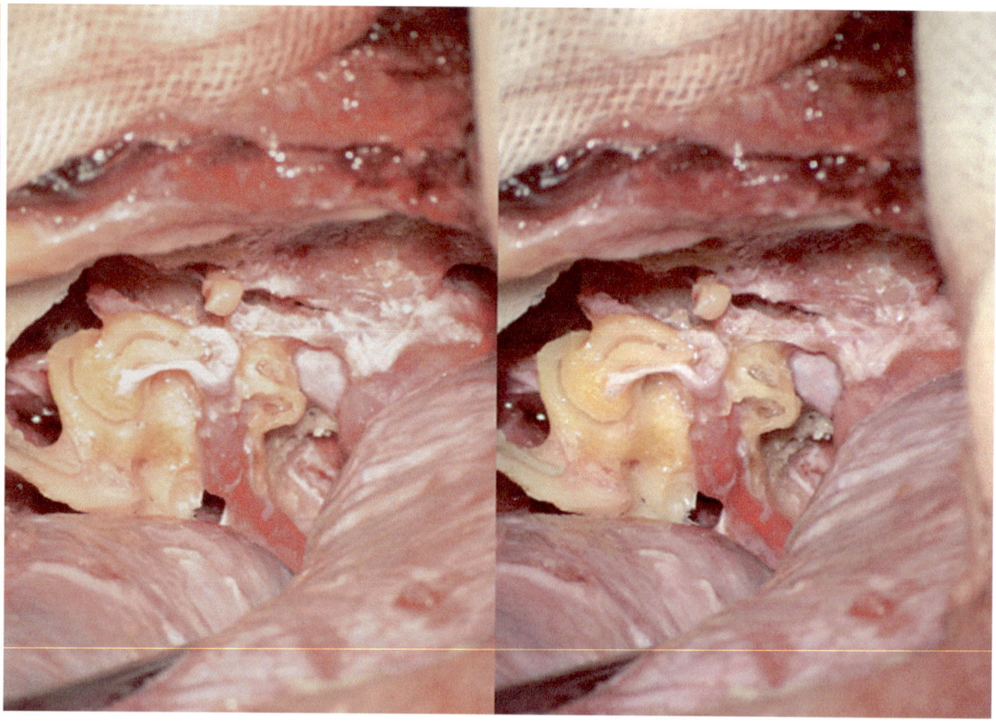

Fig. 6.20 Opening the middle turn of the cochlea (left)
The GSPN is cut at its distal end and bent back with the geniculate ganglion toward the vestibule. The bony wall of the middle turn of the cochlea is removed
Instruments: small-sized diamond burs

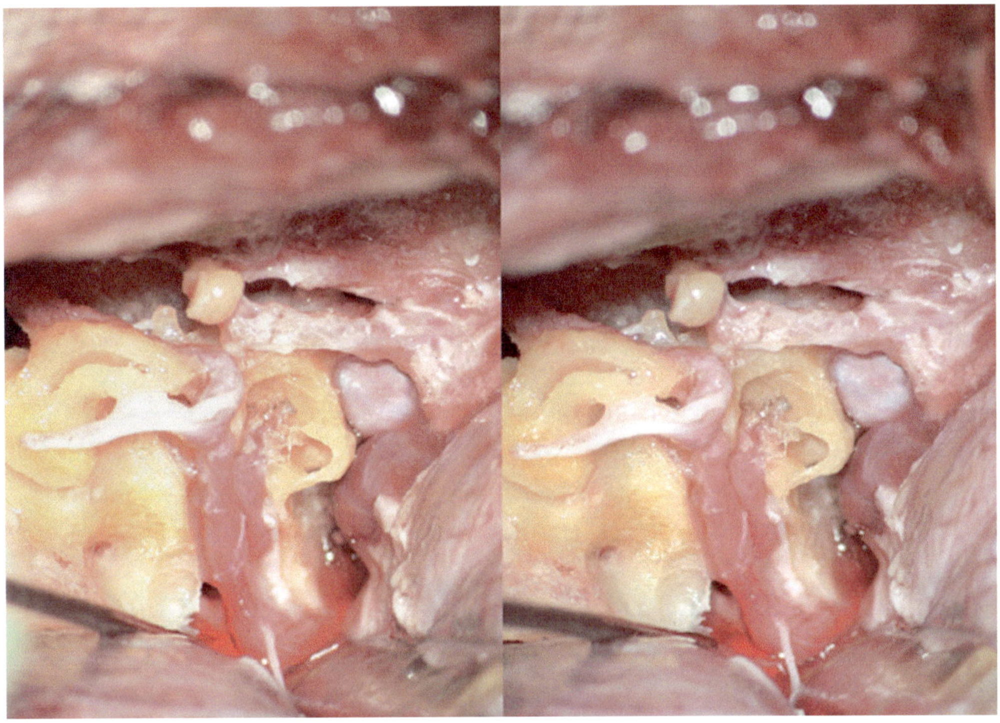

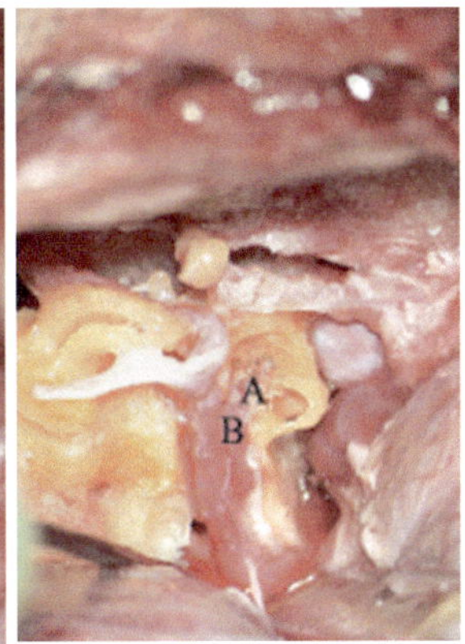

A. Cochlear modiolus
B. Cochlear nerve

Fig. 6.21 Exposing the cochlear nerve in the cochlear apex (left)
The bony wall of the middle and apex turns of the cochlea is removed to expose the cochlear apex and the cochlear nerve inside the modiolus

Instruments: small-sized diamond burs

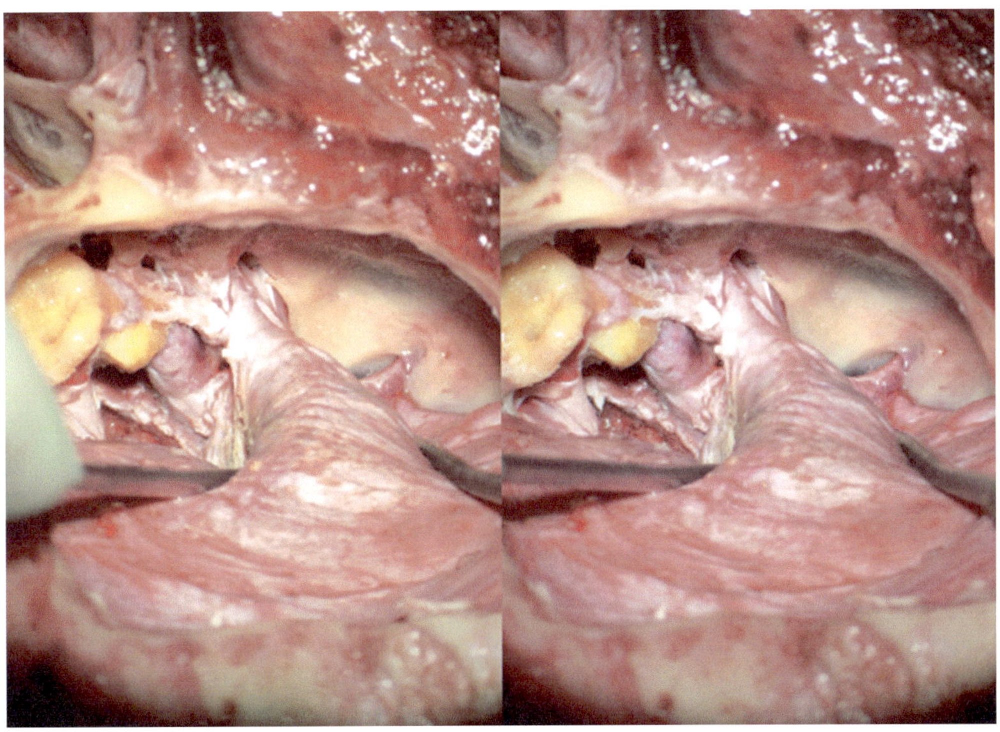

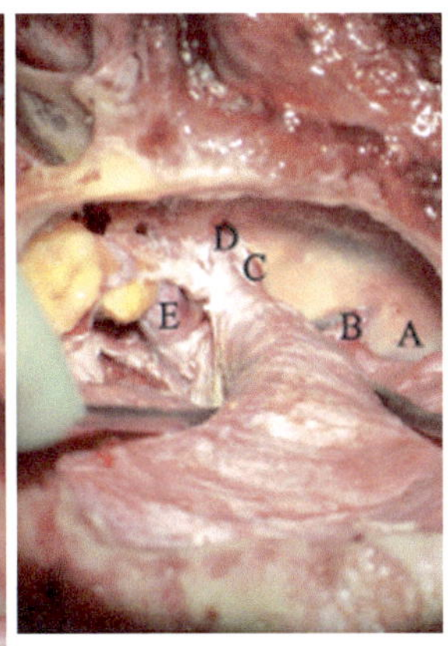

A. Sphenoid bone
B. Foramen rotundum and the maxillary division of the trigeminal nerve
C. Foramen ovale and the mandibular division of the trigeminal nerve
D. Foramen spinosum and the middle meningeal artery
E. Internal carotid artery

Fig. 6.22 Petrous apex and surrounding structures (left)
The petrous apex sits between the sphenoid and occipital bones. There are three important foramina, i.e., from medial to lateral the foramen rotundum, the foramen ovale, and the foramen spinosum, which contain the maxillary division of the trigeminal nerve, the mandibular division of the trigeminal nerve, and the middle meningeal artery, respectively
Instruments: elevator

Suggested Reading

Gulya A-J. Gulya and Schuknecht's anatomy of the temporal bone with surgical implications. New York: Informa Healthcare USA; 2007.

Han D-y. Nerve otology and lateral skull base surgery. Beijing: Science Press; 2008.

Jiang S-C, Yang W-y, Gu R. Operative surgery of otorhinolaryngology head and neck department. The complete works of operative surgery. 2nd ed. Beijing: People's Military Medical Press; 2005.

7 Retrosigmoid Approach

Yong-yi Yuan, Jun Liu, Jian-dong Zhao, Wei-qian Wang, Xue Gao, and Vincent C Cousins

Surgical Procedures Using the Retrosigmoid Approach
This approach provides access to lesions of the cerebellopontine angle (CPA). The biggest advantage of this approach is that the exposure of CPA lesions can be maximized while preserving hearing. The disadvantage is that operative complications may be severe, particularly due to retraction of the cerebellum.

Indications for the approach include:

1. Resection of acoustic neuroma
2. Vestibular nerve section (Meniere's disease)
3. Intracranial nerve microvascular decompression (glossopharyngeal neuralgia, trigeminal neuralgia, hemifacial spasm)
4. Auditory brainstem implantation
5. Brainstem and cerebellar parenchymal lesions
6. Vascular disease of the vertebrobasilar arterial system
7. Resection of other lesions in the CPA, such as cholesteatoma or meningioma

Related Anatomical Structures

1. The cerebellum ("little brain") overlies the posterior aspect of the pons and medulla oblongata and fills the greater part of the posterior fossa of the skull, separated from the occipital lobes of the cerebral hemispheres by the tentorium cerebelli. The cerebellum originates from the rhombencephalon in early gestation and has extensive afferent and efferent connections with the cerebrum, brainstem, and spinal cord. It participates in the regulation of balance, muscle tension, and coordination of voluntary movements.
2. The cerebellopontine angle (CPA) is a space that is triangular-shaped in cross-section and located anterior and lateral in the posterior cranial fossa; it is bounded medially by the pons, laterally by the petrous bone and posteriorly by the cerebellum. Important anatomical structures such as cranial nerves V to XII, the petrosal vein, and the anteroinferior and anterosuperior cerebellar arteries course through the CPA. A CPA syndrome can present due to compression and involvement of these structures by lesions such as a large acoustic neuroma or meningioma.
3. The sigmoid sinus is an intracranial venous sinus located in the sigmoid sulcus on the internal surface of the temporal bone and drains the transverse sinus into the internal jugular vein through the jugular bulb. The parietal notch is the superficial landmark of the origin of the sigmoid sinus from the transverse sinus, and the mastoid tip marks its lower genu; the line between them is the superficial landmark of its intracranial course. The sigmoid sinus is the anterior margin of the retrosigmoid approach.
4. The transverse sinus is an intracranial venous sinus that originates from the midline torcular (torcular herophili), courses in the transverse sinus sulcus which grooves the internal surfaces of the occipital and parietal bones and becomes the sigmoid sinus posterior to the temporal bone. The transverse sinus is the superior margin of the retrosigmoid approach.
5. The mastoid emissary veins are located at the occipitomastoid junction; they vary in number, exact position, and size. They course through the mastoid foramen or foramina, draining occipital veins into the sigmoid sinus.
6. The temporal line extends anteriorly to the superior margin of the zygomatic arch; the temporalis muscle attaches here. It is the superior limit of mastoid surgical procedures and is the superficial landmark of the base of the middle cranial fossa.

Y.-y. Yuan (✉) · J. Liu · J.-d. Zhao
College of Otolaryngology Head and Neck Surgery, Chinese PLA General Hospital, Beijing, China

W.-q. Wang · X. Gao
Department of Otolaryngology Head and Neck Surgery, PLA Rocket Force Characteristic Medical Center, Beijing, China

V. C. Cousins
Department of Ear Nose and Throat Surgery, Alfred Hospital, Melbourne, Australia

Department of Surgery, Monash University, Melbourne, Australia

P. Dai et al. (eds.), *Stereoscopic Anatomical Atlas of Ear Surgery*, https://doi.org/10.1007/978-981-16-0927-5_7

7. The parietal notch is the notch between the squamous and mastoid portions of the temporal bone, corresponding to the mastoid angle of the parietal bone. It is one of the superficial landmarks of the sigmoid sinus.
8. The internal auditory canal (IAC) is a passage at the middle portion of the petrous bone. It opens medially into the intracranial space through the porus and ends laterally at the internal auditory fundus, with a plate of bone separating it from the inner ear. The facial nerve, cochlear nerve, vestibular nerves, intermediate nerve, and labyrinthine artery and vein course through the canal.
9. The anterior inferior cerebellar artery originates from the basilar artery and usually bifurcates into cranial and caudal trunks, which sit anterior to the facial nerve. The cranial trunk forms a vascular loop at the IAC and gives off branches including the labyrinthine artery.
10. The posterior inferior cerebellar artery originates mostly from the ipsilateral vertebral artery, which supplies the lower part of the cerebellar hemisphere and courses along the ipsilateral lower cranial nerves.
11. The petrosal vein, also called the vein of Dandy, originates from the anterior cerebellum and drains various tributaries from the pons, cerebellum, brainstem, and fourth ventricle, which merge at the cerebellopontine cistern. It courses anterior-laterally, usually dorsal and lateral to the trigeminal nerve and along the base of the middle cranial fossa near the IAC and Meckel's cave.
12. The trigeminal nerve, or cranial nerve V, is located anterior-superiorly to the facial and cochlear nerves. It is a composite nerve with two kinds of nerve fibers: general somatic sensory fibers and special visceral motor fibers. Three main branches originate from the trigeminal or Gasserian ganglion: from anterior to posterior, the ophthalmic, maxillary, and mandibular nerves. These branches control sensation of the anterior scalp, face, nasal cavity, and oral cavity and they innervate the masticatory muscles.
13. The abducent nerve, or cranial nerve VI, is a motor nerve. It originates from the abducens nucleus of the pons, leaves laterally from the pontomedullary sulcus, and courses anteriorly into the orbit through the superior orbital fissure to control the lateral rectus muscle of the eye. Injury to this nerve results in an inability to rotate the eyeball laterally (abductor paralysis).
14. The facial nerve, or cranial nerve VII, consists of sensory, motor, and parasympathetic nerve fibers, which control taste in the anterior 2/3 of the tongue, the muscles of facial expression, and secretions of the sublingual, submandibular, and lacrimal glands.
15. The vestibulocochlear nerve, or cranial nerve VIII, is responsible for hearing and balance. It is formed by the union of the cochlear nerve and the two vestibular nerves in the IAC, before passing medially to enter the brainstem between the pons and medulla.
16. The glossopharyngeal nerve, or cranial nerve IX, originates from the medulla oblongata, courses anterior-laterally, and exits the skull through the anterior part of the jugular foramen. It consists of three kinds of nerve fibers: sensory (general somatic afferent, special visceral afferent, and general visceral afferent), motor (special visceral efferent), and parasympathetic (general visceral efferent) nerve fibers. It is responsible for taste in the posterior 1/3 of the tongue, sensation of the carotid body, and innervation of the stylopharyngeus muscle and parotid gland.
17. The vagus nerve, or cranial nerve X, originates from the medulla oblongata and exits the skull through the jugular foramen along with the glossopharyngeal and accessory nerves. It is the longest and most widely distributed cranial nerve and consists of sensory, motor, and parasympathetic nerve fibers. The vagus nerve controls most organs involved in respiration, digestion via afferent and efferent supply, as well as muscular contraction of the heart and glandular secretion.
18. The accessory nerve, or cranial nerve XI, consists of a cranial root and a spinal root and exits the skull through the jugular foramen. The cranial root, which consists of special visceral motor fibers, joins the vagus nerve, and the spinal root innervates the ipsilateral trapezius and sternocleidomastoid muscles.

Anatomy Overview

1. Skin incision: It is crucial to correctly position the incision, aiming to fully expose the scope of the intended cranial bone window. A postauricular U-shaped incision is made starting superior to the auricular attachment, extending 6 cm posteriorly, turning downward 1–2 cm inferior to the mastoid tip, and continuing anteriorly 6 cm to form a large U-shaped skin flap with an anteriorly positioned pedicle.
2. Craniotomy: This bony window, approximately 5 × 5 cm in size, is made inferior to the temporal line and posterior to the sigmoid sinus. After the correct position is selected, the four corners of the bone flap are drilled with cutting burs and diamond burs and connected in a square shape

with middle-sized cutting and diamond burs. The bone flap is elevated to expose the dura mater of the posterior cranial fossa. The transverse sinus can be observed superiorly, and the sigmoid sinus can be observed anteriorly. *Hints: When the bone flap is created, the sigmoid sinus, transverse sinus, and dura mater should not be traumatized, so its positioning should be precise. A diamond bur should be used when drilling close to these structures to minimize the risk of injury. When drilling and elevating the bone flap, dissection should be done close to the bone surface without deep probing to spare the aforementioned structures. Exposed air cells posterior to the sigmoid sinus should be sealed thoroughly with bone wax to prevent postoperative cerebrospinal fluid otorrhea/rhinorrhea.*

3. Dural incision: The incision should be made 2–3 mm away from the edges of the transverse and sigmoid sinuses, with the flap pedicled anteriorly, allowing it to be retracted anteriorly with sutures. Caution should be taken not to injure the venous sinuses and vessels of the pia mater or brain tissue.
4. Exposing the CPA: After retracting the dura flap anteriorly, the cerebellum should be gently retracted posterior-superiorly with a brain spatula. Cerebrospinal fluid (CSF) should be drained after opening the cisterna magna to reduce posterior cranial fossa pressure, allowing the cerebellum to fall medially. With the cerebellum retracted posteromedially using a brain spatula, the arachnoid can be divided to open the CPA. *Hints: Most specimens used in anatomical practice have been soaked in formalin for a long time, so the cerebellar tissue is too firm to be retracted posteriorly, limiting exposure of the CPA. In this scenario, a certain amount of cerebellum can be resected (preserving structures on its surface) so that the CPA can be fully exposed with suitable retraction. Drill burs must be held steadily to avoid injury to surrounding tissue, vessels, and nerves.*
5. Dissection of vessels and nerves of the CPA: The surgical field should be exposed superiorly as far as the cerebellar tentorium, inferiorly to the jugular foramen and foramen magnum, and medially to the brain including the cerebellar hemisphere, pons, and lateral surface of the superior medulla oblongata. Cranial nerves V–XI can be visualized clearly when approaching the brainstem and cerebellopontine cistern. The structures that course through the CPA are the vestibular nerve, facial nerve, and cochlear nerve, with the trigeminal nerve located anterior-superiorly to the facio-cochlear nerve tract and cranial nerves IX–XI located inferior to it. The labyrinthine artery from the anterior inferior cerebellar artery usually courses between the facial and cochlea-vestibular nerves.
6. Dissection of the IAC: The cochlear nerve, facial nerve, and vestibular nerve form a bundle between the IAC porus and brainstem. Bone posterior and superior to the IAC should be drilled away, starting from the IAC porus, to expose the IAC sufficiently to identify the nerves coursing through it. *Hints: Observing the IAC through the retrosigmoid approach, the relative location of individual nerves should be memorized: (1) Superior and inferior vestibular nerves are in the posterosuperior quadrant and the posteroinferior quadrant of the fundus of the IAC, respectively, while the facial and cochlear nerves are in the anterosuperior and anteroinferior quadrants, respectively. (2) The cranial nerve VIII enters the brainstem at the junction of the pons and medulla, lateral to the facial nerve.*

Purposes and Requirements of Anatomical Dissection

1. Master the use of different types and sizes of burs
2. Understand the advantages and disadvantages of surgical instruments and be able to choose the best equipment according to the surgical or dissection need
3. Locate the sigmoid sinus and transverse sinus with correct positioning of the craniotomy
4. Master safe opening of the retrosigmoid bone window
5. Understand the anatomical relationship between the cranial nerves, vessels, and adjacent structures in the CPA area
6. Understand the relative relationships between the cochlear, facial, and vestibular nerves from the brainstem to the fundus of the IAC

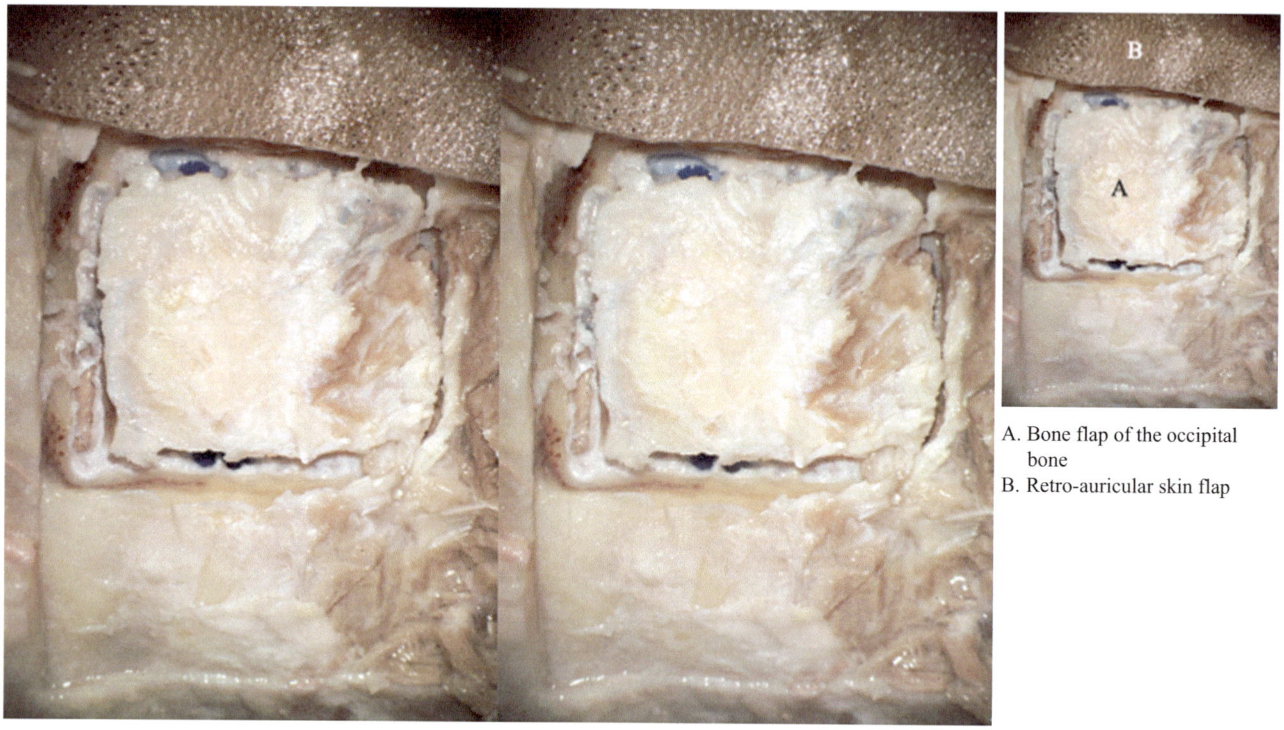

A. Bone flap of the occipital bone
B. Retro-auricular skin flap

Fig. 7.1 Craniotomy of the retrosigmoid approach (right)
For the anatomical dissection, undertake extended resection of the skin and subcutaneous tissue of the ear, retro-auricular region, and occiput region, using a large U-shaped incision in the retro-auricular region in the temporal bone specimen (making an incision from 2 cm above the auricle to 1 cm below the mastoid tip to form an anteriorly based pedicle of approximately 6 cm anteroposterior diameter). Expose the parietal notch, temporal line, mastoid tip, etc. and then make a 5 × 5 cm craniotomy in the retrosigmoid occipital bone with a posterior extension of the temporal line as the upper limit and the line between the parietal notch and mastoid tip as the anterior limit
Instruments: surgical knife, periosteal elevator, medium-sized cutting burs

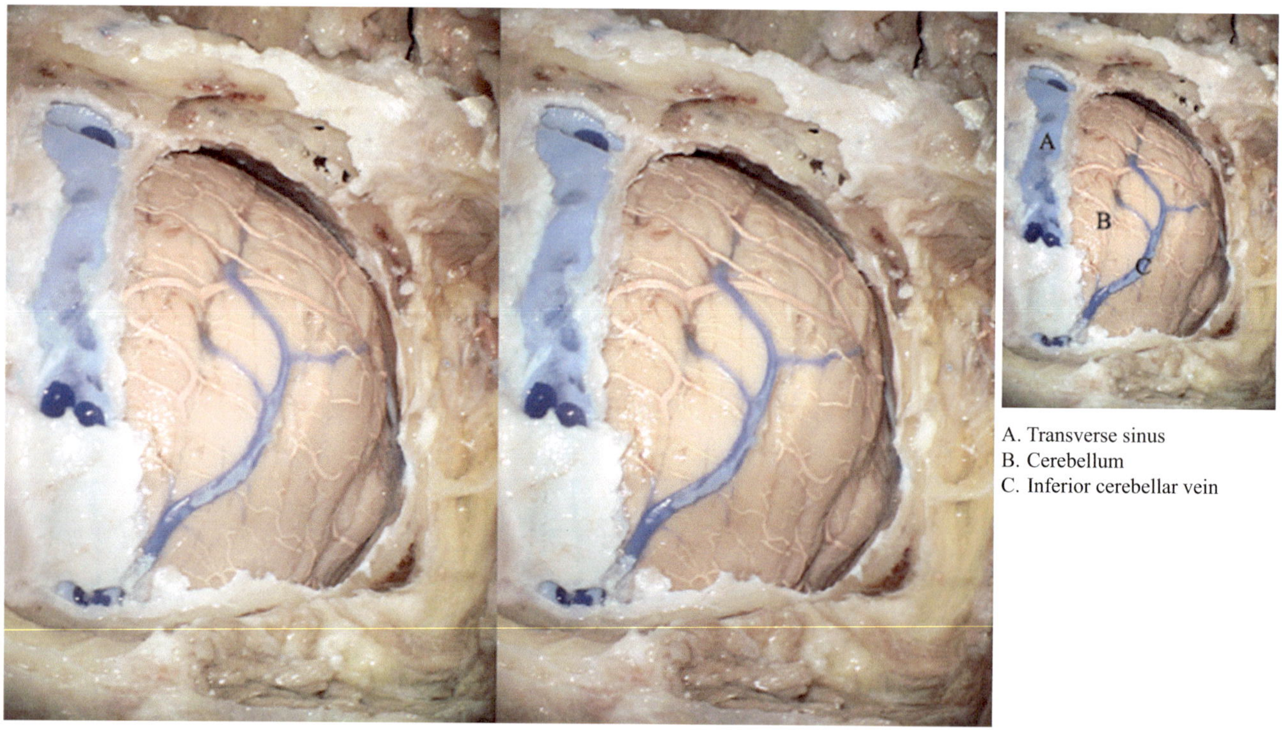

A. Transverse sinus
B. Cerebellum
C. Inferior cerebellar vein

Fig. 7.2 Exposing the cerebellum by removing the dura (right/supine)
Remove the occipital bone flap and resect the dura mater under the bone flap (or make a dural flap with an anterior pedicle) to expose the cerebellum. It is necessary to confirm the location of the sigmoid and transverse sinuses before opening the dura mater to avoid injuring them
Instruments: ophthalmic scissors, elevator

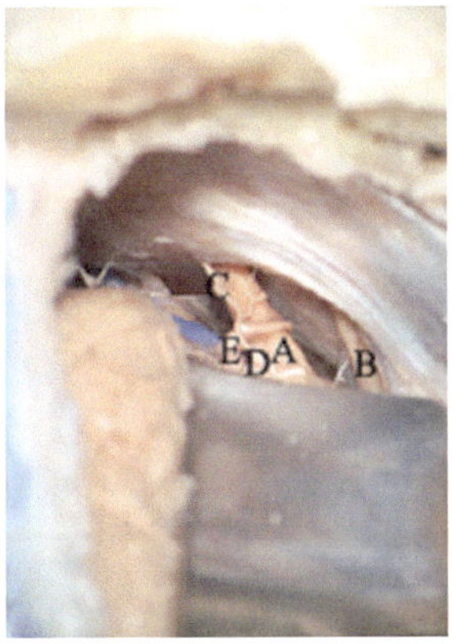

A. Acoustic-facial nerve bundle
B. Lower cranial nerves
C. Labyrinthine artery
D. Recurrent perforating artery
E. Anterior inferior cerebellar artery

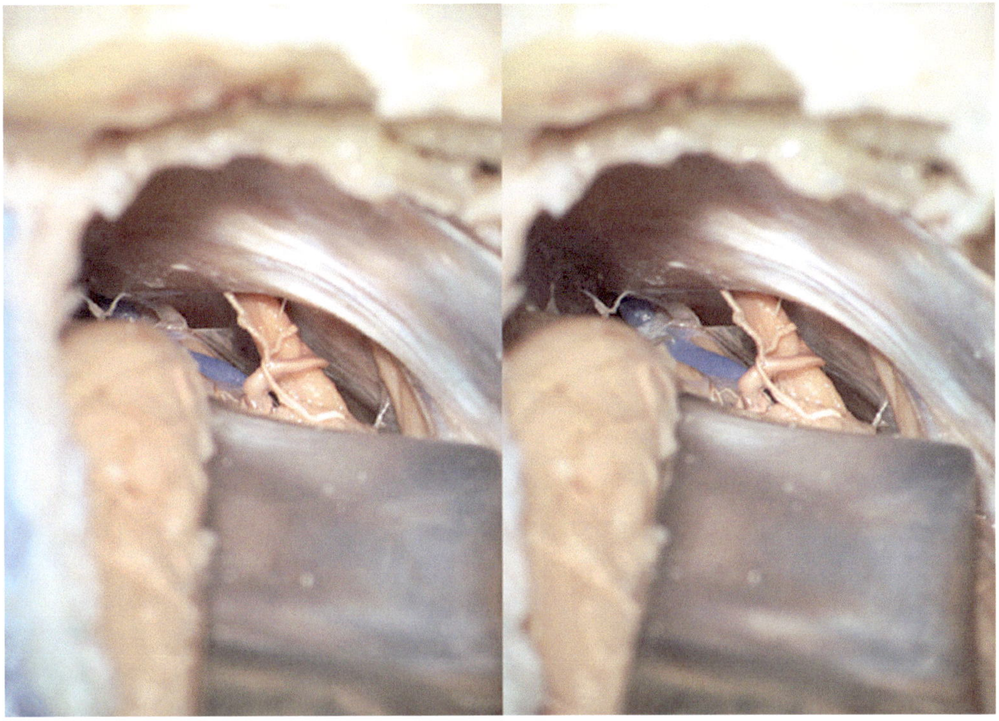

Fig. 7.3 Exposing the acoustic-facial nerve bundle in the CPA (right) The cerebellum is retracted posteriorly with a brain spatula to fully expose the CPA. Part of the cerebellum can be removed during anatomical dissection to widen the surgical field. The acoustic-facial nerve bundle is generally located in the center of the operative field, entering the IAC laterally and being in close contact with the anterior inferior cerebellar artery (AICA), which originates from the basilar artery. The anterior inferior cerebellar artery often divides into upper and lower branches in front of the basilar artery. The upper branch forms a vascular loop at the IAC and gives off the labyrinthine artery to supply the inner ear. Sometimes the upper branch gives off recurrent perforating branches, as seen in this cadaveric specimen
Instruments: brain spatula

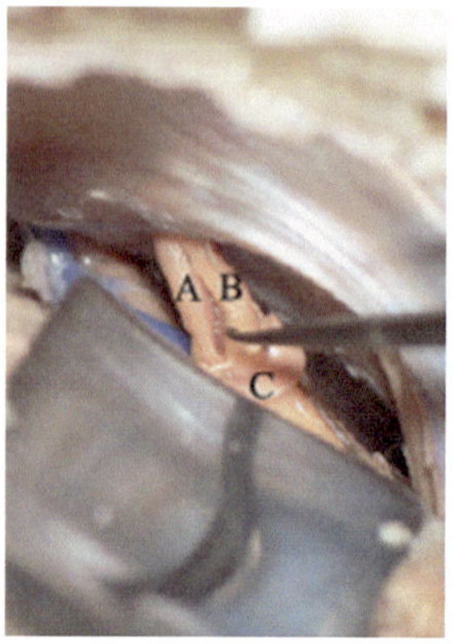

A. Vestibular nerve
B. Cochlear nerve
C. Anterior inferior cerebellar artery

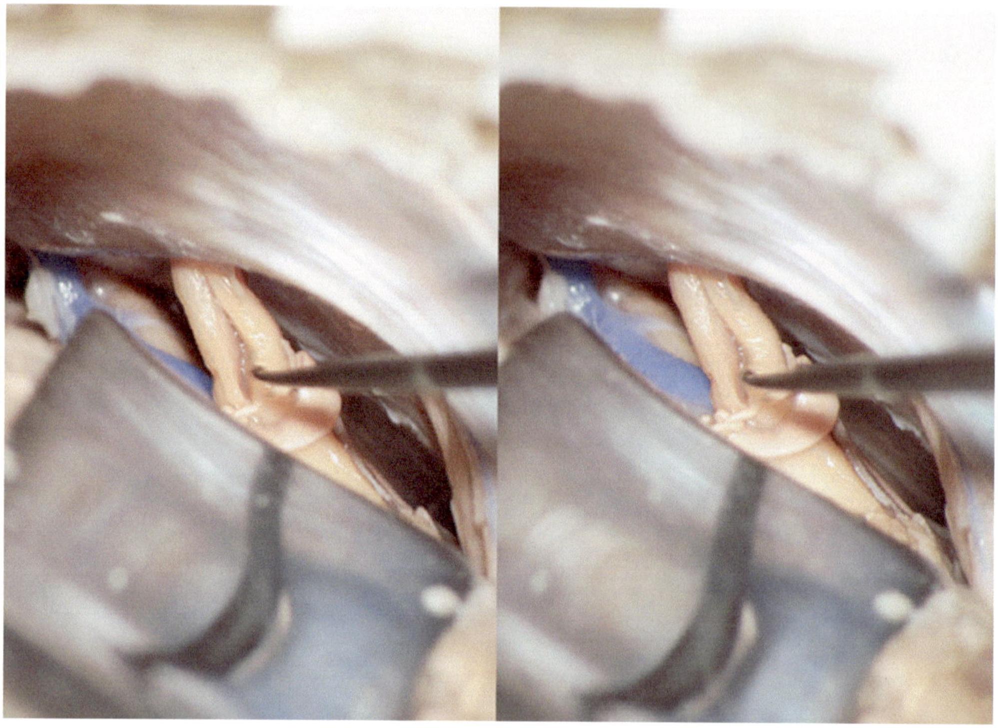

Fig. 7.4 Vestibular nerve and cochlear nerve (right)
In passing from the fundus of the IAC, IAC porus, middle part of the CPA, and the brainstem, the location of the facial nerve in the acoustic-facial nerve bundle is anterior-superior, anterior-superior, anterior, and inferior, respectively. The cochlear nerve is located inferior to the facial nerve at the fundus of the IAC, but it is relatively posterior-superior to the facial nerve at the level of the brainstem. In the above figure, using a straight needle to separate the acoustic-facial nerve bundle, we can see the vestibular nerve superiorly and the cochlear nerve inferiorly, with the anterior inferior cerebellar artery wrapping around them. The facial nerve, located in the anterior and inferior portion of the acoustic-facial nerve bundle, is not seen here
Instruments: straight micro-needle

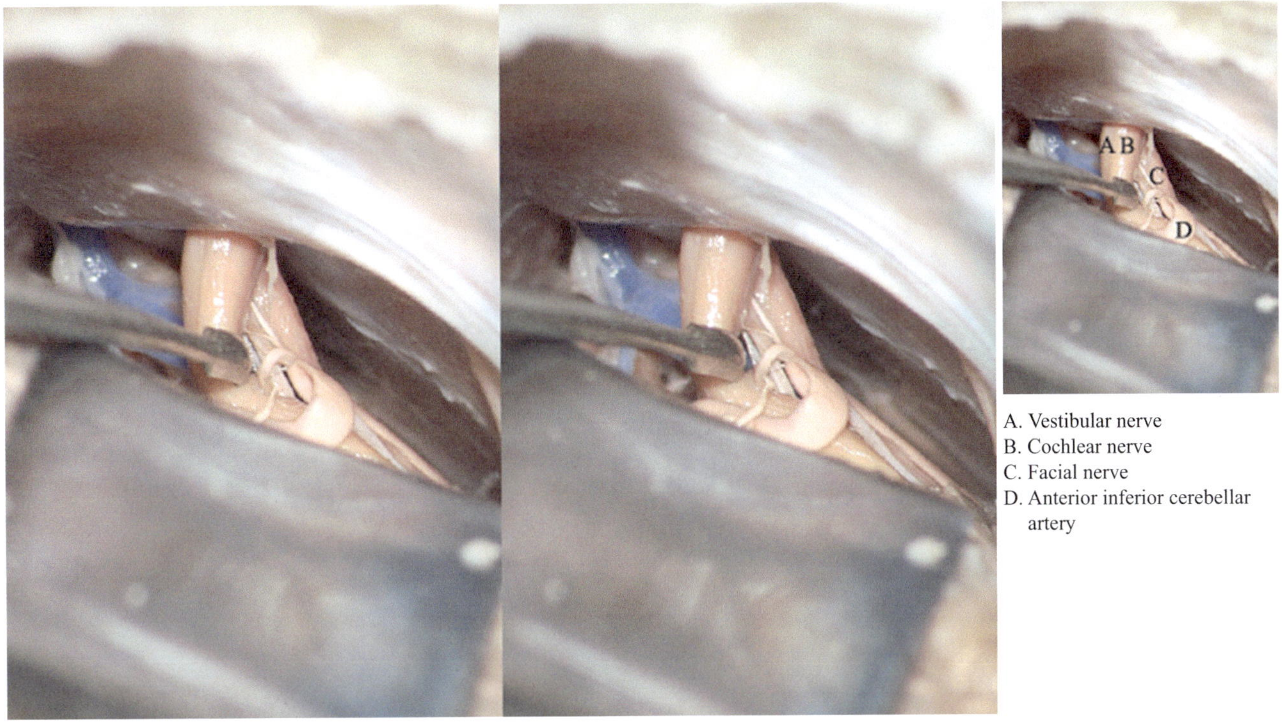

Fig. 7.5 Facial nerve (right)
The facial nerve can be exposed by separating the acoustic-facial nerve bundle using the middle ear elevator and retracting the vestibulocochlear nerve upward

Instruments: brain spatula, middle ear elevator

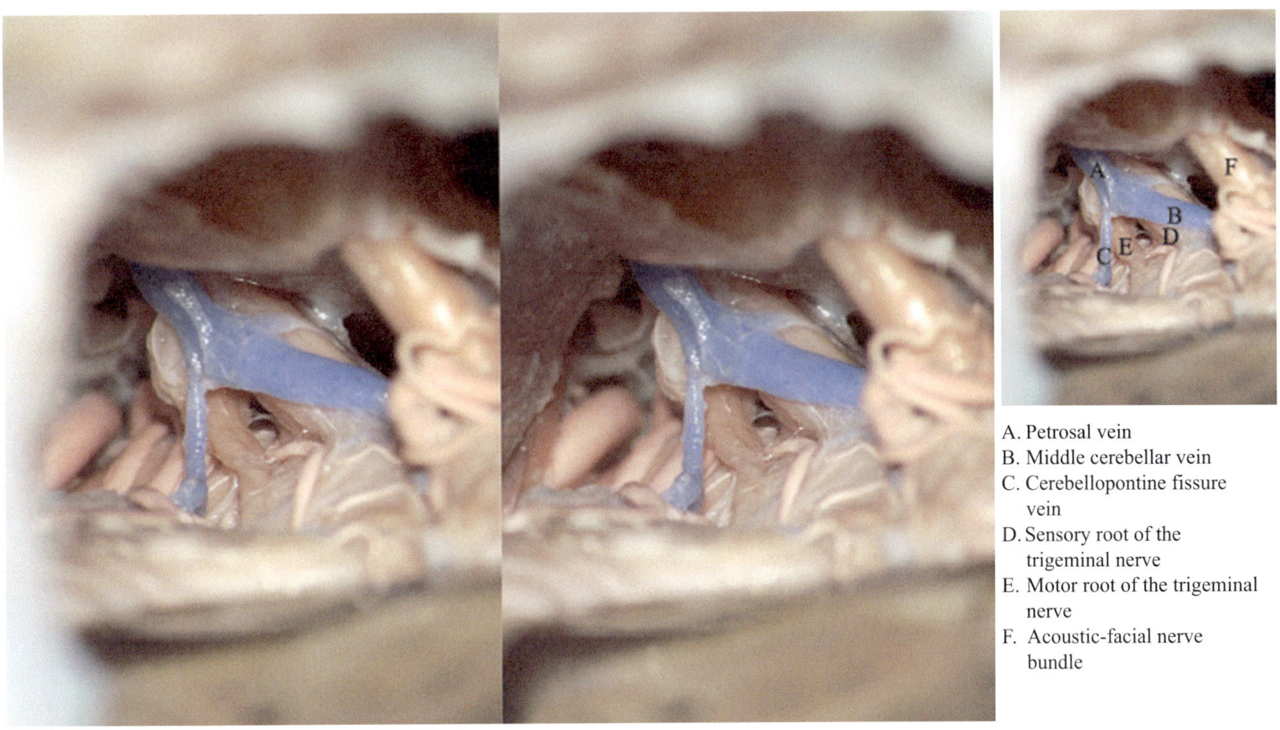

Fig. 7.6 Petrosal vein and trigeminal nerve (right)
Looking superiorly, we can see the large trigeminal nerve and petrosal vein. The trigeminal nerve is divided into a thin motor root anterosuperiorly and a large sensory root located posteriorly. The large petrosal vein (Dandy vein) is superior to the root of the trigeminal nerve and drains the middle cerebellar vein, cerebellopontine fissure vein, etc., then enters the superior petrosal sinus. If the petrosal vein is damaged during surgery, massive hemorrhage may occur. Occluding this vessel may lead to poor drainage of the cerebellar hemisphere, severe cerebellar swelling, intracranial hypertension, and other serious complications that may be life-threatening
Instruments: brain spatula, middle ear elevator

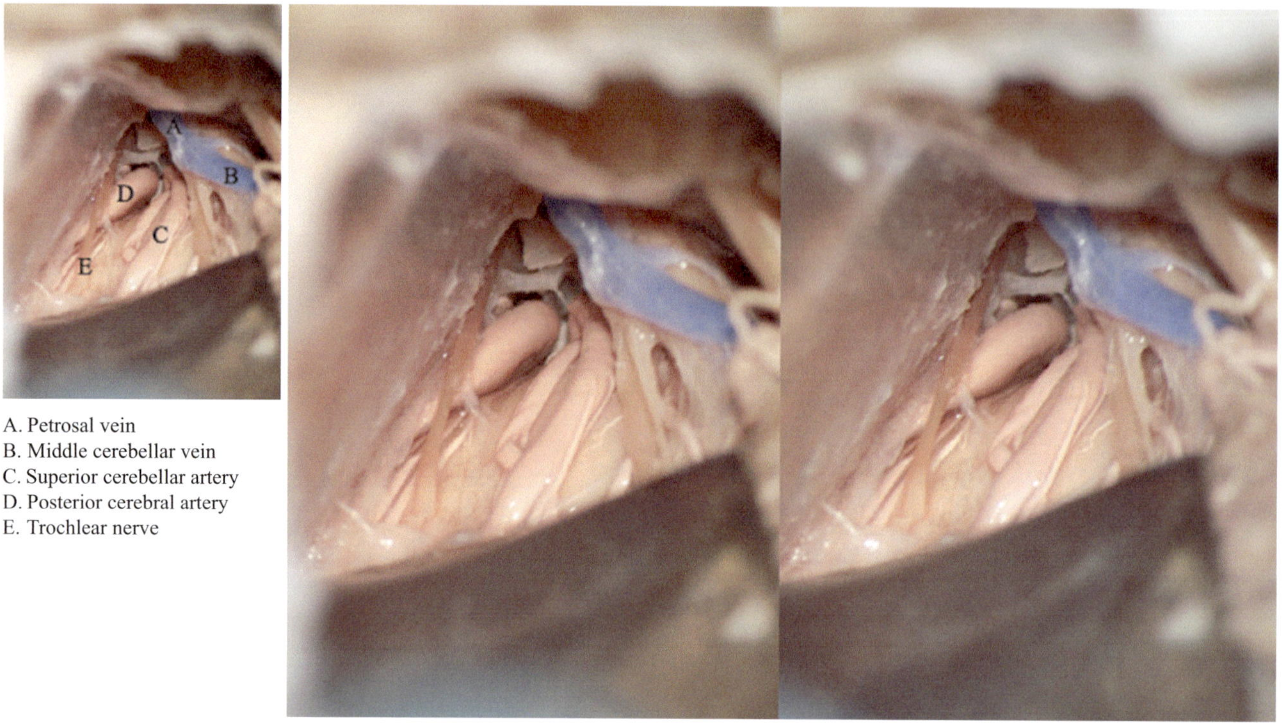

A. Petrosal vein
B. Middle cerebellar vein
C. Superior cerebellar artery
D. Posterior cerebral artery
E. Trochlear nerve

Fig. 7.7 Posterior cerebral artery, superior cerebellar artery, and trochlear nerve (right)
After dividing the cerebellopontine fissure vein and looking superior to the trigeminal nerve, we can see the posterior cerebral artery, trochlear nerve, and superior cerebellar artery. Both the posterior cerebral and superior cerebellar arteries originate from the lower part of the basilar artery and supply the posterior part of the cerebrum and the upper part of the cerebellum, respectively
Instruments: brain spatula, middle ear elevator, middle ear scissors

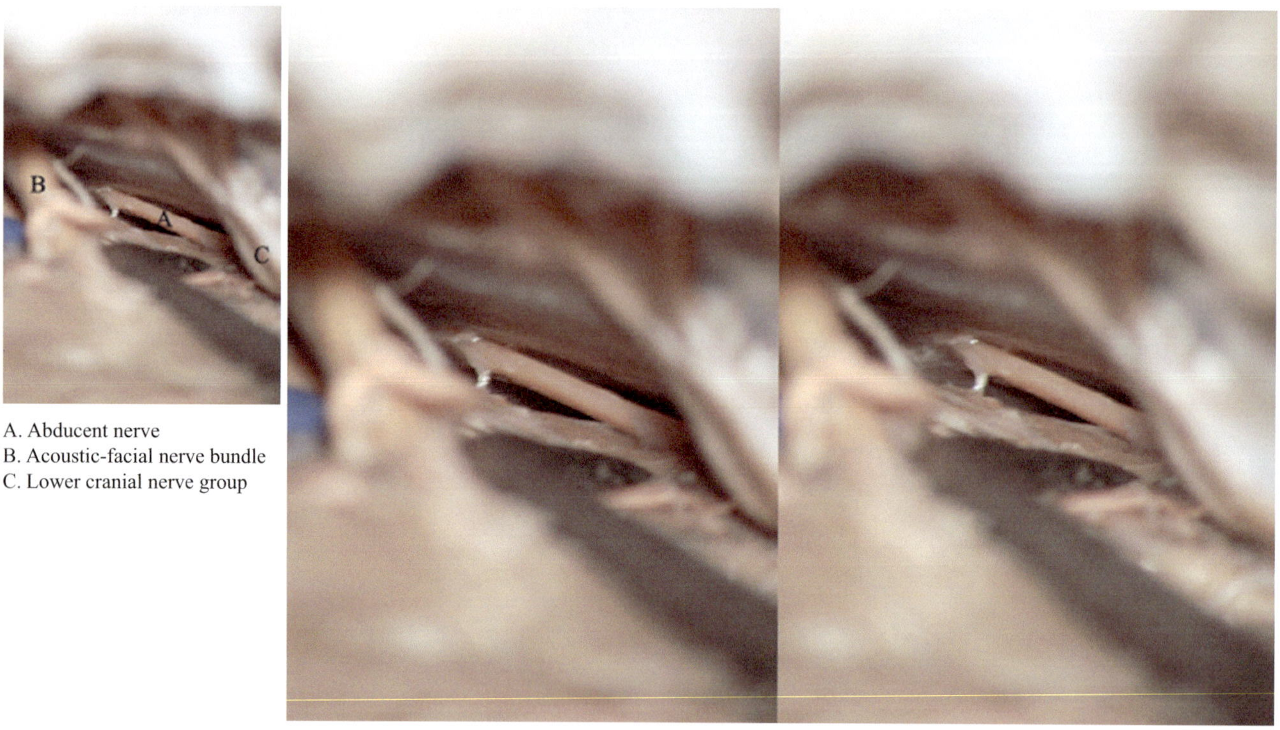

A. Abducent nerve
B. Acoustic-facial nerve bundle
C. Lower cranial nerve group

Fig. 7.8 Exposure of the abducent nerve (right)
The abducent nerve emerges from the brainstem near the midline in the ponto-bulbar sulcus and ascends in the cerebellopontine cistern. The acoustic-facial nerve bundle and the lower cranial nerve group are located superior and inferolateral to the abducent nerve, respectively
Instruments: brain spatula, middle ear elevator

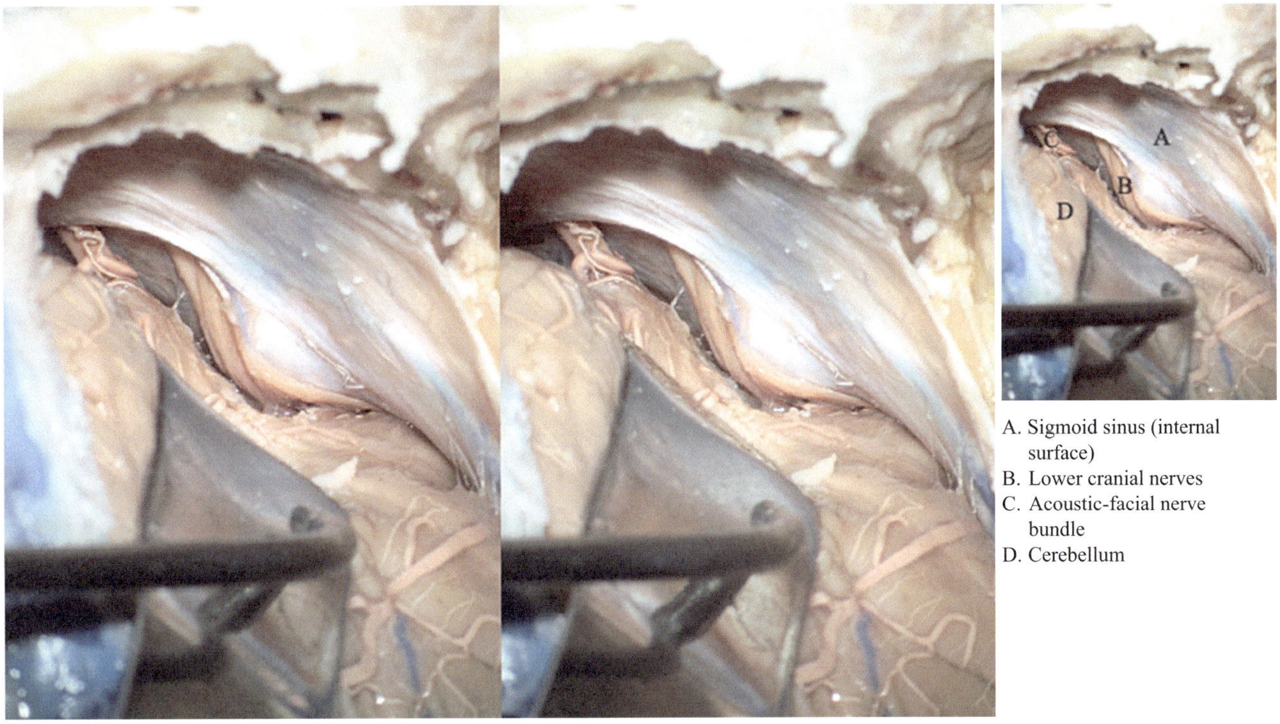

A. Sigmoid sinus (internal surface)
B. Lower cranial nerves
C. Acoustic-facial nerve bundle
D. Cerebellum

Fig. 7.9 Sigmoid sinus and lower cranial nerves (right)
When observing the lower part of the surgical field, we can see the lower cranial nerves inferior to the acoustic-facial nerve bundle and the sigmoid sinus located laterally to the cerebral dura mater. The lower cranial nerves, including the glossopharyngeal, vagus, and accessory nerves, exit the skull via the jugular foramen inferior to the jugular bulb. The hypoglossal nerve exits the skull via the hypoglossal foramen which is more anteriorly placed
Instruments: brain spatula, middle ear elevator

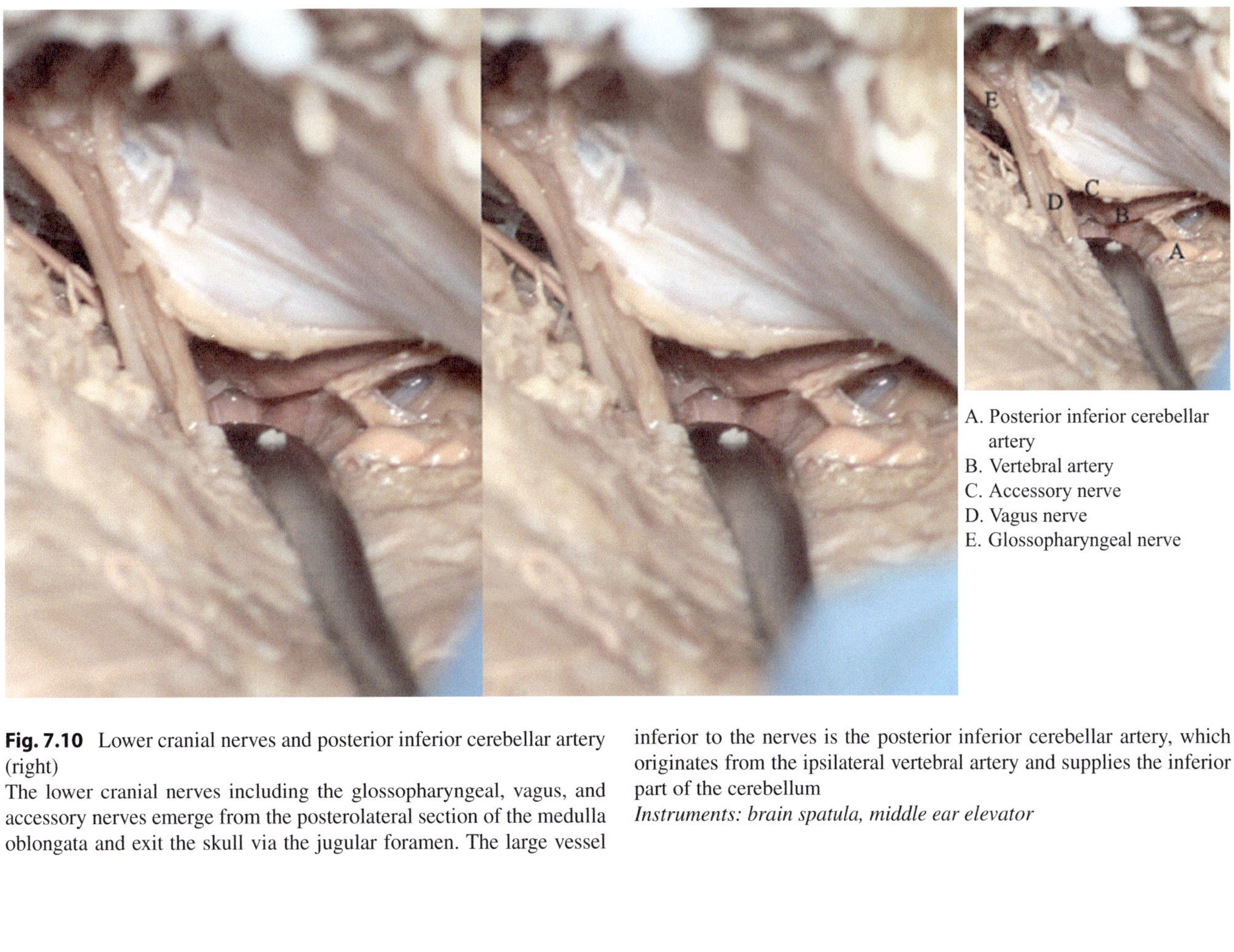

A. Posterior inferior cerebellar artery
B. Vertebral artery
C. Accessory nerve
D. Vagus nerve
E. Glossopharyngeal nerve

Fig. 7.10 Lower cranial nerves and posterior inferior cerebellar artery (right)
The lower cranial nerves including the glossopharyngeal, vagus, and accessory nerves emerge from the posterolateral section of the medulla oblongata and exit the skull via the jugular foramen. The large vessel inferior to the nerves is the posterior inferior cerebellar artery, which originates from the ipsilateral vertebral artery and supplies the inferior part of the cerebellum
Instruments: brain spatula, middle ear elevator

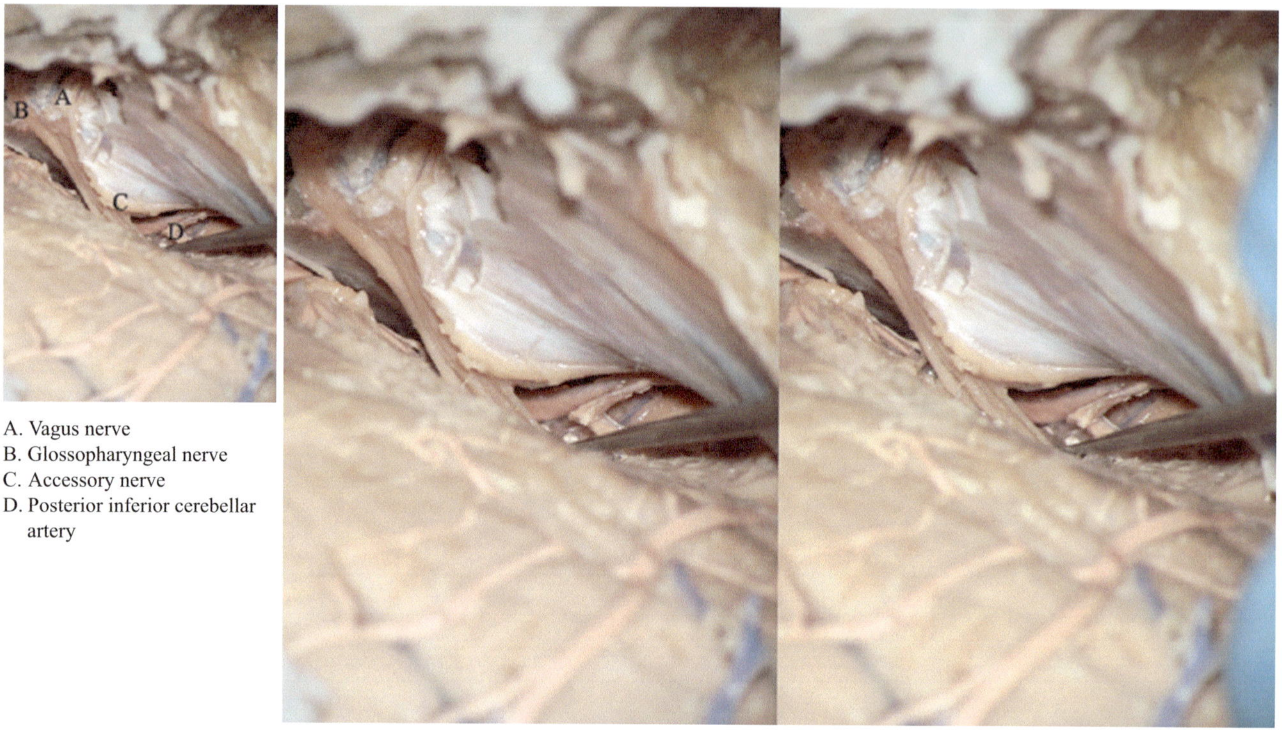

A. Vagus nerve
B. Glossopharyngeal nerve
C. Accessory nerve
D. Posterior inferior cerebellar artery

Fig. 7.11 Observation of the jugular foramen from inside the skull (right)
By excising the sigmoid sinus and jugular bulb, opening the jugular foramen, and observing the pathway of the lower cranial nerves after exiting the skull, we can see the strong association between the intracranial segments of the glossopharyngeal and vagus nerves, with the accessory nerve running inferior to them. After crossing the jugular foramen, the glossopharyngeal nerve exits the skull in front of the inferior petrosal sinus, the vagus and accessory nerves exit the skull behind the inferior petrosal sinus. Tumors in the posterior cranial fossa can compress the lower cranial nerves, causing a jugular foramen syndrome
Instruments: brain spatula, middle ear elevator

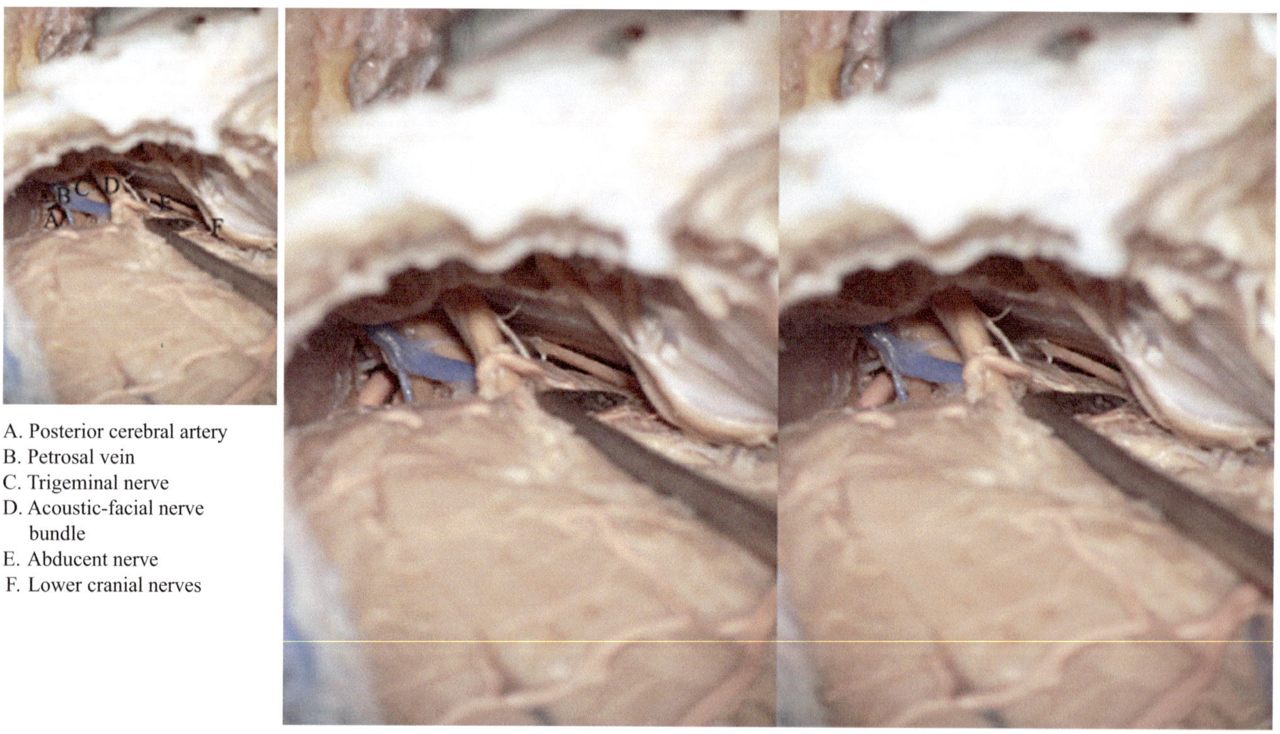

A. Posterior cerebral artery
B. Petrosal vein
C. Trigeminal nerve
D. Acoustic-facial nerve bundle
E. Abducent nerve
F. Lower cranial nerves

Fig. 7.12 Overview of the CPA (right)
Retracting the cerebellum backward using a brain spatula to explore the CPA from top to bottom, we can see the structures of the posterior cerebral artery, the petrosal vein, trigeminal nerve, the acoustic-facial nerve bundle, abducent nerve, and the lower cranial nerves
Instruments: brain spatula, middle ear elevator

Suggested Reading

Brackmann D-E, Shelton C, Arriaga M-A. Otologic surgery. 3rd ed. Philadelphia: Elsevier Medicine; 2009.

Huang M-z, Wang J-b, Kong W-j. Practical otolaryngology head and neck surgery. 2nd ed. Beijing: People's Health Publishing House; 2008.

Jiang S-c, Yang W-y, Gu R. Otorhinolaryngology—head and neck surgery. 2nd ed. Beijing: People's Medical Publishing House; 2007.

Kong W-j. Otorhinolaryngology head and neck surgery. Beijing: People's Health Publishing House; 2005.

Sanna M, Khrais T, Falcioni M, et al. The temporal bone: a manual for dissection and surgical approaches. New York: Thieme; 2005.

Yang W-y, Zhai S-q. Head and neck anatomy and temporal bone surgery. Beijing: People's Medical Publishing House; 2002.

8 Infratemporal Fossa Approach

Xue Gao, Sha-sha Huang, Ying Fu, Ping Gu,
and Yue-shuai Song

Surgical Procedures Using the Infratemporal Fossa Approach

Infratemporal Fossa Approach, Type A

This is essentially a jugular foramen approach and is a routine operation for lateral skull base surgery. Surgical access includes the jugular foramen, labyrinth, petrous apex, posterior part of the infratemporal fossa, vertical segment of the internal carotid artery, and upper part of the internal jugular venous space. This pathway can expose a wider operative field after re-routing the facial nerve, to allow removal of the tympanic bone and the styloid process. Operations that can be performed by an infratemporal fossa approach include:

1. Excision of types C and D glomus jugulare tumors
2. Excision of lower cranial nerve Schwannoma and meningioma
3. Excision of cholesteatoma of petrous bone and petrous apex
4. Excision of lower clivus chordoma
5. Excision of facial nerve Schwannoma
6. Excision of malignant tumor of infratemporal fossa
7. Excision of invasive meningioma of the infratemporal fossa

X. Gao (✉)
Department of Otolaryngology Head and Neck Surgery, PLA Rocket Force Characteristic Medical Center, Beijing, China

S.-s. Huang
College of Otolaryngology Head and Neck Surgery, Chinese PLA General Hospital, Beijing, China

Y. Fu
Department of Otorhinolaryngology, Qilu Hospital (Qingdao), Cheeloo College of Medicine, Shandong University, Qingdao, China

P. Gu
Department of Otolaryngology Head and Neck Surgery, Shenzhen Children's Hospital, Shenzhen, China

Y.-s. Song
Department of Otolaryngology Head and Neck Surgery, Beijing Friendship Hospital, Capital Medical University, Beijing, China

This chapter mainly demonstrates the surgical approach of Type A.

Infratemporal Fossa Approach, Type B

This is a widened infratemporal fossa, extralabyrinthine approach, extending the type A approach inward and anteriorly. The facial nerve is not displaced. Surgical access includes the petrous apex, occipital clivus, and superior part of the infratemporal fossa. Operations that can be performed by this approach include:

1. Excision of inferior petrosal cholesteatoma
2. Excision of clival tumor
3. Excision of giant cell tumor of petrous bone
4. Excision of nasopharyngeal carcinoma
5. Excision of Eustachian tube tumor and pharyngeal fistula

Infratemporal Fossa Approach, Type C

This is a further extension of the type B approach, removing the sphenoid wing and dividing the maxillary nerve if necessary. This approach can expose the nasopharynx, pterygopalatine fossa, Eustachian tube, parasellar region, and sphenoid sinus. Operations that can be performed by this approach include:

1. Excision of tumors in the infratemporal fossa and Eustachian tube
2. Excision of nasopharyngeal carcinoma after failed radiotherapy
3. Excision of nasopharyngeal angiofibroma in the pterygopalatine fossa and infratemporal fossa
4. Excision of anterior infratemporal tumor invading the parasellar region

Related Anatomical Structures

1. Infratemporal fossa: an irregular space located deep to the zygomatic arch and body of the mandible and posterior to the maxilla. The outer wall of the infratemporal fossa is the ascending ramus of the mandible and condy-

P. Dai et al. (eds.), *Stereoscopic Anatomical Atlas of Ear Surgery*, https://doi.org/10.1007/978-981-16-0927-5_8

lar process. The inner boundary is the lateral pterygoid plate and petrous apex. Anteriorly is the posterior wall of the maxillary sinus, posteriorly is the mandibular ligament, and above are the greater wing of the sphenoid bone and temporal fossa. Below is the attachment of the medial pterygoid muscle near the angle of the mandible. The infratemporal fossa contains the inferior part of the temporal muscle, medial and lateral pterygoid muscles, maxillary artery, pterygoid venous plexus, mandibular nerve, lingual nerve, and inferior alveolar nerve.

2. Parotid glands: the largest of the three paired salivary glands. Each parotid is located in front of the external auditory canal (EAC) and sits between the mandibular ramus and mastoid, resembling a pyramid with its apex medial and base lateral. The parotid gland is wrapped in the parotid fascia which is part of the investing layer of the deep cervical fascia; the whole gland can be divided into superficial and deep lobes. The main trunk of the facial nerve enters the parotid gland through its posterior wall from the stylomastoid foramen and passes between the superficial and deep lobes, where it divides into superior and inferior divisions and the parotid plexus (pes anserinus), which then forms five sets of terminal branches that pass out of the anterior wall of the parotid gland to the muscles of facial expression.
3. Clivus: forms the central part of the anterior wall of the posterior cranial fossa, making an angulated surface extending from the pituitary sella to the foramen magnum.
4. Carotid sheath: the connective tissue sheath that passes from the cranial base superiorly to the mediastinum inferiorly, wrapping around the internal carotid artery, internal jugular vein, and vagus nerve. It is closely attached to the prevertebral fascia and skull base.
5. Styloid process: located at the lower part of the tympanic bone, lateral to the jugular fossa and carotid artery. The distal end of the styloid process gives attachment to the stylopharyngeus, styloglossus, and stylohyoid muscles and the stylohyoid and stylomandibular ligaments. The styloid process passes forward and downward due to the pull of these muscles and ligaments during development. Accordingly, it must be resected for access to the internal carotid artery and jugular vein in the infratemporal fossa approach.
6. Jugular foramen: an opening in the skull between the occipital and petrosal bones, containing the IX, X, and XI cranial nerves, the internal jugular vein, and a branch of the occipital artery.
7. Glomus jugularis (jugular glomus body): resembles the carotid body, located at the top of the jugular bulb with a size of approximately 0.5 mm × 0.5 mm × 0.25 mm, and which may be duplicated.
8. Glomus jugulare tumor: an angioma-like tumor arising in the body of the jugular glomus.
9. Mastoid emissary foramen: at the junction of the occipital and mastoid bones, either single or multiple, of variable position and size. Veins pass through the mastoid foramen draining the occipital vein into the sigmoid sinus.
10. Lower cranial nerves: general designation of IX (glossopharyngeal), X (vagus), XI (accessory), and XII (hypoglossal) cranial nerves. These nerve roots sit close together. The XII cranial nerve passes out of the skull via the hypoglossal foramen. The IX, X, XI cranial nerves exit the skull via the jugular foramen. Paralysis of the lower cranial nerves may lead to symptoms of dyspnea, hoarseness, dysphagia, cough, and difficulty elevating the shoulders.

Anatomical Overview

The type A infratemporal fossa approach is a routine surgical approach in lateral skull base surgery. It provides access to the tympanic bone and petrous pyramid, mastoid, jugular foramen, and neck. It is necessary to have a good knowledge of temporal bone anatomy to carry out surgery of the infratemporal fossa.

1. Incision. Make a large "?-shaped" incision starting from a point 4–5 cm above the attachment of the auricle. The distance between the middle of the incision and the posterior sulcus is 3–4 cm. The incision should extend below the mastoid tip, curving anteriorly and then extending vertically to the upper neck. The incision must be large enough to provide adequate surgical exposure and will indirectly allow the surgical cavity to become wide and relatively shallow while large amounts of soft tissue are separated during the procedure.
2. Exploration of the facial nerve trunk. The facial nerve trunk turns anteriorly with an approximate 105-degree angle after exiting the skull through the stylomastoid foramen, then enters the parotid gland 1 cm further forward. The distance between the facial nerve trunk and the skin surface is about 1.5 cm. In anatomical dissection, the facial nerve is exposed along its long axis with ophthalmic scissors between the mastoid tip and the lower part of the tympanic bone. The approach to the facial nerve usually uses four anatomical landmarks to locate the trunk of the nerve as it leaves the stylomastoid foramen: (a) the anteroinferior angle of the cartilage of the EAC forms a "pointer" to the position of the facial nerve; (b) the suture between the tympanic and mastoid parts of the temporal bone is a constant landmark found just medial to the pointer and palpation leads to the stylomastoid foramen lying as much as 1 cm deeper; (c) the stylomastoid foramen sits just in front of the anterior

upper edge of the posterior belly of the digastric muscle; (d) the styloid process can be followed superiorly from tip to base where it sits lateral to the foramen. The facial nerve passes forwards and down across the styloid. *Hints: (1) Before the separation of the soft tissue, it is necessary to determine the location of the facial nerve trunk by multiple anatomical landmarks and various positioning methods. (2) The direction of separation of soft tissue must be parallel to the facial nerve trunk to avoid transection of the nerve. (3) Any cord-like structure cannot be dissected blindly; it must be separated carefully, and its identification confirmed during initial exploration of the facial nerve trunk. (4) If it is difficult to determine the position of the facial nerve trunk by dissection outside the mastoid, a mastoid approach can be used to identify the facial nerve and follow its course out through the stylomastoid foramen.*

3. Extended mastoid exposure. A canal-wall-down mastoidectomy is performed and the extent of bone removal should include bone over the sigmoid sinus from front to back and from 2 cm above the temporal line. The remaining skin of the EAC is removed along with the tympanic membrane (with care not to traumatize the ossicular chain). Remove the scutum to the anterior wall of the EAC, remove the inferior wall of the EAC and expose the hypotympanum. A new canal is drilled in the root of the zygoma and the anterior wall of the epitympanum to accommodate the re-routed facial nerve.
4. Removal of the contents of the tympanic cavity. Separate the incudostapedial joint, cut the tendons of the tensor tympani muscle and stapedius muscles. Remove the tympanic membrane, malleus, chorda tympani, incus, and superstructure of the stapes leaving the footplate in a normal position. *Hints: Separation of the incudostapedial articulation should be performed before removing the contents of the tympanic cavity to avoid pulling out the whole stapes and to protect the function of the inner ear.*
5. Amputation of mastoid tip and styloid process. Remove the bone on the top and posterior parts of the digastric ridge and lateral part of the stylomastoid foramen to separate the mastoid tip from the mastoid. The muscles and connective tissues attached to the mastoid tip are sharply dissected away and the mastoid tip is amputated using a rongeur. The muscles attached to the styloid process are sharply dissected away from it and the styloid process is then removed with a rongeur, Full exposure of the main trunk of the facial nerve and the internal carotid artery can then be achieved.
6. Anterior transposition (re-routing) of facial nerve. The infratemporal fossa approach type A requires exposure of the jugular bulb by anterior transposition of the facial nerve. The facial nerve is skeletonized from the stylomastoid foramen back to the geniculate ganglion. Furthermore, the temporal and cervical branches should be freed outside the stylomastoid foramen. The eggshell bone covering the nerve is carefully removed using a double-curved raspatory. The tympanic and mastoid segments of the nerve are carefully elevated, and a tunnel is created in the parotid gland to accommodate the transposed nerve to allow the gland to be sutured over the nerve. The soft tissues surrounding the facial nerve at the level of the stylomastoid foramen are left on the nerve to protect it then sutured to the soft tissues of the parotid gland anteriorly. *Hints: (1) Do not remove the scutum beyond the anterior wall of the EAC, to avoid damage to the temporomandibular joint and allow drilling of a new canal in the anterior wall of the epitympanum for the re-routed facial nerve. (2) Be careful to preserve the greater superficial petrosal nerve (GSPN) when removing bone lateral to the geniculate ganglion. Keeping the bone superior and medial to the geniculate ganglion will help preserve the blood supply of the facial nerve and yield better post-operative function of the nerve. (3) A soft-tissue cuff is left around the facial nerve at the level of the stylomastoid foramen. This tissue can be sutured with parotid tissue in the anterior wall of the surgical cavity.*
7. Exposure of jugular vein and jugular bulb. The jugular bulb is located at the inferior end of the sigmoid sinus. Removing the remaining bone around the vertical portion of the empty facial nerve canal allows full exposure of the jugular bulb. Care should be taken not to penetrate the thin vein wall of the jugular bulb by controlling the speed and force of the bur. During surgery for glomus jugulare tumors, more bleeding will be seen when closer to the jugular bulb. Before removing the jugular bulb, the internal jugular vein in the upper neck should be dissected and double-ligated, and the lumen of the sigmoid sinus above compressed with packing.
8. Exposure of internal carotid artery. The internal carotid artery is located anteromedial to the promontory and posteroinferior to the tympanic opening of the Eustachian tube. The tympanic opening of the Eustachian tube and the promontory can help to localize the horizontal and vertical segments of the internal carotid artery. Using a medium-sized diamond bur, the tympanic bone is drilled away along the direction of the vertical portion of the internal carotid artery to expose the vessel. After removal of the jugular bulb, the internal carotid artery will be exposed. *Hints: (1) Avoid damage to the jugular bulb, internal jugular vein, and cochlea. (2) The dense soft-tissue layer between the internal carotid artery, the internal jugular vein, and the jugular bulb at the entrance of the artery into the carotid foramen should be separated using sharp dissection techniques along the*

direction of the artery. (3) The vagus nerve runs between the internal carotid artery and jugular vein, and the accessory and glossopharyngeal nerves usually run medial to the jugular bulb. Care should be taken to preserve these nerves during the surgical dissection.

9. Anatomy of jugular foramen. Open the cavity of the jugular bulb after packing the sigmoid sinus above and ligating the internal jugular vein below, then pack the opening of the inferior petrosal sinus in the deep wall of the bulb, which may be multiple. Parts of the sigmoid sinus and the internal jugular vein are then carefully dissected to expose the jugular foramen. The inferior petrosal sinus and cranial nerves IX, X, and XI pass through the medial part of the jugular foramen and posterior to the internal carotid artery. The glossopharyngeal nerve is usually located at the medial side of the jugular bulb and exits the jugular foramen anterior to the inferior petrosal sinus separately. The vagus and accessory nerves exit the jugular foramen posterior to the inferior petrosal sinus.
10. Anatomy of the lower cranial nerves. Incise the dura of the lower part of the posterior cranial fossa to open the cerebellopontine angle region and expose the cranial nerves IX, X, and XI passing through the jugular foramen. Tracing the lower cranial nerves outside the jugular foramen: (1) The glossopharyngeal nerve crosses the internal carotid artery and reaches the root of the tongue through the medial part of the hyoglossus muscle. (2) The vagus nerve passes downward between the internal jugular vein and internal carotid artery. (3) The accessory nerve continues downward and laterally, passing over the jugular vein, and enters the trapezius muscle after leaving the deep surface of the sternocleidomastoid muscle. The accessory nerve innervates the sternocleidomastoid and trapezius muscles. (4) The hypoglossal nerve passes through the hypoglossal canal alone, continuing downwards between the jugular vein and internal carotid artery, and reaches the superficial side of the hyoglossus muscle. The hypoglossal nerve innervates all the intrinsic and extrinsic lingual muscles.

Purposes and Requirements of Anatomical Dissection

1. Master the anatomic and surgical scope of the infratemporal fossa approach.
2. Master the surgical steps of the infratemporal fossa approach, type A.
3. Master the spatial relationships between the structures of the infratemporal fossa, parotid gland, and carotid sheath.
4. Master the technique of transposition of the facial nerve in the temporal bone.
5. Master the technique of separating the internal carotid artery.
6. Master the technique of sigmoid sinus obliteration, jugular bulb resection, and internal jugular vein ligation and control of bleeding from the inferior petrosal sinus.
7. Master the anatomy of the lower cranial nerves.

The opening of the inner ear structures in the following images is for anatomical dissection and not a routine part of the infratemporal approaches.

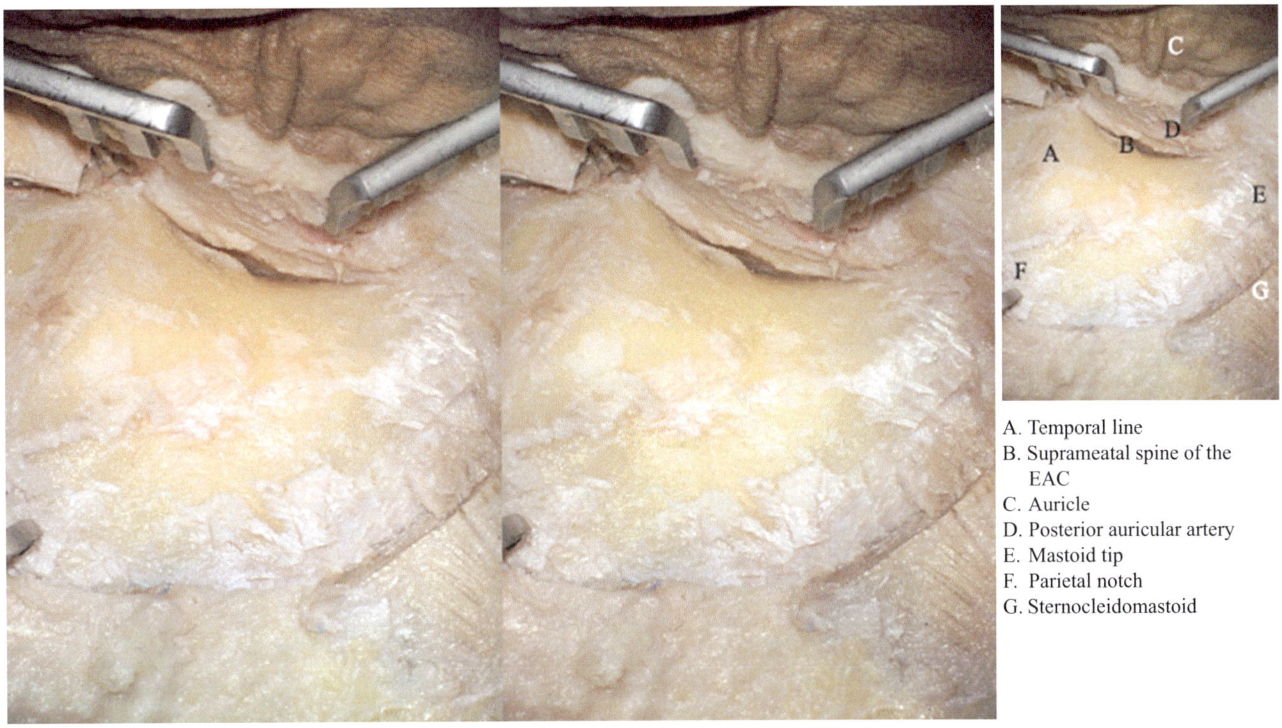

A. Temporal line
B. Suprameatal spine of the EAC
C. Auricle
D. Posterior auricular artery
E. Mastoid tip
F. Parietal notch
G. Sternocleidomastoid

Fig. 8.1 Exposure of bony landmarks of mastoid (right)
A curved retroauricular incision has been made. The skin, subcutaneous tissues, and periosteum are elevated from the mastoid cortex. The exposure extends up to the temporal line, down to the mastoid tip, forward to the posterior wall of the EAC, and back to the parietal notch and posterior edge of the mastoid
Instruments: surgical knife, periosteal elevator, mastoid retractor

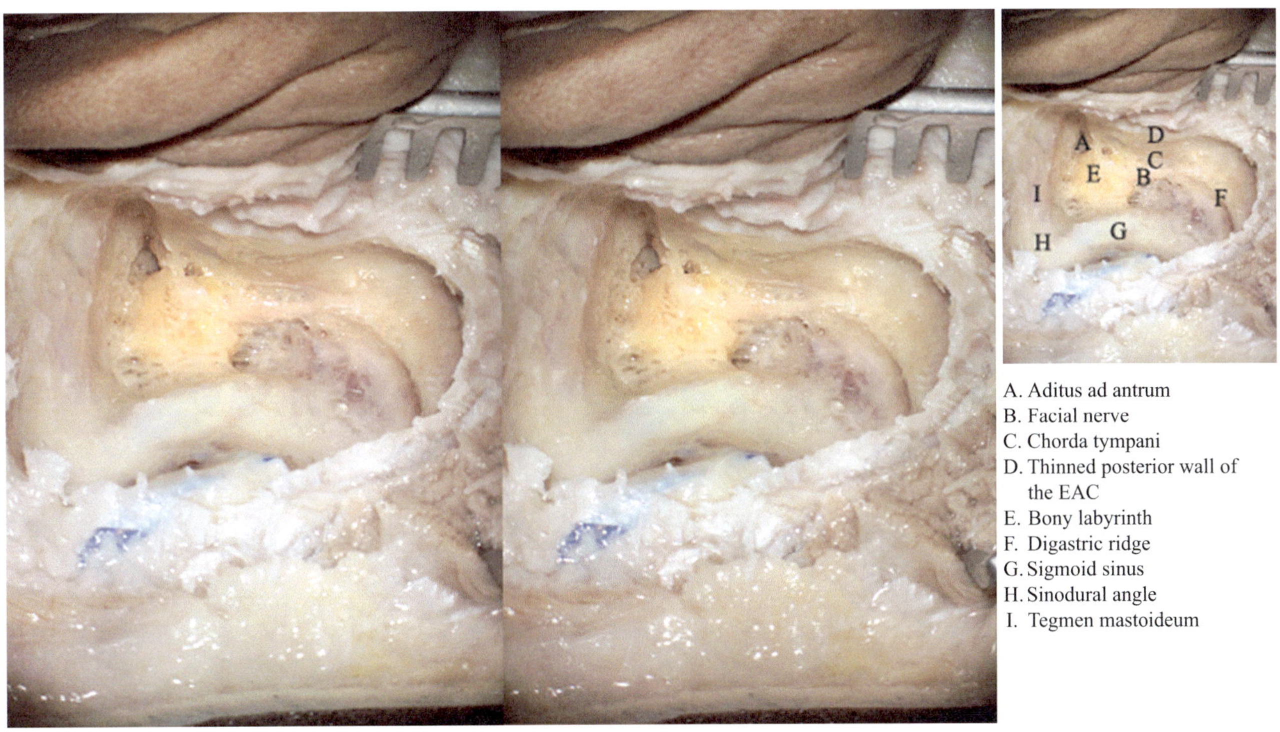

A. Aditus ad antrum
B. Facial nerve
C. Chorda tympani
D. Thinned posterior wall of the EAC
E. Bony labyrinth
F. Digastric ridge
G. Sigmoid sinus
H. Sinodural angle
I. Tegmen mastoideum

Fig. 8.2 Extensive mastoidectomy (right)
The limits of removal of the mastoid cortex are: 2 cm above the temporal line, down to the mastoid tip, and forward to the posterior wall of the EAC. An extensive mastoidectomy is performed by thinning the posterior wall of the EAC, outlining the sigmoid sinus, the tegmen mastoideum, the sinodural angle, and the digastric muscle ridge. The mastoid cavity is enlarged, and the bony labyrinth outlined
Instruments: large- and medium-sized cutting burs, medium-sized diamond burs

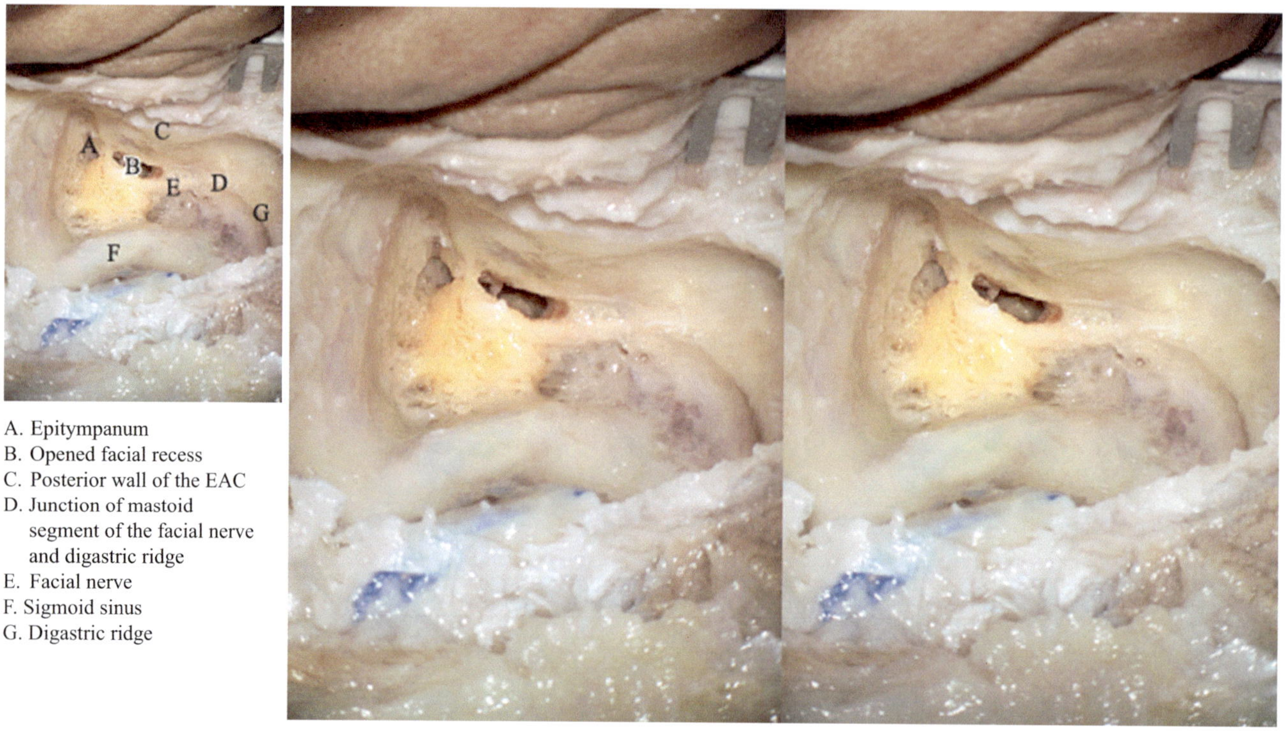

Fig. 8.3 Open the facial recess (right)
The short process of the incus and lateral semicircular canal is identified as landmarks for opening the facial recess. Expose the promontory of the tympanic cavity and the incudostapedial joint. Care should be taken not to injure the facial nerve, chorda tympani, and the lateral semicircular canal. The surgeon should avoid touching the intact ossicular chain with activated drills
Instruments: small-sized cutting burs, diamond burs

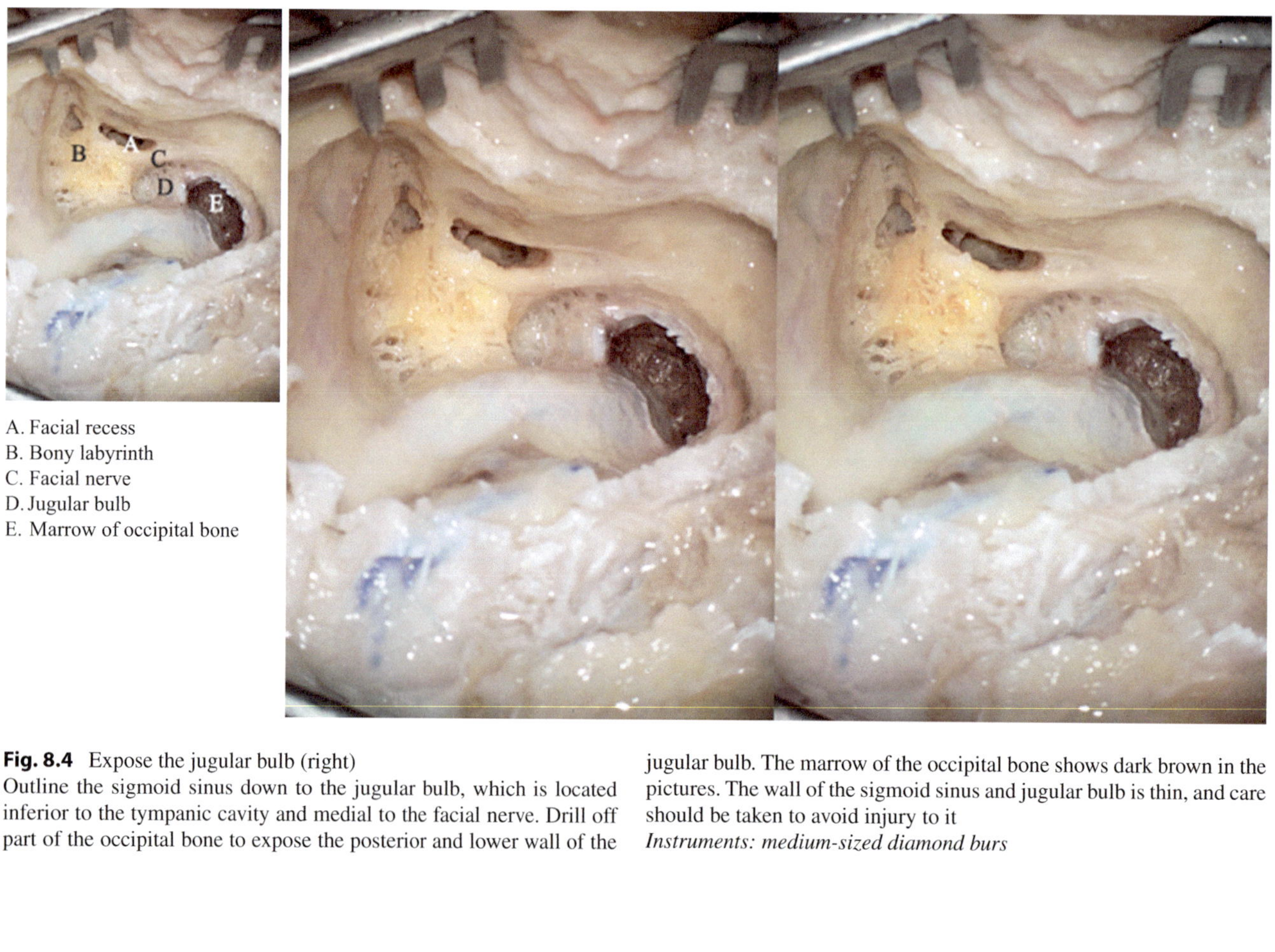

Fig. 8.4 Expose the jugular bulb (right)
Outline the sigmoid sinus down to the jugular bulb, which is located inferior to the tympanic cavity and medial to the facial nerve. Drill off part of the occipital bone to expose the posterior and lower wall of the jugular bulb. The marrow of the occipital bone shows dark brown in the pictures. The wall of the sigmoid sinus and jugular bulb is thin, and care should be taken to avoid injury to it
Instruments: medium-sized diamond burs

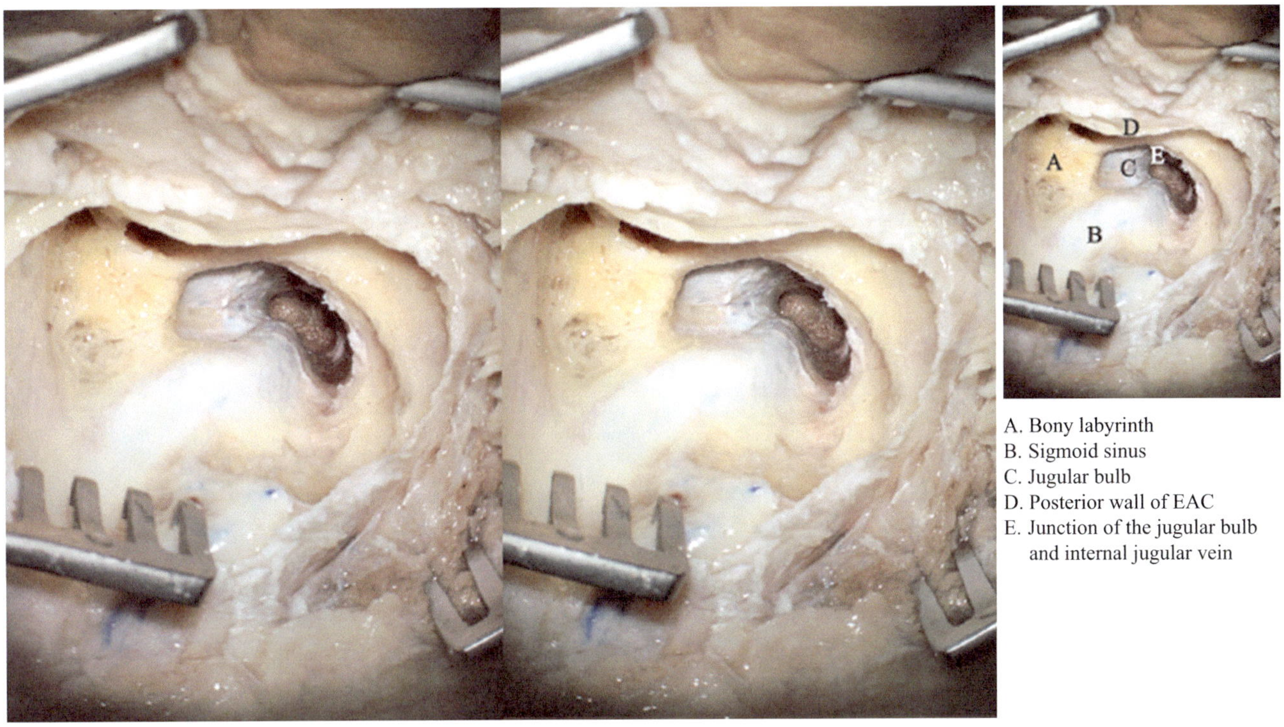

A. Bony labyrinth
B. Sigmoid sinus
C. Jugular bulb
D. Posterior wall of EAC
E. Junction of the jugular bulb and internal jugular vein

Fig. 8.5 Delicately outline the jugular bulb (right)
Delicately outline the jugular bulb and observe the continuity of the sigmoid sinus, the jugular bulb, and internal jugular vein

Instruments: diamond burs

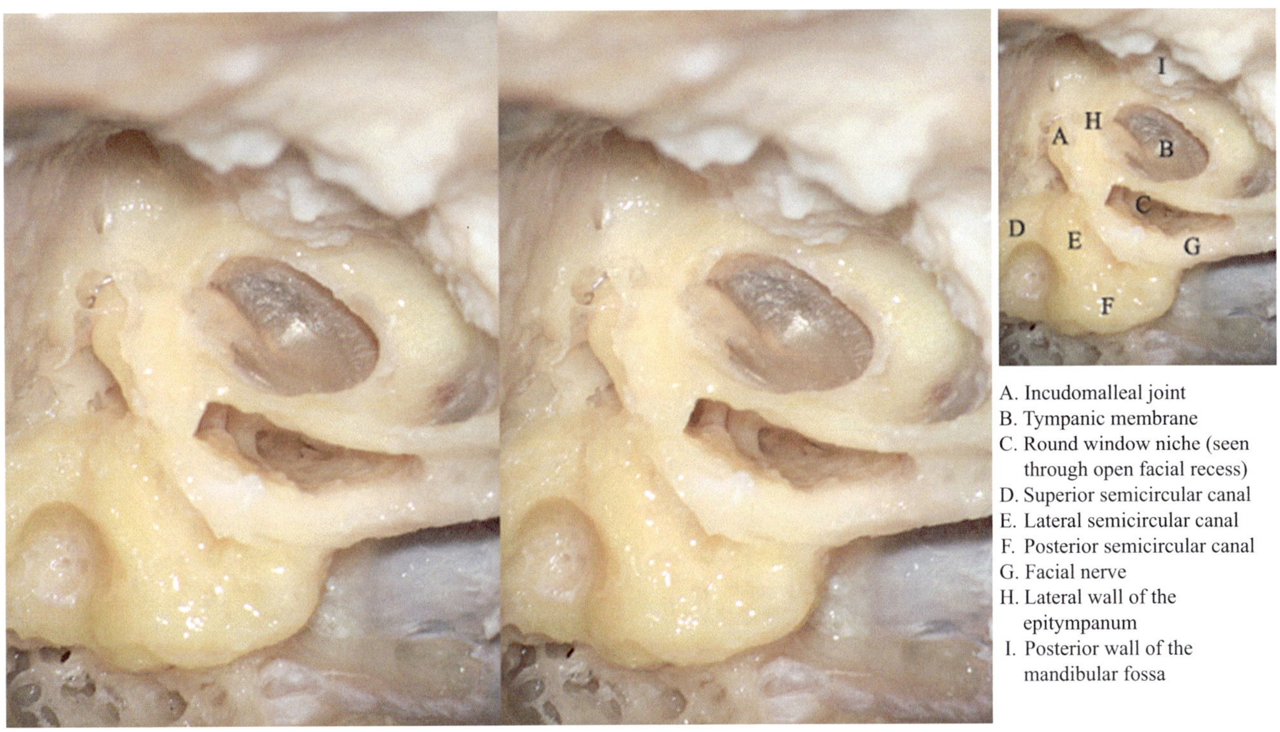

A. Incudomalleal joint
B. Tympanic membrane
C. Round window niche (seen through open facial recess)
D. Superior semicircular canal
E. Lateral semicircular canal
F. Posterior semicircular canal
G. Facial nerve
H. Lateral wall of the epitympanum
I. Posterior wall of the mandibular fossa

Fig. 8.6 Resect the bony EAC (right)
Resect the bony EAC then outline the tegmen tympani above and the posterior wall of the mandibular fossa in front. Drill off the tympanic bone to the level of the tympanic membrane. Observe the incudomalleal joint medial to the lateral wall of the epitympanum. Leave a thin bone plate between the anterior wall of the EAC and the mandibular fossa. Observe the sharp angle between the tympanic membrane and the anteroinferior wall of the EAC. Locate the canaliculus of the chorda tympani inside the posterior wall of the EAC
Instruments: medium-sized cutting burs, diamond burs

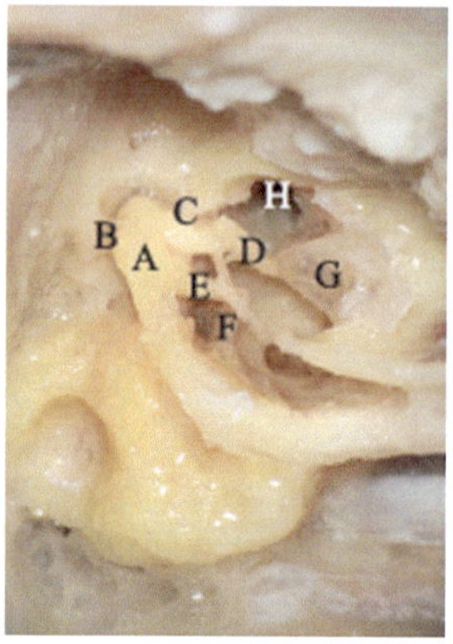

A. Body of incus
B. Superior ligament of malleus
C. Lateral ligament of malleus
D. Handle of malleus
E. Long process of incus
F. Stapes
G. Tympanic membrane (reflected downwards)
H. Tympanic opening of the Eustachian tube

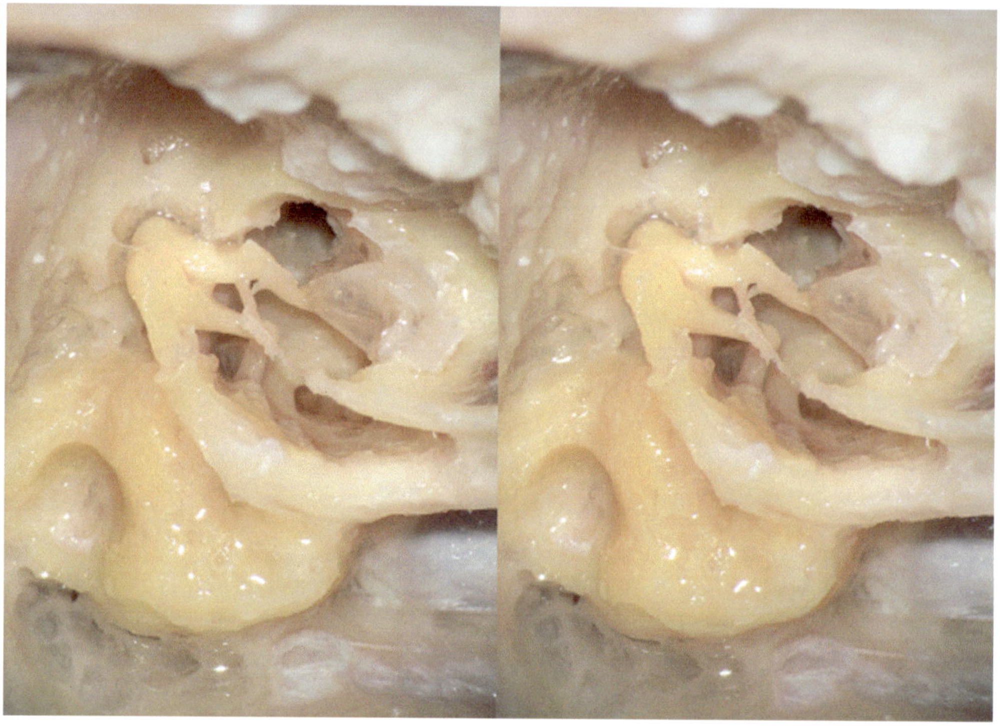

Fig. 8.7 Remove the bone bridge and strip down the tympanic membrane (right)
Drill off the lateral wall of the epitympanum and remove the bone bridge to expose the ossicular chain and the epitympanum. Observe the intact ossicular chain, superior and lateral ligaments of the malleus, round window niche, facial nerve, chorda tympani, and tympanic opening of the Eustachian tube
Instruments: medium-sized cutting burs, small-sized diamond burs, middle ear elevator

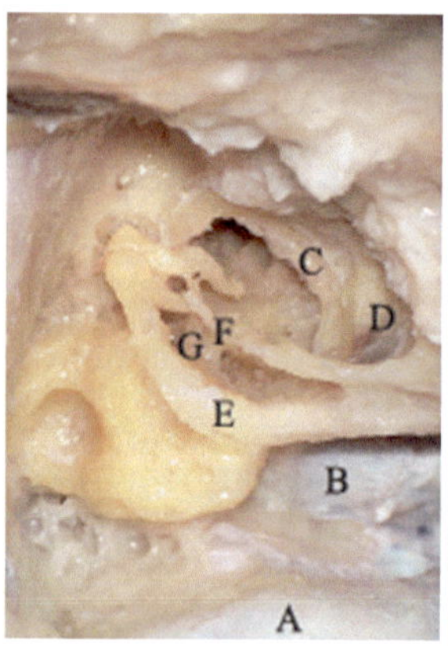

A. Sigmoid sinus
B. Jugular bulb
C. Tympanic sulcus
D. Remnants of the tympanic bone
E. Facial nerve
F. Chorda tympani
G. Pyramidal eminence

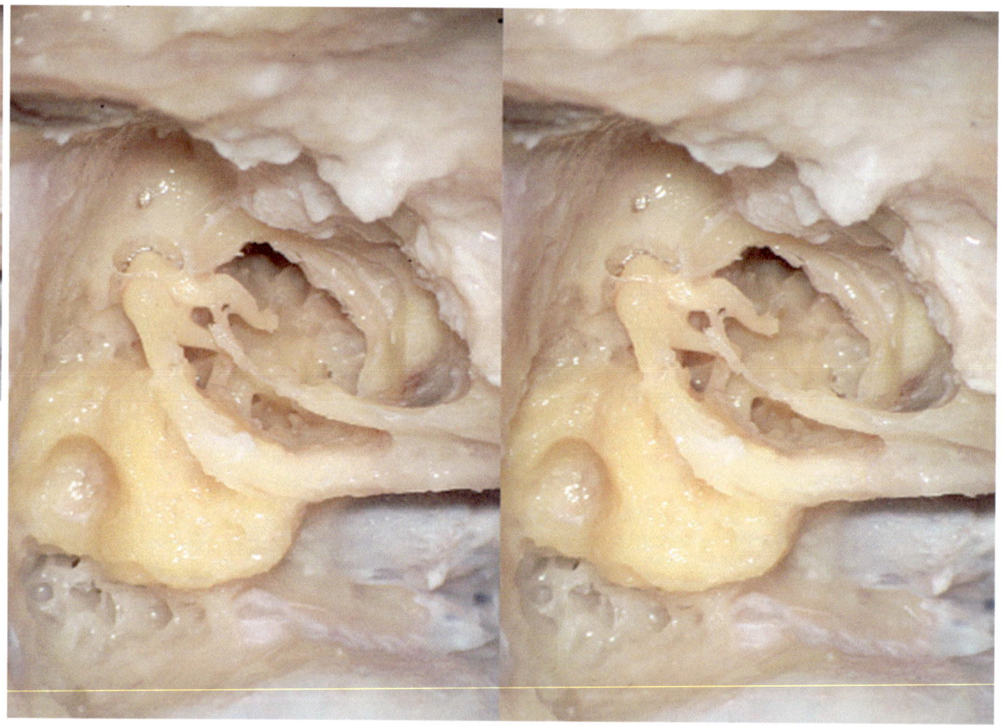

Fig. 8.8 Resect the tympanic membrane and expose the mesotympanum (right)
Separate the tympanic annulus from the tympanic sulcus and resect the tympanic membrane to expose the mesotympanum fully. The stapes, pyramidal eminence, and round window niche are seen through the facial recess. The lower medial wall of the mesotympanum is composed of irregular cells and bone ridges
Instruments: middle ear elevator, cupped forceps

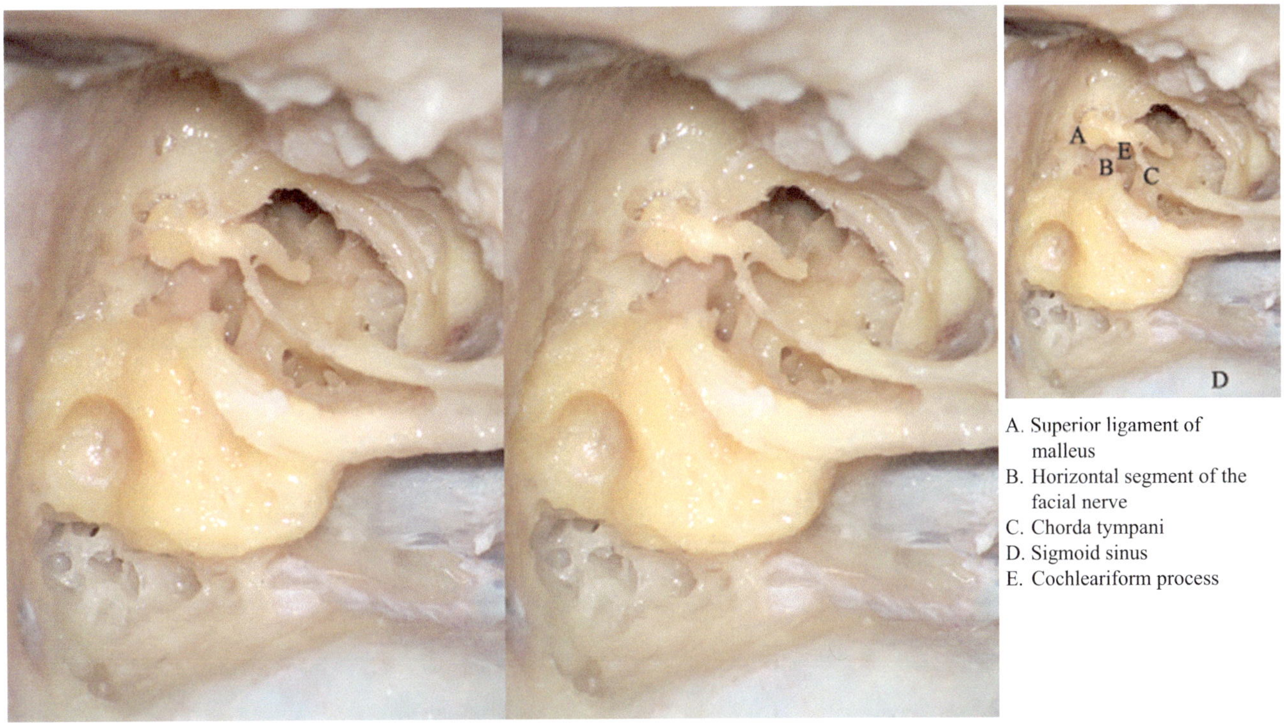

A. Superior ligament of malleus
B. Horizontal segment of the facial nerve
C. Chorda tympani
D. Sigmoid sinus
E. Cochleariform process

Fig. 8.9 Remove incus and expose the horizontal segment of the facial nerve (right)
Separate the incudostapedial and incudomalleal joints with a right-angle hook. Remove the incus and expose the horizontal segment of the facial nerve, stapes, and cochleariform process

Instruments: right-angle hook

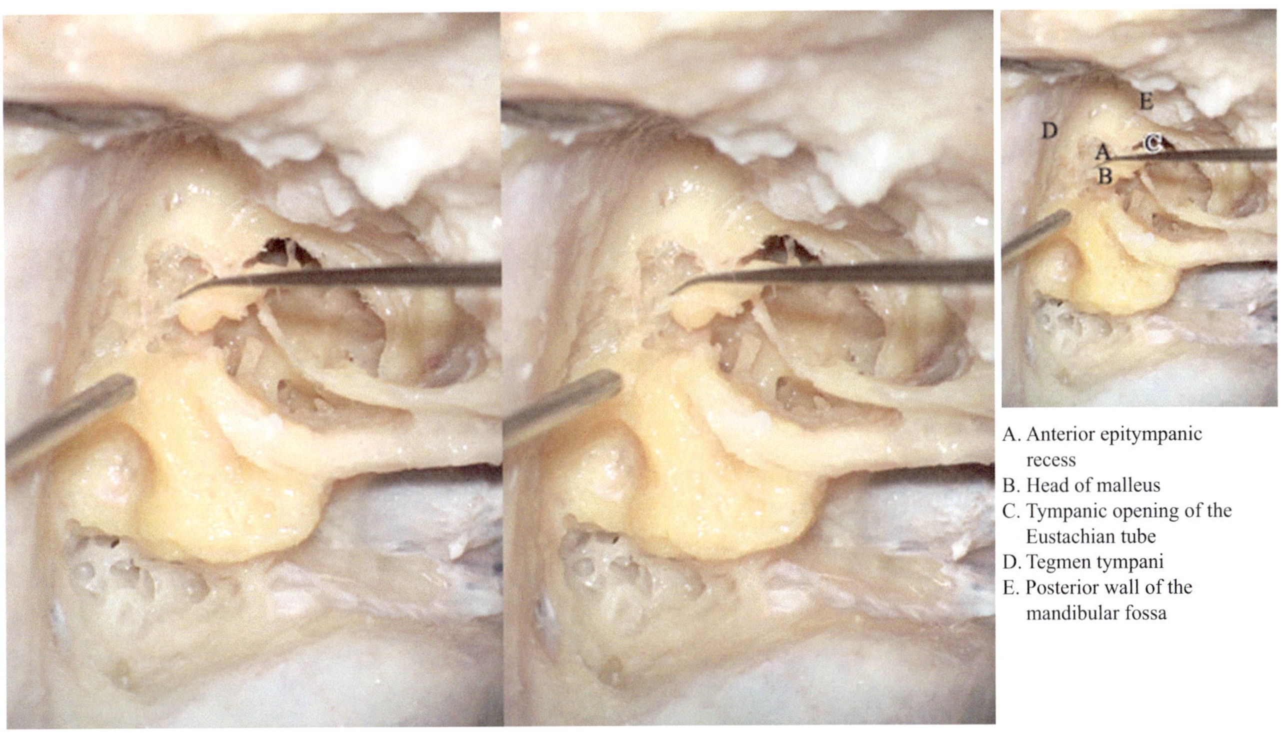

A. Anterior epitympanic recess
B. Head of malleus
C. Tympanic opening of the Eustachian tube
D. Tegmen tympani
E. Posterior wall of the mandibular fossa

Fig. 8.10 Expose the anterior epitympanic recess (right)
Retract the head of the malleus with a right-angle hook and expose the anterior epitympanic recess (a site that is often involved in cholesteatoma cases)

Instruments: right-angle hook, suction apparatus

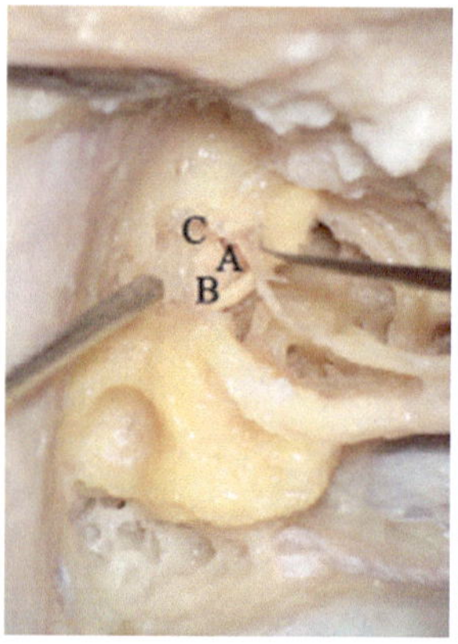

A. Cochleariform process
B. Horizontal segment of the facial nerve
C. Anterior epitympanic recess

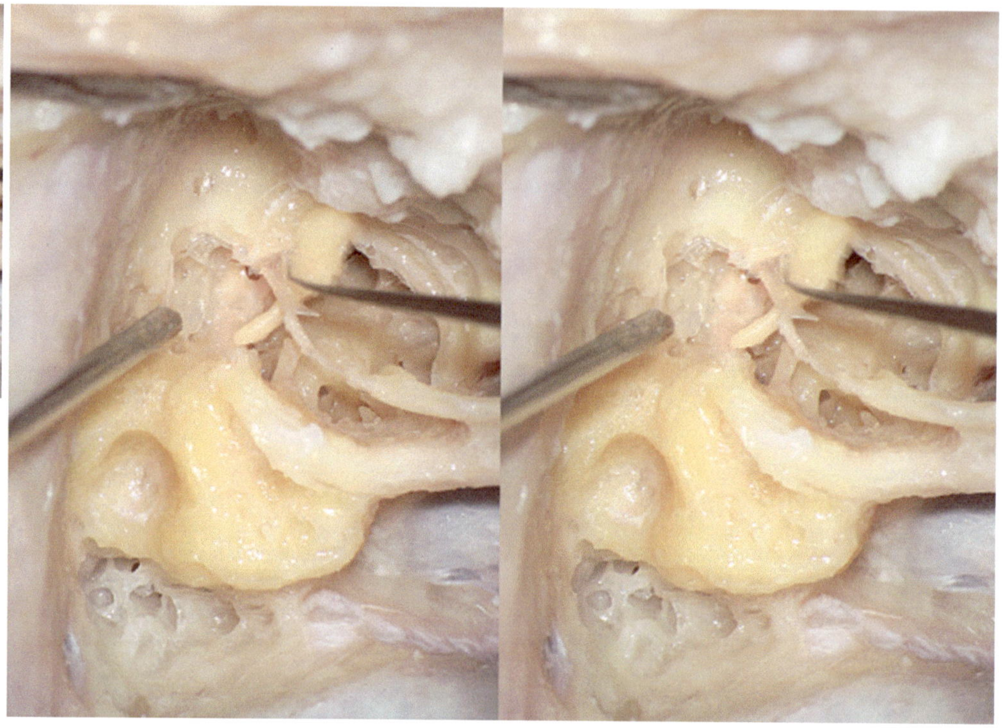

Fig. 8.11 Dislocate the malleus and explore the anterior epitympanic recess (right)
Pull down the head of the malleus with a right-angle hook and fully expose the epitympanum and anterior epitympanic recess. Observe the pink horizontal segment of the facial nerve and white cochleariform process
Instruments: right-angle hook, suction apparatus

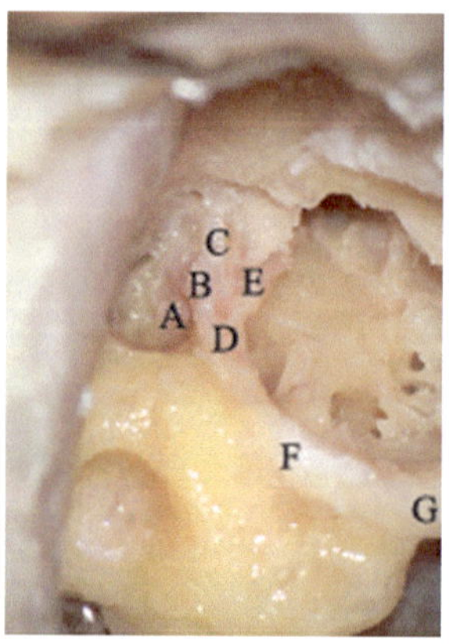

A. Labyrinthine segment of the facial nerve
B. Geniculate ganglion
C. GSPN
D. Horizontal segment of the facial nerve
E. Cochleariform process
F. Pyramid segment of the facial nerve
G. Mastoid segment of the facial nerve

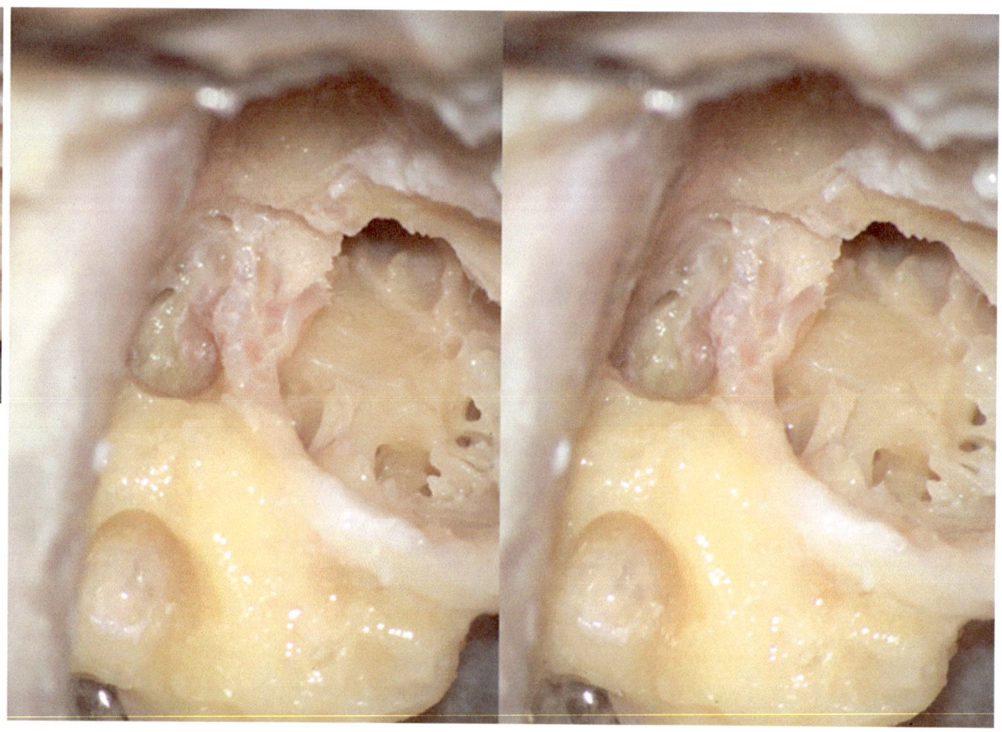

Fig. 8.12 Expose the geniculate ganglion and labyrinthine segment of the facial nerve (right)
Resect the chorda tympani, cut the tensor tympani tendon and remove the malleus. Drill off the bone above the horizontal segment of the facial nerve to expose the geniculate ganglion and the labyrinthine segment of the facial nerve. Observe the GSPN passing forward from the geniculate ganglion
Instruments: small-sized diamond burs

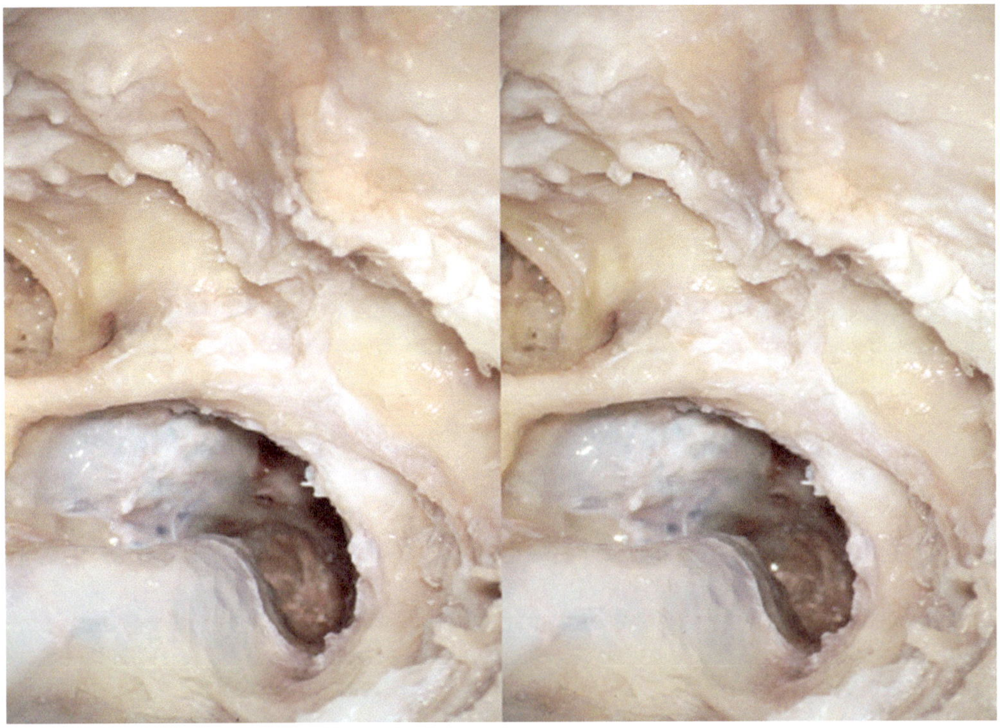

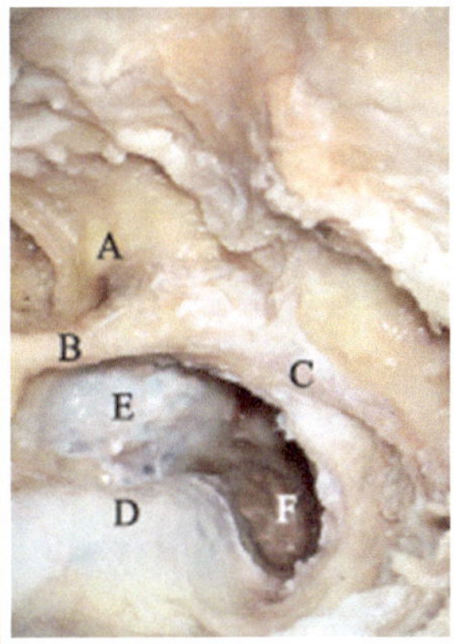

A. Remnants of the tympanic bone
B. Mastoid segment of the facial nerve
C. Digastric ridge
D. Sigmoid sinus
E. Jugular bulb
F. Occipital bone

Fig. 8.13 Junction of the sigmoid sinus and the jugular bulb (right)
The sigmoid sinus is located at the back of the mastoid. The location of the jugular bulb is variable. The jugular bulb is usually medial to the mastoid segment of the facial nerve and below the tympanic cavity. It can be exposed by working along the lower segment of the sigmoid sinus. Care should be taken when outlining the jugular bulb to avoid injury to the posterior semicircular canal and vertical segment of the facial nerve

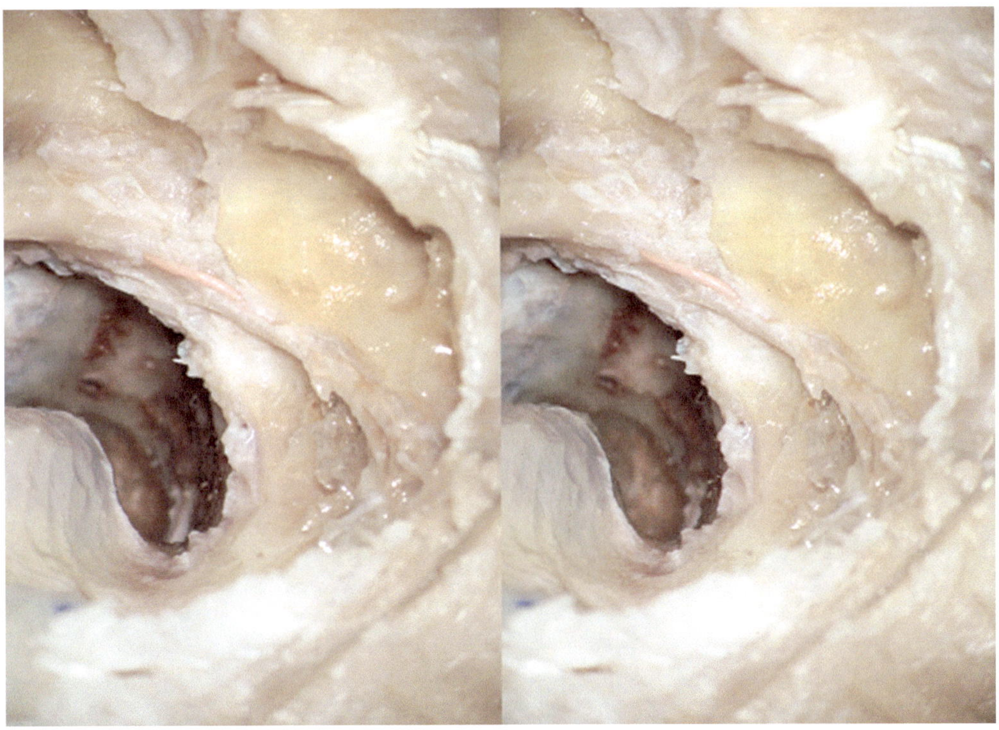

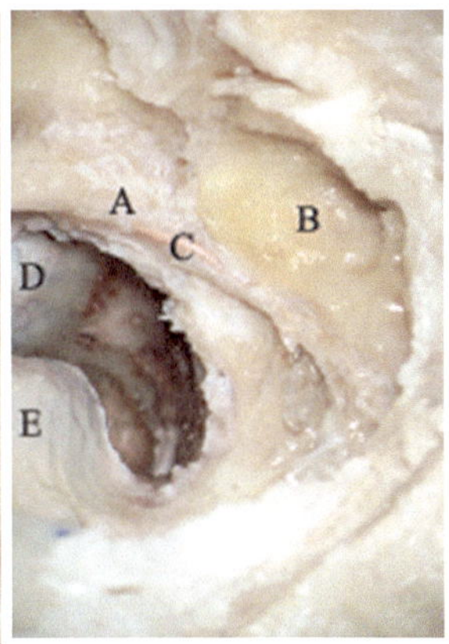

A. Stylomastoid foramen
B. Mastoid tip
C. Stylomastoid artery
D. Jugular bulb
E. Sigmoid sinus

Fig. 8.14 Stylomastoid artery (right)
There are two notches located medial to the mastoid tip that accommodate the posterior belly of the digastric muscle and the occipital artery. Open the digastric muscle ridge and identify the stylomastoid artery medial to the digastric muscle
Instruments: medium-sized cutting burs, right-angle hook

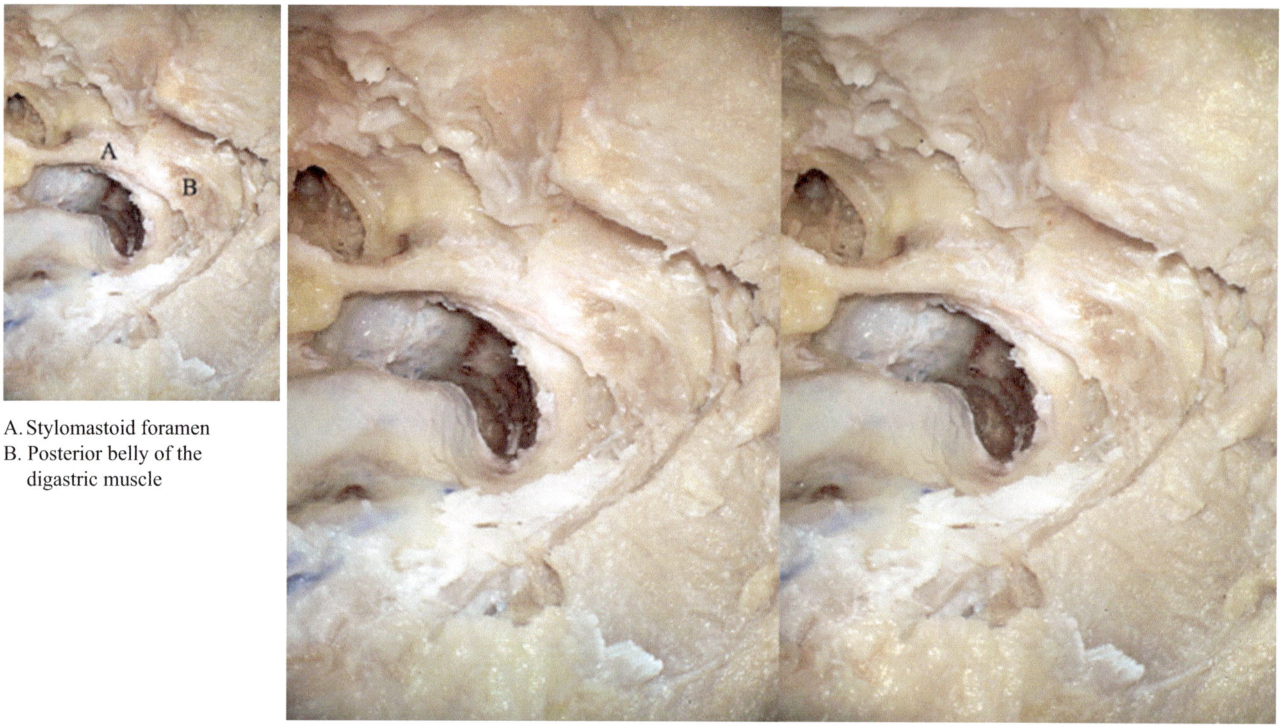

A. Stylomastoid foramen
B. Posterior belly of the digastric muscle

Fig. 8.15 Excise the mastoid tip (right)
Drill off the tympanic bone, the posterior wall of the mastoid, and bone around the posterior belly of the digastric muscle with medium-sized diamond burs, then excise the mastoid tip

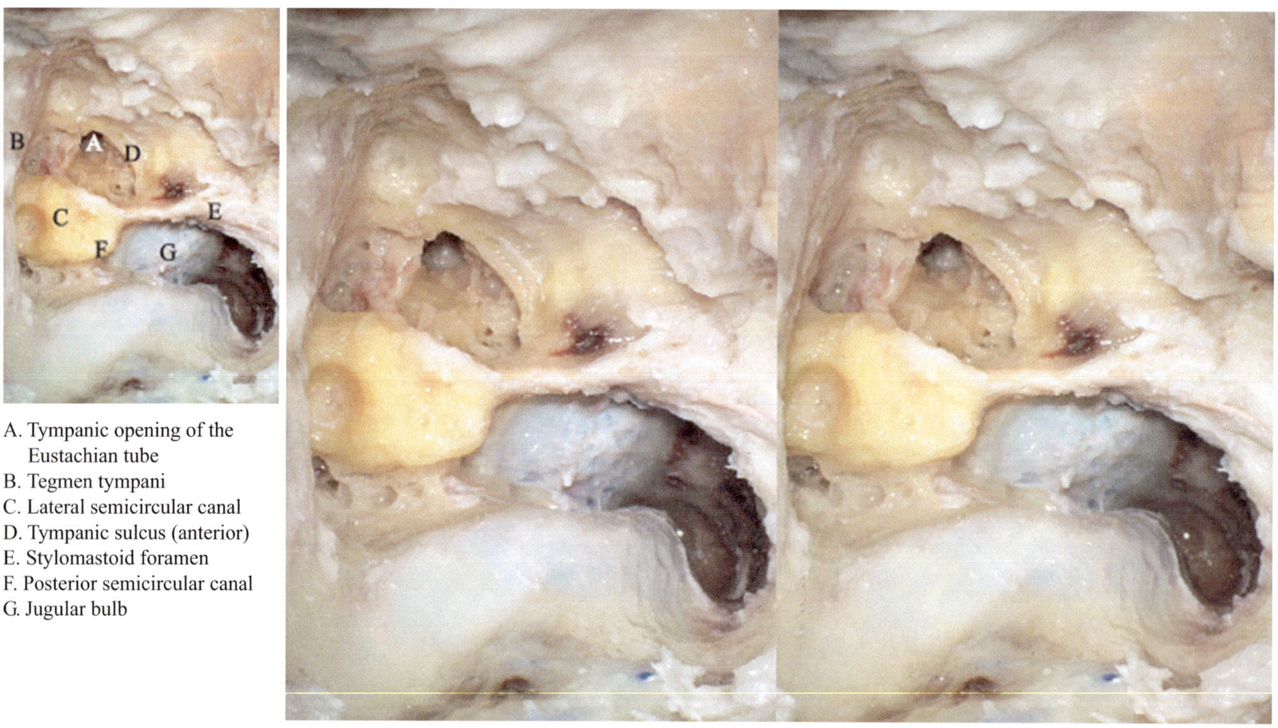

A. Tympanic opening of the Eustachian tube
B. Tegmen tympani
C. Lateral semicircular canal
D. Tympanic sulcus (anterior)
E. Stylomastoid foramen
F. Posterior semicircular canal
G. Jugular bulb

Fig. 8.16 Full view of the facial nerve in the temporal bone (right)
The facial nerve is transposed in the type A infratemporal fossa approach, while in the type B and C infratemporal fossa approaches it can be left in its normal position. When transposing it, the facial nerve must be mobilized from the stylomastoid foramen to the geniculate ganglion. In some cases with well-pneumatized mastoids, the labyrinthine segment of the facial nerve can be partly observed without excision of any of the labyrinth
Instruments: medium-sized diamond burs, surgical knife

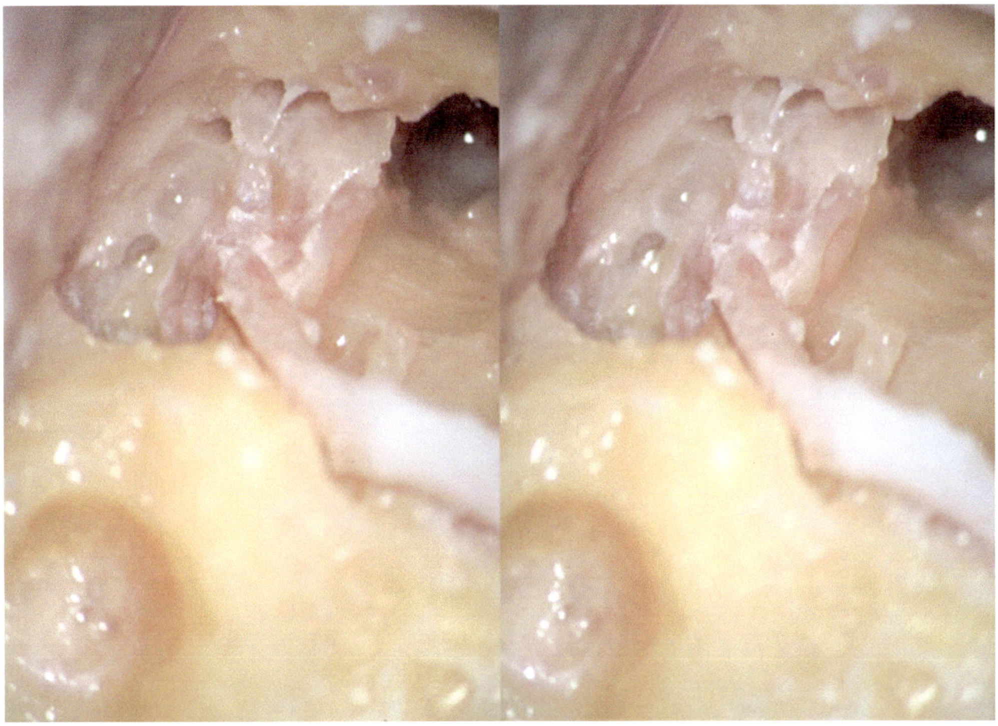

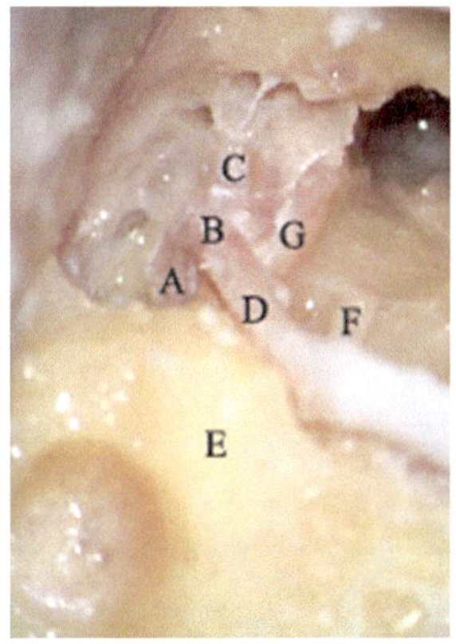

A. Labyrinthine segment of the facial nerve
B. Geniculate ganglion
C. GSPN
D. Horizontal segment of the facial nerve
E. Lateral semicircular canal
F. Stapes
G. Cochleariform process

Fig. 8.17 Dissect the pyramid and mastoid segments of the facial nerve (right)
Outline the bony canal of the facial nerve in the temporal bone in a spiral fashion until only a thin bone shell is left, then remove the bone shell with a right-angle hook. (The spiral approach refers to exposure of the nerve posteriorly in the mastoid segment, laterally at the second genu, and inferiorly along the horizontal segment which allows preservation of other important structures close to the nerve). Once the facial nerve is exposed for 1/2–2/3 of its circumference, separate it from the canal with a middle ear elevator. The epineurium should not be incised. To avoid any injury, the facial nerve should not be elevated before adequate opening of its bony canal
Instruments: medium- and small-sized diamond burs, right-angle hook, middle ear elevator

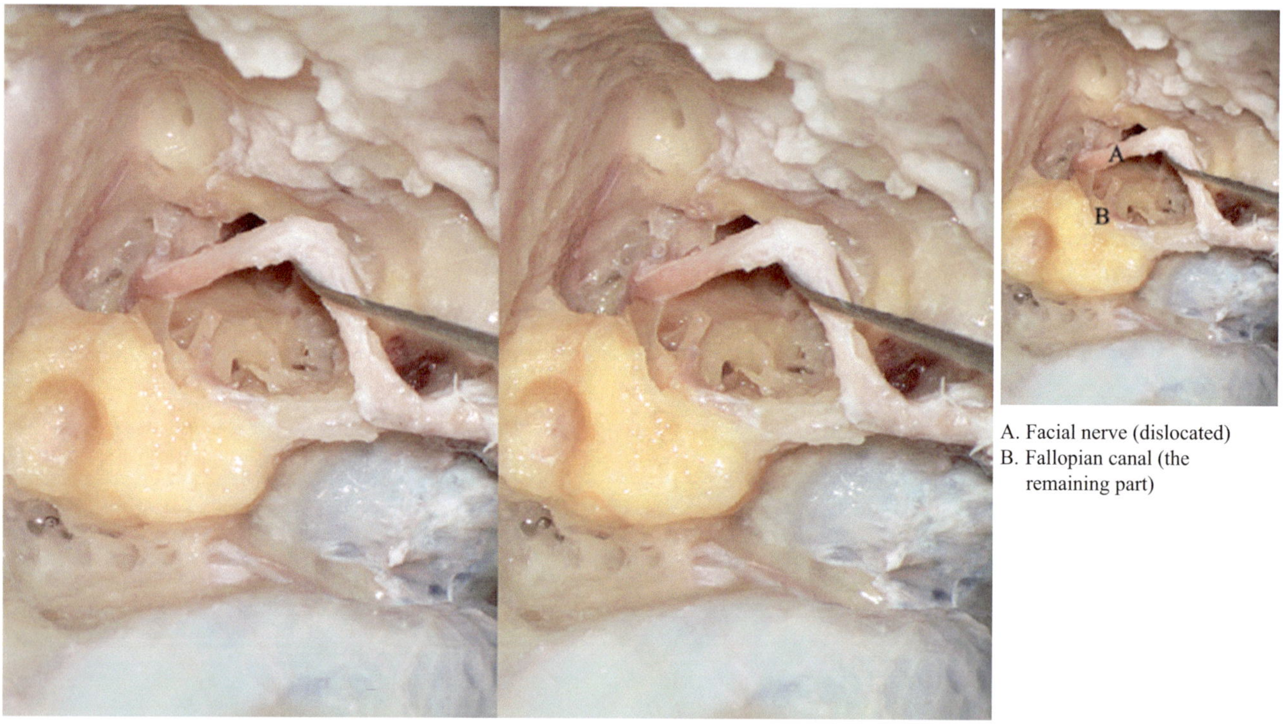

A. Facial nerve (dislocated)
B. Fallopian canal (the remaining part)

Fig. 8.18 Dislocate the facial nerve from its bony canal (right)
Free the facial nerve along its bony canal from the stylomastoid foramen to the geniculate ganglion. Create a groove in the bone on the anterior bony wall of the epitympanum to accommodate the repositioned facial nerve. No bony fragments should be left outside the geniculate ganglion to avoid penetrating the facial nerve when repositioning it. Retaining the bone medial to the geniculate ganglion is helpful to protect the blood supply and reduce the incidence of postoperative facial-nerve paralysis
Instruments: medium- and small-sized diamond burs, right-angle hook, middle ear elevator

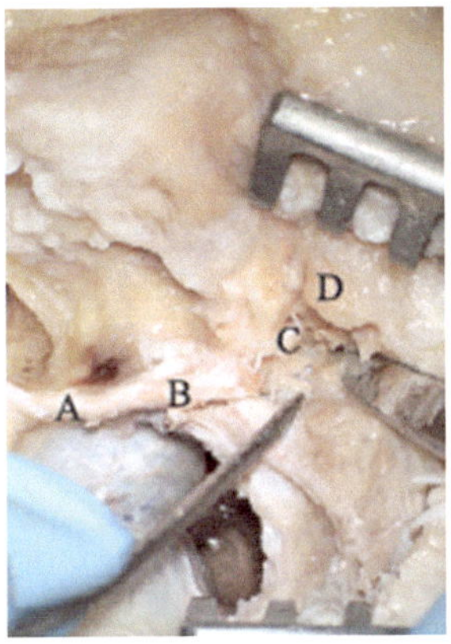

A. Mastoid segment of the facial nerve
B. Facial nerve at the stylomastoid foramen level
C. Main trunk of the extratemporal facial nerve
D. Parotid gland

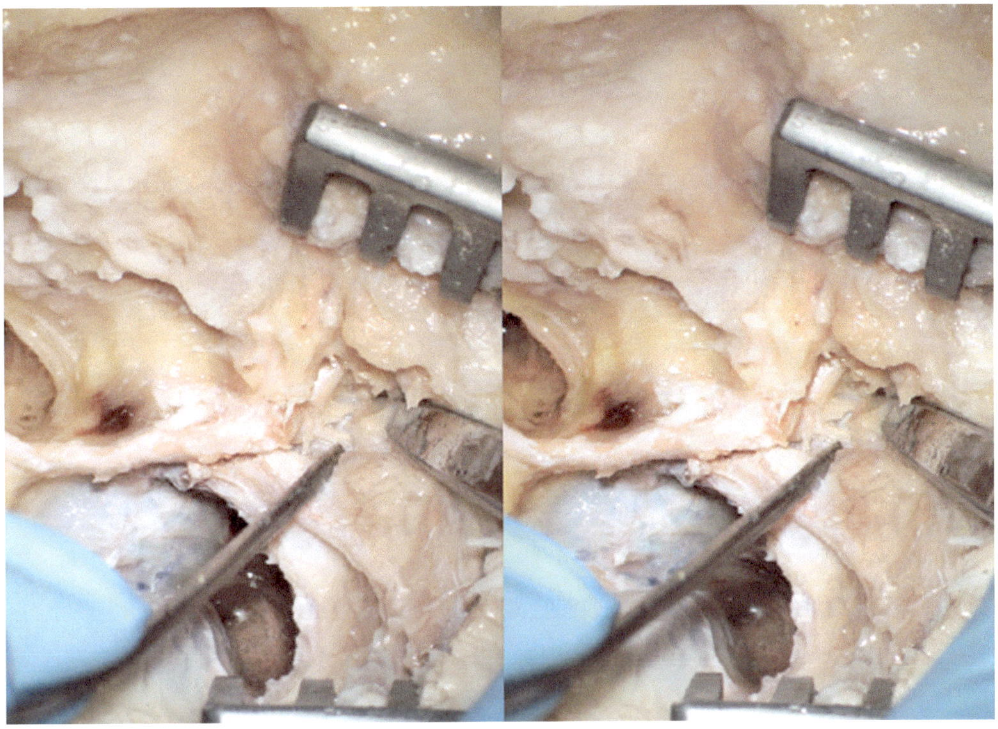

Fig. 8.19 Exploration of the main trunk of the extratemporal facial nerve (right)
Using ophthalmic scissors, the soft tissue anterior to the stylomastoid foramen can be removed layer by layer parallel to the course of the facial nerve. The extratemporal facial nerve is explored and the main trunk is freed for approximately 1 cm to reduce stretching of the nerve during its transpositioning

Hints: When exploring the extratemporal facial nerve, the direction of separation should be parallel to the direction of the facial nerve fibers to prevent facial nerve injury
Instruments: ophthalmic scissors, ophthalmic forceps

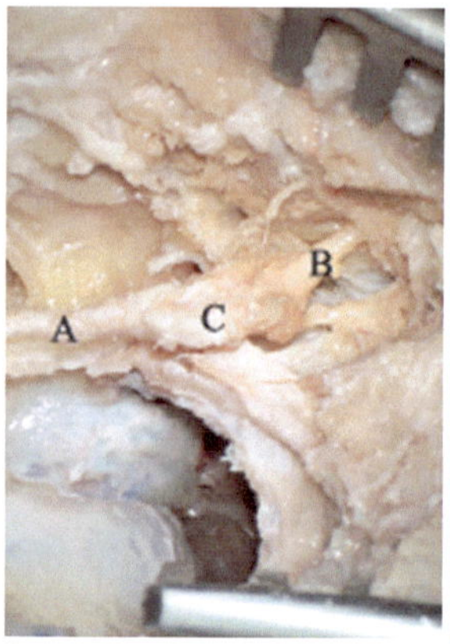

A. Mastoid segment of the facial nerve
B. Main trunk of the extratemporal facial nerve
C. Facial nerve and its surrounding connective tissue at the stylomastoid foramen

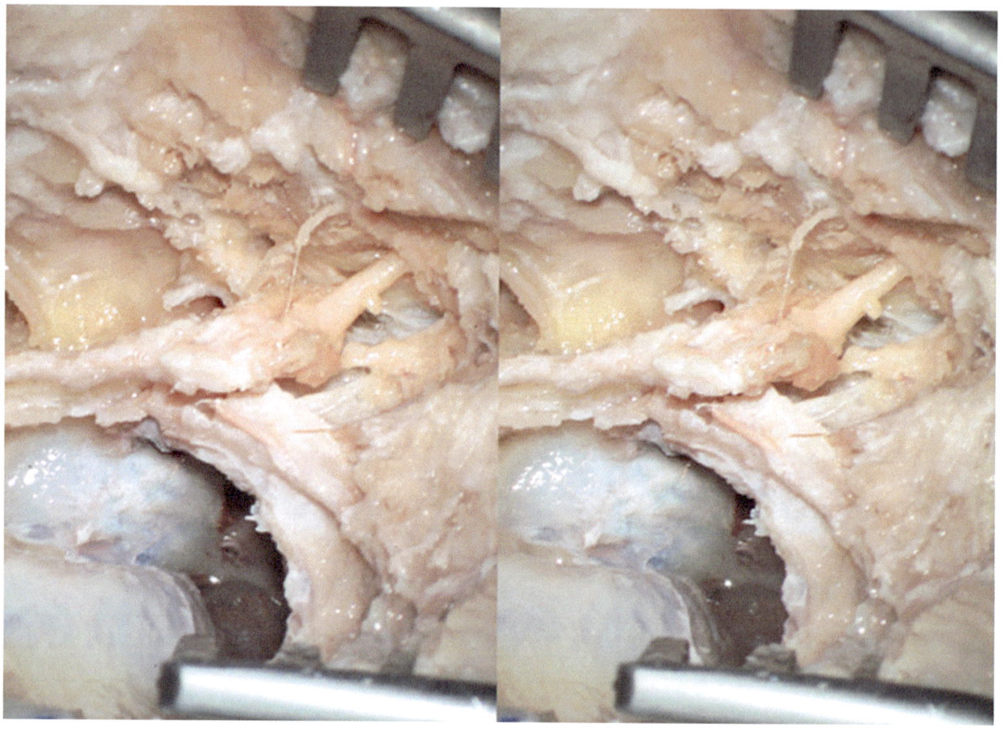

Fig. 8.20 Dissection of the facial nerve at the stylomastoid foramen level (right)
The connective tissue surrounding the stylomastoid foramen is tightly connected to the facial nerve and contains vasa vasorum. It can be used to fix the facial nerve in the parotid and protect its blood supply. Therefore, the facial nerve at the level of the stylomastoid foramen and the attached soft tissue should be dissected and re-routed anteriorly together
Instruments: ophthalmic scissors, ophthalmic forceps

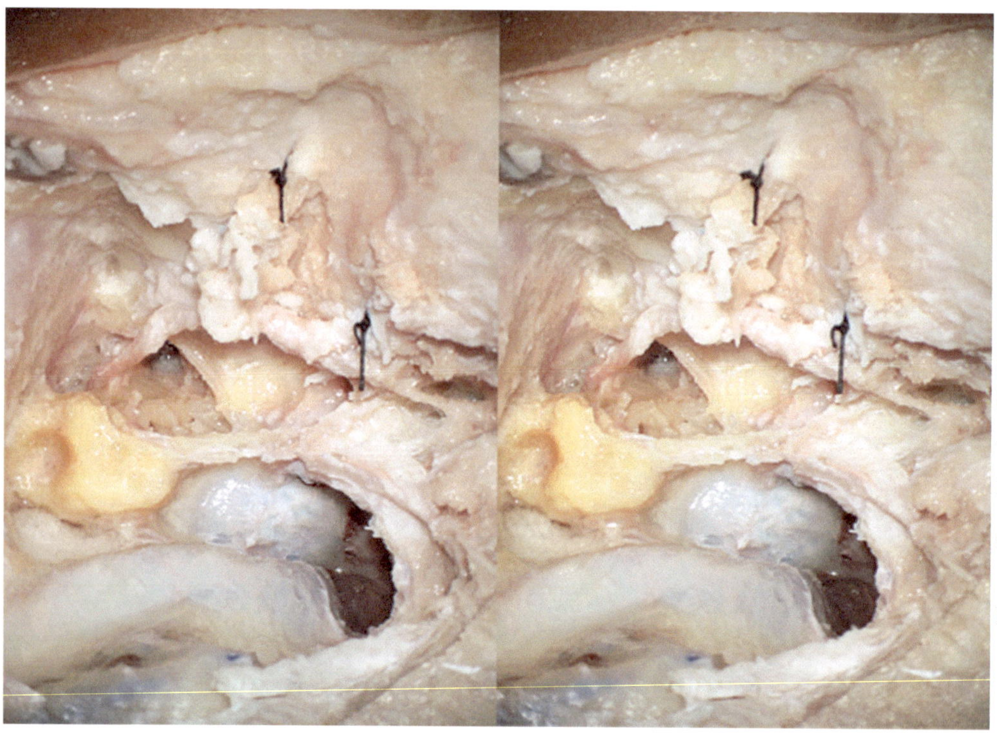

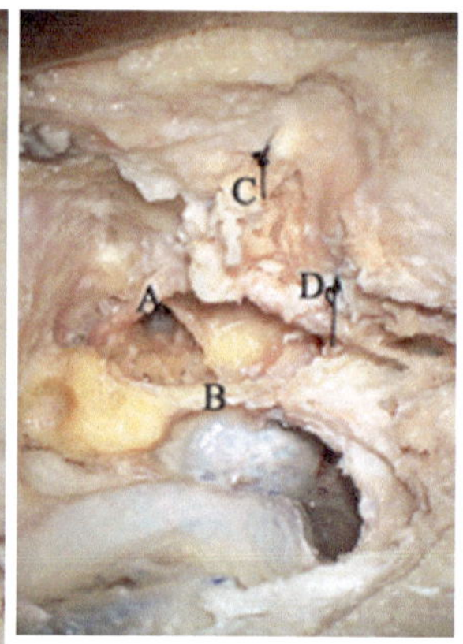

A. Rerouted part of the facial nerve
B. Fallopian canal (the remaining part)
C. Stylomastoid soft tissues are used to fix the facial nerve
D. Soft tissues surrounding the stylomastoid foramen are fixed in the anterior wall of the cavity

Fig. 8.21 Rerouting of the facial nerve (right)
Transfer the tympanic segment of the facial nerve to the newly formed bony groove anterolateral to the epitympanum. A tunnel is created in the tissues of the parotid gland, the mastoid segment of the facial nerve is transferred to the soft tissue tunnel, and the facial nerve is fixed to the anterior wall of the cavity using sutures. Then the soft tissues surrounding the facial nerve at the level of the stylomastoid foramen are sutured to the soft tissues of the anterior wall of the cavity, and anterior rerouting of the facial nerve is completed
Hints: (1) Do not penetrate or suture the facial nerve. (2) Ensure that the rerouted facial nerve is tension-free
Instruments: needle holder, round suture needle, suture

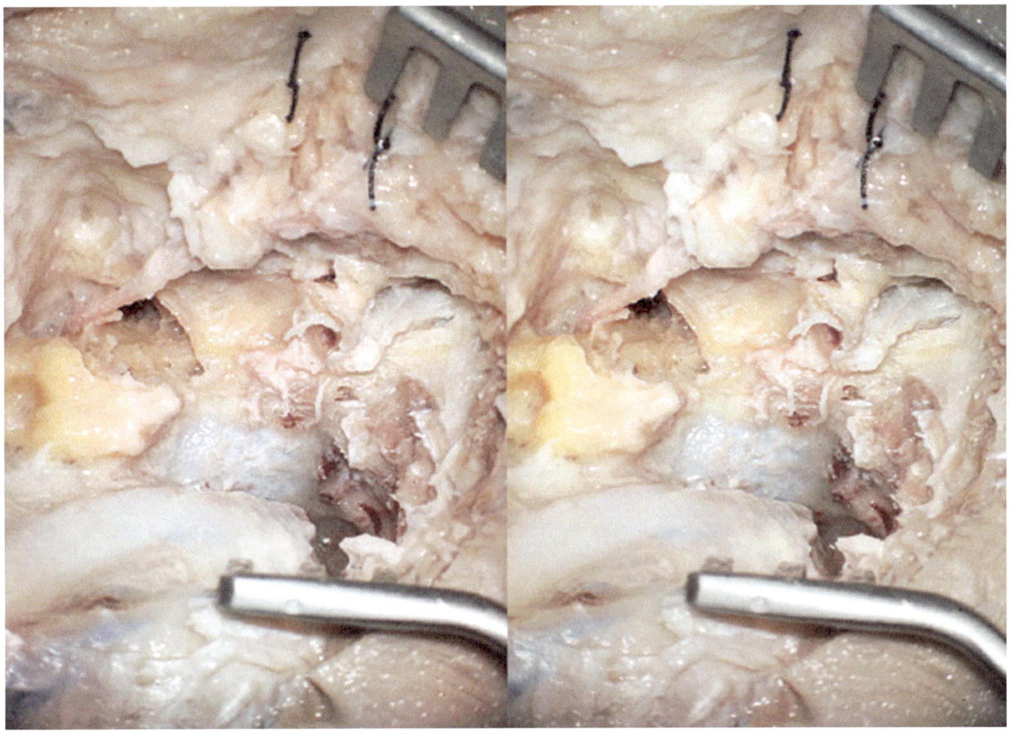

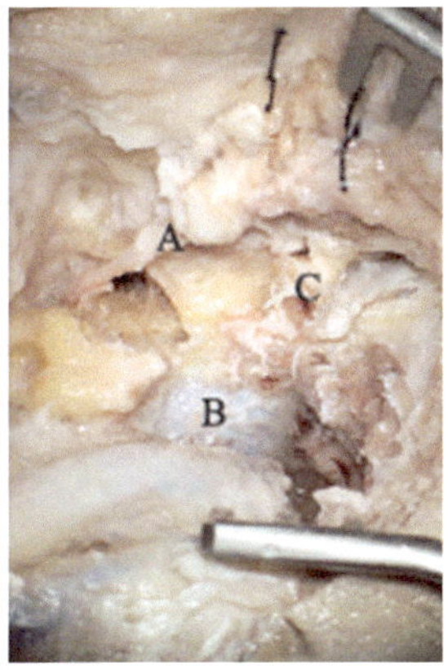

A. Rerouted part of the facial nerve
B. Jugular bulb
C. Styloid process

Fig. 8.22 Removing the fallopian canal and freeing the styloid process (right)
The remaining part of the fallopian canal is removed; the styloid process is explored with ophthalmic scissors; the bone in front of the stylomastoid foramen is drilled away with a medium-sized cutting bur; the root of the styloid process can be seen; the muscles of the styloid are resected and the styloid process is freed
Instruments: ophthalmic scissors, cutting bur

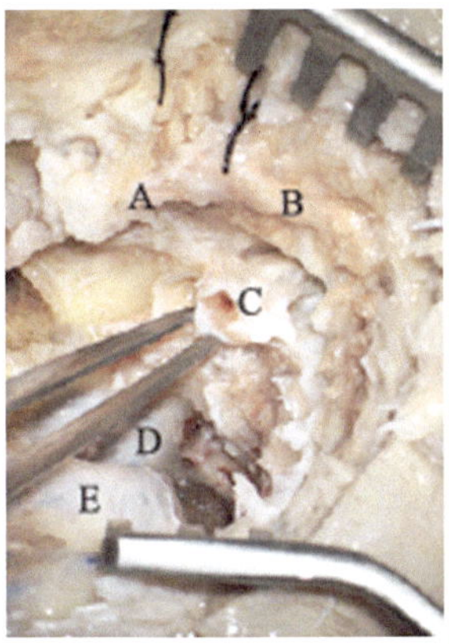

A. Rerouted part of the facial nerve
B. Main trunk of the extratemporal facial nerve
C. Styloid process
D. Jugular bulb
E. Sigmoid sinus

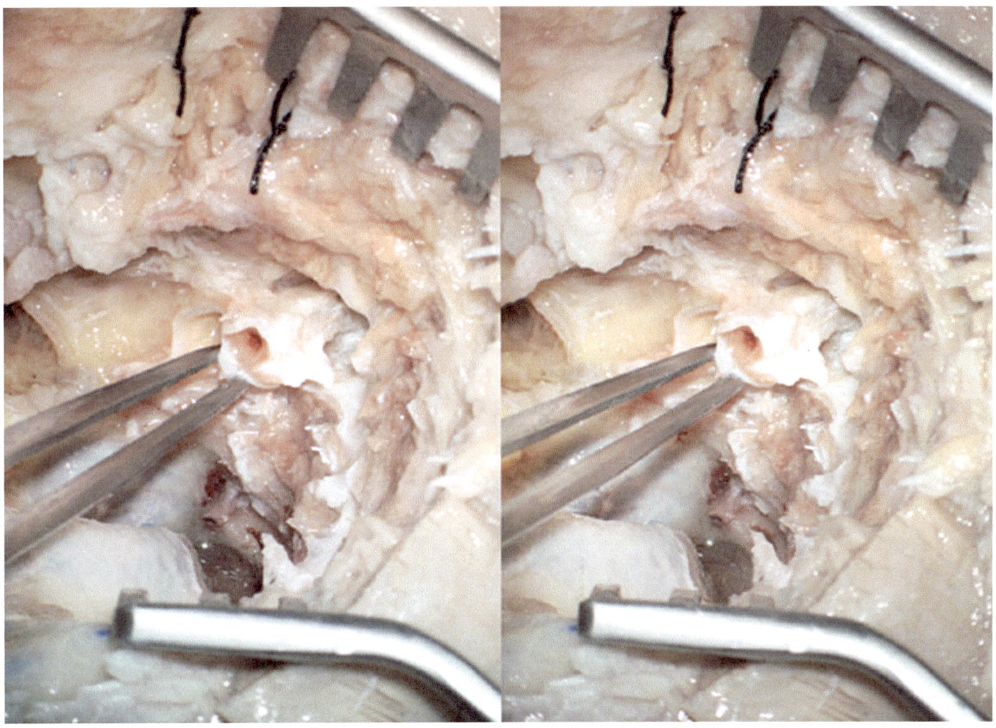

Fig. 8.23 Resection of the styloid process (right)
The freed styloid process is being held by non-toothed forceps; the bone marrow cavity is clearly visible
Instruments: non-toothed forceps

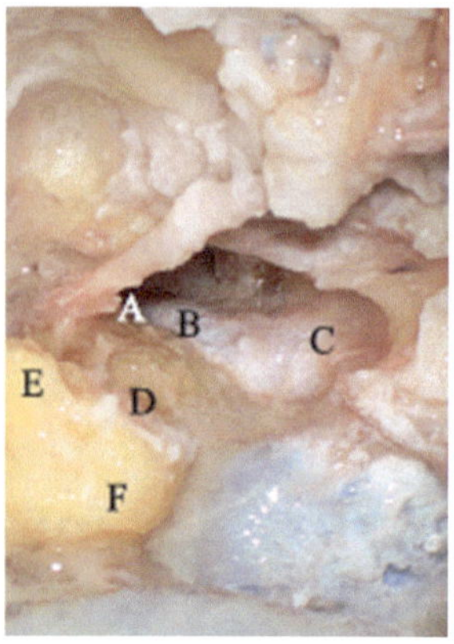

A. Remaining part of the Eustachian tube
B. Horizontal segment of the internal carotid artery
C. Vertical segment of the internal carotid artery
D. Round window niche
E. Lateral semicircular canal
F. Posterior semicircular canal

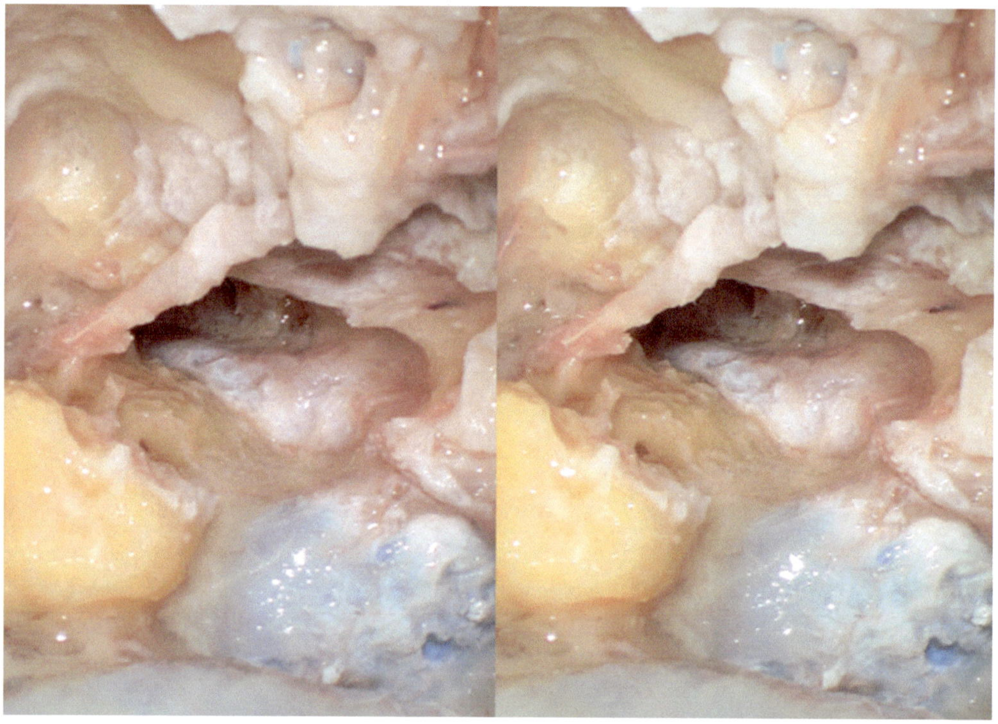

Fig. 8.24 Internal carotid artery canal (right)
The internal carotid artery enters the canal in the petrous portion of the temporal bone, curving and continuing as the horizontal segment anteroinferior to the cochlea, exiting the petrous bone anterior to the foramen lacerum, and then it curves superiorly on its way to the cavernous sinus. After removing the shell of bone anteroinferior to the cochlea and inferior to the Eustachian tube, the internal carotid artery is clearly visible
Instruments: medium-sized diamond burs

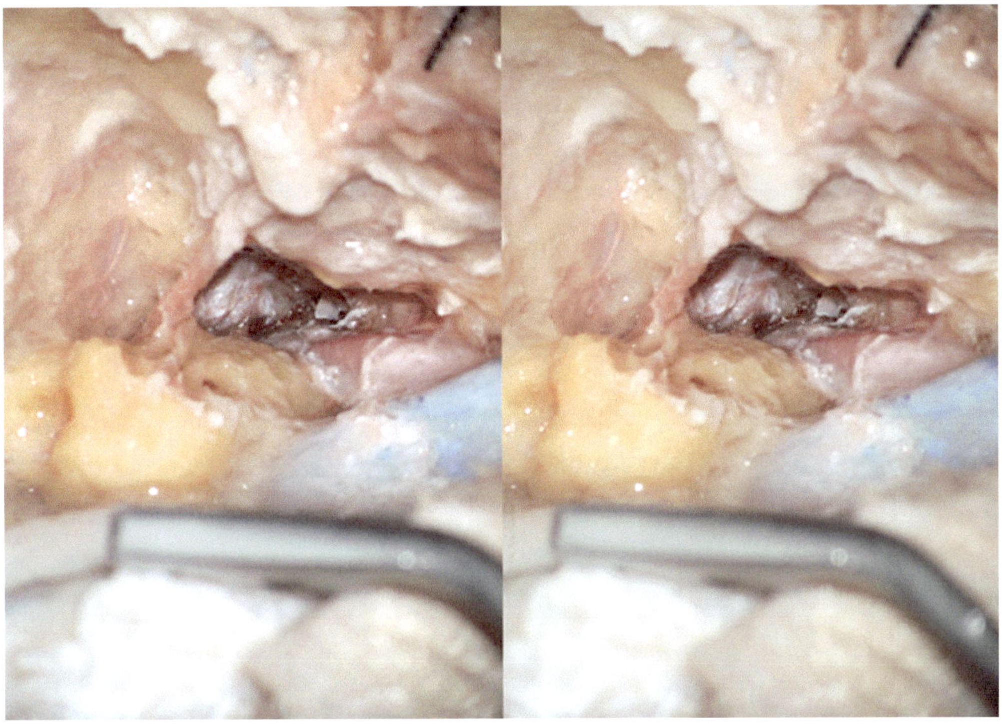

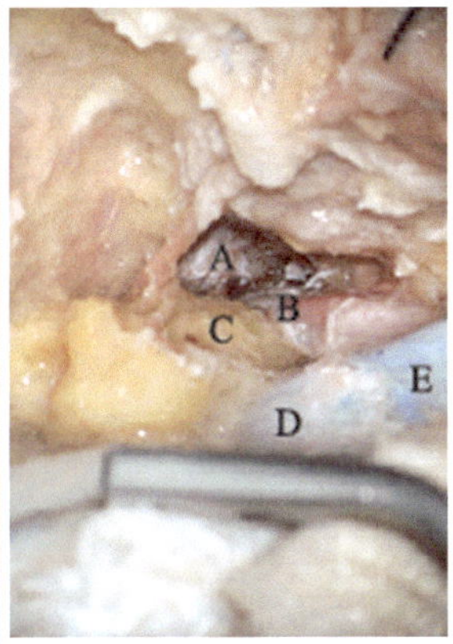

A. Middle cranial fossa dura
B. Horizontal segment of the internal carotid artery
C. Promontory
D. Jugular bulb
E. Internal jugular vein

Fig. 8.25 Horizontal segment of the internal carotid artery (right)
The bone anterosuperior to the horizontal segment of the internal carotid artery is removed with a medium-sized diamond bur to expose that section of the artery. *Hints: (1) The cochlea is closely related to the internal carotid artery; to avoid unnecessary opening of the cochlea, care should be taken not to drill the bone posterior to the internal carotid artery. (2) The horizontal segment of the internal carotid artery and the middle cranial fossa dura are separated by only a thin bony shell. To avoid injuring the middle fossa dura, drilling of the area superior to the horizontal segment of the internal carotid artery must be carried out very carefully. (3) The thin plate of bone separating the Eustachian tube from the internal carotid artery may be dehiscent for up to 5 mm in 2% of cases*
Instruments: medium-sized diamond burs

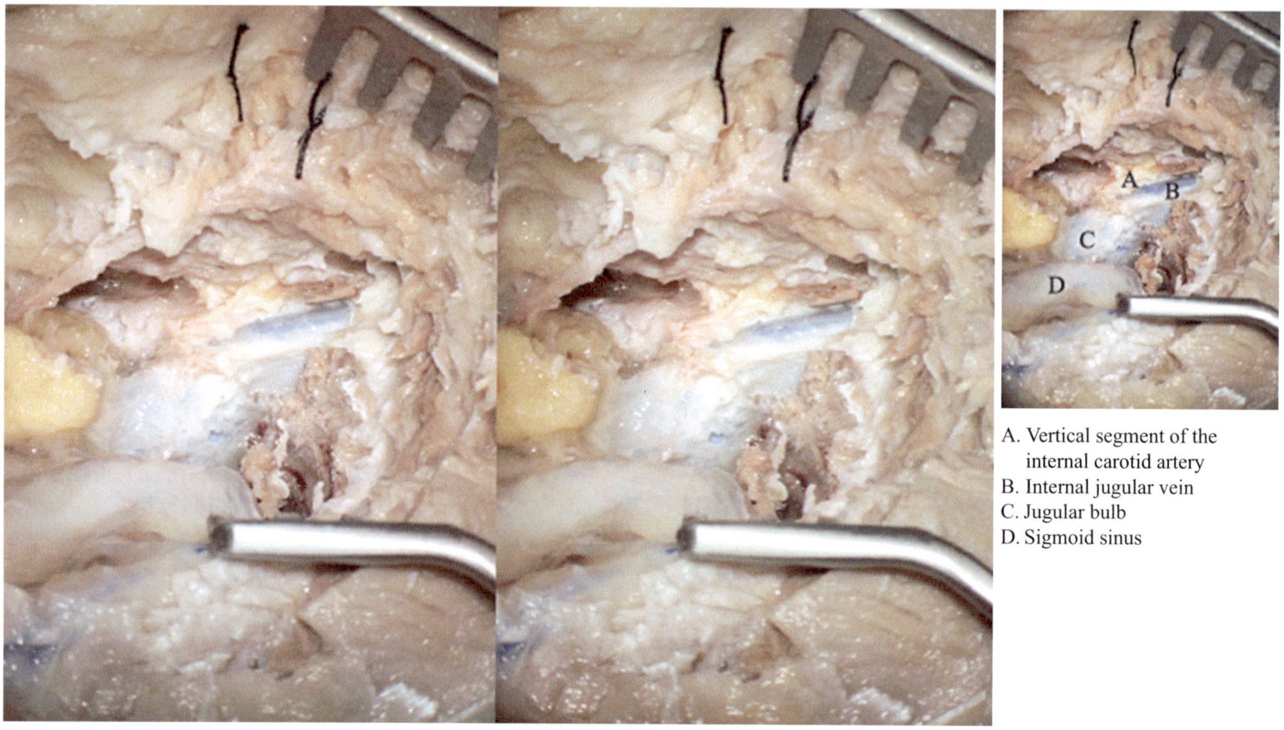

A. Vertical segment of the internal carotid artery
B. Internal jugular vein
C. Jugular bulb
D. Sigmoid sinus

Fig. 8.26 Internal jugular vein and vertical segment of the internal carotid artery (right)
The bone is removed down along the jugular bulb, the jugular foramen is opened, and the internal jugular vein is revealed. The bone anteromedial to the jugular bulb and along the direction of the vertical segment of the internal carotid artery is drilled away from superior to inferior layer by layer, exposing the vertical segment of the internal carotid artery. *Hints: Because of the close relationship between the carotid sheath and the skull base, it is difficult to separate. Dissection can be conducted along the long axes of the internal jugular vein and internal carotid artery, or the internal jugular vein and internal carotid artery can be separated in the neck (below the skull base) and traced superiorly*
Instruments: medium-sized diamond burs, ophthalmic scissors, ophthalmic forceps

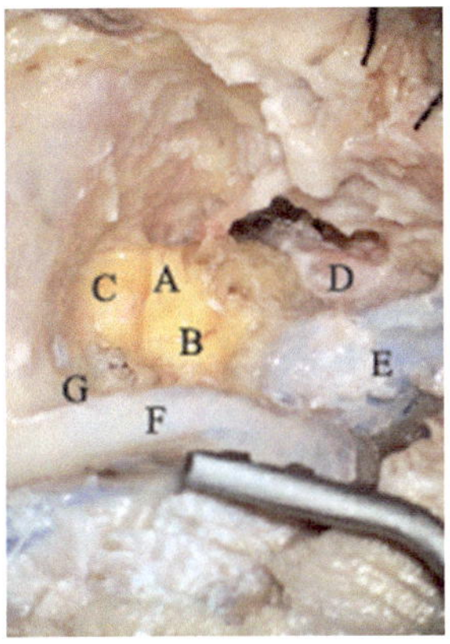

A. Lateral semicircular canal
B. Posterior semicircular canal
C. Superior semicircular canal
D. Internal carotid artery
E. Jugular bulb
F. Sigmoid sinus
G. Sinodural angle

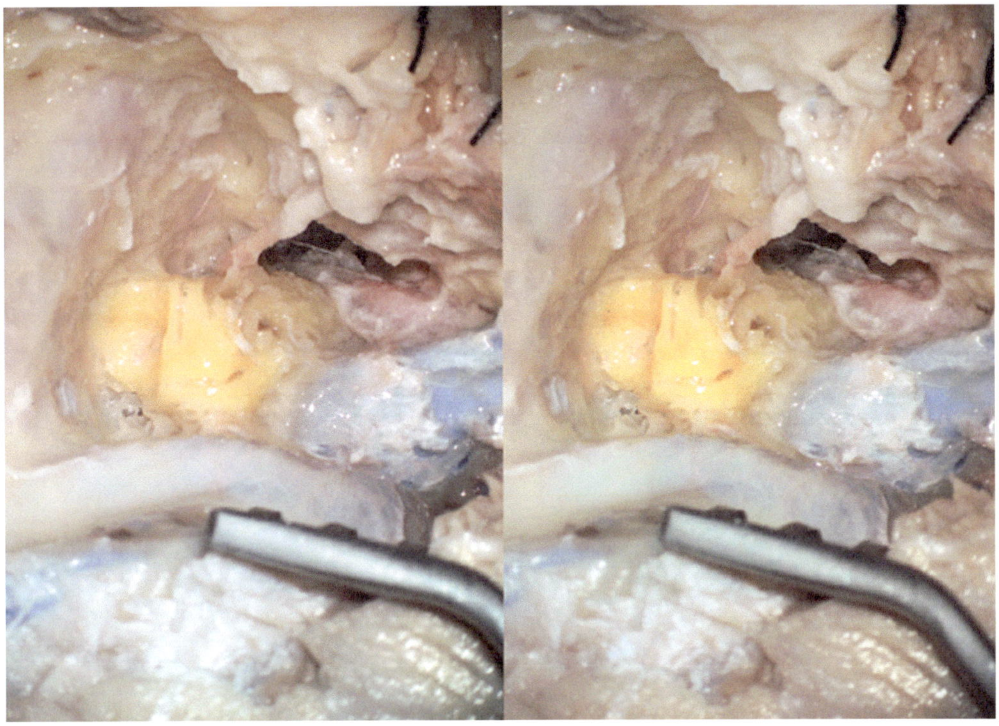

Fig. 8.27 Open the three semicircular canals (right)
A smaller diamond bur is used to drill the three semicircular canals until the "blue line" of semicircular canals can be seen. A right-angle hook is used to open the semicircular canals

Instruments: small-sized diamond burs, right-angle hook

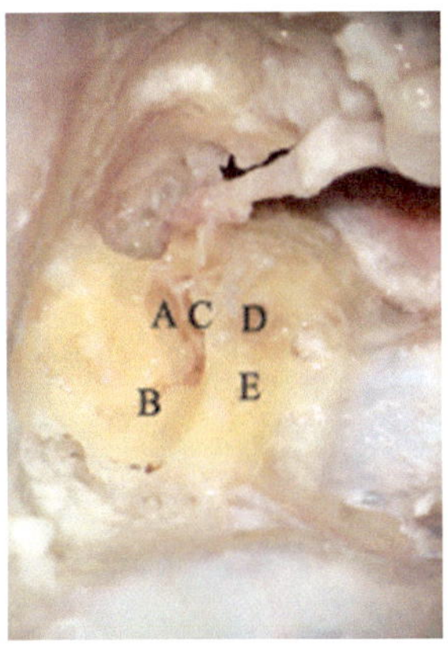

A. Ampulla of the lateral semicircular canal
B. Common crus
C. Stapes footplate and oval window
D. Round window membrane
E. Posterior semicircular canal

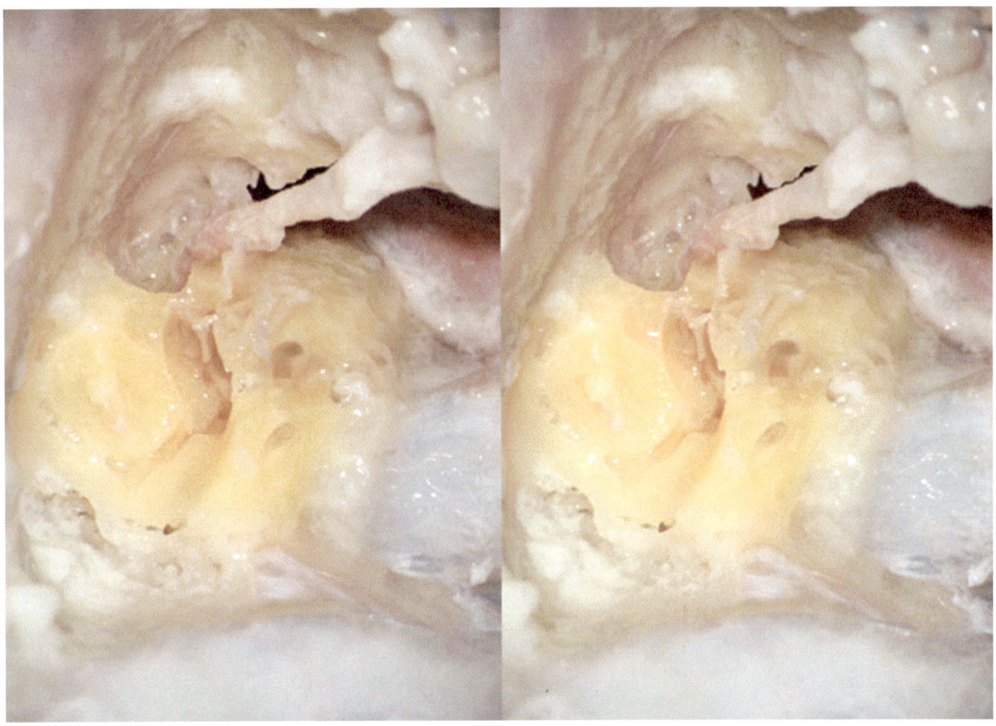

Fig. 8.28 Open the vestibule, exposing the common crus (right)
The lateral wall of the vestibule, and the superior and lateral semicircular canals are drilled out. The vestibule is opened, and the stapes are kept intact. The stapes footplate and the annular ligament in the oval window can be seen. The common crus can be traced along the superior and posterior semicircular canals. The opening where the common crus enters the vestibule can be seen. *Hints: (1) In the infratemporal fossa approach type A, only the superstructure of the stapes is removed so as not to cause injury to the inner ear. (2) To display the anatomy of the temporal bone comprehensively, dissection of the jugular foramen area and the trans labyrinthine approach is carried out simultaneously*
Instruments: small- and medium-sized diamond burs

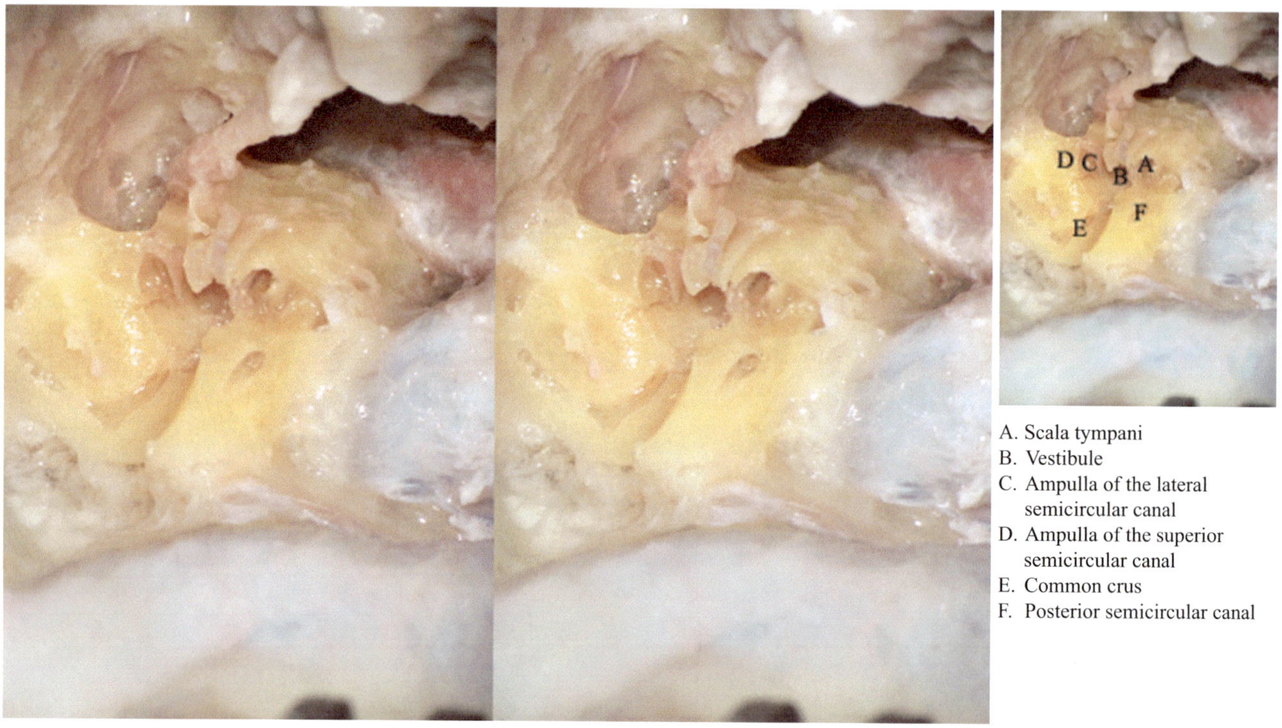

A. Scala tympani
B. Vestibule
C. Ampulla of the lateral semicircular canal
D. Ampulla of the superior semicircular canal
E. Common crus
F. Posterior semicircular canal

Fig. 8.29 Open the basal turn of the cochlea (right)
The vestibule receives the perilymph in the scala vestibuli, and the ductus reuniens connects the saccule and the membranous cochlear canal. The scala vestibuli, the scala tympani, and the bony spiral lamina can be seen after opening the lateral wall of the vestibule and the round window membrane
Instruments: small-sized diamond burs, right-angle hook

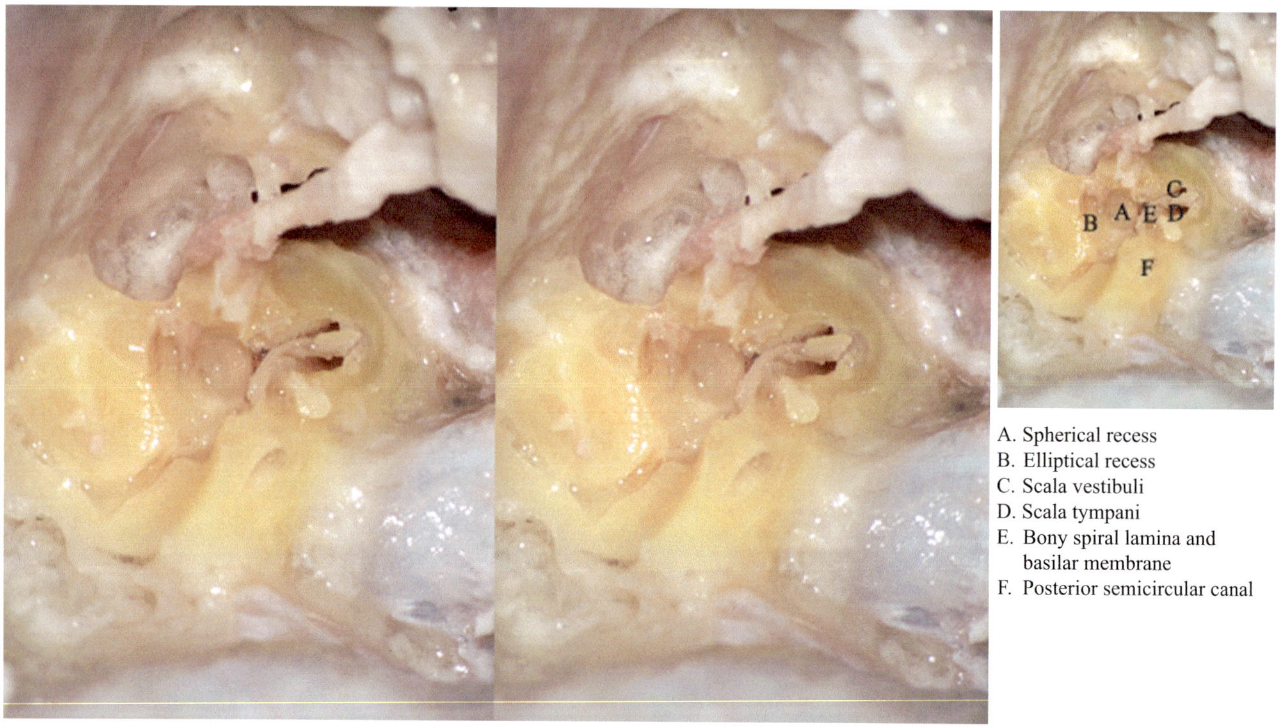

A. Spherical recess
B. Elliptical recess
C. Scala vestibuli
D. Scala tympani
E. Bony spiral lamina and basilar membrane
F. Posterior semicircular canal

Fig. 8.30 Medial wall of the vestibule and the basal turn of the cochlea (right)
There are two recesses in the medial wall of the vestibule: the anteroinferior spherical recess and the posterosuperior elliptical recess. Between them is the crest of the vestibule. The cochlea is located anteroinferior to the vestibule and the basal turn of the cochlea projects into the tympanic cavity, forming the bulge of the promontory
Instruments: small-sized diamond burs, right-angle hook

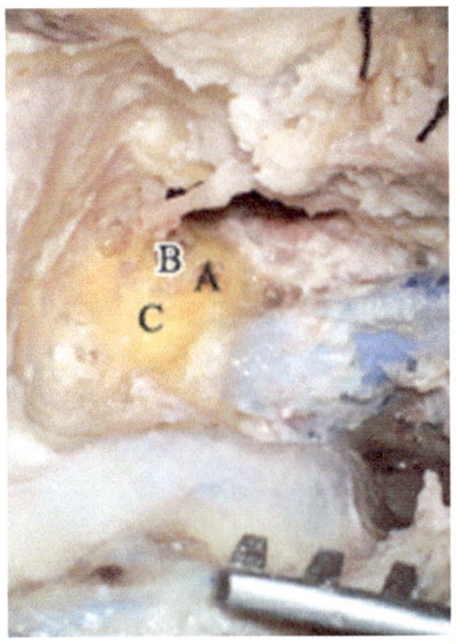

A. Basal turn of the cochlea
B. Apical and middle turn of the cochlea
C. Medial wall of the vestibule

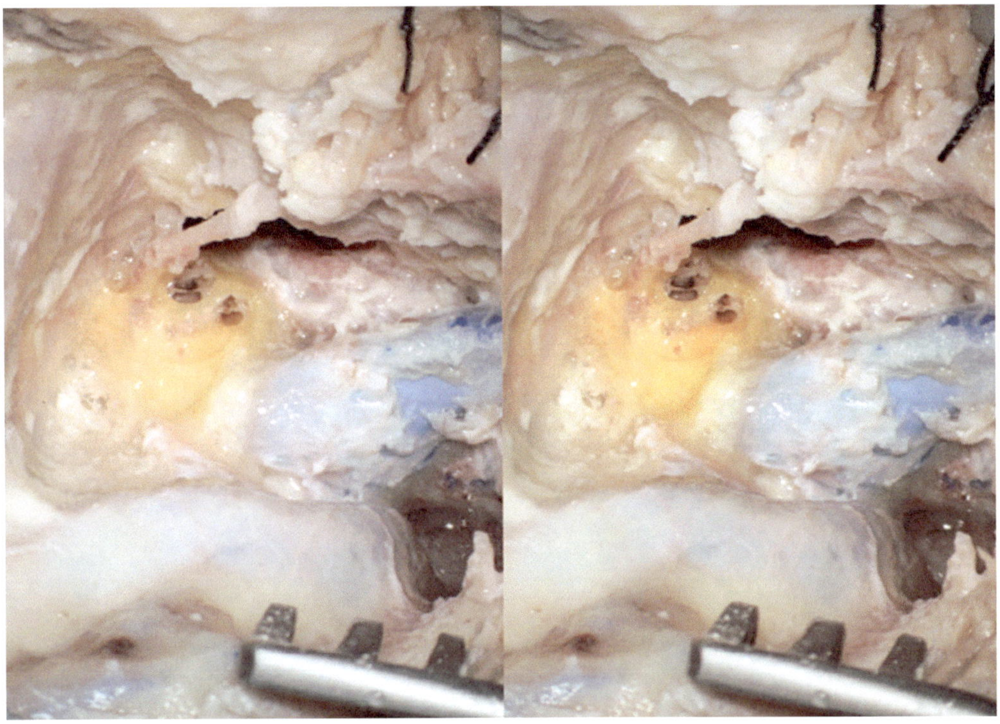

Fig. 8.31 Resection of the vestibule, opening the cochlea (right)
The lateral wall of the cochlea is drilled out along its direction of rotation. The right-sided cochlea is shown in the picture above; the direction of its rotation is the same as the index finger direction of a fist made with the right hand. The internal auditory canal (IAC) is located medial to the vestibule, and the medial wall of the vestibule is part of the lateral wall of the IAC
Instruments: medium- and small-sized diamond burs

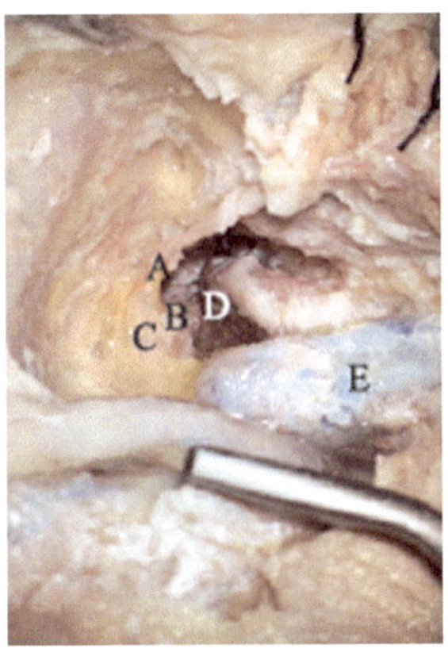

A. Labyrinthine segment of the facial nerve
B. End of the cochlear nerve
C. IAC
D. Horizontal segment of the internal carotid artery
E. Internal jugular vein

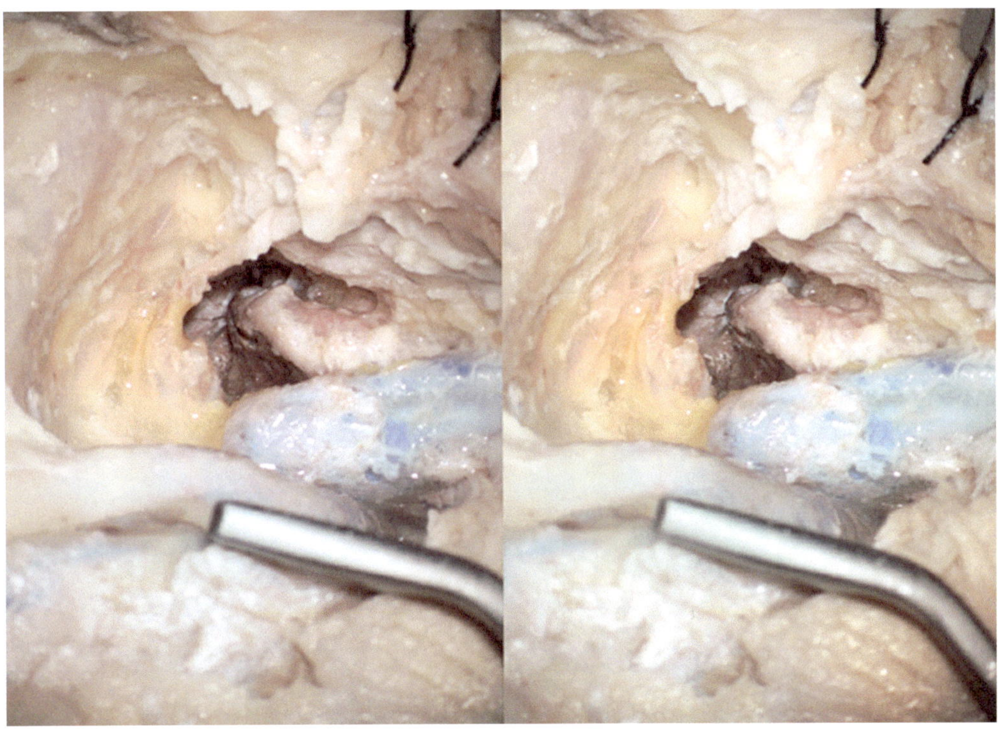

Fig. 8.32 Skeletonized IAC and the internal carotid artery (right)
Once the cochlea has been drilled out, the labyrinthine segment of the facial nerve can be seen. The bone posterior to the horizontal segment of the internal carotid artery is drilled away to expose that part of the artery. The IAC is skeletonized after bone medial to the vestibule has been removed. The labyrinthine segment of the facial nerve runs above the upper borders of the cochlea and the vestibule. The internal carotid artery is located anteroinferior to the basal turn of the cochlea, separated from it by a thin plate of bone
Instruments: medium-sized diamond burs

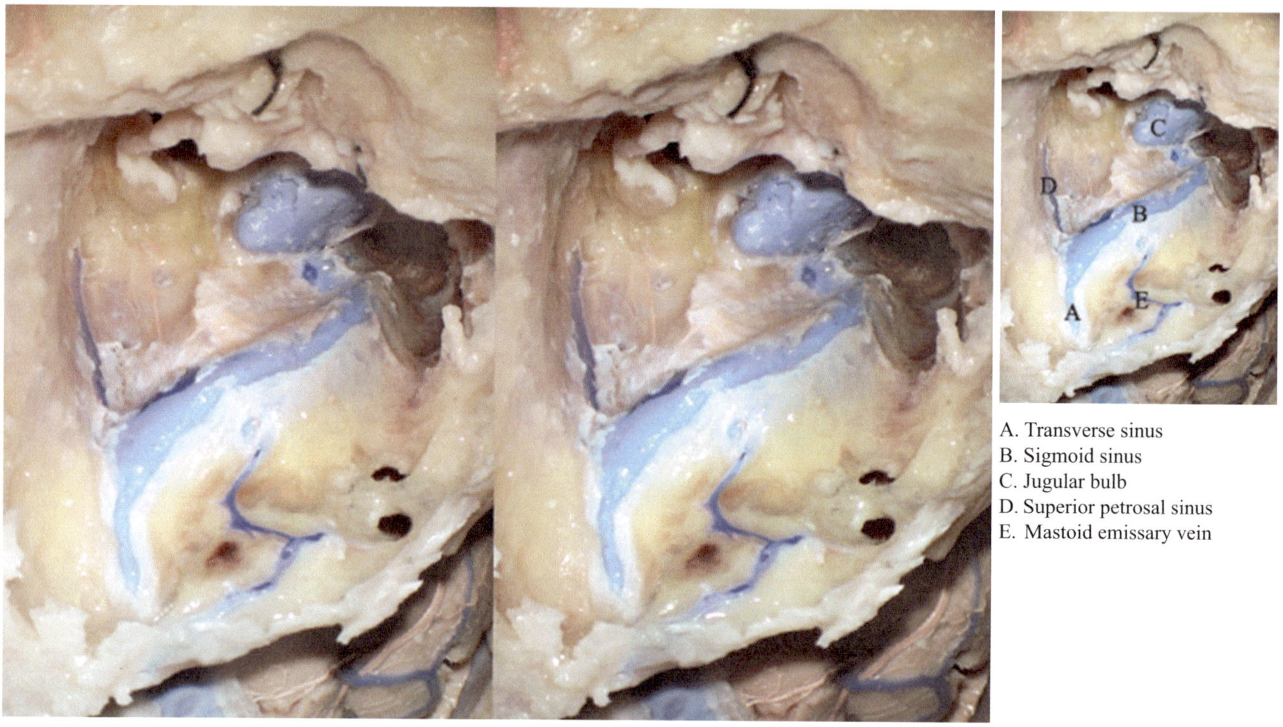

A. Transverse sinus
B. Sigmoid sinus
C. Jugular bulb
D. Superior petrosal sinus
E. Mastoid emissary vein

Fig. 8.33 Transverse sinus, sigmoid sinus, and jugular bulb (right)
The sigmoid sinus is located between the inner and outer layers of the dura. It starts at the end of the transverse sinus and expands at its lower end to form the jugular bulb. The sigmoid sinus receives the superior petrosal sinus at its origin and the mastoid emissary vein in its mid portion; the inferior petrosal sinus opens into the jugular bulb and/or internal jugular vein. A view of the vascular cavity containing blue material (a mixture of self-curing denture material and oil paint) after removal of the bone covering the sigmoid sinus and transverse sinus and the vessel wall
Instruments: large-sized cutting burs, medium-sized diamond burs

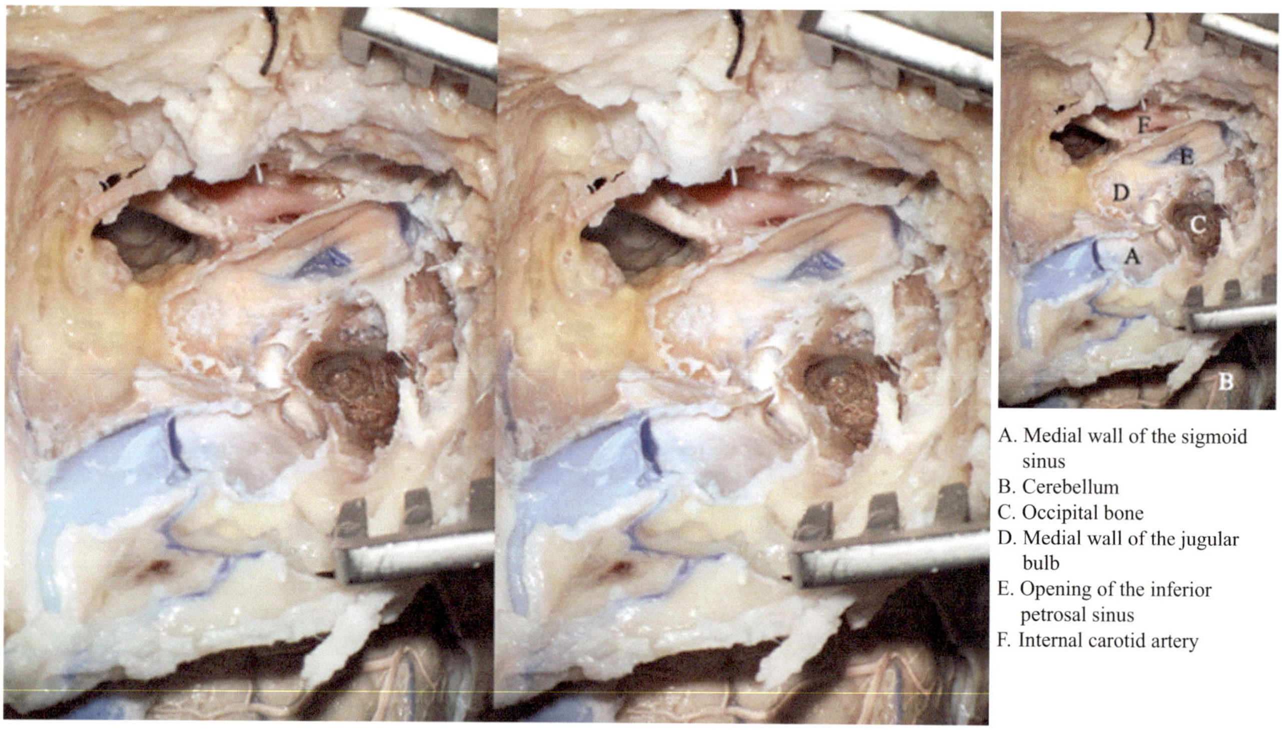

A. Medial wall of the sigmoid sinus
B. Cerebellum
C. Occipital bone
D. Medial wall of the jugular bulb
E. Opening of the inferior petrosal sinus
F. Internal carotid artery

Fig. 8.34 Medial wall of the sigmoid sinus and the jugular bulb (right)
The jugular bulb and the filling in the lower end of the sigmoid sinus are removed to show the inner wall of the blood vessel. The jugular bulb can be seen receiving the inferior petrosal sinus
Instruments: medium-sized cutting burs

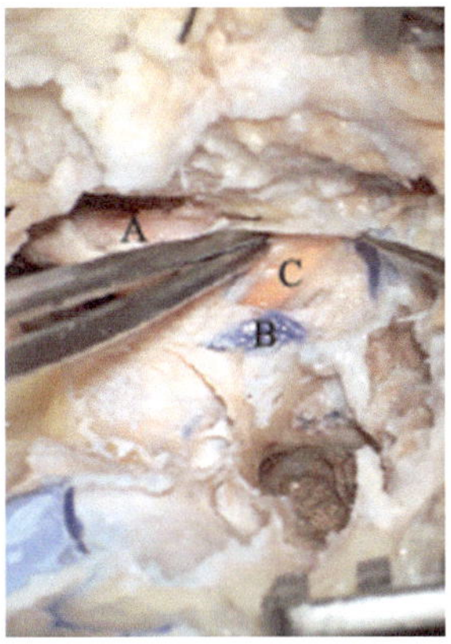

A. Internal carotid artery
B. Inferior petrosal sinus
C. Glossopharyngeal nerve

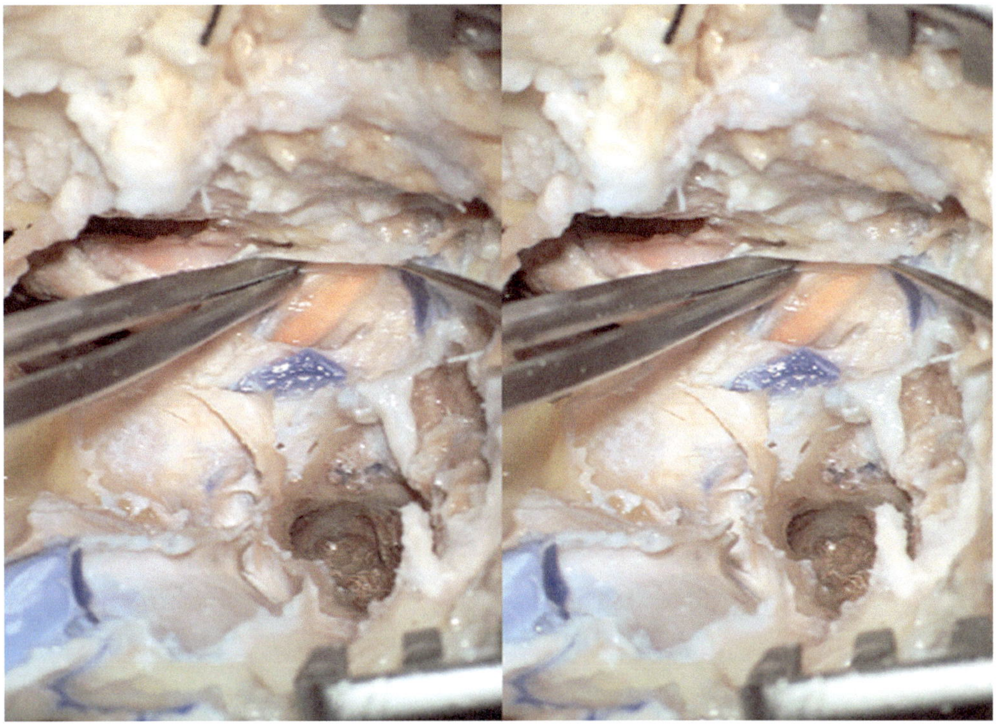

Fig. 8.35 Glossopharyngeal nerve (right)
The glossopharyngeal nerve is a mixed nerve, exiting the brainstem from the posterior olivary sulcus and accompanying the vagus nerve to enter the jugular foramen. The glossopharyngeal nerve exits the skull via the jugular foramen medial to the jugular bulb and anterior to the inferior petrosal sinus. The tympanic nerve, the carotid sinus branch, and the tonsillar branches are the main branches of the glossopharyngeal nerve. The vagus nerve also exits the skull via the jugular foramen, along with the accessory nerve, posterior to the inferior petrosal sinus
Instruments: ophthalmic scissors, septal raspatory, straight micro-needle

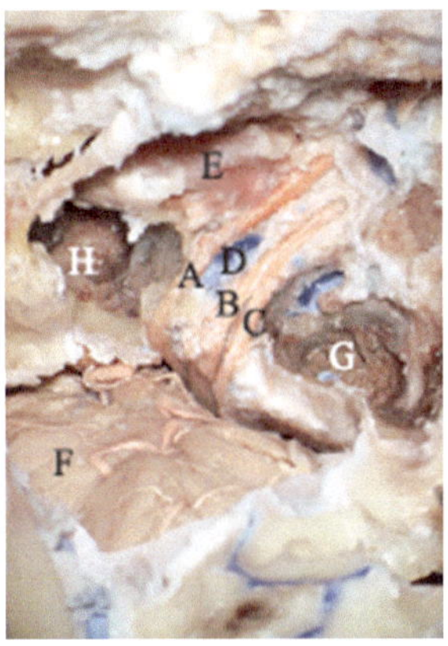

A. Glossopharyngeal nerve
B. Vagus nerve
C. Accessory nerve
D. Inferior petrosal sinus
E. Internal carotid artery
F. Cerebellum
G. Occipital bone
H. Petrous apex

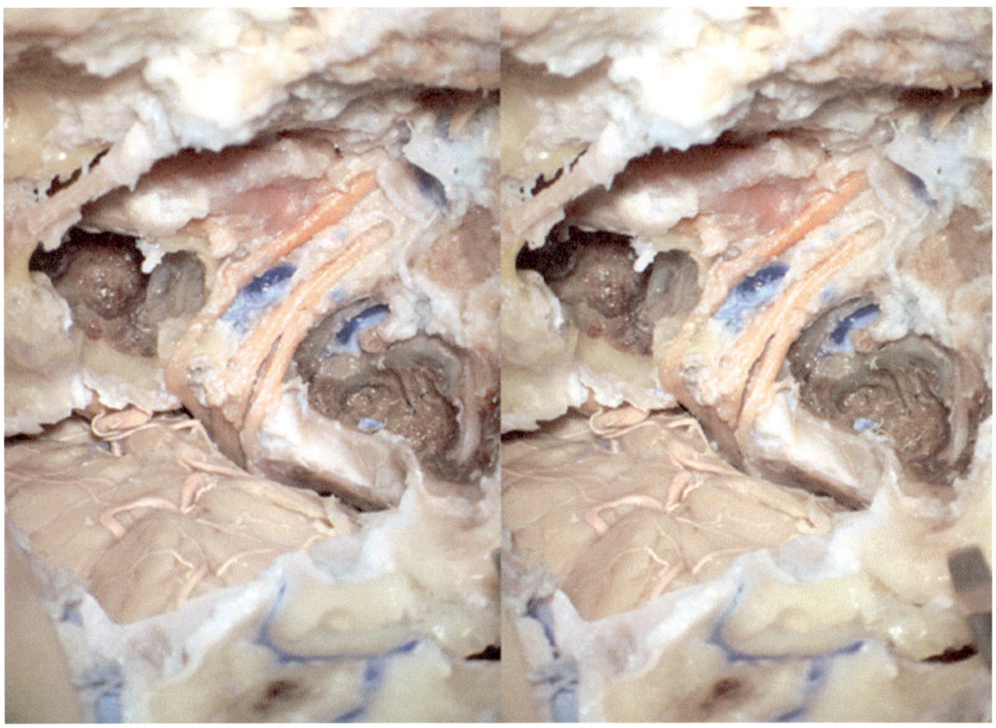

Fig. 8.36 Lower cranial nerves (right)
The lower cranial nerves are visible after removal of the posterior fossa dura and the medial wall of the jugular bulb. The vagus nerve together with the accessory nerve can be seen exiting the skull via the jugular foramen, posterior to the inferior petrosal sinus, and medial to the jugular bulb. The glossopharyngeal nerve exits the skull anterior to the inferior petrosal sinus

Suggested Reading

Dai P, Han D-y, Cousins VC, et al. Stereo operative atlas of micro ear surgery. Singapore: Springer; 2017.

Sanna M, Saleh E, Khrais T, et al. Atlas of microsurgery of the lateral skull base. 2nd ed. New York: Thieme; 2008.

Sharma R, Sirohi D. Proximal and distal facial nerve exploration during superficial parotidectomy. J Maxillofac Oral Surg. 2010;9(2):150–4.

Stereoscopic Virtual Anatomy of Temporal Bone

9

Sha-sha Huang, Yi-chen Wan, De-jun Zhang, Xiao-hong Li, Chang Guo, and Yue-shuai Song

The original data used in this chapter comes from *3-D Viewer of the Human Temporal Bone Mode* (Haobing Wang et al., Eaton-Peabody Lab, Massachusetts Eye & Ear Infirmary), and permission for the secondary development has been obtained from Dr. Haobing Wang.

Virtual Anatomy: Transcanal Approach

Yi-chen Wan and Sha-sha Huang

S.-s. Huang (✉) · C. Guo
College of Otolaryngology Head and Neck Surgery, Chinese PLA General Hospital, Beijing, China

Y.-c. Wan
Department of Otolaryngology Head and Neck Surgery, Peking University International Hospital, Beijing, China

D.-j. Zhang
Department of Otolaryngology Head and Neck Surgery, The Second Hospital of Jilin University, Changchun, China

X.-h. Li
Department of Otolaryngology Head and Neck Surgery, Beijing Children's Hospital, Capital Medical University, Beijing, China

Y.-s. Song
Department of Otolaryngology Head and Neck Surgery, Beijing Friendship Hospital, Capital Medical University, Beijing, China

P. Dai et al. (eds.), *Stereoscopic Anatomical Atlas of Ear Surgery*, https://doi.org/10.1007/978-981-16-0927-5_9

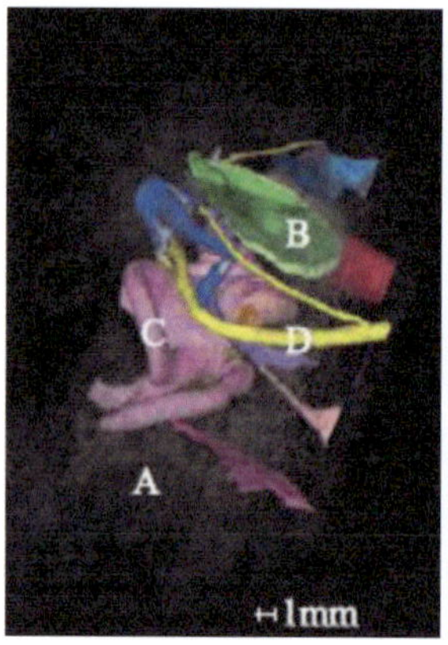

A. Temporal bone (semi-transparent)
B. Tympanic membrane
C. Lateral semicircular canal
D. Mastoid segment of the facial nerve

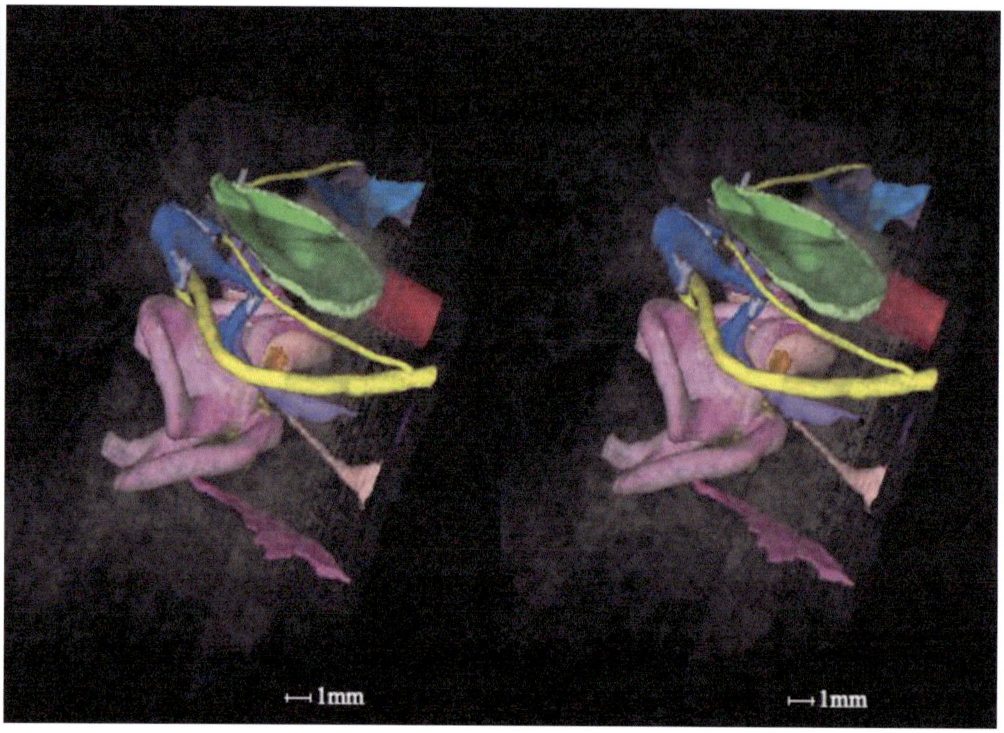

Fig. 9.1 Scenography of temporal bone (right, lateral)
Simulating a postauricular approach; observe the spatial relationships between the different structures of the temporal bone

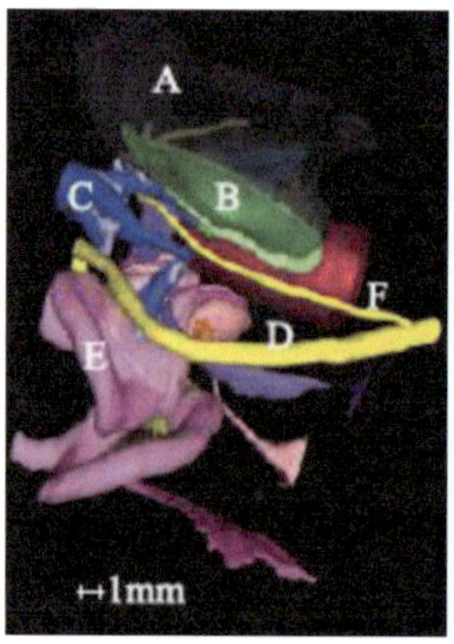

A. Bony part of the EAC
B. Tympanic membrane
C. Incus
D. Mastoid segment of the facial nerve
E. Lateral semicircular canal
F. Chorda tympani

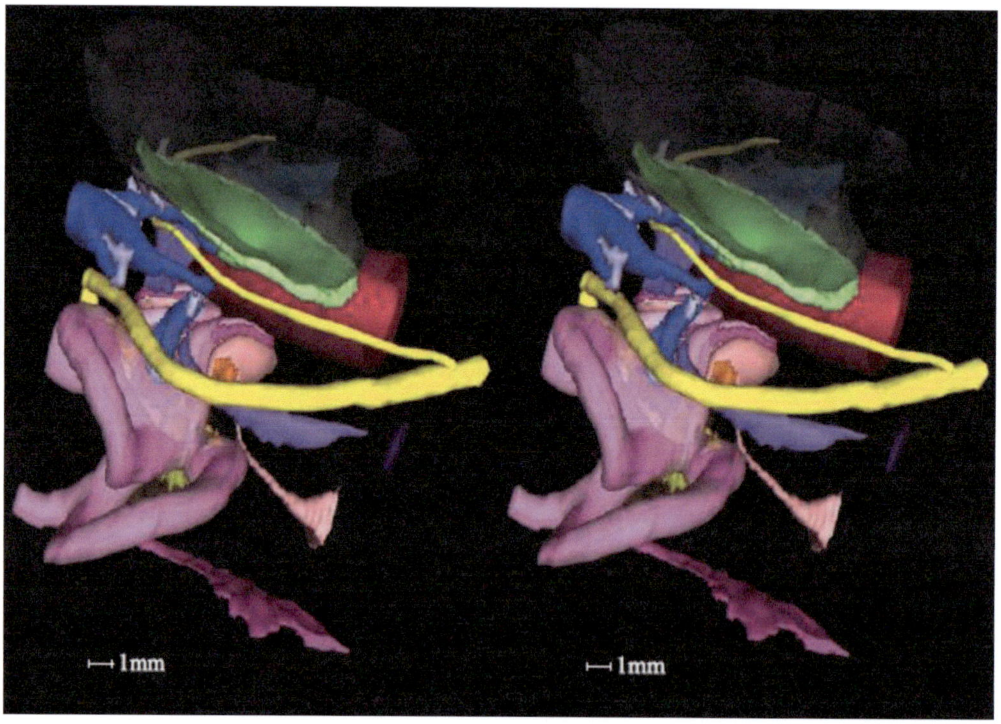

Fig. 9.2 Part of temporal bone removed (right)
Remove part of the temporal bone with the inner structures preserved, so the bony part of the external auditory canal (EAC), tympanic membrane, chorda tympani, and ossicles can be revealed. The posterior tympanotomy opening into the facial recess is a triangular space bounded anteriorly by the chorda tympani, and posteriorly by the mastoid segment of the facial nerve. Due to the proximity of the chorda tympani and the posterior wall of the EAC, the latter needs to be drilled down to a thin layer to give a better exposure of the facial recess

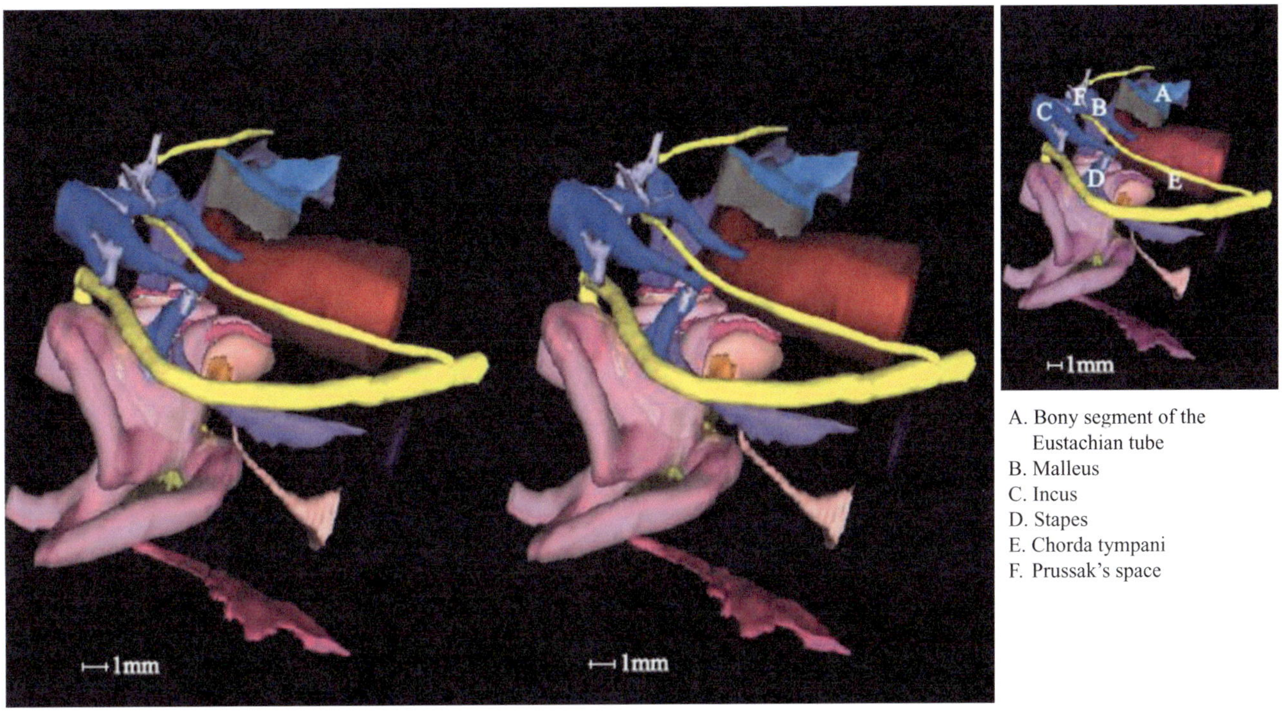

A. Bony segment of the Eustachian tube
B. Malleus
C. Incus
D. Stapes
E. Chorda tympani
F. Prussak's space

Fig. 9.3 Tympanic membrane and bony part of the EAC removed (right)
Remove the tympanic membrane and bony part of the EAC to reveal the three ossicles. The bony segment of the Eustachian tube (lateral 1/3) is located superiorly in the anterior wall of the tympanic cavity, while the semicanal for the tensor tympani muscle is superior to it and the internal carotid artery (ICA) is inferior to it. Prussak's space, also known as the superior recess of the tympanic membrane, is a space between the lateral process of the malleus, neck of the malleus, lateral ligament of the malleus, and pars flaccida of the tympanic membrane, and is a site predisposed to the formation of cholesteatoma

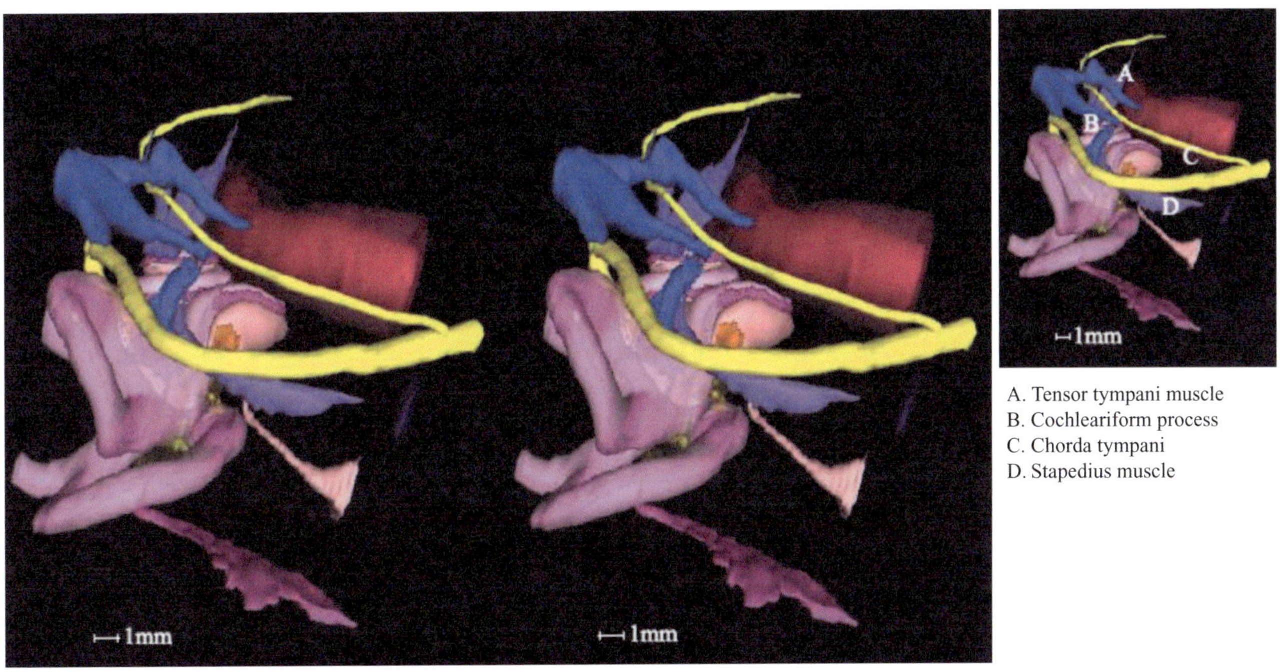

A. Tensor tympani muscle
B. Cochleariform process
C. Chorda tympani
D. Stapedius muscle

Fig. 9.4 Tympanic membrane and bony part of the EAC removed (right)
The tensor tympani muscle resides in its own semicanal. The tensor tympani tendon passes through the cochleariform process, at approximately 90° and attaches to the upper part of the handle of the malleus. The stapedius muscle, which is innervated by the stapedius branch of the facial nerve, is located deep in the bony canal medial to the facial nerve. The tendon of the stapedius muscle enters the tympanic cavity through the pyramidal eminence and attaches to the neck of the stapes. The cochleariform process, pyramidal eminence, and the facial nerve are closely related; the former two structures are almost always located in the same position and are thus important landmarks for locating the facial nerve during surgery

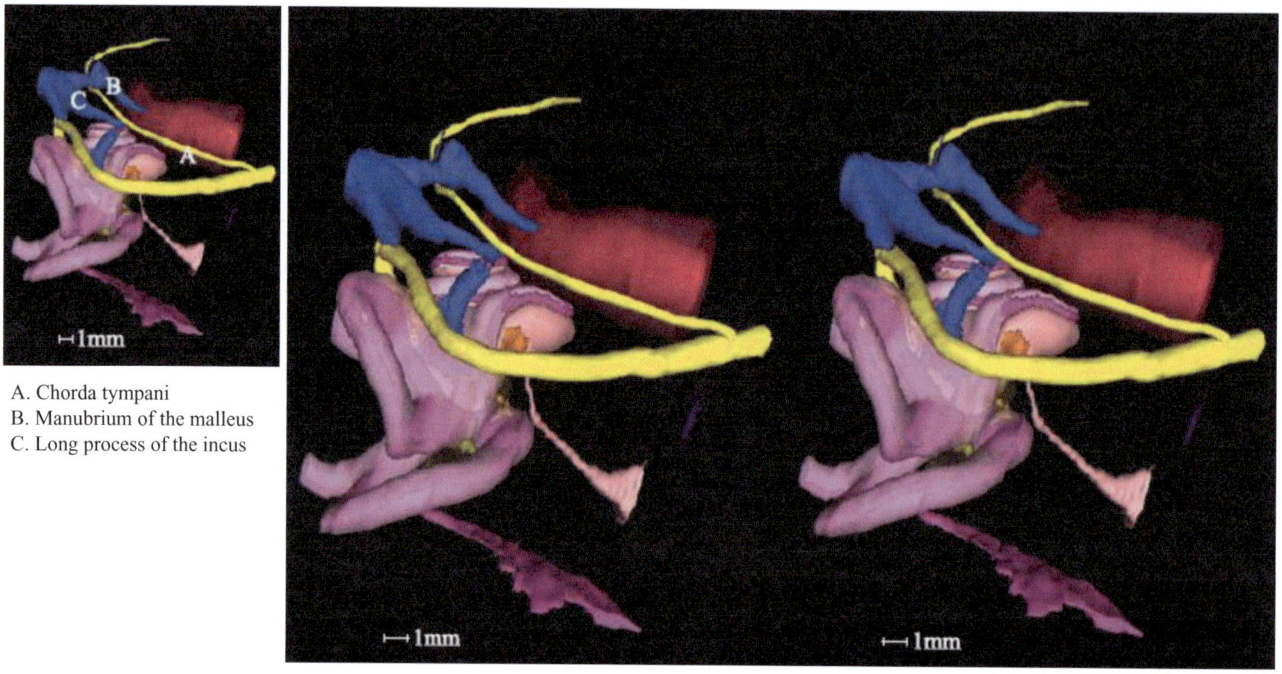

A. Chorda tympani
B. Manubrium of the malleus
C. Long process of the incus

Fig. 9.5 Stapedius muscle and tensor tympani muscle removed (right)
The chorda tympani is a branch given off by the facial nerve in the lower half of the mastoid segment, usually 6 mm or so before the facial nerve reaches the stylomastoid foramen. The chorda tympani runs up and forward to pass through its posterior canaliculus into the middle ear space. It leaves the canaliculus above the tympanic ring, crossing forward through the tympanic cavity between the manubrium of the malleus and the long process of the incus and leaves the tympanic cavity via its anterior canaliculus (medial part of the petrotympanic fissure) in the anterior wall of the tympanic cavity to enter the infratemporal fossa. Gustatory fibers of the chorda tympani transmit taste stimuli from the anterior 2/3 of the tongue, while its parasympathetic fibers innervate the sublingual and submandibular glands

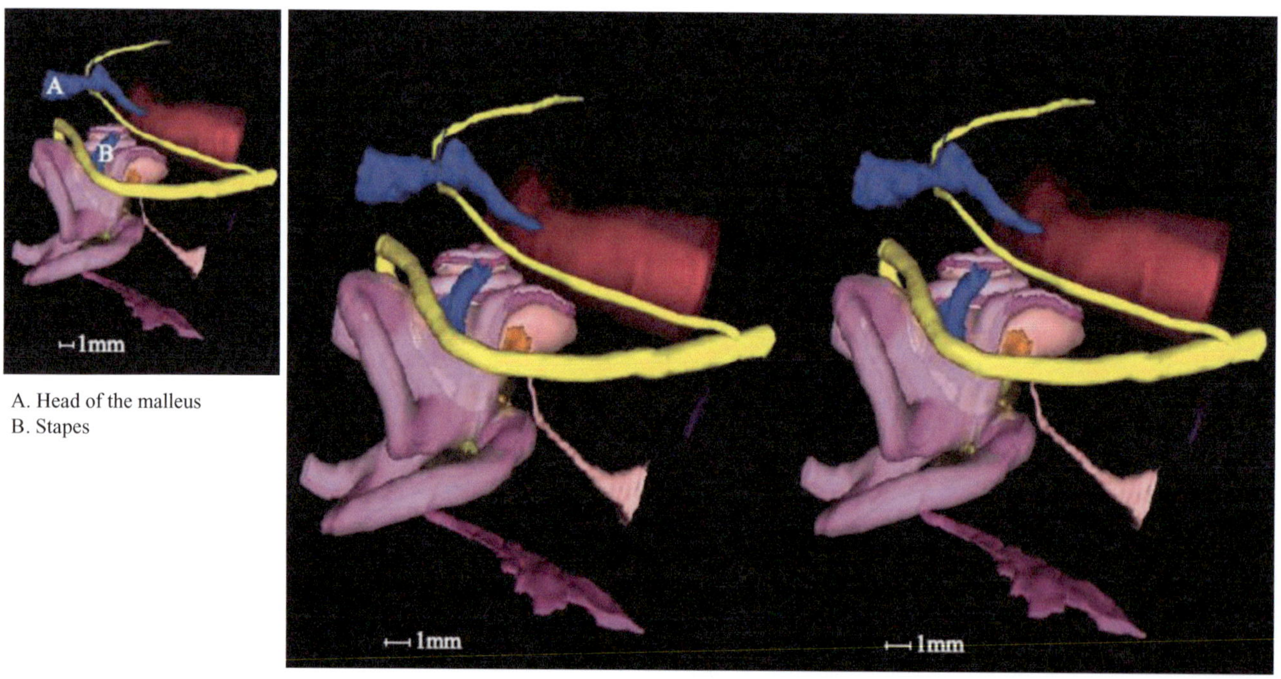

A. Head of the malleus
B. Stapes

Fig. 9.6 Incus removed (right)
The head of the malleus and the body of the incus articulate at the incudomalleal joint. The short process of the incus resides in the incudal fossa. The end of the long process of the incus is called the lenticular process and forms the incudostapedial joint with the head of the stapes

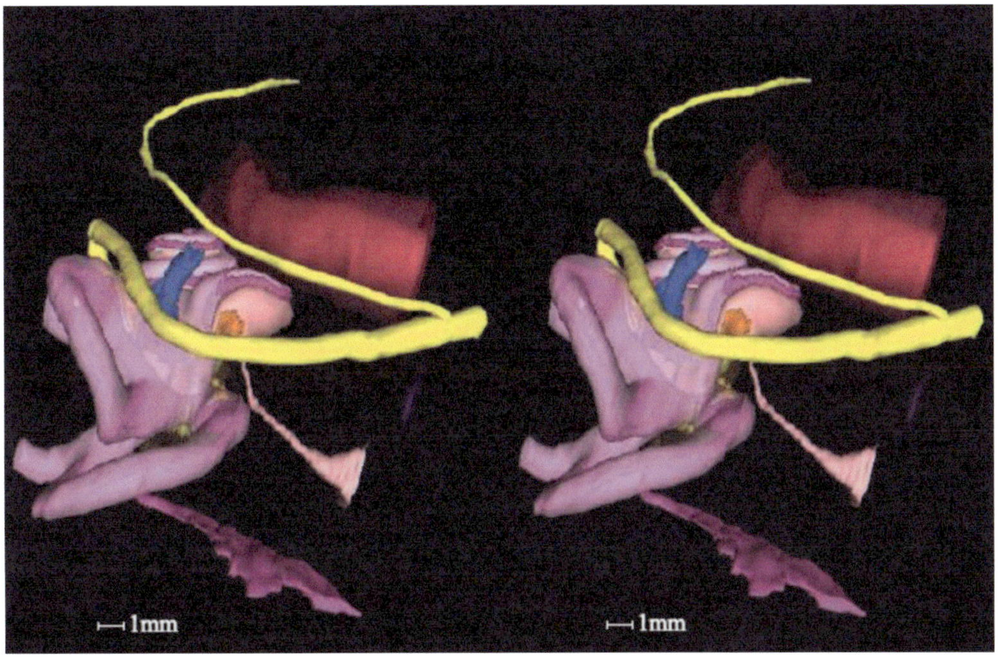

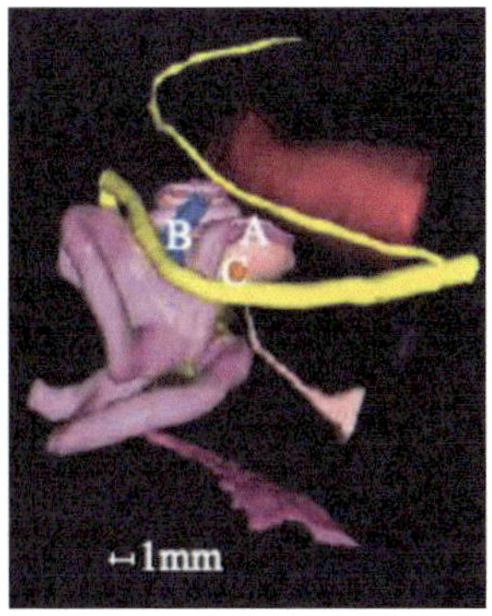

A. Promontory
B. Stapes
C. Round window

Fig. 9.7 Malleus removed (right)
When the malleus is removed, the full course of tympanic segment and geniculate ganglion of the facial nerve are exposed

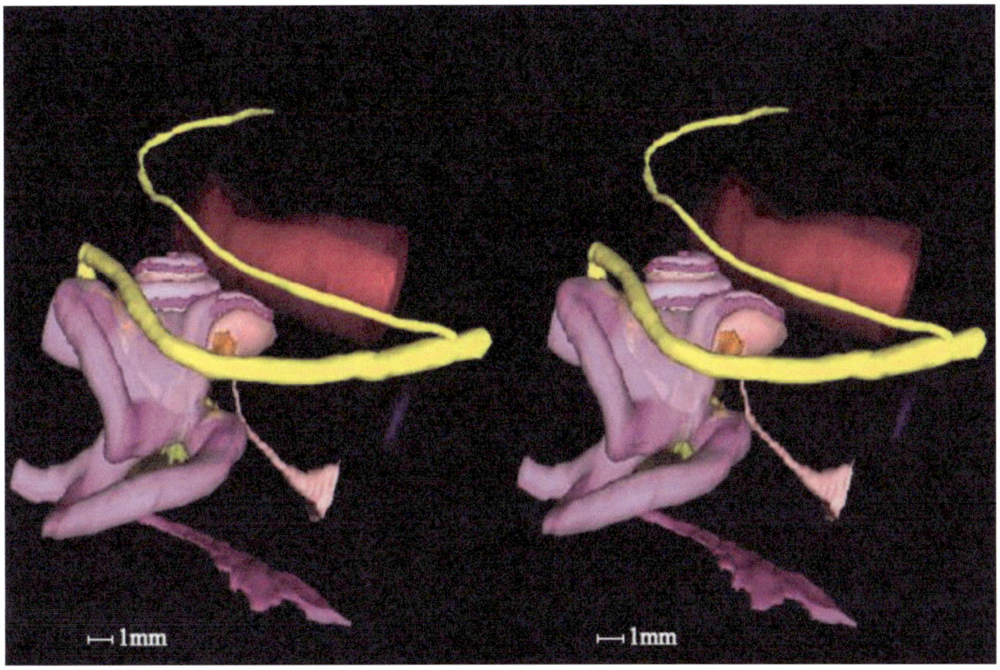

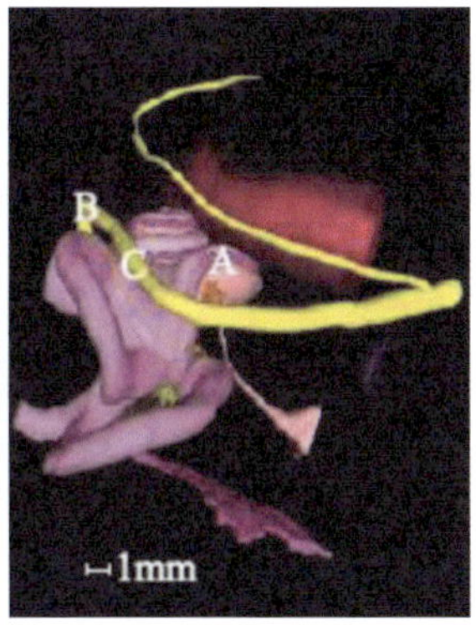

A. Basal turn of the cochlea
B. Geniculate ganglion of the facial nerve
C. Tympanic (horizontal) segment of the facial nerve

Fig. 9.8 Stapes removed (right)
The entire ossicular chain is eliminated when the stapes is removed. The part protruding from the basal turn of the cochlea into the tympanic cavity is called the promontory. The small depression posterior-superior to the promontory is the oval window, and the structure posterior to the promontory is the round window

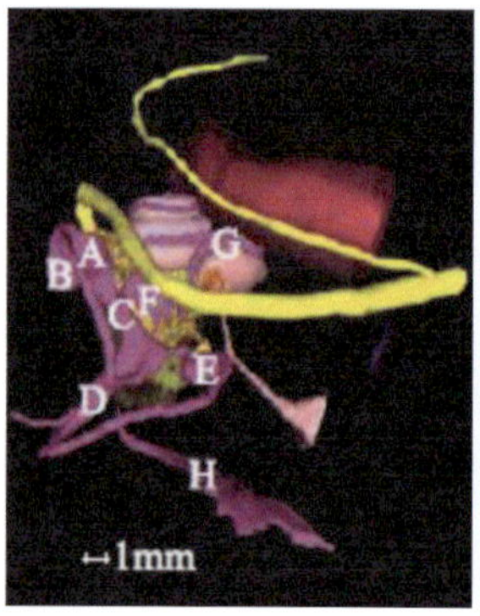

A. Ampulla of the lateral semicircular canal
B. Ampulla of the superior semicircular canal
C. Utricle
D. Common crus
E. Ampulla of the posterior semicircular canal
F. Saccule
G. Cochlear duct
H. Endolymphatic duct and the endolymphatic sac

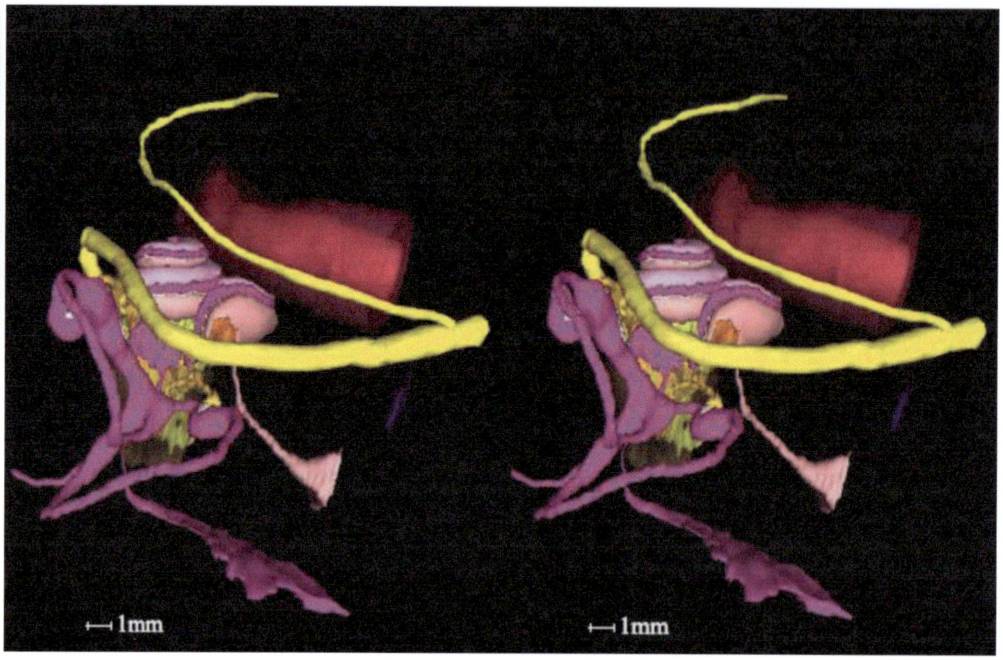

Fig. 9.9 Bony semicircular canals and vestibule removed (right)
The labyrinthine component of the inner ear is divided into the osseous labyrinth and the membranous labyrinth. Once the osseous semicircular canals and the bony wall of the vestibule are removed, the membranous labyrinth, including the saccule and utricle, are exposed. The cochlear duct is also called the scala media, and it nests between the scala vestibuli and scala tympani. The J-shaped endolymphatic duct (the long limb is adjacent to the endolymphatic sac, while the short limb is in proximity with the vestibule) sits deep to the common crus, connecting the endolymphatic sac to the saccule and utricle

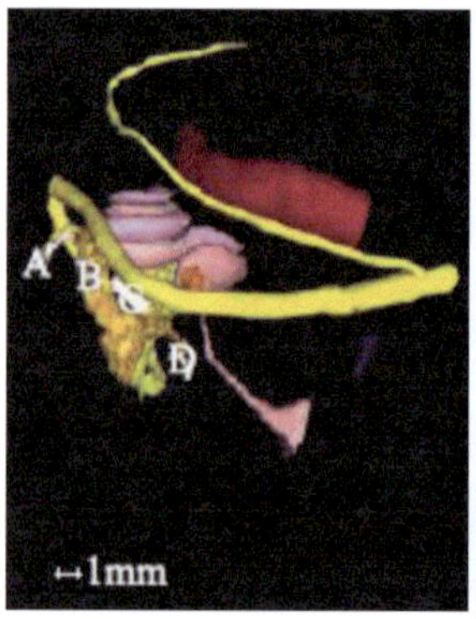

A. Nerve terminal distributed to the ampullae of the superior and lateral semicircular canals
B. Macula of the utricle
C. Macula of the saccule
D. Nerve terminal distributed to the ampulla of the posterior semicircular canal

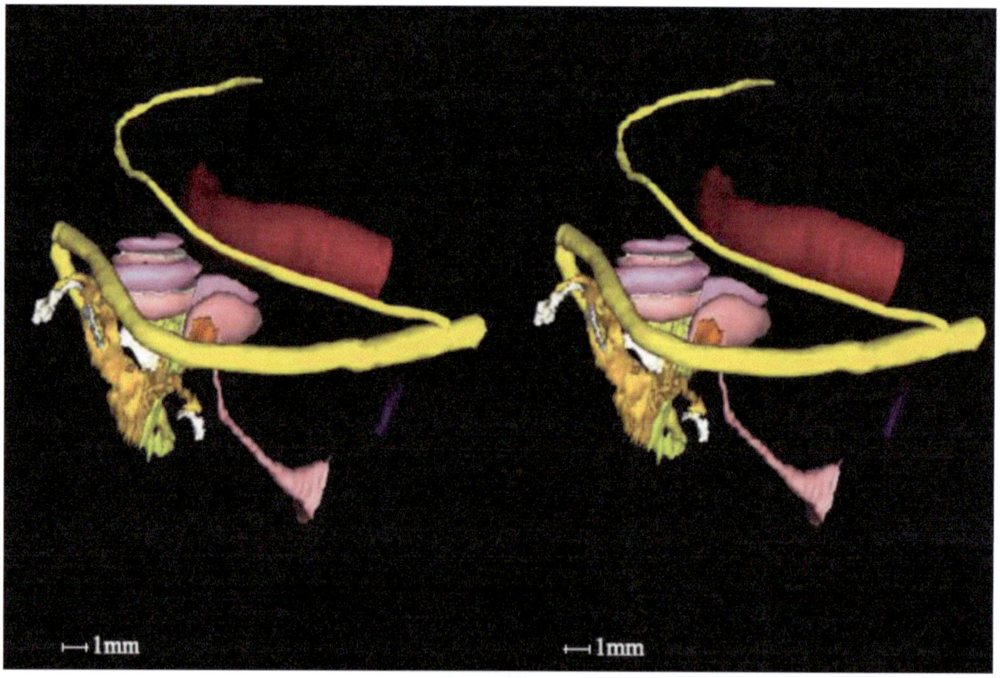

Fig. 9.10 Membranous labyrinth removed (right)
After removing the membranous labyrinth, the vestibular nerve endings, which innervate the membranous labyrinth, can be observed. The superior vestibular nerve endings dominate the ampullae of the superior and lateral semicircular canal as well as the macula of the utricle, and the inferior vestibular nerve endings innervate the posterior semicircular canal and the macula of the saccule

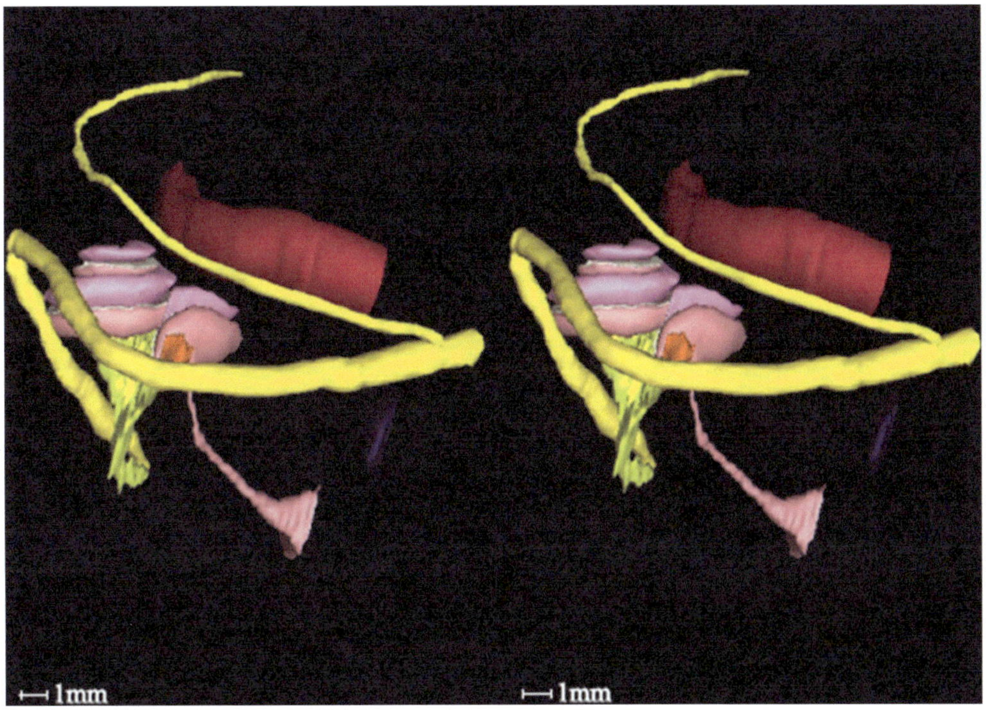

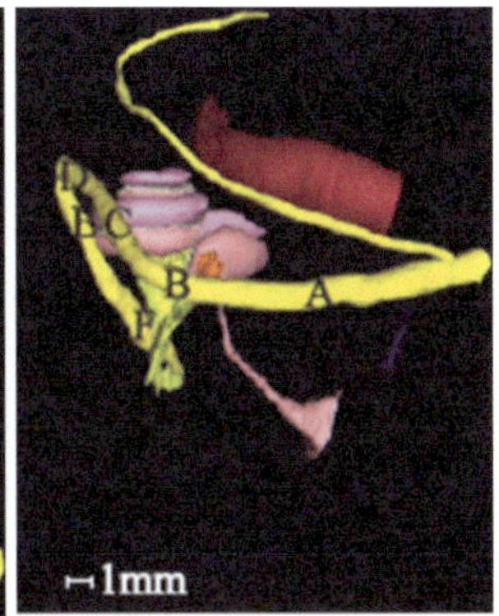

A. Mastoid segment of the facial nerve
B. Pyramidal segment of the facial nerve
C. Horizontal segment of the facial nerve
D. Geniculate ganglion
E. Labyrinthine segment of the facial nerve
F. IAC segment of the facial nerve

Fig. 9.11 Vestibular nerve removed (right)
The labyrinthine segment and internal auditory canal (IAC) segment of the facial nerve is located in front of the vestibular nerve. When the latter is removed, the full course of the facial nerve is exposed. The anatomical structures that can be helpful in locating the facial nerve include the digastric ridge, stylomastoid foramen, short process of the incus, eminence of the lateral semicircular canal, pyramidal eminence, oval window, cochleariform process, anterior epitympanic recess, sinus tympani, GSPN, eminence of the superior semicircular canal, horizon crest, vertical crest, nervus intermedius, vestibulocochlear nerve, anterior inferior cerebellar artery, and labyrinthine artery

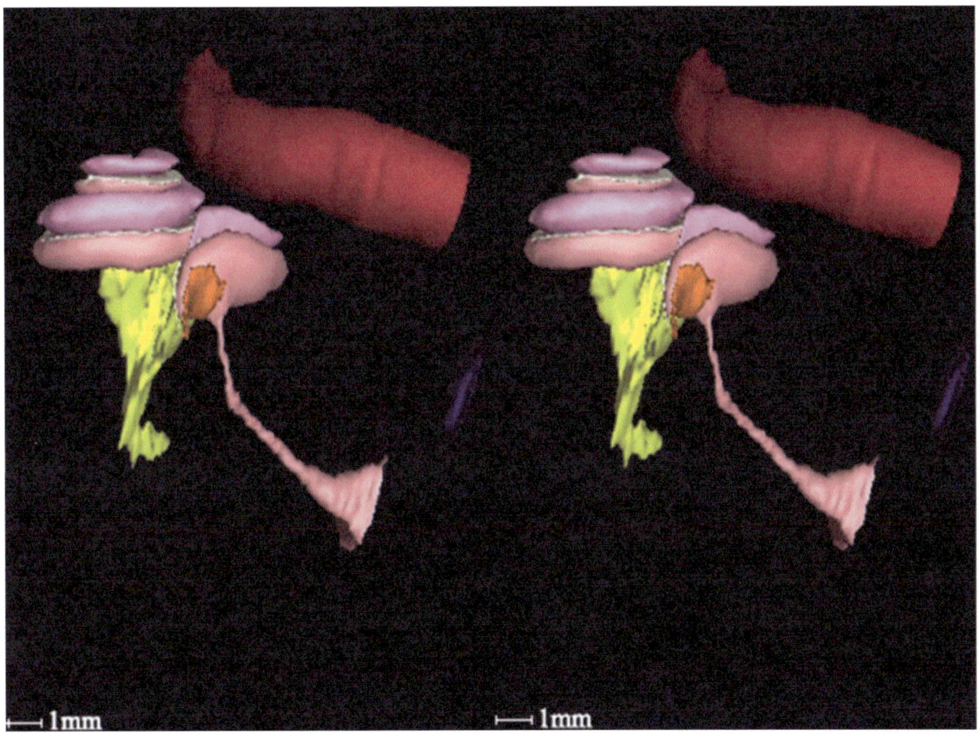

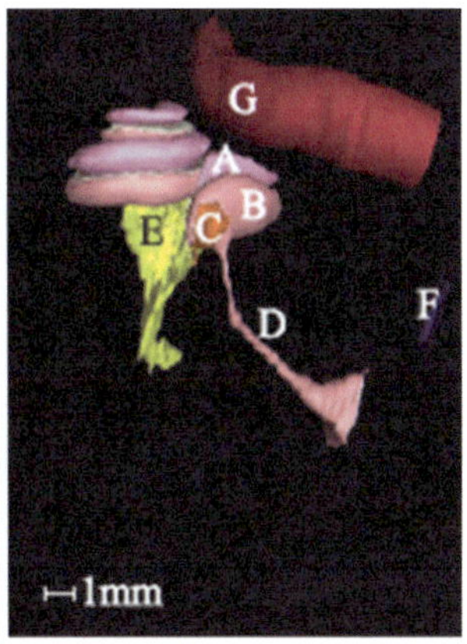

A. Scala vestibuli
B. Scala tympani
C. Round window
D. Cochlear aqueduct
E. Cochlear nerve
F. Top of the jugular bulb
G. Internal carotid artery (ICA)

Fig. 9.12 Facial nerve removed (right)
After removing the facial nerve, inside the IAC, we can see the cochlear nerve extending into the canal of the modiolus. The cochlear aqueduct runs a long distance, its internal opening is medial and inferior to the round window, and the external opening is medial to the jugular bulb. The internal carotid artery sits close to the cochlea, with its vertical segment joining the horizontal segment beneath the cochlea

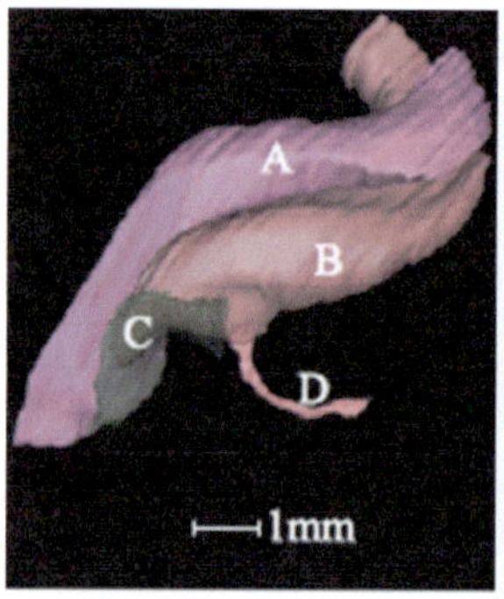

A. Scala vestibuli
B. Scala tympani
C. Round window
D. Cochlear aqueduct

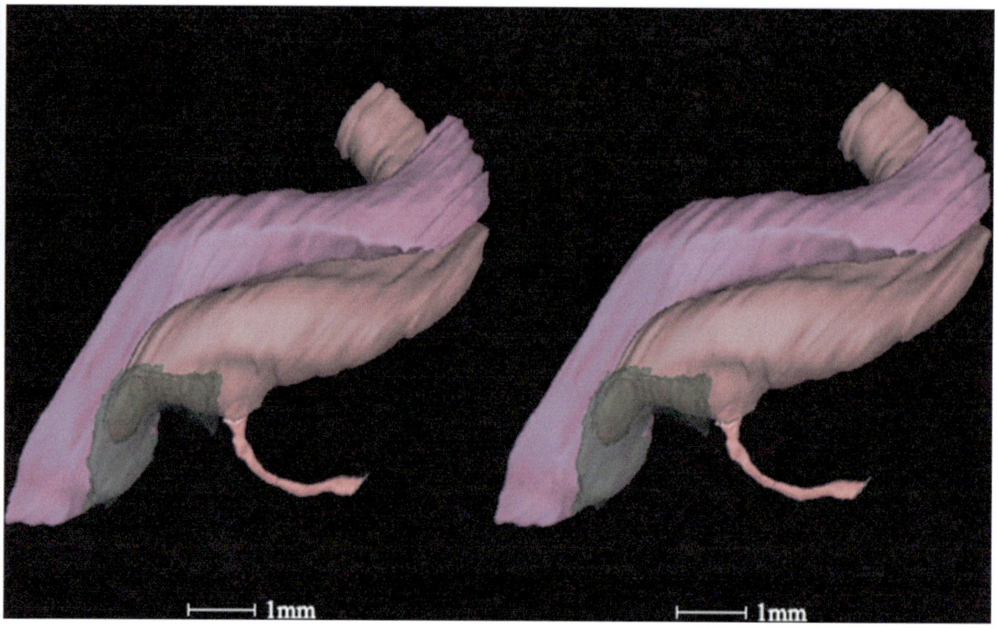

Fig. 9.13 Round window (right)
The round window is a blind terminal of the scala tympani, sealed by a membrane inside the round window niche. The medial end of the cochlear aqueduct opens medial and inferior to the round window

Virtual Anatomy: Retro Auricular Approach

De-jun Zhang

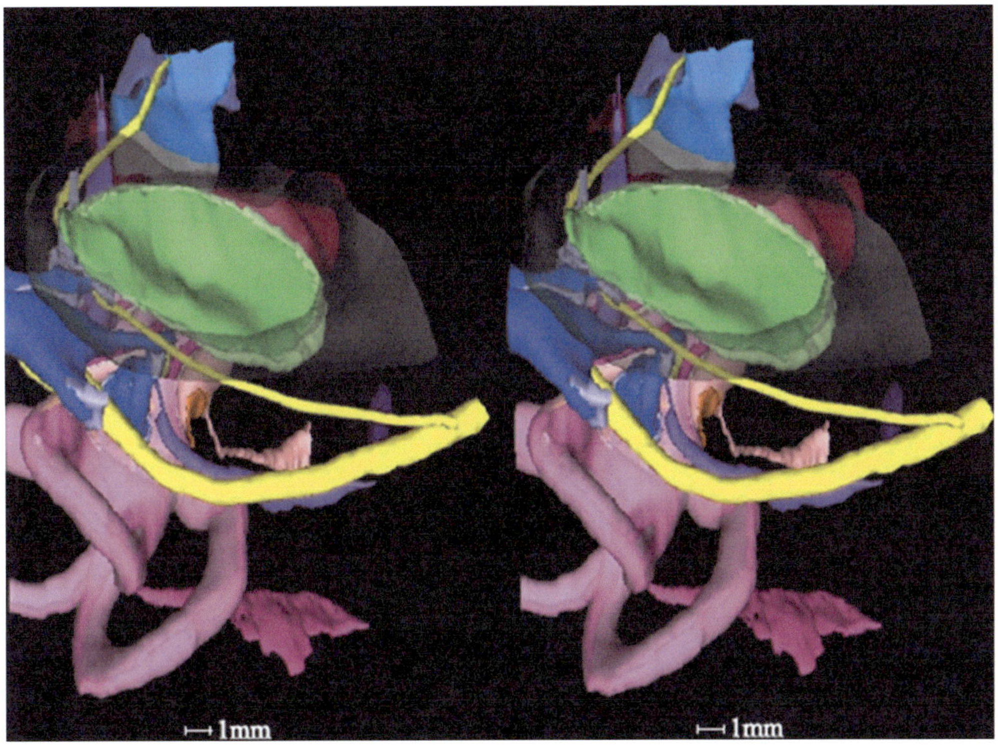

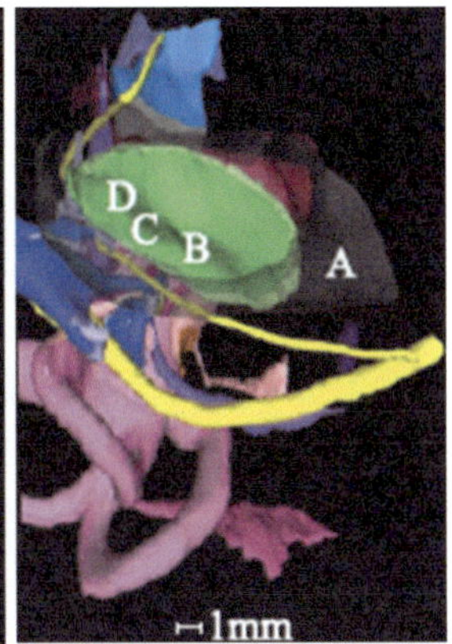

A. Inferior wall of the EAC
B. Umbo
C. Malleal stria
D. Malleal lateral process (prominence)

Fig. 9.14 Tympanic membrane (right)
The umbo (the tip of manubrium), posterior malleal stria, and malleal prominence (the lateral process of malleus) can be seen through the EAC

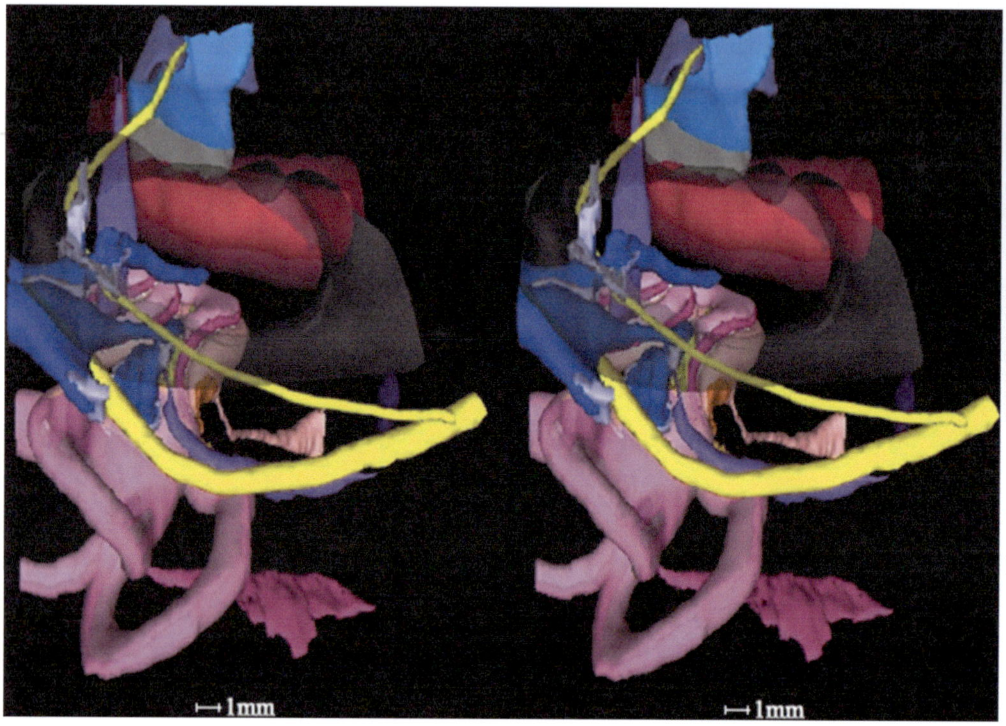

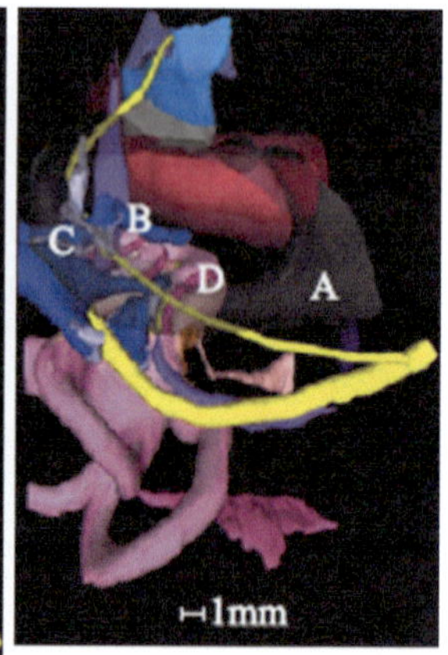

A. Inferior wall of the EAC
B. Manubrium (handle of malleus)
C. Posterior-superior wall of the EAC
D. Basal turn of the cochlea

Fig. 9.15 Removed tympanic membrane (right)
The head and neck of the malleus and most of the incus covered by the posterosuperior wall of the EAC (tympanic scutum) can be observed through the reconstructed bony canal. It is necessary to remove part of the lateral wall of the epitympanum when performing the transcanal approach to explore the epitympanum

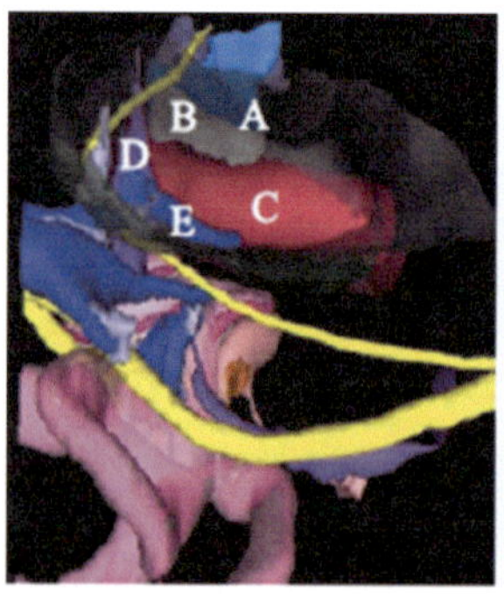

A. Anterior wall of the EAC
B. Tympanic orifice of the Eustachian tube
C. Internal carotid artery
D. Tensor tympani muscle
E. Handle of malleus (manubrium)

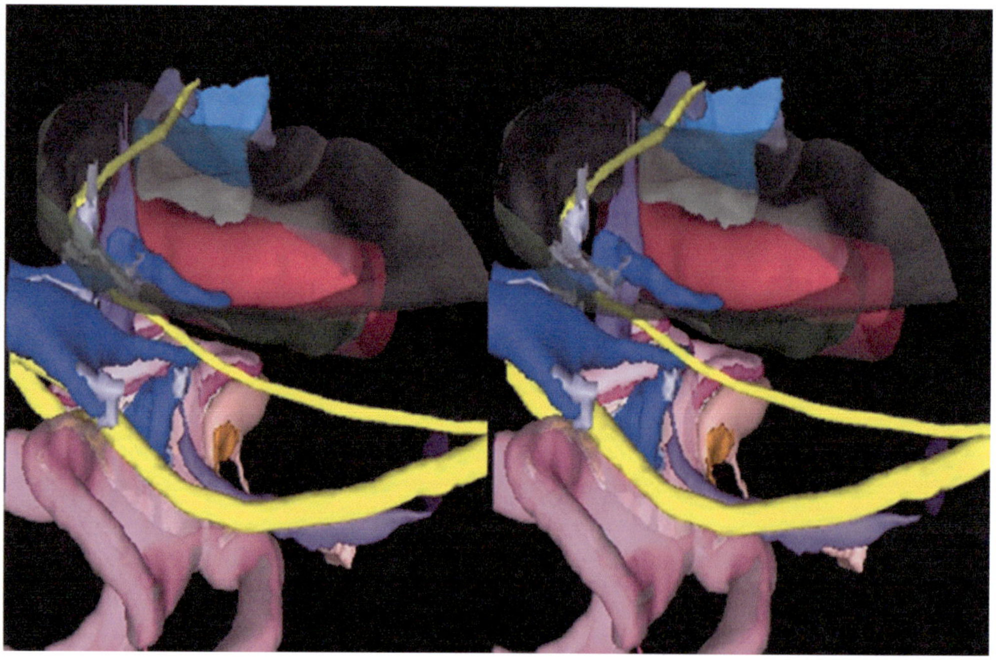

Fig. 9.16 Anterior tympanic cavity (right)
The Tensor tympani muscle (located in the semicanal for the tensor tympani muscle), the tympanic orifice of the Eustachian tube, and the internal carotid artery (surrounded by its bony wall) can be seen through the anterior tympanic cavity

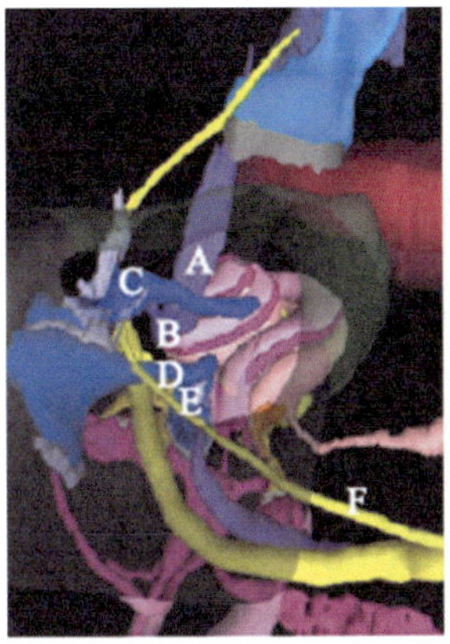

A. Tensor tympani muscle
B. Cochleariform process
C. Lateral process of the malleus
D. Long process of the incus
E. Stapes
F. Chorda tympani

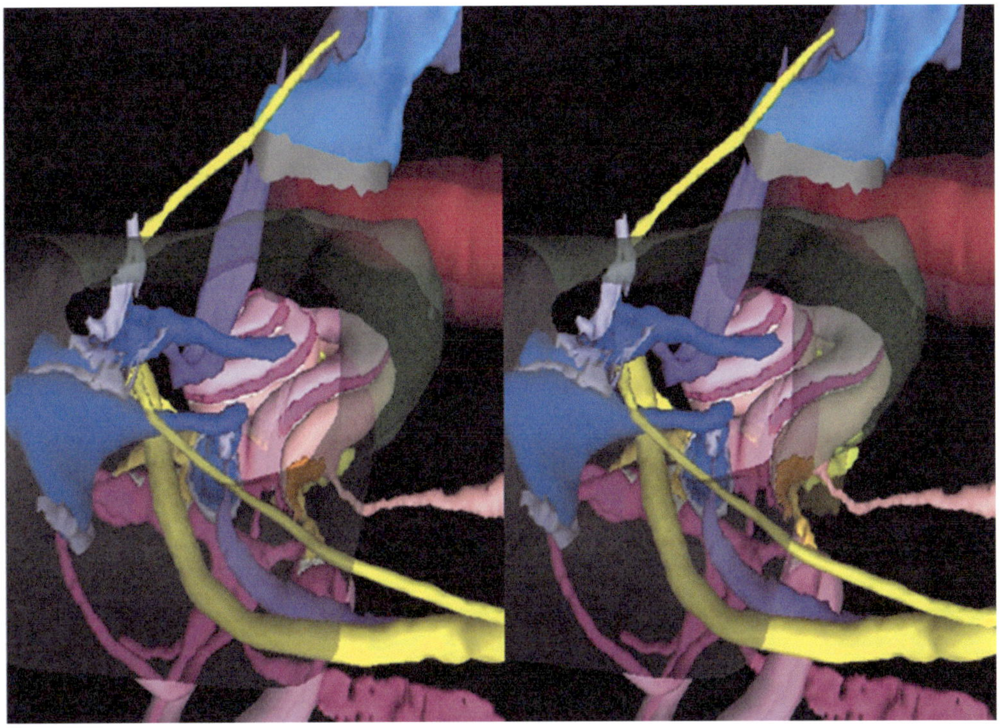

Fig. 9.17 Superior tympanic cavity (right)
The tensor tympani tendon attaches to the upper part of the handle of malleus after it emerges from the cochleariform process. The cochleariform process is anteroinferior to the tympanic segment of the facial nerve. The tympanic segment of the facial nerve runs superior to the stapes and the oval window. The chorda tympani, emerging from the posterosuperior wall of the tympanic cavity, crosses the tympanic cavity between the long process of the incus and the manubrium

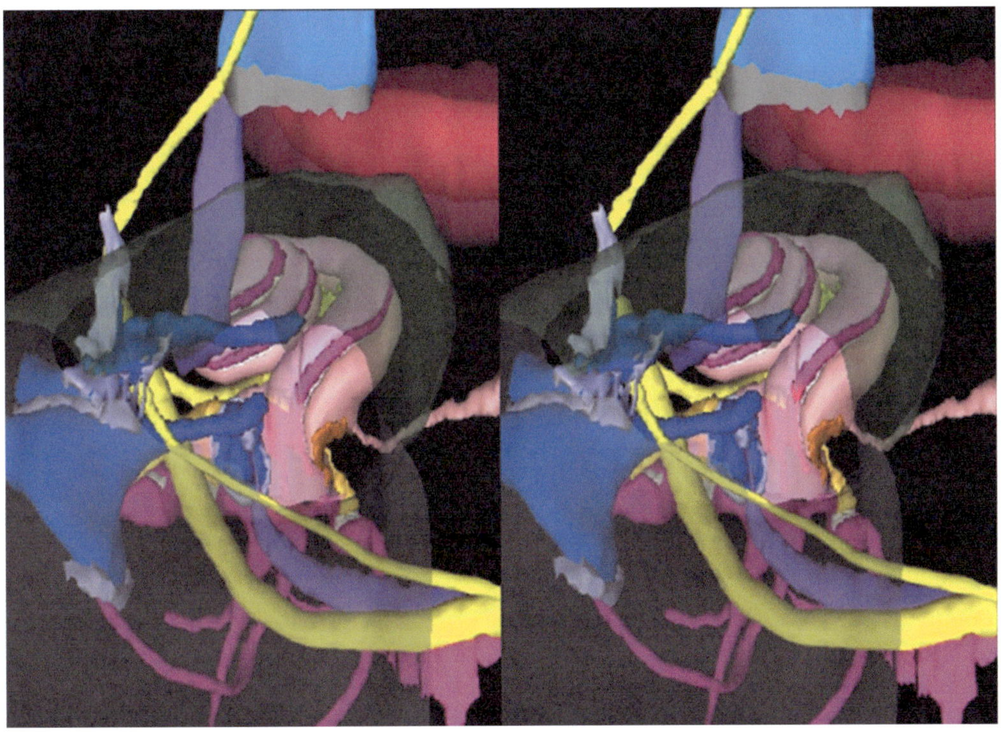

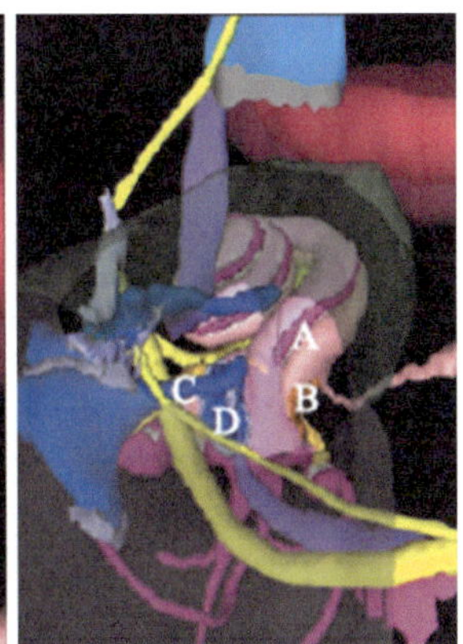

A. Basal turn of the cochlea
B. Round window
C. Long process of the incus
D. Stapes

Fig. 9.18 Posterior tympanic cavity (right)
Observed through the posterior tympanic cavity: the basal turn of the cochlea, the posterosuperior part of the promontory, the oval window, and the round window, which lies in the depression seen posteriorly. The oval window is sealed by the stapes footplate and annular ligament. The round window lies deep within the round window niche and cannot be observed easily

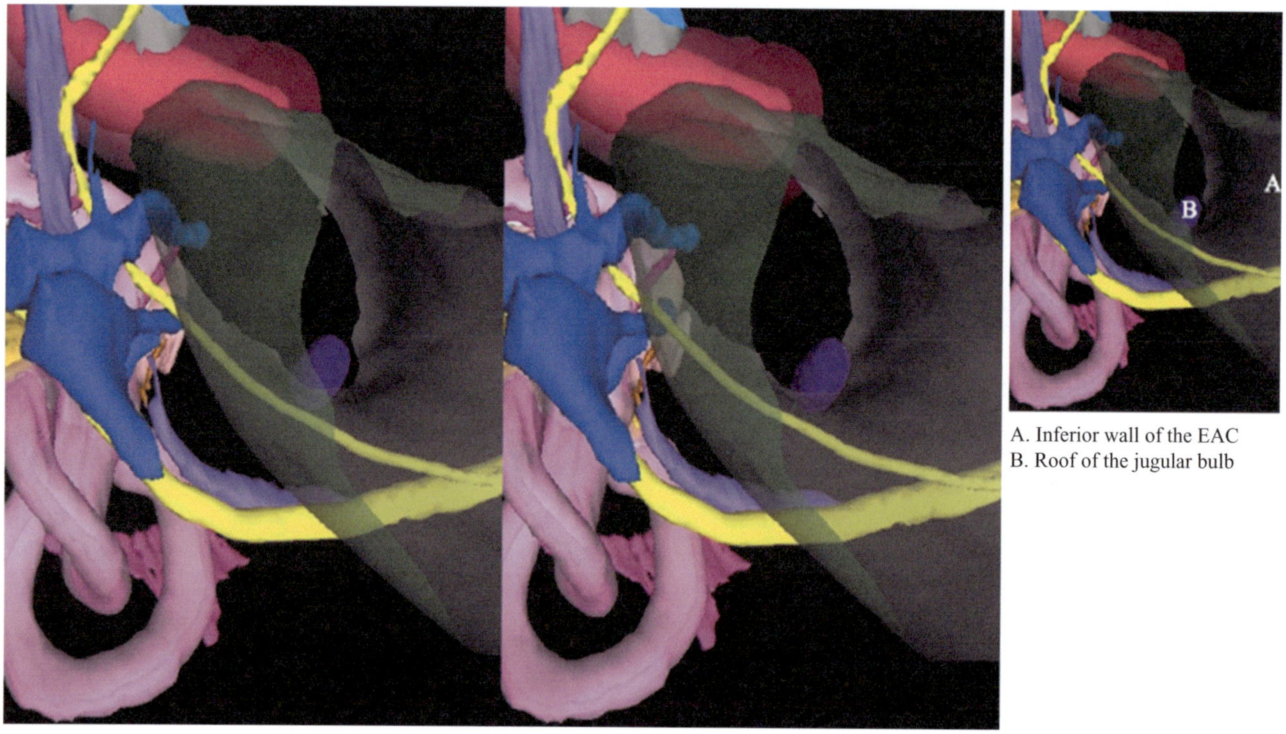

A. Inferior wall of the EAC
B. Roof of the jugular bulb

Fig. 9.19 Inferior tympanic cavity (right)
The inferior tympanic cavity is separated by an irregular bony wall from the jugular bulb postero-inferiorly. The inferior wall of the tympanum is also called the jugular wall. In some cases, the jugular wall is dehiscent. When the high- or finger-like jugular bulb protrudes into the middle ear cavity through the dehiscence of the jugular wall, it can cause pulsatile tinnitus or conductive hearing loss. The jugular body, a chemoreceptor similar to the carotid body, is located at the dome of the jugular bulb. Glomus jugulare tumors arise from this chemoreceptor

Virtual Anatomy: Middle Cranial Fossa Approach

Xiao-hong Li

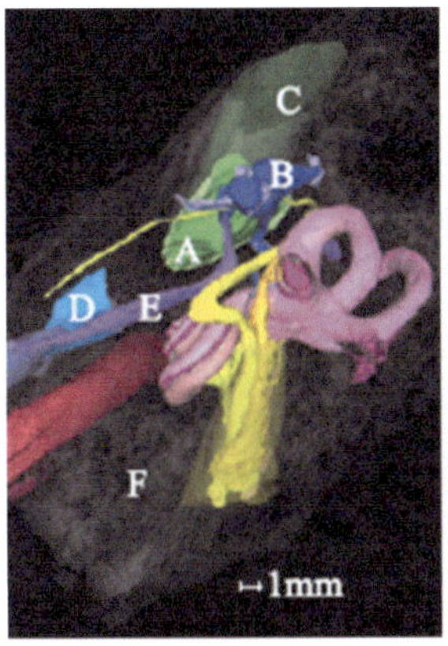

A. Tympanic membrane
B. Ossicular chain
C. Bony wall of EAC
D. Bony part of Eustachian tube
E. Tensor tympani muscle
F. Temporal bone (anterior petrous apex)

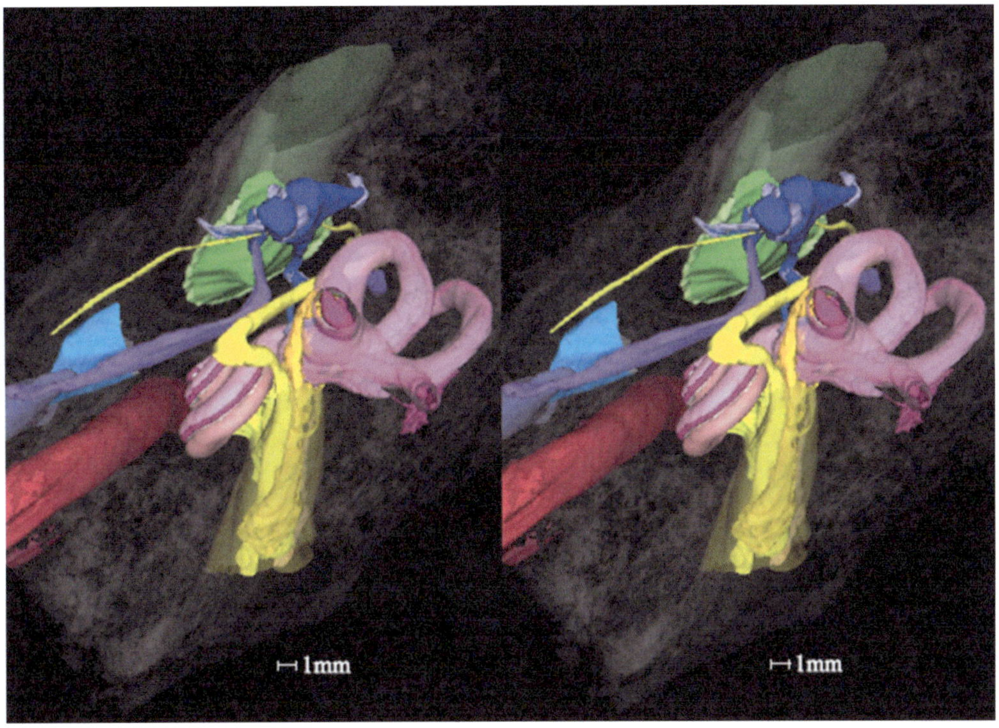

Fig. 9.20 General view of the temporal bone (right)
A superior view of the components in the temporal bone via a middle cranial fossa approach

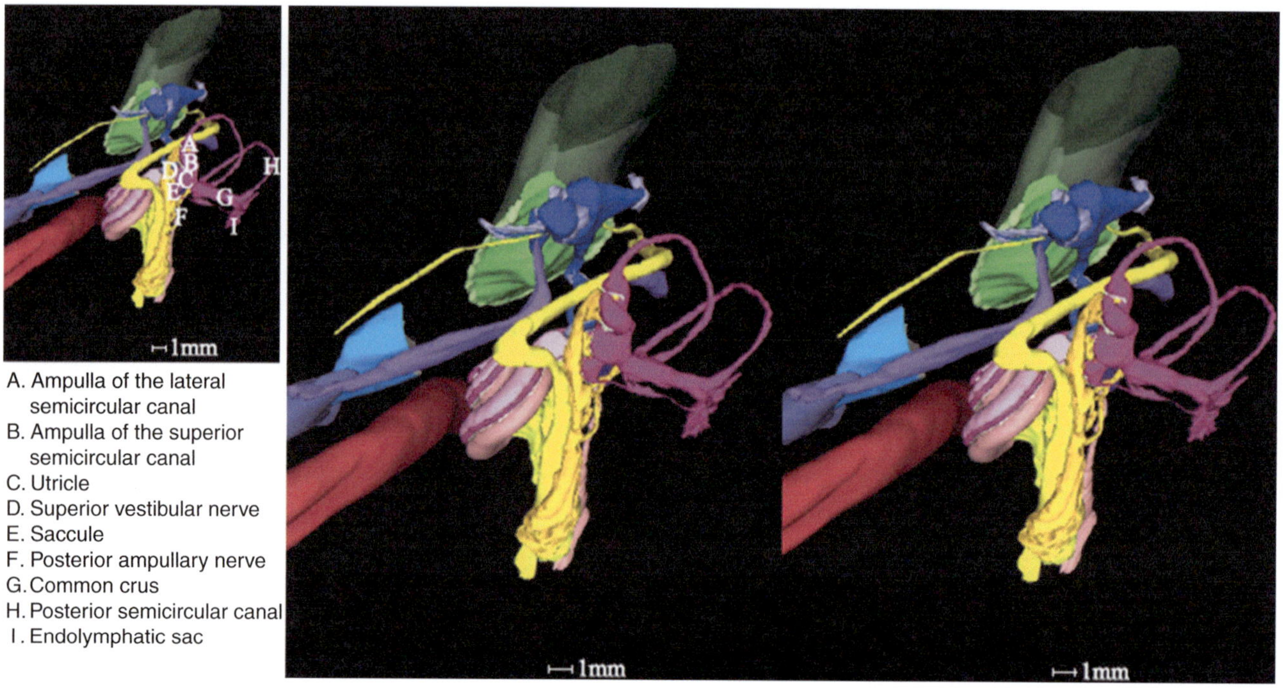

Fig. 9.21 Removal of the adjacent bone of important structures in the temporal bone (right)
The three semicircular canals are orthogonally related to one another, and the combined mass of the three semicircular canals is known as the solid angle. The superior vestibular nerve innervates the crista of the superior and lateral semicircular canals, as well as the utricular macula. The inferior vestibular nerve innervates the saccular macula. The course of the posterior ampullary nerve can also be seen. The posterior ampullary nerve, which innervates the ampulla of the posterior semicircular canal, separates from the main trunk of the inferior vestibular nerve. Note the rotation of the facial, cochlear, and vestibular nerves as they traverse the IAC. Note the relationship between the facial nerve, the cochleariform process, and the lateral semicircular canal

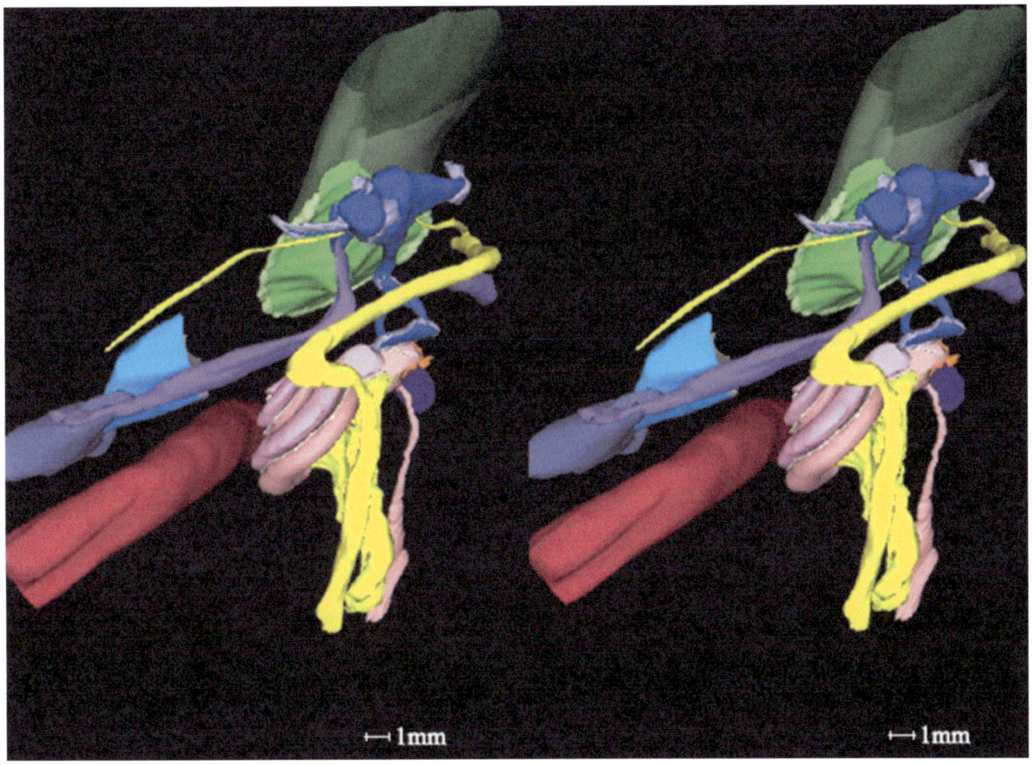

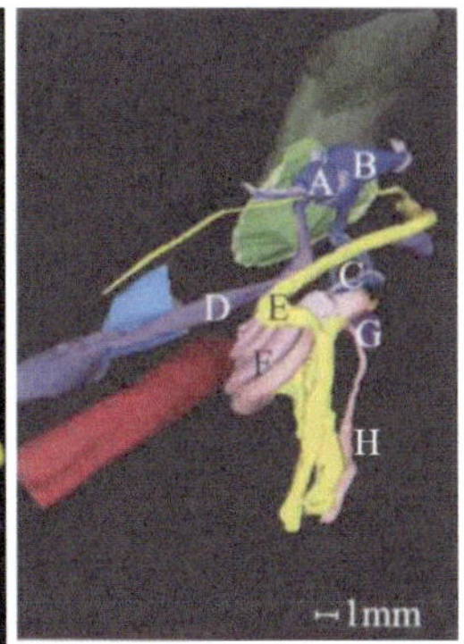

A. Malleus
B. Incus
C. Stapes footplate
D. Tensor tympani muscle
E. Geniculate ganglion
F. Cochlea
G. Dome of the jugular bulb
H. Cochlear aqueduct

Fig. 9.22 View after removal of the membranous labyrinth and vestibular nerve (right)
The stapes footplate, lodged in the oval window, can be seen after removal of the membranous labyrinth and vestibular nerve. The course of the cochlear aqueduct also can be seen. It starts from the scala tympani of the basal turn just inferior to the round window membrane and extends to its external opening inferior to the IAM and medial to the jugular bulb

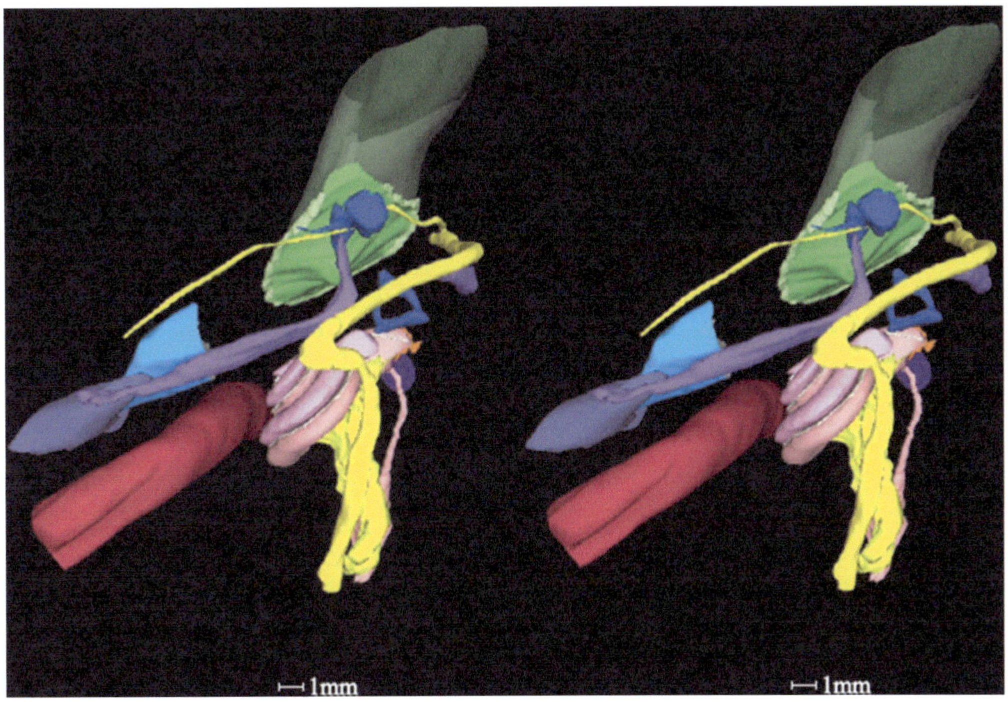

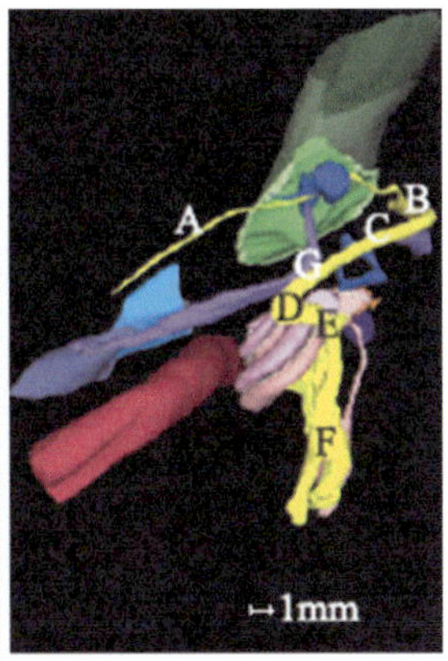

A. Chorda tympani
B. Vertical segment of the facial nerve
C. Horizontal segment of the facial nerve
D. Geniculate ganglion
E. Labyrinthine segment of the facial nerve
F. IAC segment of the facial nerve
G. Cochleariform process

Fig. 9.23 View after removal of the incus (right)
Note the course of the facial nerve. It is advisable to identify all the segments of the facial nerve and the virtual location of the anatomic "pointers" to the nerve, including the short process of the incus, the lateral and posterior semicircular canals, the pyramidal eminence, the oval window, the cochleariform process, the anterior epitympanic recess, the sinus tympani, the greater and lesser superficial petrosal nerves, the transverse crest, and Bill's bar

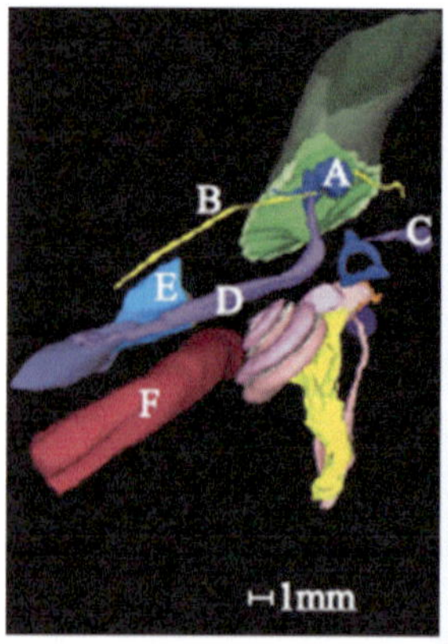

A. Prussak's space and malleus head
B. Chorda tympani
C. Stapedius muscle
D. Tensor tympani muscle
E. Bony part of the Eustachian tube
F. Internal carotid artery

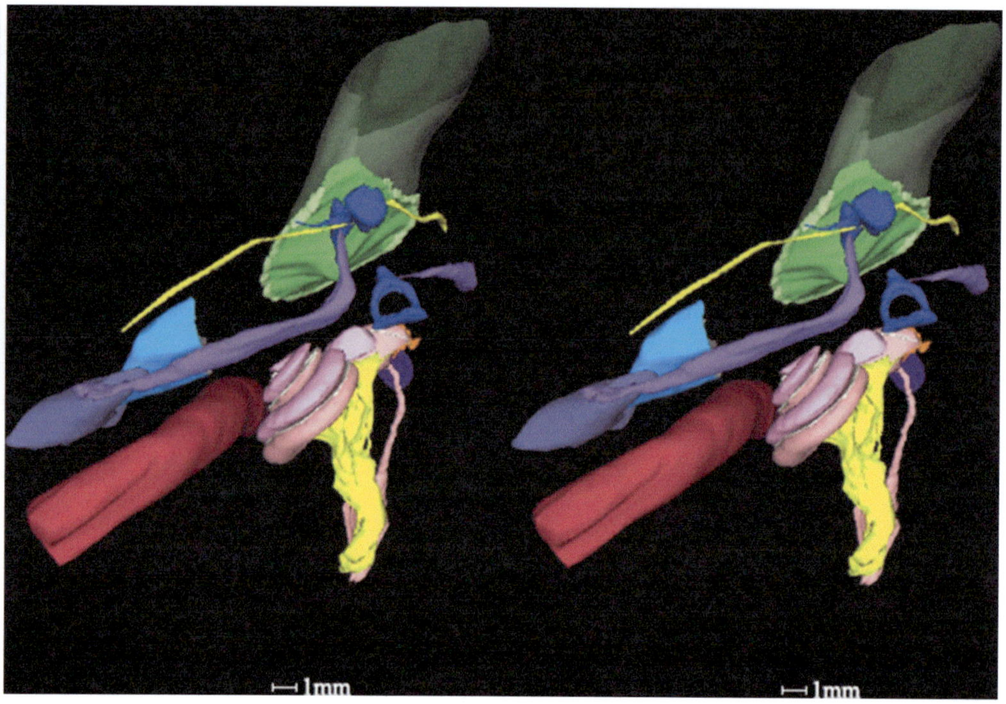

Fig. 9.24 View after Removal of the Facial Nerve (right)
Note Prussak's space, which is located medial to the pars flaccida and lateral to the neck of the malleus. The stapedius muscle and stapedius tendon can be seen posterior to the stapes. In a superior view via a middle cranial fossa approach, the Eustachian tube and tensor tympani muscle are both parallel to the horizontal segment of the internal carotid artery. The junction of the vertical and horizontal parts of the internal carotid artery sits anterior to the cochlea. The modiolus points in an anterolateral direction from the base toward the apex

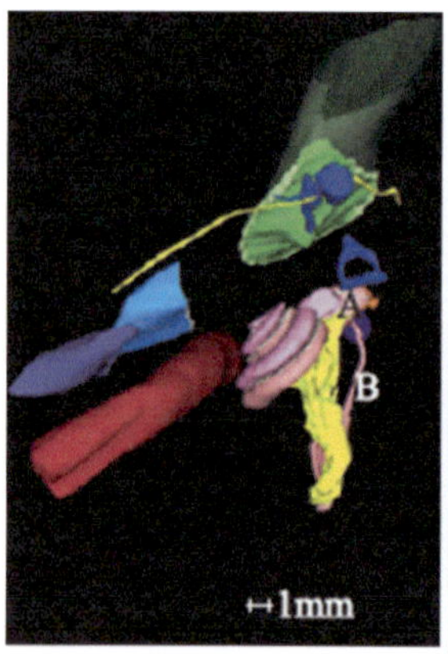

A. Basal turn of the cochlea
B. Cochlear aqueduct

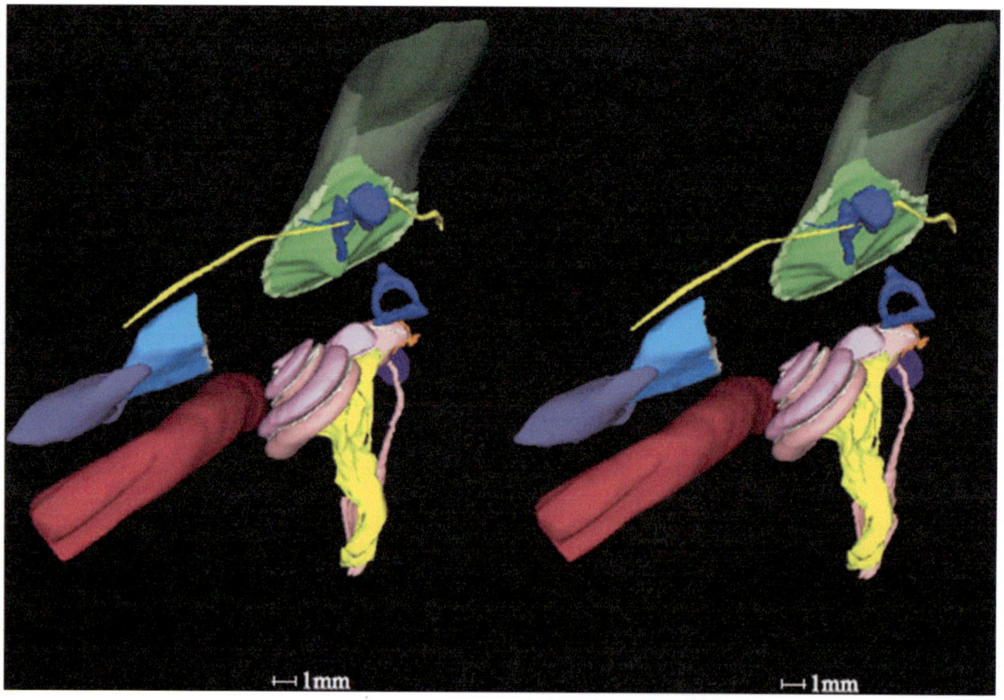

Fig. 9.25 View after removal of the Tensor tympani muscle and stapedius muscle (right)
Note the cochlear (auditory) nerve. The cochlear nerve arises from the spiral ganglion neurons and the nerve fibers leave the cochlea in a sequential manner. The fibers from the most apical turn of the cochlea joining in the center of the nerve bundle code low-frequency sounds, whereas the fibers from the basal end joining on the outside of the bundle code high-frequency sounds. The cochlear aqueduct extends from the scala tympani of the basal turn to the subarachnoid space in a posteromedial direction

Temporal Bone-Related Structures

Chang Guo and Yue-shuai Song

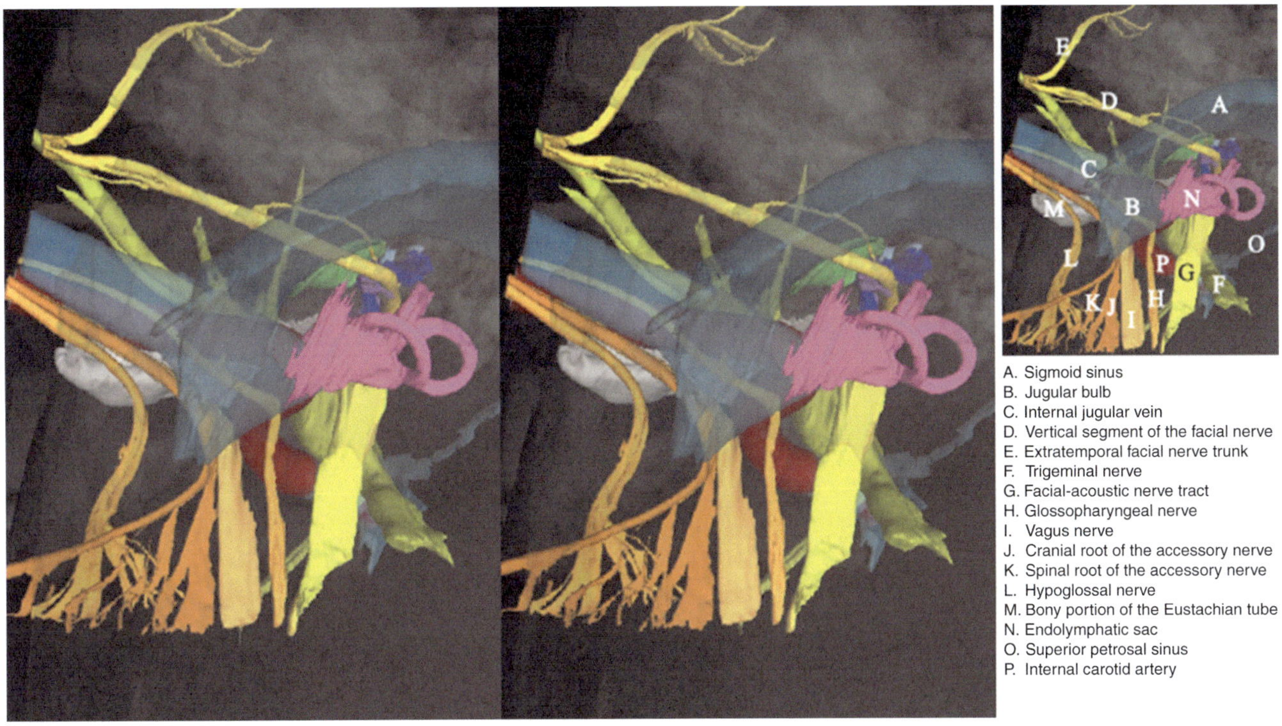

A. Sigmoid sinus
B. Jugular bulb
C. Internal jugular vein
D. Vertical segment of the facial nerve
E. Extratemporal facial nerve trunk
F. Trigeminal nerve
G. Facial-acoustic nerve tract
H. Glossopharyngeal nerve
I. Vagus nerve
J. Cranial root of the accessory nerve
K. Spinal root of the accessory nerve
L. Hypoglossal nerve
M. Bony portion of the Eustachian tube
N. Endolymphatic sac
O. Superior petrosal sinus
P. Internal carotid artery

Fig. 9.26 Observing the temporal bone from the rear of the sigmoid sinus (left, simulated retro sigmoid approach)
The IV–XI cranial nerves can be exposed through a retro sigmoid approach. Exposure of the XII cranial nerve, which is located in the lowest position, is difficult to see through this approach

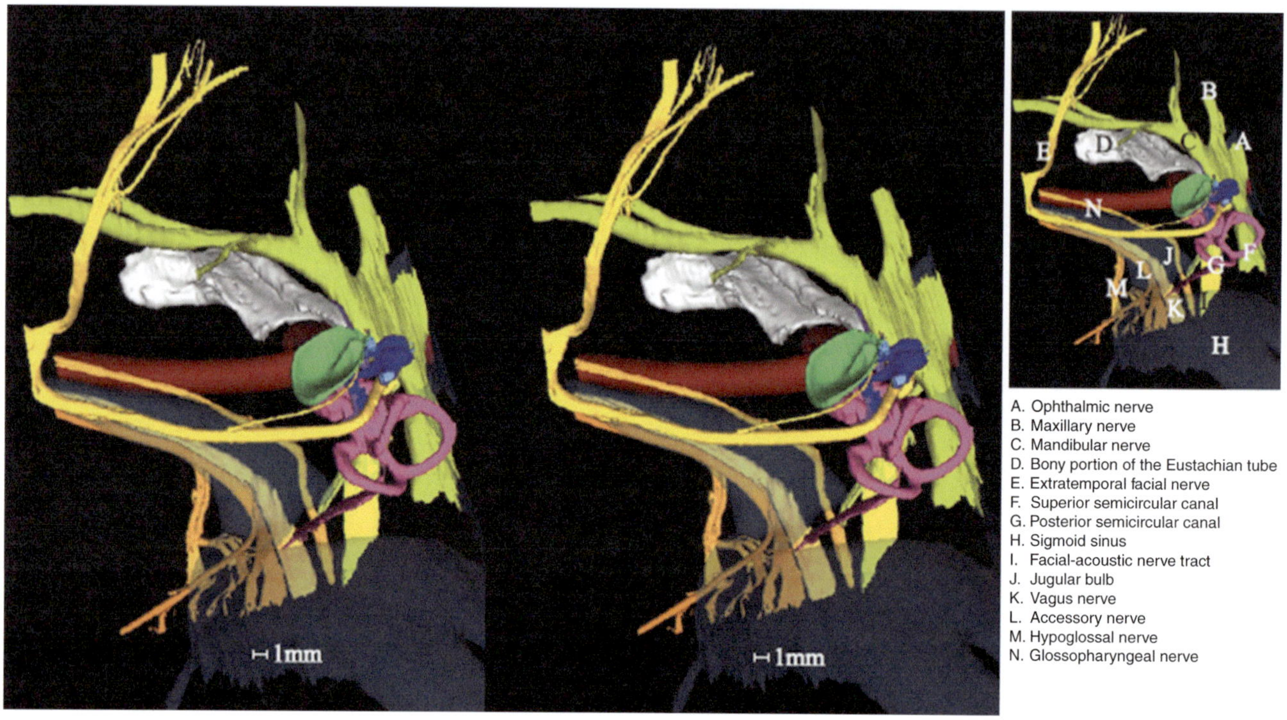

Fig. 9.27 Observing the temporal bone from a posterolateral to an anteromedial view (left)
The trigeminal nerve exits from the brainstem and travels anterolaterally to the trigeminal ganglion and gives rise to three divisions: the first division (ophthalmic nerve) travels anteriorly to the supraorbital fissure, the second division (maxillary nerve) enters the pterygopalatine fossa through the foramen rotundum, the third division (mandibular nerve) enters the inferior temporal fossa via the foramen ovale

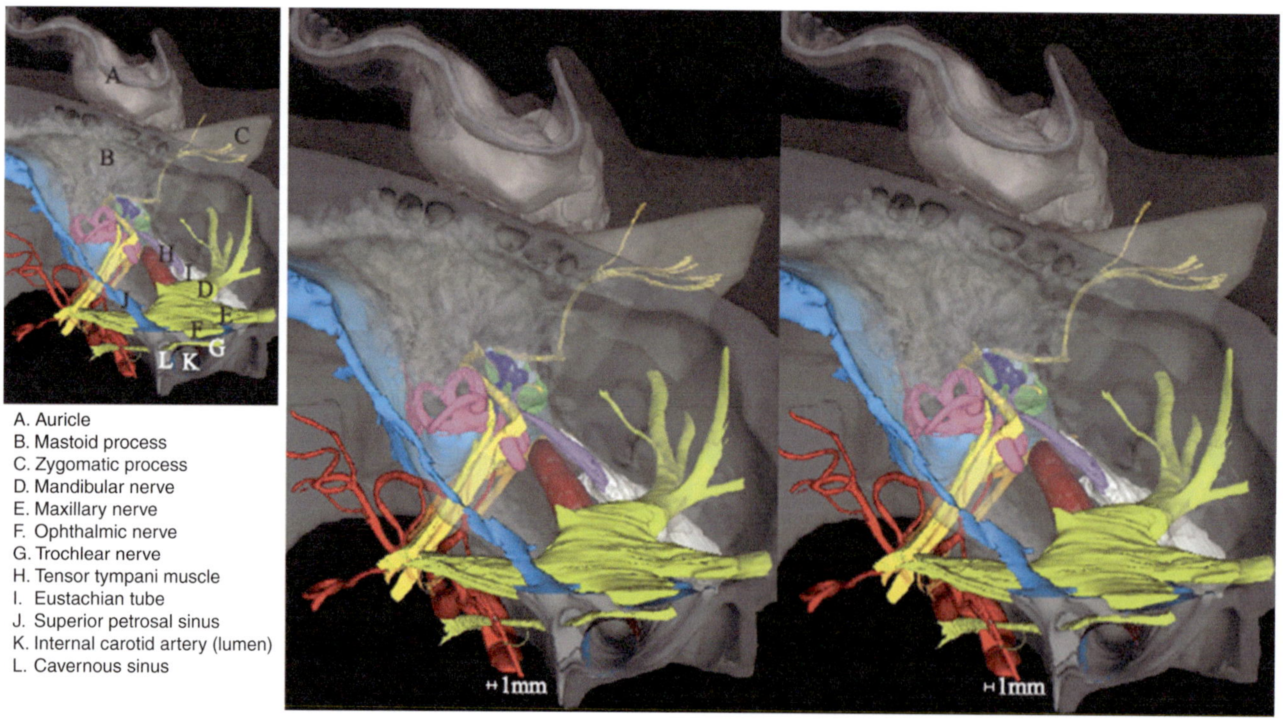

Fig. 9.28 Superior view of the temporal bone (left, simulated middle cranial fossa approach)

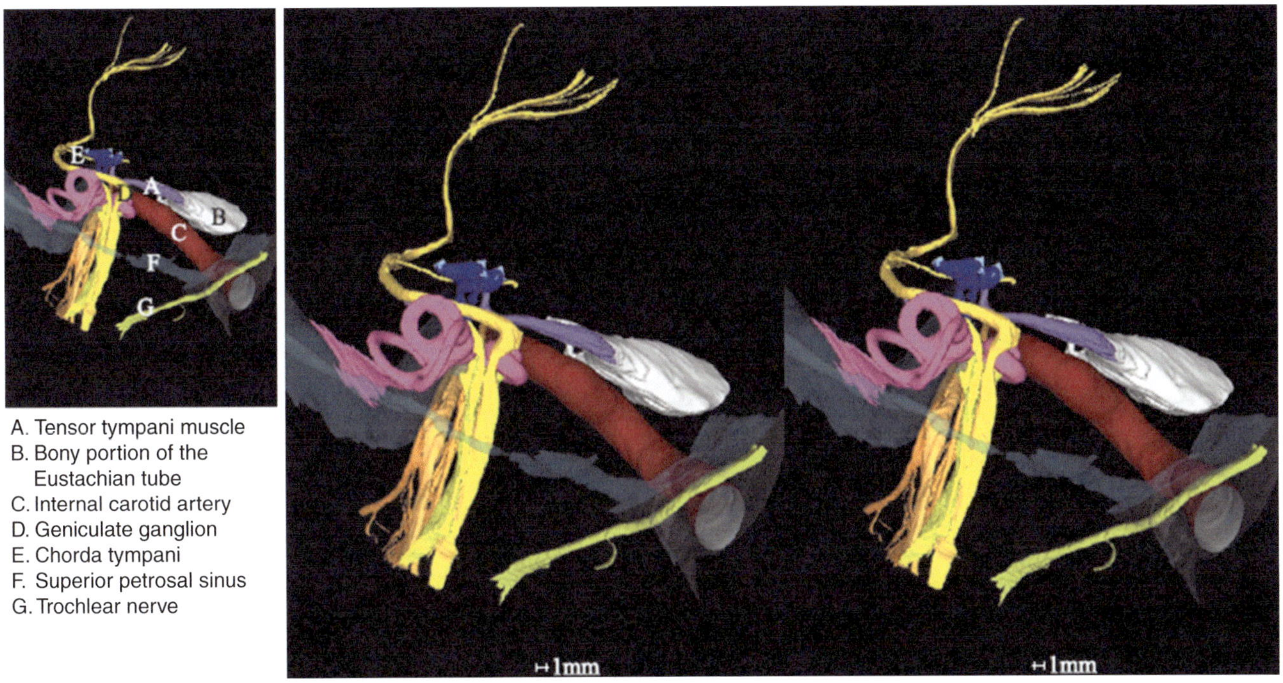

Fig. 9.29 Superior view of the temporal bone after removal of the trigeminal (left)

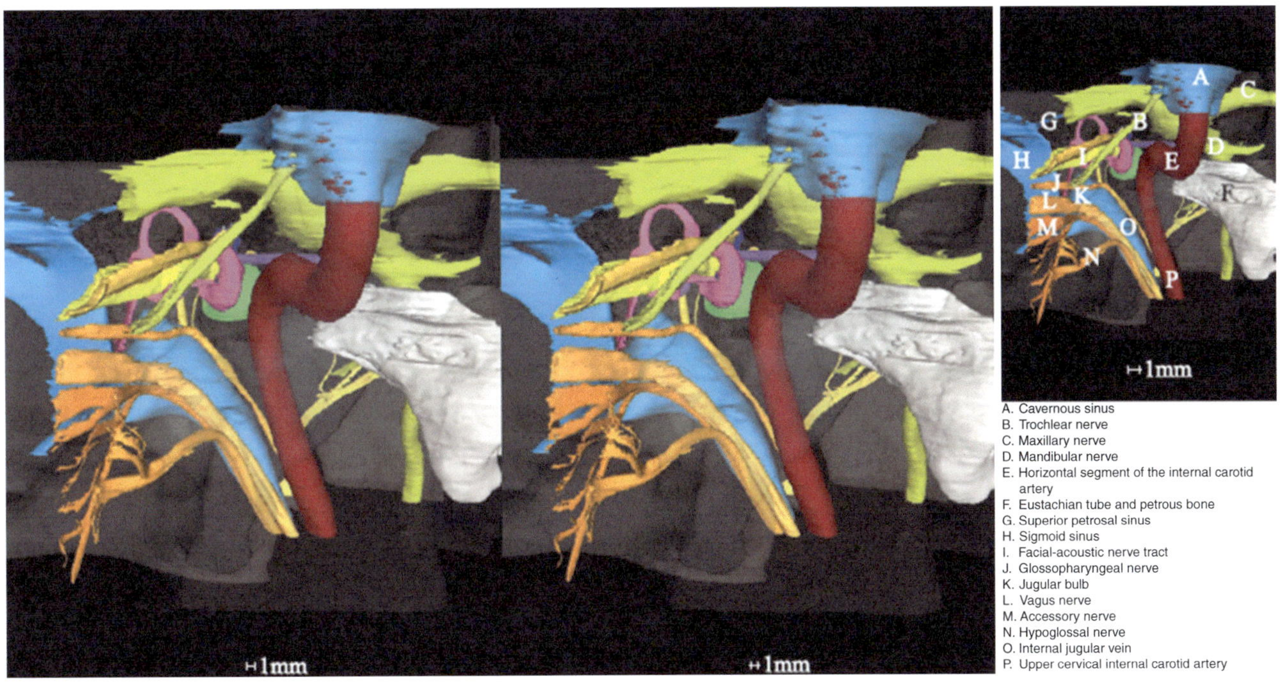

Fig. 9.30 Observing the temporal bone from the intracranial to the extracranial position (erect position)

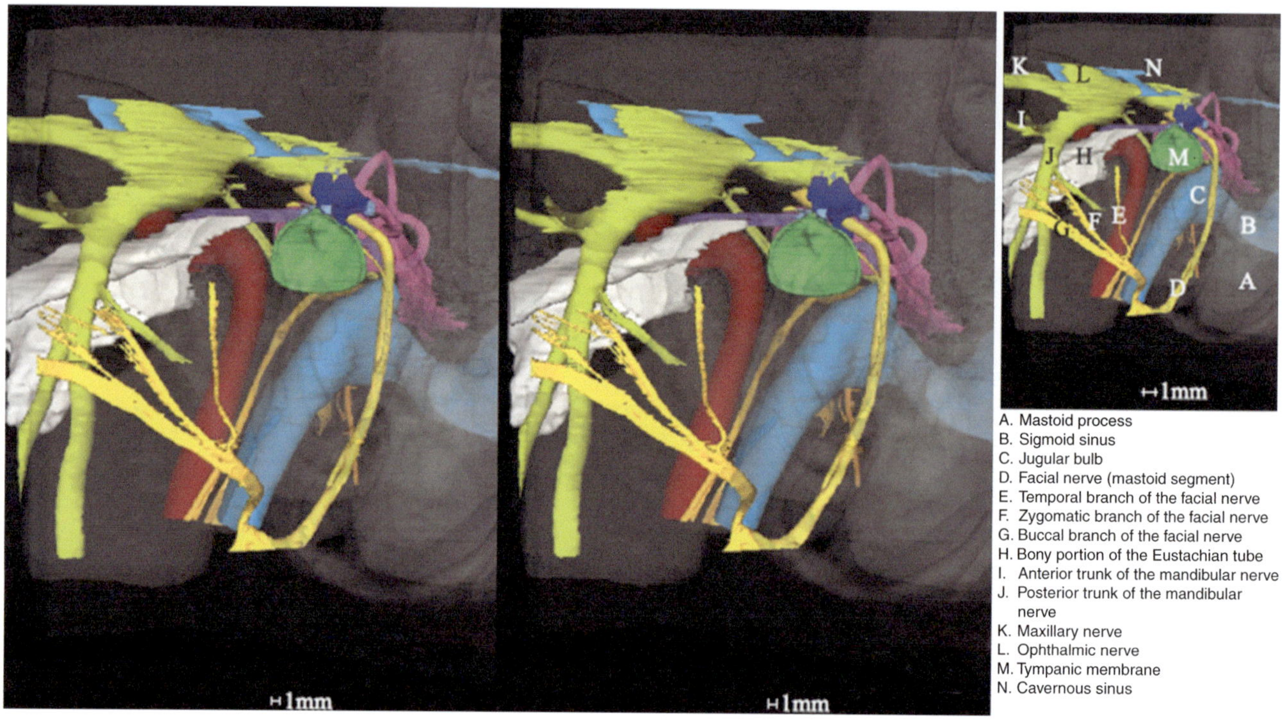

Fig. 9.31 Observing the temporal bone from the extracranial to the intracranial position (erect position)

Suggested Reading

3-D virtual models of the human temporal bone and related structures. 2020. https://research.meei.harvard.edu/Otopathology/3dmodels/download.html.

Li P-m, Wang H-b, Northrop C, et al. Anatomy of the round window and hook region of the cochlea with implications for cochlear implantation and other endocochlear surgical procedures. Otol Neurotol. 2007;28(5):641–8.

MIX
Papier aus verantwortungsvollen Quellen
Paper from responsible sources
FSC® C105338
FSC
www.fsc.org

If you have any concerns about our products,
you can contact us on
ProductSafety@springernature.com

In case Publisher is established outside the EU,
the EU authorized representative is:
Springer Nature Customer Service Center GmbH
Europaplatz 3, 69115 Heidelberg, Germany

Printed by Libri Plureos GmbH
in Hamburg, Germany